Surgical Treatment of Colorectal Cancer

Nam Kyu Kim • Kenichi Sugihara
Jin-Tung Liang
Editors

Surgical Treatment of Colorectal Cancer

Asian Perspectives on Optimization and Standardization

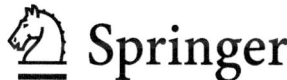 Springer

Editors
Nam Kyu Kim
Department of Surgery
Yonsei University College of Medicine
Seoul
South Korea

Kenichi Sugihara
Department of Surgery
Tokyo Medical and Dental University
Tokyo
Japan

Jin-Tung Liang
Department of Surgery
National Taiwan University Hospital and
College of Medicine
Taipei City
Taiwan

Associate Editors
Jin Cheon Kim
Asan Medical Center
Ulsan University College of Medicine
Seoul
South Korea

Wai Lun Law
Department of Surgery
Queen Mary Hospital
The University of Hong Kong
Hong Kong
China

Jin Gu
Department of Surgery
Peking University Cancer Hospital
Beijing
China

ISBN 978-981-13-3846-5   ISBN 978-981-10-5143-2   (eBook)
https://doi.org/10.1007/978-981-10-5143-2

We dedicate this book to the patients who were treated for colorectal cancer and participated in research program delineated in this text.

좋은 수술에는 왕도는 없다. 인간 해부학 지식을 바탕으로 한 수술 치료 원칙만 있다.

There is no royal road to good surgery, only principle of surgery based on human anatomy exist.

良質の手術を習得する近道はない。ただ、解剖に基づいた手術を心掛けるのみ.

完美手術無捷徑,其要旨在於遵守人體解剖學所呈現的外科基本原理.

達至良好外科手術是沒有捷徑的 。然而,手術的原則是基於人體解剖學的知識.

外科的成功沒有捷径,只有基于現代人体解剖的外科原則.

ليس هناك طريق ملكي لعملية جراحية جيدة ولكن فقط مبدأ الجراحة على أساس التشريح البشري لابد ان يكون حاضرا

अच्छी सर्जरी के लिए शाही सड़क नहीं है, लेकिन केवल मानव शरीर रचाना विज्ञान के आधार पर सर्जरी का सिद्धांत है

Không có con đường thật sự để đưa đến cuộc phẫu thuật tốt, chỉ có nguyên tắc duy nhất là dựa vào giải phẫu cơ thể con người hiện tại

Preface

In the past, colorectal cancer was the most prevalent digestive tract cancer in western countries, and there have been abundant studies conducted regarding the epidemiology, early detection, and treatment of the disease. In the past decade, along with the economic growth in the Eastern countries, eating habits of people and their lifestyle have shifted toward westernization, and the proportion of obese population has dramatically increased. As a result, colorectal cancer has been threatening the Asian population as the most frequently occurring digestive tract cancer. Colorectal cancer is already the most prevalent digestive tract cancer in Hong Kong, Taiwan, Singapore, part of China, Philippines, and Thailand, and although stomach cancer is the most common digestive tract cancer in Korea, Japan, and most of China, it is predicted that the prevalence of colorectal cancer will exceed in the near future.

The experience and studies of colorectal cancer and the epidemiology, cause, early detection, and treatment of the disease have been mainly dependent on the clinical and basic research conducted in the United States and Europe. However, the treatment status, results, and the problems faced by the Asian population cannot be mutual to that of Western countries. In order to properly reciprocate to the growing population of colorectal cancer patients in Asia, a pivotal conference was held in Bangkok, Thailand, in 2011, with colorectal cancer surgeons playing the key role. In May 2012, professors of major university hospitals in Korea, Japan, Taiwan, Singapore, Hong Kong, China, Malaysia, Thailand, Philippines, India, and Saudi Arabia gathered in Seoul, Korea, for the first joint conference. The object of the conference was to share the experience and knowledge encountered during the treatment of colorectal patients in the Asia-Pacific area. In order to achieve the proposed goals, mutual exchange of information and cooperation on the prevention, diagnosis, and treatment of colorectal cancer and general problems that follow are needed. Through interchange of needed education, we aimed to improve the quality of the treatment in the Asia-Pacific area. This book describes extensively the fundamental surgical principles of colorectal cancer, the current status on minimally invasive surgery, and the multidisciplinary approach in cases of cancer metastases or recurrence. The title and contents in each chapter are composed of themes that were discussed and deliberated at the meetings. We hope that the readers will not only master the very specialized techniques but also learn about the current treatment status in the Asia-Pacific area. This book is intended to be the cornerstone of treatment for the increasing colorectal cancer patients in Asia and act to standardize the future treatment protocol and to optimize the treatment results. This book is a treasure house of knowledge and experience of the founding members, who are willing to provide their wisdom to the younger generation of surgeons.

Furthermore, we wish to spread our will to the Middle East, India, Pakistan, Vietnam, Mongolia, Bangladesh, Sri Lanka, and Myanmar and hope that the patients there will receive optimal treatment in the future.

Seoul, South Korea   Nam Kyu Kim
Tokyo, Japan   Kenichi Sugihara
Taipei City, Taiwan   Jin-Tung Liang

Acknowledgments

I would like to thank the esteemed Professor Kenichi Sugihara, Professor Jin Cheon Kim, and Professor Jin Gu, my proud colleague, Professor Jin Tung Liang and Professor Wai Lun Law for all your efforts as the main editors. Also, I thank Professor Min Soo Cho, Jenny Chun of Springer Nature, Kate Hong and Yeon Sill Choi of SY convention, who helped me immensely with the editing of this book.

Contents

Part IV   Standard Surgical Techniques in Rectal Cancer Surgery

Part V   Anatomic Consideration for Colon Cancer Surgery

**Part VI   Standard Surgical Concepts and Techniques
in Colon Cancer Surgery**

List of Editors and Associate Editors

Editors

Nam Kyu Kim Department of Surgery, Yonsei University College of Medicine, Seoul, South Korea

Kenichi Sugihara Department of Surgery, Tokyo Medical and Dental University, Tokyo, Japan

Jin-Tung Liang Department of Surgery, National Taiwan University Hospital and College of Medicine, Taipei City, Taiwan

Associate Editors

Jin Cheon Kim Asan Medical Center, Ulsan University College of Medicine, Seoul, South Korea

Wai Lun Law Department of Surgery, Queen Mary Hospital, The Univeristy of Hong Kong, Hong Kong, China

Jin Gu Department of Surgery, Peking University Cancer Hospital, Beijing, China

Contributors

Albert Chan Department of Surgery, The University of Hong Kong, Queen Mary Hospital, Hong Kong, China

William Tzu-Liang Chen Division of Colorectal Surgery, Department of Surgery, Minimally Invasive Surgery Center, China Medical University Hospital, Taichung City, Taiwan

Min Soo Cho Department of Surgery, Yonsei University College of Medicine, Seoul, South Korea

Qingyang Feng Colorectal Cancer Center, Zhongshan Hospital, Fudan University, Shanghai, China

Jin Gu Department of Colorectal Surgery, Peking University Cancer Hospital, Beijing, People's Republic of China

Yojiro Hashiguchi Department of Surgery, Teikyo University, Tokyo, Japan

Koya Hida Department of Surgery, Kyoto University Graduate School of Medicine, Kyoto, Japan

Nobuaki Hoshino Department of Surgery, Kyoto University Graduate School of Medicine, Kyoto, Japan

Jung Wook Huh Department of Surgery, Samsung Medical Center, Sungkyunkwan University School of Medicine, Seoul, South Korea

Masaaki Ito Department of Colorectal Surgery, National Cancer Center Hospital East, Kashiwa, Chiba Prefecture, Japan

Sun Ha Jee Graduate School of Public Health, Yonsei University, Seoul, South Korea

Seung-Yong Jeong Department of Surgery, Seoul National University College of Medicine, Seoul, South Korea

Colorectal Cancer Center, Seoul National University Cancer Hospital, Seoul, South Korea

Cancer Research Institute, Seoul National University, Seoul, South Korea

Hiroyasu Kagawa Division of Colon and Rectal Surgery, Shizuoka Cancer Center Hospital, Shizuoka, Japan

Yukihide Kanemitsu Department of Colorectal Surgery, National Cancer Centre Hospital, Tokyo, Japan

Jeonghyun Kang Department of Surgery, Yonsei University College of Medicine, Seoul, South Korea

Sung-Bum Kang Department of Surgery, Seoul National University College of Medicine, Seoul National University Bundang Hospital, Seongnam, South Korea

Sung Il Kang Department of Surgery, Seoul National University College of Medicine, Seoul National University Bundang Hospital, Seongnam, South Korea

Dae Joon Kim Department of Thoracic and Cardiovascular Surgery, Yonsei University College of Medicine, Seoul, South Korea

Hee Cheol Kim Department of Surgery, Samsung Medical Center, Sungkyunkwan University School of Medicine, Seoul, South Korea

Hoguen Kim Department of Pathology, Yonsei University College of Medicine, Seoul, South Korea

Honsoul Kim Department of Radiology, Yonsei Cancer Center, Yonsei University College of Medicine, Seoul, South Korea

Ji Yeon Kim Department of Surgery, Division of Colorectal Surgery, Chungnam National University School of Medicine, Daejeon, South Korea

Jin Cheon Kim Division of Colon and Rectal Surgery, Department of Surgery, University of Ulsan College of Medicine and Asan Medical Center, Seoul, South Korea

Nam Kyu Kim Department of Surgery, Yonsei University College of Medicine, Seoul, South Korea

Seon-Hahn Kim Colorectal Division, Korea University Anam Hospital, Seoul, South Korea

Korea University College of Medicine, Seoul, South Korea

Yusuke Kinugasa Department of Gastrointestinal Surgery, Tokyo Medical Dental University, Tokyo, Japan

Woong Sub Koom Department of Radiation Oncology, Yonsei University College of Medicine, Seoul, South Korea

Wai Lun Law Department of Surgery, The Univeristy of Hong Kong, Queen Mary Hospital, Hong Kong, People's Republic of China

In Kyu Lee Department of Surgery, College of Medicine, Seoul St. Mary's Hospital, The Catholic University of Korea, Seoul, South Korea

Jong Min Lee Department of Surgery, Yonsei University College of Medicine, Seoul, South Korea

Kang Young Lee Department of Surgery, Yonsei University College of Medicine, Seoul, South Korea

Jin-Tung Liang Department of Surgery, National Taiwan University Hospital, Taipei City, Taiwan

Joon Seok Lim Department of Radiology, Yonsei Cancer Center, Yonsei University College of Medicine, Seoul, South Korea

Seok-Byung Lim Division of Colon and Rectal Surgery, Department of Surgery, University of Ulsan College of Medicine and Asan Medical Center, Seoul, South Korea

Cheng-Jen Ma Kaohsiung Medical University and Hospital, Kaohsiung, Taiwan

In Ja Park Department of Colon and Rectal Surgery, University of Ulsan College of Medicine and Asan Medical Center, Seoul, South Korea

Ji Won Park Department of Surgery, Seoul National University College of Medicine, Seoul, South Korea

Colorectal Cancer Center, Seoul National University Cancer Hospital, Seoul, South Korea

Cancer Research Institute, Seoul National University, Seoul, South Korea

Sohee Park Graduate School of Public Health, Yonsei University, Seoul, South Korea

Youn Young Park Department of Surgery, Uijeongbu St. Mary's Hospital, College of Medicine, The Catholic University of Korea, Seoul, South Korea

Amar Chand Doddama Reddy Division of Colorectal Surgery, Department of Surgery, Minimally Invasive Surgery Center, China Medical University Hospital, Taichung City, Taiwan

Zhao Ren Rui Jin Hospital, Shanghai Jiaotong University School of Medicine, Shanghai, China

Yoshiharu Sakai Department of Surgery, Kyoto University Graduate School of Medicine, Kyoto, Japan

Takaki Sakurai Department of Diagnostic Pathology, Kyoto University Graduate School of Medicine, Kyoto, Japan

Nieun Seo Department of Radiology, Yonsei Cancer Center, Yonsei University College of Medicine, Seoul, South Korea

Kenichi Sugihara Graduate School, Tokyo Medical and Dental University, Tokyo, Japan

Zhang Tao Rui Jin Hospital, Shanghai Jiaotong University School of Medicine, Shanghai, China

James Wei Tatt Toh Colorectal Division, Korea University Anam Hospital, Seoul, South Korea

Korea University College of Medicine, Seoul, South Korea

Colorectal Division, Department of Surgery, Westmead Hospital, Sydney, NSW, Australia

Hideki Ueno Department of Surgery, National Defense Medical College, Saitama, Japan

Hiroyuki Uetake Graduate School, Tokyo Medical and Dental University, Tokyo, Japan

Jaw-Yuan Wang Kaohsiung Medical University and Hospital, Kaohsiung, Taiwan

Ye Wei Colorectal Cancer Center, Zhongshan Hospital, Fudan University, Shanghai, China

Jianmin Xu Colorectal Cancer Center, Zhongshan Hospital, Fudan University, Shanghai, China

Shinichi Yamauchi Graduate School, Tokyo Medical and Dental University, Tokyo, Japan

Seung Yoon Yang Department of Surgery, Yonsei University College of Medicine, Seoul, South Korea

Hideaki Yano Division of Colorectal Surgery, Department of Surgery, National Center for Global Health and Medicine, Tokyo, Japan

Jeremy Yip Division of Colorectal Surgery, Department of Surgery, Queen Mary Hospital, University of Hong Kong, Hong Kong, China

Chang Sik Yu Department of Colon and Rectal Surgery, University of Ulsan College of Medicine and Asan Medical Center, Seoul, South Korea

Andee Dzulkarnaen Zakaria Colorectal Division, Korea University Anam Hospital, Seoul, South Korea

Korea University College of Medicine, Seoul, South Korea

Department of Surgery, School of Medical Sciences, Universiti Sains Malaysia, Kubang Kerian, Kelantan, Malaysia

Dexiang Zhu Colorectal Cancer Center, Zhongshan Hospital, Fudan University, Shanghai, China

Part I

Essential Basic Considerations in Colorectal Cancer

Epidemiology of Colorectal Cancer in Asia-Pacific Region

Sohee Park and Sun Ha Jee

Abstract

Colorectal cancer is the third most common cancer with about 1.36 million new cases and 694,000 deaths worldwide. Over the past two decades, colorectal cancer incidence has been drastically increasing in countries of the Asia-Pacific region, such as the Republic of Korea, Singapore, the Philippines, Thailand, and China. There is large geographic variation in colorectal cancer incidence and mortality throughout the world. The Republic of Korea has the highest colorectal cancer incidence (45 per 100,000). While the incidence of colorectal cancer has been stabilizing in parts of Northern and Western Europe and the USA, the rates have rapidly increased in economically developed Asia-Pacific countries such as Australia, New Zealand, Japan, Korea, and Singapore. The 5-year survival was estimated to be ranging from 28.1% to 66.0% for colon cancer patients and 39.7–65.9% for rectal cancer patients diagnosed during 2005–2009 in Asian countries.

A sharp increase in the incidence of colorectal cancer in Asian developed countries may be attributable to economic growth and environ-

mental factors such as a Western lifestyle. Lifestyle-related risk factors of colorectal cancer include smoking, alcohol drinking in men, high consumption of red meat and processed meat, body fatness, abdominal fatness, and physical inactivity. Colorectal cancer has clearly become an emerging health threat in Asia-Pacific regions and is dramatically increasing in its incidence. Prevention and treatment programs for colorectal cancer control should be actively implemented and evaluated in this region.

Keywords

Colorectal cancer incidence · Epidemiology · Geographic variation · Risk factor · Lifestyle

1.1 Trends of Colorectal Cancer Incidence and Mortality

Colorectal cancer is the third most common cancer with about 1.36 million new cases and 694,000 deaths worldwide. Colorectal cancer ranks the third in cancer incidence of men (746,000 cases, 10.0% of the total cancer incident cases) and the second in women (614,000 cases, 9.2% of the total cancer incident cases) [1]. Approximately 55% of the newly diagnosed colorectal cancer cases occur in more developed regions. Colorectal cancer is the fourth leading cause of cancer deaths (8.5% of the total) in the

S. Park (✉) · S. H. Jee
Graduate School of Public Health,
Yonsei University, Seoul, South Korea
e-mail: soheepark@yuhs.ac

© Springer Nature Singapore Pte Ltd. 2018
N. K. Kim et al. (eds.), *Surgical Treatment of Colorectal Cancer*,
https://doi.org/10.1007/978-981-10-5143-2_1

world. Unlike incident cases, more colorectal cancer deaths occur in less developed regions of the world (52%) which implies a worse survival in these regions [1].

The Republic of Korea has the highest colorectal cancer incidence in the world according to the GLOBOCAN 2012 estimates, with an age-standardized incidence rate of 45.0 per 100,000 person-years, followed by Slovakia (42.7 per 100,000), Hungary (42.3 per 100,000), Denmark (40.5 per 100,000), and the Netherlands (40.2 per 100,000). Most of the countries listed in the top 20 highest colorectal cancer incidence rates are in Northern Europe, but it is notable that Asia-Pacific countries such as the Republic of Korea, Singapore, Japan, Australia, and New Zealand are also included (Table 1.1). The colorectal cancer

incidence rate in the Republic of Korea is remarkably high compared with that of other Asian countries (13.7 per 100,000) and the USA (25.0 per 100,000). Despite its rapid increase of incidence rate (20.4 in 1999 and 36.2 in 2009, average percent change of 6.2%), the 5-year survival improved dramatically from 58.0% to 76.3% over the last two decades in Korea [2, 3]. Both early detection through nationwide cancer screening and advancement of cancer treatment may have contributed to the improved survival in colorectal cancer patients in the Republic of Korea. However, most recent statistics of Korea show that the colorectal cancer incidence began to decrease after year 2010 with annual percent change of −4.6% [3].

Table 1.1 Top 20 countries with highest colorectal cancer incidence rates in the world

Population	Number of incident cases	Crude incidence rates	Age-standardized incidence rates[a]
Republic of Korea	33,773	69.5	**45.0**
Slovakia	3963	72.3	**42.7**
Hungary	8442	84.8	**42.3**
Denmark	4832	86.4	**40.5**
The Netherlands	13,918	83.3	**40.2**
Czech Republic	8336	78.9	**38.9**
Norway	3913	78.9	**38.9**
Australia	15,869	69.2	**38.4**
New Zealand	3018	67.6	**37.3**
Slovenia	1621	79.5	**37.0**
Belgium	8683	80.5	**36.7**
Israel	4033	52.4	**35.9**
Canada	23,769	68.5	**35.2**
Ireland	2560	55.9	**34.9**
Italy	48,110	78.9	**33.9**
Singapore	2662	50.6	**33.7**
Spain	32,240	68.9	**33.1**
Croatia	3209	73.1	**32.9**
Serbia	5513	56.0	**32.6**
Japan	112,675	89.1	**32.2**

Data were generated from GLOBOCAN 2012 estimates [1]
[a]Age-standardized rates were based on the world population (per 100,000 person-years)

1.1.1 Temporal Trends

Over the past two decades, colorectal cancer incidence has been drastically increasing in countries of the Asia-Pacific region, such as Singapore, the Philippines, Thailand, the Republic of Korea, and China (Fig. 1.1). While colorectal cancer incidence of Japanese men appeared to decrease since 1993, most countries in Fig. 1.1 shows significantly increasing trend in Asia. Similarly increasing trends are observed in Western and Northern European countries such as Denmark, England, Finland, and Slovakia, while decreasing trend has been observed in the USA, Australia, and France [4].

1.1.2 Geographic Variations

While colorectal cancer affects men and women almost equally, there is large geographic variation in colorectal cancer incidence and mortality throughout the world [5]. Colorectal cancer is known to be common in developed countries and be associated with Western lifestyle [6]. There is a large variation in colorectal cancer incidence rates (Fig. 1.2). The age-standardized colorectal incidence rate in more developed regions is 29.2 per 100,000 in contrast to 11.7 per 100,000 in less developed regions, and there is 37-fold dif-

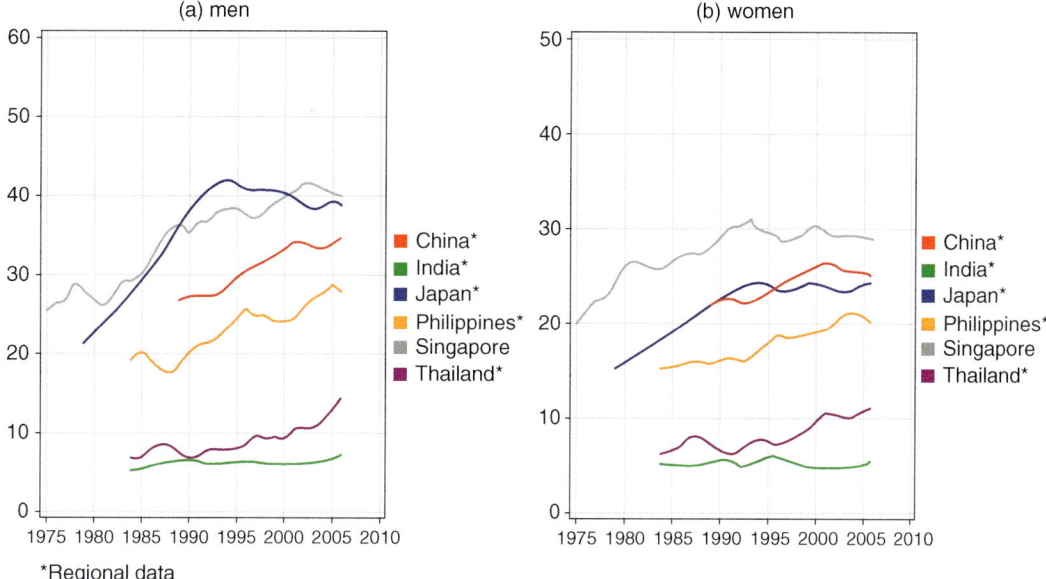

Fig. 1.1 Trend of colorectal cancer incidence in selected Asian countries. (**a**) Men. (**b**) Women. Source: GLOBOCAN 2012, http://globocan.iarc.fr/old/FactSheets/cancers/colorectal-new.asp

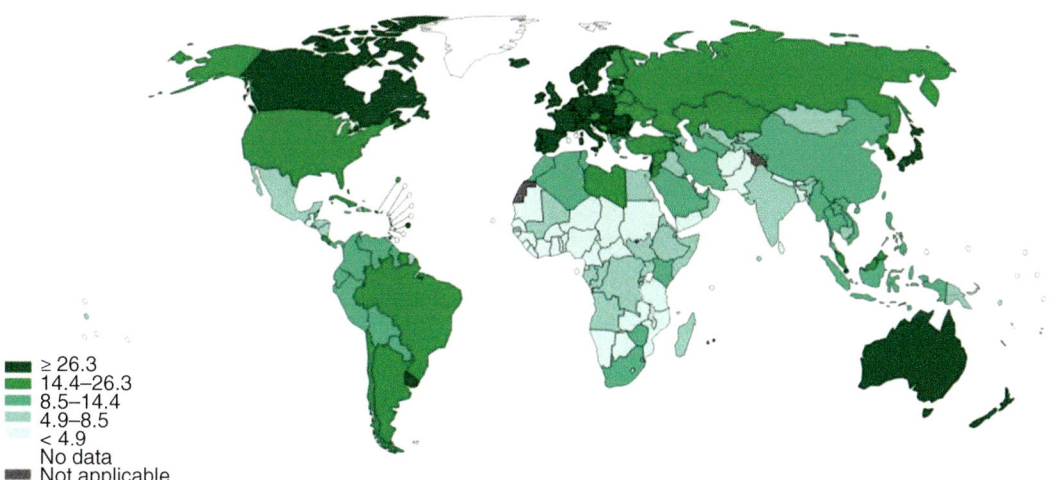

Fig. 1.2 Estimated colorectal cancer incidence rates in the world, age-standardized rates per 100,000 person-years. Source: GLOBOCAN 2012, http://globocan.iarc.fr

ference in the rate of the Republic of Korea (highest, 45.0 per 100,000) and Mozambique (lowest, 1.2 per 100,000) [4].

In contrast to a large discrepancy in colorectal cancer incidence across regions, there is less difference in colorectal cancer mortality. The age-standardized colorectal cancer mortality rate in more developed regions is 11.6 per 100,000 compared with 6.6 per 100,000 in less developed

regions. Hungary has the highest colorectal cancer mortality (20.8 per 100,000) and Mozambique has the lowest (0.9 per 100,000) [4].

While the incidence of colorectal cancer has been stabilizing in parts of Northern and Western Europe and the USA, the rates have rapidly increased in economically developed Asia-Pacific countries including Australia, New Zealand, Japan, Korea, and Singapore.

Through investigating the trends of colorectal cancer by subsite, substantial variation in subsite distribution of colorectal cancer in Asian countries was observed, and it was suggested that increase in overall colorectal cancer incidence may be mainly due to the increase in colon cancer, but not rectal cancer [7].

1.1.3 Survival of Colorectal Cancer Patients

According to the recent global study (CON-CORD-2), the 5-year survival in Asia was estimated ranging from 28.1% to 66.0% for colon cancer patients and 39.7–65.9% for rectal cancer patients diagnosed during 2005–2009 [8]. Table 1.2 summarizes the age-standardized incidence rates and 5-year survival for colorectal cancer in selected countries. In particular, 5-year survival estimates of the Republic of Korea and Japan appear to be similar to those of Australia and the USA.

It was also shown that the 5-year survival has risen for both colon and rectal cancers in most developed countries and regions, such as North America, Europe, and Oceania, and parts of East Asia including the Republic of Korea and urban region of China [8].

1.2 Risk Factors

A sharp increase in the incidence of colorectal cancer in Asian developed countries may be attributable to economic growth and environmental factors such as a Western lifestyle. Lifestyle-related risk factors of colorectal cancer include smoking, alcohol drinking in men, high consumption of red meat and processed meat, body fatness, abdominal fatness, and physical inactivity. These factors were mostly classified as having a convincing evidence for their association with significantly increased risk of colorectal cancer after being evaluated by expert groups of the World Cancer Research Foundation (WCRF) and American Institute for Cancer Research [9]. The WCRF report showed that foods containing dietary fiber, garlic, non-starchy vegetables, fruits, foods containing folate and selenium, soy products, and green tea may have a protective effect against colorectal cancer risk, but the level of evidence was weaker (Table 1.3).

An update of the WCRF report was recently published from a comprehensive search on foods and beverages and their association with colorectal cancer during the period of January 1, 2010, to May 31, 2015. This reevaluation confirmed that red and processed meat consumption and alcohol drinking are still significant risk factors for colorectal cancer [10]. There was insufficient evidence for the association with colorectal cancer risk for the consumption of fruits, legumes, poultry, coffee, and tea.

Table 1.2 Age-standardized incidence rates and 5-year survival for colorectal cancer in selected countries

Population	Age-standardized incidence rates (per 100,000)	5-year survival	
		Colon cancer	Rectal cancer
Republic of Korea	45.0	66.0	65.9
Japan	32.2	64.4	60.3
China	14.2	54.6	53.2
Malaysia	18.3	53.3	42.5
Indonesia	12.8	28.1	58.0
Thailand	12.4	50.4	39.7
Australia	38.4	64.2	64.2
New Zealand	37.3	61.6	60.8
USA	25.0	64.7	64.0
UK	30.2	53.8	56.6

Age-standardized rates of colorectal cancer are from GLOBOCAN 2012 [4], and 5-year survival estimates for cancer patients diagnosed in 2005–2009 are from CONCORD-2 [8]

1.2.1 Smoking

While many studies have reported a 20–60% increase in risk of colorectal cancer associated with active smoking, neither the International

Table 1.3 List of factors associated with colorectal cancer

Level of evidence	Increase RISK	Decrease RISK	Evidence source
Convincing	Smoking	Physical activity (colon)	WCRF
	Alcohol drinking (men)		WCRF
	Red meat		WCRF
	Processed meat		WCRF
	Body fatness		WCRF
	Abdominal fatness		WCRF
Probable	Alcohol drinking (women)	Foods containing dietary fiber	WCRF
		Garlic	WCRF
		Non-starchy vegetables	
		Fruits	WCRF
		Foods containing folate	
		Selenium	
		Soy products	
		Green tea	
		Milk	WCRF-update
		Whole grain	
		Fish	
Less convincing		Vegetables	WCRF-update
Not associated	Coffee	Fruits	WCRF-update
	Tea		

WCRF World Cancer Research Fund [9]; WCRF-update [10]

Agency for Research on Cancer nor the US Surgeon General has classified smoking as a convincing risk factor for colorectal cancer because of concern about residual confounding [11]. A large prospective cohort study of over 180,000 subjects showed that the incidence of colorectal cancer was significantly higher among current smokers (hazard ratios (HR) = 1.27, 95% CI: 1.06–1.52) and among former smokers (HR = 1.23, 95% CI: 1.11–1.36) compared with nonsmokers, even in the analysis after controlling for 13 potential confounding factors including screening [11]. Studies

in Korea and Japan also showed elevated risk of colorectal cancer among smokers compared to nonsmokers [12, 13].

1.2.2 Alcohol Drinking

Alcohol drinking is a known risk factor for colorectal cancer with convincing evidence. There was a significant dose-response relationship (RR = 1.07, 95% CI: 1.05–1.09, per 10 g/day increment) [10]. In a pooled analysis of Korean data, there was an elevated risk of colorectal cancer (RR = 1.12 in men and RR = 1.19 in women for average alcohol consumption of 28.53 g/day in men and 6.38 g/day in women, respectively). Even light drinking (≤1 drink/day) was shown to be associated with the increased incidence of male colorectal cancer in a meta-analysis [14].

1.2.3 Meat Consumption

High consumption of red meat and processed meat possibly increases risk of colorectal cancer or colon cancer in both Japanese and Korean populations [15, 16]. An updated WCRF report reinforced the evidence that high intake of red and processed meat and alcohol increases the risk of colorectal cancer [10]. In particular, red and processed meat consumption showed a significant dose-response relationship with colorectal cancer risk (RR = 1.12, 95% CI: 1.04–1.21, per 100 g/day increment).

However, dietary fat and its association with colorectal cancer may be still controversial. A meta-analysis of 13 prospective cohort studies showed that dietary fat may not be associated with increased risk of colorectal cancer [17].

1.2.4 Obesity and Physical Inactivity

Obesity and physical inactivity were found to increase the colorectal cancer risk. Both body fatness and abdominal fatness were shown to have convincing evidence to increase the colorectal cancer.

According to the WCRF evaluation, most of the cohort studies out of 60 studies showed that body fatness increased the risk of colorectal cancer. Meta-analysis showed that summary effect estimate of 1.03 (85% CI: 1.02–1.04) per 1 kg/m^2 increment of body mass index [9]. Abundant and consistent epidemiological evidence exists that greater body fatness is a cause of colorectal cancer.

1.2.5 Fruits and Vegetables

Based on the update of WCRF report, vegetables (RR = 0.98, 95% CI: 0.96–0.99, 100 g/day increment) were inversely associated with the risk of colorectal cancer [10]. However, there does not seem to be sufficient evidence for the protective effect of fruits on colorectal cancer. The studies conducted in Japanese and Korean population showed inconsistent results. A recent study on Japanese population showed that there was insufficient evidence to support an association between vegetable intake and colorectal cancer risk [18]. Furthermore, a meta-analysis on Korean population showed that vegetables and soybeans were not significantly associated with colorectal cancer risk [16].

1.2.6 Soy Product and Green Tea Consumption

Soy intake and green tea consumption represent a protective Asian diet that has drawn much attention recently. Soy product consumption was inversely associated with the incidence of overall GI cancer (0.857; 95% CI: 0.766, 0.959) and the gastric cancer subgroup (0.847; 95% CI: 0.722, 0.994) but not the colorectal cancer subgroup [19]. Green tea consumption is not associated with colorectal cancer prevention [20]. Furthermore, with an increment of 1 cup/day of green tea consumption, there was a protective effect on colorectal cancer risk (OR = 0.98, 95% CI = 0.96–1.01, in men; OR = 0.68, 95% CI = 0.56–0.81, in women) [21].

Regarding coffee consumption, compared to nondrinkers, ORs of less than 1 cup/day, 1–2 cups/day,

and 3 or more cups/day for colorectal cancer were 0.88 (95% CI: 0.77–1.00), 0.90 (95% CI: 0.80–1.01), and 0.78 (95% CI: 0.65–0.92), respectively (p for trend = 0.009) [22].

1.2.7 Dairy Product and Whole Grains

Milk and whole grains may have a protective role against colorectal cancer. High consumption of dairy product (RR = 0.87, 95% CI: 0.83 = 0.90, per 400 g/day increment) and total milk (RR = 0.94, 95% CI: 0.92–0.96, per 200 g/day increment) were associated with lowering colorectal cancer risk [10].

1.2.8 Migrant Studies

Migrant studies implied that patterns of cancer among migrant groups often change faster than they do among people that remain in their home country. For instance, one migrant study revealed that colorectal cancer incidence in US-born Japanese men and women had 40–50% higher colorectal incidence rates than foreign-born Japanese men and women [23]. Such findings may suggest that changing into a Western lifestyle increases the risk of colorectal cancer.

Table 1.4 summarizes the PAF estimates of each risk factor for colorectal cancer incidence in Korea, Japan, and China. When comparing these three countries, PAF estimates for smoking and alcohol drinking seem to be quite high in Japanese population. According to the estimated population attributable fraction (PAF) in Korea, approximately 17% of colorectal cancer incidence was attributable to risk factors including smoking, alcohol drinking, overweight and obesity, and physical inactivity [24].

Colorectal cancer has clearly become an emerging health threat in the Asia-Pacific region and is dramatically increasing in its incidence. Prevention and treatment programs for colorectal cancer control should be actively implemented and evaluated in this region.

Table 1.4 Population attributable fraction (%) of lifestyle-related factors for colorectal cancer in Korea, Japan, and China

	Republic of Korea		Japan		China	
Population	Men	Women	Men	Women	Men	Women
Smoking	1.50	0.02	20.4	4.5	–	–
Alcohol drinking	8.57	4.23	32.9	2.1	2.06	0.15
Excess body weight	6.75	6.60	5.2	4.0	1.39[a] (0.65)	NA[a] (1.80)
Physical inactivity	0.78	0.87	3.2	3.9	–	–

PAF estimates for Korea [12, 24–26]; Japan [13]; China [27, 28]
[a]Colon (Rectum)

References

1. Ferlay J, Soerjomataram I, Dikshit R, Eser S, Mathers C, Rebelo M, et al. Cancer incidence and mortality worldwide: sources, methods and major patterns in GLOBOCAN 2012. Int J Cancer. 2015;136(5):E359–86.
2. Jung KW, Park S, Kong HJ, Won YJ, Lee JY, Seo HG, et al. Cancer statistics in Korea: incidence, mortality, survival, and prevalence in 2009. Cancer Res Treat. 2012;44(1):11–24.
3. Jung KW, Won YJ, CM O, Kong HJ, Lee DH, Lee KH. Cancer statistics in Korea: incidence, mortality, survival, and prevalence in 2014. Cancer Res Treat. 2017;49(2):292–305.
4. Ferlay JSI, Ervik M, Dikshit R, Eser S, Mathers C, Rebelo M, Parkin DM, Forman D, Bray F. GLOBOCAN 2012 v1.0, cancer incidence and mortality worldwide: IARC cancerbase No. 11. Lyon: International Agency for Research on Cancer; 2013. Available from: http://globocan.iarc.fr
5. Center MM, Jemal A, Smith RA, Ward E. Worldwide variations in colorectal cancer. CA. 2009;59(6):366–78.
6. Park S, Bae J, Nam BH, Yoo KY. Aetiology of cancer in Asia. Asian Pac J Cancer Prev. 2008;9(3):371–80.
7. Park HM, Woo H, Jung SJ, Jung KW, Shin HR, Shin A. Colorectal cancer incidence in 5 Asian countries by subsite: an analysis of cancer incidence in five continents (1998-2007). Cancer Epidemiol. 2016;45:65–70.
8. Allemani C, Weir HK, Carreira H, Harewood R, Spika D, Wang XS, et al. Global surveillance of cancer survival 1995-2009: analysis of individual data for 25,676,887 patients from 279 population-based registries in 67 countries (CONCORD-2). Lancet. 2015;385(9972):977–1010.
9. World Cancer Research Fund and American Institute for Cancer Research. Food, Nutrition. Physical activity, and the prevention of cancer: a global perspective. Washington DC: AICR; 2007.
10. Vieira AR, Abar L, Chan D, Vingeliene S, Polemiti E, Stevens C, et al. Foods and beverages and colorectal cancer risk: a systematic review and meta-analysis of cohort studies, an update of the evidence of the WCRF-AICR continuous update project. Ann Oncol. 2017;28(8):1788–802.
11. Hannan LM, Jacobs EJ, Thun MJ. The association between cigarette smoking and risk of colorectal cancer in a large prospective cohort from the United States. Cancer Epidemiol Biomark Prev. 2009;18(12):3362–7.
12. Park S, Jee SH, Shin HR, Park EH, Shin A, Jung KW, et al. Attributable fraction of tobacco smoking on cancer using population-based nationwide cancer incidence and mortality data in Korea. BMC Cancer. 2014;14:406.
13. Inoue M, Sawada N, Matsuda T, Iwasaki M, Sasazuki S, Shimazu T, et al. Attributable causes of cancer in Japan in 2005--systematic assessment to estimate current burden of cancer attributable to known preventable risk factors in Japan. Ann Oncol. 2012;23(5):1362–9.
14. Choi YJ, Myung SK, Lee JH. Light alcohol drinking and risk of cancer: a meta-analysis of cohort studies. Cancer Res Treat. 2017. https://doi.org/10.4143/crt.2017.094.
15. Pham NM, Mizoue T, Tanaka K, Tsuji I, Tamakoshi A, Matsuo K, et al. Meat consumption and colorectal cancer risk: an evaluation based on a systematic review of epidemiologic evidence among the Japanese population. Jpn J Clin Oncol. 2014;44(7):641–50.
16. Woo HD, Park S, Oh K, Kim HJ, Shin HR, Moon HK, et al. Diet and cancer risk in the Korean population: a meta-analysis. Asian Pac J Cancer Prev. 2014;15(19):8509–19.
17. Liu L, Zhuang W, Wang RQ, Mukherjee R, Xiao SM, Chen Z, et al. Is dietary fat associated with the risk of colorectal cancer? A meta-analysis of 13 prospective cohort studies. Eur J Nutr. 2011;50(3):173–84.
18. Kashino I, Mizoue T, Tanaka K, Tsuji I, Tamakoshi A, Matsuo K, et al. Vegetable consumption and colorectal cancer risk: an evaluation based on a systematic review and meta-analysis among the Japanese population. Jpn J Clin Oncol. 2015;45(10):973–9.
19. Lu D, Pan C, Ye C, Duan H, Xu F, Yin L, et al. Meta-analysis of soy consumption and gastrointestinal cancer risk. Sci Rep. 2017;7(1):4048.
20. Wang ZH, Gao QY, Fang JY. Green tea and incidence of colorectal cancer: evidence from prospective cohort studies. Nutr Cancer. 2012;64(8):1143–52.
21. Chen Y, Wu Y, Du M, Chu H, Zhu L, Tong N, et al. An inverse association between tea consumption and colorectal cancer risk. Oncotarget. 2017;8(23):37367–76.

22. Senda Nakagawa H, Ito H, Hosono S, Oze I, Tanaka H, Matsuo K. Coffee consumption and the risk of colorectal cancer by anatomical subsite in Japan: results from the HERPACC studies. Int J Cancer. 2017;141(2):298–308.

23. Flood DM, Weiss NS, Cook LS, Emerson JC, Schwartz SM, Potter JD. Colorectal cancer incidence in Asian migrants to the United States and their descendants. Cancer Causes Control. 2000;11(5):403–11.

24. Shin HR, Shin A, Jung KW, et al. Attributable causes of cancer in Korea in the year 2009. Goyang: National Cancer Center; 2014.

25. Park S, Kim Y, Shin HR, Lee B, Shin A, Jung KW, et al. Population-attributable causes of cancer in Korea: obesity and physical inactivity. PLoS One. 2014;9(4):e90871.

26. Park S, Shin HR, Lee B, Shin A, Jung KW, Lee DH, et al. Attributable fraction of alcohol consumption on cancer using population-based nationwide cancer incidence and mortality data in the Republic of Korea. BMC Cancer. 2014;14:420.

27. Liang H, Wang J, Xiao H, Wang D, Wei W, Qiao Y, et al. Estimation of cancer incidence and mortality attributable to alcohol drinking in China. BMC Public Health. 2010;10:730.

28. Wang D, Zheng W, Wang SM, Wang JB, Wei WQ, Liang H, et al. Estimation of cancer incidence and mortality attributable to overweight, obesity, and physical inactivity in China. Nutr Cancer. 2012;64(1):48–56.

A Multidisciplinary Approach for Advanced Colorectal Cancer

2

Nam Kyu Kim and Youn Young Park

Abstract

As the incidence of colorectal cancer and difficult cases demanding complex clinical decisions have increased and multimodal treatment strategies have been much developed, the need for a multidisciplinary team (MDT) approach is increasing for treating colorectal cancer patients in that MDT approach would allow more tailored treatment for complex or advanced colorectal cancer patients. In this chapter, the background of increasing need of MDT and its impacts on various aspects are dealt with, and the factors affecting the efficacy of MDT clinics are reviewed. This chapter will help you to establish the basic concept of MDT and to review evidences advocating its positive impacts as well as some debate issues.

Keywords

Multidisciplinary team (MDT) · Colorectal cancer

N. K. Kim(✉)
Department of Surgery, Yonsei University College of Medicine, Seoul, South Korea
e-mail: namkyuk@yuhs.ac

Y. Y. Park
Department of Surgery, Uijeongbu St. Mary's Hospital, College of Medicine, The Catholic University of Korea, Seoul, South Korea

Colorectal cancer is the fourth leading cause of cancer mortality and the second most common malignancy worldwide [1]. In Korea, the incidence rate of colorectal cancer has increased rapidly and was predicted to be the most common cancer among men for the first time in 2016 [2]. Although early detection rates of colorectal cancer are increasing since a mass screening system has been established, around 70% of newly diagnosed colorectal cancer patients still demonstrate advanced tumors that are not primarily resectable, and synchronous liver metastases are present in approximately 30% of them [3, 4]. As surgical techniques such as the introduction of total mesorectal excision (TME), complete mesocolic excision (CME) with central vessel ligation (CVL), and the use of minimally invasive surgery (MIS) have advanced and various chemotherapeutic agents and radiation techniques have developed, the era of multimodal treatments has been established in colorectal cancer. With the use of multimodal treatments, available treatment regimens with various therapeutic orders have been more complicated in an effort to achieve higher R0 resection rates in advanced colorectal cancer. Owing to these attempts to convert initially unresectable tumors to resectable tumors, a fine boundary of operability no longer exists. In this context, a multidisciplinary team (MDT) approach is integral to achieve a highly tailored therapy for better oncological and clinical outcomes. MDT care has increasingly been imple-

© Springer Nature Singapore Pte Ltd. 2018
N. K. Kim et al. (eds.), *Surgical Treatment of Colorectal Cancer*,
https://doi.org/10.1007/978-981-10-5143-2_2

mented throughout Asian countries including South Korea, where the colorectal cancer incidence is rapidly increasing; thereby, the number of difficult cases that need more complex clinical decisions is increasing simultaneously.

2.1 Definition and Team Composition

Before we discuss the necessity of MDT, a review of the terms of a multidisciplinary team (MDT) approach must precede. The MDT approach is a form of teamwork; therefore, it is easier for us to understand the term teamwork in healthcare first. In a concept analysis, Andreas et al. proposed it as a dynamic process involving two or more healthcare professionals with complementary backgrounds and skills, sharing common health goals and exercising concerted physical and mental efforts in assessing, planning, or evaluating patient care [5]. The term multidisciplinary is often used interchangeably with interdisciplinary, interprofessional, and multiprofessional in reports on MDT [6]. These generally refer to any healthcare teams including a range of health service workers with the majority being from professional groups. Therefore, when focusing on cancer care treatment, MDTs include a surgical oncologist, a medical oncologist, a radiation oncologist, physicians, nurses, pharmacists, social workers, and other groups with specialty training such as primary care, palliative care, and hospice care [7]. In colorectal cancer care, MDTs mainly include a surgical oncologist, a medical oncologist, a radiation oncologist, a radiologist, a gastroenterologist, hepatobiliary surgeons, coordinators, and nurses.

The MDT approach can be understood as an evolved and more structural form of a tumor board, which brings together any professionals in charge of the planned treatments for cancer patients in a complicated situation. Fennell et al. pointed out that differentiating elements between the tumor board and MDT are the use of team structure and involvement of the patients [8]. Therefore, within the team structure, collaboration and communication with each team member and a patient-oriented approach are essential for MDT.

2.2 Increasing Need for Clinical MDTs and a Brief Introduction to Our Experience of a MDT

One of the main reasons why the MDT approach is growing is that the increasing specialization and complexity of skills and knowledge from a single physician is not enough to deal with the complex needs of some patients [9]. An increasing number of elderly patients with more complex comorbidities and the recent move toward the continuous improvement of the patients' quality of life throughout the treatment pathway are also the key reasons [9].

In our institution, the tumor board for very complicated colorectal cancer cases started 15 years ago. It evolved to form a structured team and has been running as a face-to-face MDT clinic since 2013. Since the Korean government began to reimburse the costs of MDT clinics from 2014 and with the motivation of Korean Cancer Association and Korean Society of Surgical Oncology members, more referral hospitals have started MDT clinics (Fig. 2.1). According to reimbursement coverage in Korea, at least four specialists should attend a MDT clinic, which are mainly surgeons, medical oncologists, radiation oncologists, and radiologists. An additional gastroenterologist and pathologist can also attend. A total of 531 MDT clinics within all departments were held in 2014, with the number of cases continuing to increase after starting insurance coverage, reaching 1098 cases. Among them, colorectal MDT clinics were held most frequently and consisted of over 30% of the total cases (Fig. 2.2). This rapid increase indicates that many clinical practitioners actually want to discuss complicated cases with interdisciplinary professionals in order to obtain better treatment plans and outcomes. MDT clinics have fulfilled not only the physician's but also the patient satisfaction; the survey on patient satisfaction in our institution in 2014 showed that 97% of the patients were satisfied with the explanation of their treatment plan after MDT clinics and 99.3% of them fully trusted the decisions made by the MDT clinic (Fig. 2.3). As human resources are of great importance for successful MDT meetings, a coordinator has had a role in arranging an appropriate time for the meeting, making sure the clinic runs smoothly.

Cost code	Category	Insurance fee	General fee	fee for international patients
AI101	MDT fees(4 person)	113,210	114,210	175,000
AI102	MDT fees(5 person)	141,510	142,510	215,000

(Unit : won)

Fig. 2.1 Multidisciplinary team (MDT) fees have been assigned by the government insurance policy since 1 Aug 2014 in South Korea

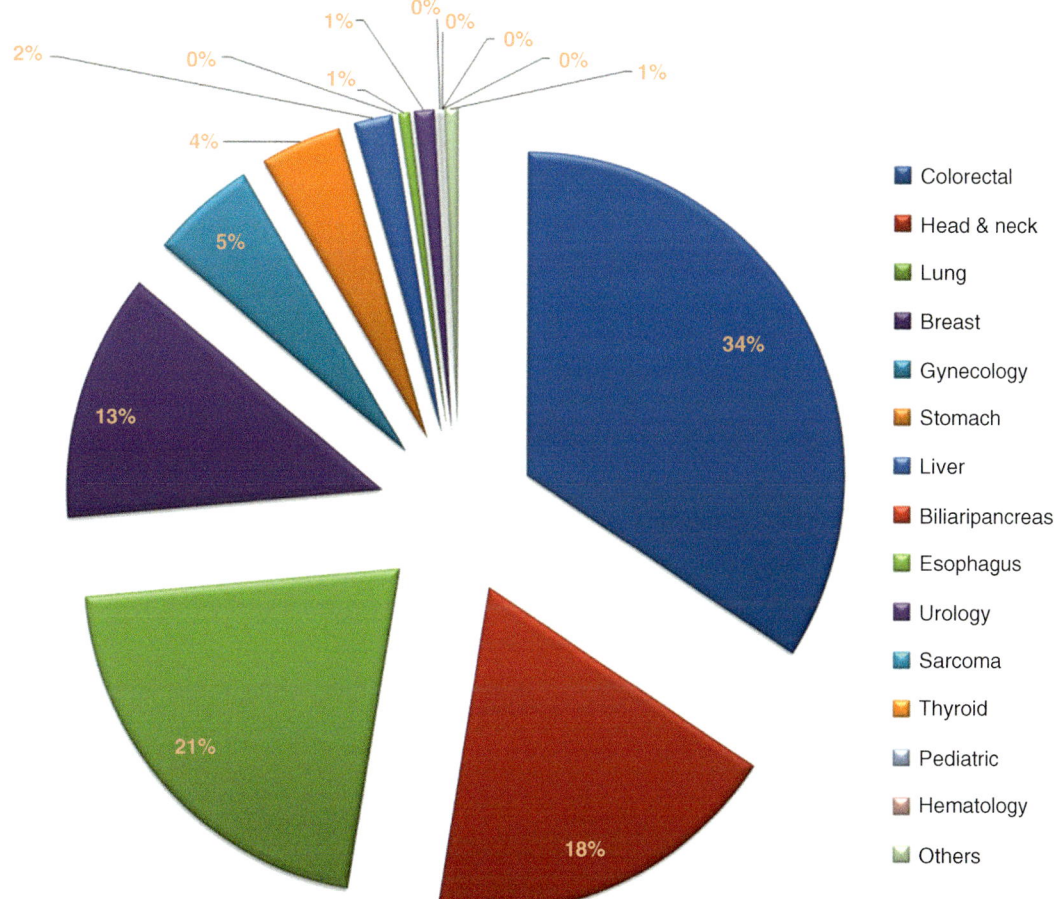

Fig. 2.2 Percentage of patient enrollment in multidisciplinary team (MDT) clinic in the Yonsei University Healthcare System

In addition to human resources, hardware has also had an important role in arranging regular MDT meetings and improving workflow. Hardware for MDT clinics includes space for regular MDT meetings equipped with personal computers for each participant to get access to electronic medical records (EMRs), a large screen to review imaging work-ups, and telemedicine for some surgeons who cannot physically come to the clinic due to their operation schedule (Fig. 2.4). Initially, the colorectal MDT clinic used for stage 4 or recurrent cases; however, indications are getting broader to include locally advanced cancer cases requiring consideration of various available treatment options and

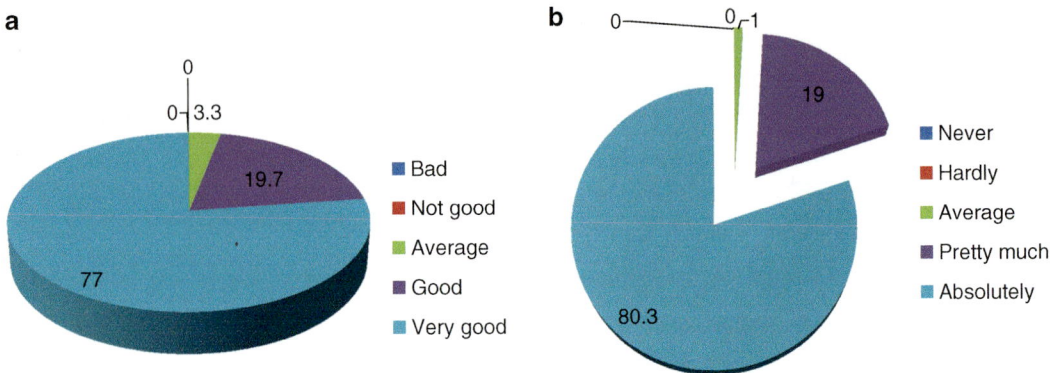

Fig. 2.3 (**a**) Patient satisfaction with the explanation of the treatment plan after a multidisciplinary team (MDT) meeting. (**b**) Degree of patients' MDT meeting

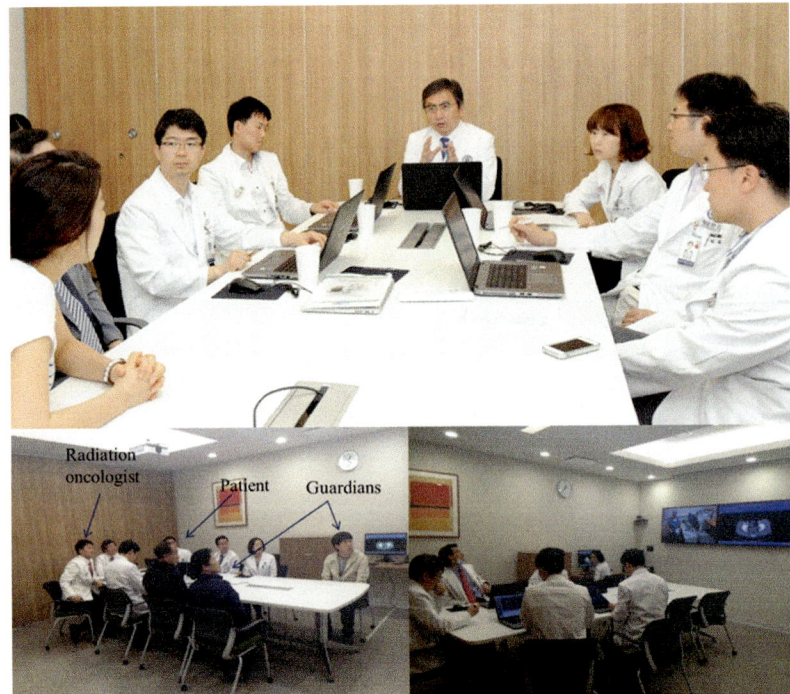

Fig. 2.4 Pictures showing the multidisciplinary team (MDT) meeting in a separate room equipped with personal computers, monitors to redraw images, and telemedicine and the presence of a patient

response evaluation along their treatment pathway, reflecting the complexity of personalized therapy in colorectal cancers.

2.3 Impact of MDT

Studies on the impact of MDT on patient outcome, including decision-making for the treatment plan, perioperative outcome, and long-term survival outcome, have been sporadically reported. Results have been inconclusive due to the accompanying evolutions of new therapeutic techniques and the development of chemotherapeutic agents for cancer patients [10]. Nevertheless, a majority of healthcare providers agree that interactive and high-quality communication and cooperation among multidisciplinary specialists is key to achieving the most desirable decision for individuals in complicated situations of varying degrees, resulting in a better patient outcome [11]. Previous researchers have shown evidence of MDT as an independent favorable prognostic factor in some aspects, which will be briefly discussed.

2.3.1 Changes in Decision-Making and Subsequent Treatment Plans

Benjamin et al. reviewed articles reporting changes in decision-making through MDT clinics. In their systematic review, six studies showed that MDT clinics changed the decision made in 2–52% of cases [12]. The greatest changes resulting from MDTs were reported by Ganesan et al.; pre-MDT diagnosis of ovarian cancer was alliterated in 52% of cases after involvement of the MDT clinic, including changes in histopathology or regarding histopathological grading, and the MDT clinic finally modified 22% of the patients' treatment plans [13]. Chang et al. reported changes in pathological results after MDT clinics, resulting in changes in treatment plans [14]. Snelgrove et al. also showed that MDT clinics lead to a change in the treatment plan in 29% of primary rectal cancer patients [15]. Page et al. introduced the example of a pancreatic cancer MDT clinic [16]; 25% of the patients with pancreatic cancer had a change in their treatment plan after MDT clinics. They explained that these changes were mainly due to reinterpretation of the imaging results between radiologists and surgeons, underscoring the importance of MDT discussion in treatment planning [16].

2.3.2 Increasing Adherence to Treatment Guidelines

In addition to changes in the diagnosis or pathological reinterpretation, some studies showed that MDT clinics improved the implementation rates of treatment guidelines. Forrest et al. reported that the rate of chemotherapy administration increased from 7% to 23%, resulting in a survival benefit in inoperable small cell lung cancer patients. Furthermore, MacDermid et al. found that MDT clinics increased the prescription rate, resulting in an improved 3-year survival

rate for advanced colorectal cancer patients [17, 18]. Abraham et al. also reported that a tumor board is the most important factor for increasing adherence to the National Comprehensive Cancer Network (NCCN) guidelines for colorectal cancer [19]. Indeed, Freeman et al. reported that MDT conferences for esophageal cancer showed not only adherence to the guidelines but also enhanced care including staging work-up and a decrease in the mean number of days between diagnosis and treatment [20]. An interesting report from Menon et al. suggested that undesired outcomes in colorectal cancer occurred in Europe due to unwarranted variations of treatments [21]. These variations affected the patients' clinical outcomes, but they cannot be understood just by patient-related risk factors or preference. Therefore, they proposed MDT clinics to improve the accuracy of the diagnosis and to decide a more adequate clinical pathway to reduce these unwarranted variations [21].

2.3.3 Improvement of Surgical Outcomes

Especially in colorectal cancer, it is preferred to treat patients according to a more stratified risk adjustment according to tumor location, associated symptoms, and clinical staging based on image findings to achieve curative resection. Some studies showed how MDT clinics could affect the surgical outcomes of colorectal cancer patients. Burtons et al. found that 26% of patients who underwent surgery without a MDT conference had a positive circumferential margin (CRM) compared with 1% for patients whose magnetic resonance imaging results were discussed at a MDT conference [22]. Similarly, Richardson et al. reported that the MDT approach improved the completeness of a TME and the subsequent outcomes [23]. Kontovounisios et al. reported high rates of complete resection of over 90% with low morbidity and mortality in locally advanced primary and recurrent colorectal cancer patients through MDT clinics [24], and Wille-Jørgensen et al. reported reduced perioperative mortality rates in primary rectal cancer patient clinics [24, 25].

2.3.4 Impact on Patient Satisfaction and Quality of Life

As mentioned above, MDT clinics resulted in 97% of the patients satisfied with the explanation of their treatment plan and 99.3% trusted the treatment decisions, as shown in a survey conducted in 2014 at our institute. Frost et al. reported that breast cancer patients whose data were discussed in MDT outpatient clinics had higher levels of satisfaction with their health, physician, and nursing care than those who received a medical–oncology consultation in the hospital [26]. In an interesting study conducted by Mark et al., predictive factors of satisfaction in patients with gastrointestinal or head and neck cancers in a MDT clinic setting were analyzed [27]. They found that the level of overall satisfaction was higher in females, providing greater attention to how patients cope with disease. Discussing a patients' psychosocial status in relation to their diagnoses and bringing it to the MDT members' attention were also predictive factors of improved patient satisfaction [27].

2.3.5 Impact on Survival

The survival benefit of the MDT clinic has been reported in several cancers including hepatocellular carcinoma, esophageal cancer, ovarian cancer, lung cancer, head and neck cancer, and rectal cancer [18, 22, 28–32]. Yopp et al. reported a markedly increased median survival from 4.8 months to 13.2 months in hepatocellular carcinoma patients after beginning MDT clinics [28]. Similarly, the survival benefit after inception of MDT for colorectal cancer patients has been reported in some literatures [17, 33, 34]. Studies on the survival benefit of the MDT clinic for just stage IV colorectal cancer patients are very limited. Lan et al. compared stage IV colorectal cancer patients who participated in MDT clinics to those who did not [34]. They analyzed a total of 1075 patients with stage IV disease between 2001 and 2010; their MDT clinics began in 2007 [34]. They found a significantly improved survival rate in patients with stage IV disease, and the 3-year survival rate increased

from 25.6% to 38.2%; the MDT clinic was an independent prognostic factor. These results suggested that the MDT clinic had increased the referral rate of metastasectomy through intensive cooperation between different specialists [34].

2.3.6 Impact on Research and Evidence-Making Process and Education

Besides improving patient outcome, MDT can also be a live educational resource for trainees not only for specific knowledge or updated treatment strategies concerning a disease but also for attaining communication and cooperation skills between different specialties, understanding the medicolegal responsibilities, and involving the patients' psychosocial aspect [35–37]. Moreover, MDT can provide insight into disease progression patterns in infrequent cases leading to clinical trials based on establishing better treatment strategies; this results in an evidence-making process. For example, in our institution, repetitive review of marginally resectable rectal cancer patients with resectable systemic metastasis enabled us to have an insight into the early failure of systemic control during long-course standard chemoradiation for local control. Thereby, it led us to start an observational study and clinical trials to improve treatment protocols for those patients. As a result, three papers have been published supporting upfront chemotherapy followed by short-course chemoradiation and a consecutive delayed operation [38–40]. Therefore, team members could be convinced that past experiences and time dedicated to the MDT approach could be beneficial to both the team member and the patient and could aid in establishing better treatment guidelines in the future.

2.4 Debate on Efficacy of MDT

Much of the published data confirms the MDT clinic's positive impact; however, there is also a study that has suggested no differences in the management of patients when a MDT clinic is held

[12, 18, 29, 41–46]. Riedel et al. retrospectively investigated the efficacy of a MDT clinic for lung cancer patients using both the time to diagnosis and time to definitive therapy as surrogates of its efficacy. They reported that there was no difference among patients who were and were not discussed by the MDT and concluded that the tumor board did not influence the quality of cancer care and may be an unnecessary allocation of resources [43]. Although the MDT approach has been widely adopted owing to patients' needs and the start of reimbursement in many referral hospitals, there must be further investigations into the efficacy of MDT in various aspects such as time to decision-making or surgery, referral sequence, improvement of quality of life, and survival. Moreover, it should be investigated how those factors are affected in terms of the structure of the MDT, which includes range of participants, the process of communication and cooperation, leadership, team climate, and infrastructures such as place, computers, monitors, electrical recording system, and telemedicine system.

2.5 Factors Affecting the Efficacy of MDT Clinics

2.5.1 Time Pressure and Inadequate Information

MDTs are mostly operated in large referral hospitals. Those hospitals usually load a lot of work onto each healthcare provider. MDT members in those large centers are likely to have little time to work up their cases to be discussed in advance. Macaskill et al. reported that over 50% of MDT meetings are held during lunchtime and 26.5% during breakfast time [37]. Sidhom et al. found that 69% of MDT members have failed to adequately work up patients before a MDT meeting, 45% of which were due to inadequate time and resources [35]. A high workload and consequent time pressure can lead to a reduction in the attendance rate of MDT members, resulting in them receiving inadequate information about cases and engaging in hasty decision-making [47–49]. In up to 16% of cases discussed in MDT meetings, the decisions are not implemented because of an inappropriate treatment for the underlying disease(s) and decision-making contradictory to the patients' choice [48, 50–54].

2.5.2 Leadership and Team Culture

Although MDTs are mostly led by surgeons, there is a report suggesting that leadership rotation can reduce conflicts between the different disciplines, leading to improvement of teamwork [37, 55]. Besides leadership, good team culture is essential for a free and open discussion in a MDT meeting, and it is associated with a high level of interdependency and cooperation [6]. Susan et al. conducted a qualitative content analysis to draw characteristics of effective MDT teamwork and proposed ten competency statements required for a highly functional MDT [9].

Competencies of an interdisciplinary team [9]:

1. Identifies a leader who establishes a clear direction and vision for the team while listening and providing support and supervision to the team members.
2. Incorporates a set of values that clearly provide direction for the team's service provision; these values should be visible and consistently portrayed.
3. Demonstrates a team culture and interdisciplinary atmosphere of trust where contributions are valued and consensus is fostered.
4. Ensures appropriate processes and infrastructures are in place to uphold the vision of the service (e.g., referral criteria, communications infrastructure).
5. Provides quality patient-focused services with documented outcomes and utilizes feedback to improve the quality of care.
6. Utilizes communication strategies that promote intra-team communication, collaborative decision-making, and effective team processes.
7. Provides sufficient team staffing to integrate an appropriate mix of skills, competencies, and personalities to meet the needs of patients and enhance smooth functioning.
8. Facilitates recruitment of staff who demonstrates interdisciplinary competencies including

team functioning, collaborative leadership, communication, and sufficient professional knowledge and experience.

9. Promotes role interdependence while respecting individual roles and autonomy.
10. Facilitates personal development through appropriate training, rewards, recognition, and opportunities for career development.

2.5.3 Infrastructures and Decision Support System

Infrastructures for MDT meeting include facilities like meeting rooms, personal computers, a projecting system for image review, and an electronic medical record system (EMR). According to the results from a survey of 2054 cancer MDT members in the UK on the key features of an effective MDT, 78% and 96% of the respondents rated the physical environment such as meeting room equipped with a projecting system for image and specimen reviews and EMR with available picture archiving and communications with a real-time documentation system (PACS), respectively [11]. With the advancement of new technology beyond these basic infrastructures, there is an increased focus on the importance of telemedicine and a clinical decision supporting system. Approximately 30% of colorectal cancer MDTs have telemedicine equipment in the UK [56]. Some studies showed that telemedicine did not have a negative impact on outcomes; however, it meant that the number of cases discussed in one meeting was reduced [48, 57, 58]. Decision support systems such as a web-based program to support adjuvant decision-making of a MDT for breast cancer patients were evaluated by Epstein et al. [59]; the program was used to predict the 10-year risks and benefits. Decisions concerning adjuvant treatment were changed in 12.7% of cases; therefore, they concluded that it can help to compare the added value of different treatments and provides more balanced information [59]. Séroussi et al. reported that use of OncoDoc2, a clinical decision supporting system implementing a local reference guideline on breast cancer management, at a MDT meeting increased the decision compliance rate with the reference guideline from 79% to 93% [60].

2.5.4 Feedback on MDT Performance

Harris et al. and Lamb et al. suggested tools to assess MDT performance [61, 62]. The former consists of ten subdomains rated on a 10-point scale from very poor to very good, including MDT meeting attendance, leadership and chairing in MDT meetings, teamwork and culture, personal development and training, physical environment available for use in MDT meetings, organization and administration during meetings, post-meeting coordination services, patient-centered care, and the clinical decision-making process [61]. The latter consists of nine subdomains rated on a 5-point scale, including the adequacy of case history information, radiological information, and pathological information, ability of MDT chair, and level of contribution (nil, vague, or precise) of surgeons, oncologists, radiologists, histopathologists, and clinical nurse specialists [62]. They found that these tools could provide a feasible and reliable way to enhance MDT performance; however, further validation and refinement is required for each.

2.6 Future Perspectives

A MDT clinic requires some infrastructure such as an adequate place and certain equipment, an allocated time, a coordinator, etc.; thus, it involves financial costs. Therefore, we need relevant studies examining whether this system is cost-beneficial or not [63]. Additionally, we should evaluate proper candidates who can benefit from a MDT clinic. Meanwhile, changes in staging, diagnosis, and treatment plans through MDT meetings truly lead to improved oncologic outcomes, quality of life, and patient satisfaction. Moreover, it is time to examine the potential benefit of artificial intelligence for discussing and reaching an optimal decision for different individuals with complex situations in a MDT meeting.

Conclusion

Multimodal therapy is now used for colorectal cancer management owing to the evolution of imaging tools, sphincter-saving surgical techniques, and development of chemotherapeutic regimens and nonsurgical treatment options. Due to its complexity and the diversity of treatment options, MDT can provide improved accuracy in decision-making and more optimal treatment plans, resulting in better surgical and oncologic outcomes and increased patient satisfaction. Moreover, MDT clinics can give educational opportunities for trainees and can provide a new insight into the nature of the disease, leading to clinical trials for more optimal treatment strategies. The efficacy of a MDT is associated with time pressure, leadership, and team culture; therefore, these factors should be assessed using the available tools for analyzing MDT performance or peer reviewed to enhance MDT performance. Further research could investigate the effects of team composition and patient involvement on the impact on the decision process including meeting time and duration, subtypes of leadership and team cultures, and the role of nursing personnel on decision-making. In Korea, we are only beginning to determine the effects of a MDT clinic. We must conduct basic studies on how this system affects patient and team satisfaction; furthermore, cost-benefit analysis should also be carried out in the future.

References

1. Jemal A, Siegel R, Ward E, Murray T, Xu J, Thun MJ. Cancer statistics, 2007. CA Cancer J Clin. 2007;57(1):43–66.
2. Jung KW, Won YJ, CM O, Kong HJ, Cho H, Lee JK, et al. Prediction of cancer incidence and mortality in Korea, 2016. Cancer Res Treat. 2016;48(2):451–7.
3. McMillan DC, McArdle CS. Epidemiology of colorectal liver metastases. Surg Oncol. 2007;16(1):3–5.
4. Simmonds PC, Primrose JN, Colquitt JL, Garden OJ, Poston GJ, Rees M. Surgical resection of hepatic metastases from colorectal cancer: a systematic review of published studies. Br J Cancer. 2006;94(7):982–99.
5. Xyrichis A, Ream E. Teamwork: a concept analysis. J Adv Nurs. 2008;61(2):232–41.
6. Thylefors I, Persson O, Hellstrom D. Team types, perceived efficiency and team climate in Swedish cross-professional teamwork. J Interprof Care. 2005;19(2):102–14.
7. Taplin SH, Weaver S, Salas E, Chollette V, Edwards HM, Bruinooge SS, et al. Reviewing cancer care team effectiveness. J Oncol Pract. 2015;11(3):239–46.
8. Fennell ML, Das IP, Clauser S, Petrelli N, Salner A. The organization of multidisciplinary care teams: modeling internal and external influences on cancer care quality. J Natl Cancer Inst Monogr. 2010;2010(40):72–80.
9. Nancarrow SA, Booth A, Ariss S, Smith T, Enderby P, Roots A. Ten principles of good interdisciplinary team work. Hum Resour Health. 2013;11(1):19.
10. Fleissig A, Jenkins V, Catt S, Fallowfield L. Multidisciplinary teams in cancer care: are they effective in the UK? Lancet Oncol. 2006;7(11):935–43.
11. Taylor C, Munro AJ, Glynne-Jones R, Griffith C, Trevatt P, Richards M, et al. Multidisciplinary team working in cancer: what is the evidence? Br Med J. 2010;340:c951.
12. Lamb BW, Brown KF, Nagpal K, Vincent C, Green JS, Sevdalis N. Quality of care management decisions by multidisciplinary cancer teams: a systematic review. Ann Surg Oncol. 2011;18(8):2116–25.
13. Ganesan P, Kumar L, Hariprasad R, Gupta A, Dawar R, Vijayaraghavan M. Improving care in ovarian cancer: the role of a clinico-pathological meeting. Natl Med J India. 2008;21(5):225–7.
14. Chang JH, Vines E, Bertsch H, Fraker DL, Czerniecki BJ, Rosato EF, et al. The impact of a multidisciplinary breast cancer center on recommendations for patient management: the University of Pennsylvania experience. Cancer. 2001;91(7):1231–7.
15. Snelgrove RC, Subendran J, Jhaveri K, Thipphavong S, Cummings B, Brierley J, et al. Effect of multidisciplinary cancer conference on treatment plan for patients with primary rectal cancer. Dis Colon Rectum. 2015;58(7):653–8.
16. Page AJ, Cosgrove D, Elnahal SM, Herman JM, Pawlik TM. Organizing a multidisciplinary clinic. Chin Clin Oncol. 2014;3(4):43.
17. MacDermid E, Hooton G, MacDonald M, McKay G, Grose D, Mohammed N, et al. Improving patient survival with the colorectal cancer multi-disciplinary team. Color Dis. 2009;11(3):291–5.
18. Forrest LM, McMillan DC, McArdle CS, Dunlop DJ. An evaluation of the impact of a multidisciplinary team, in a single centre, on treatment and survival in patients with inoperable non-small-cell lung cancer. Br J Cancer. 2005;93(9):977–8.
19. Abraham NS, Gossey JT, Davila JA, Al-Oudat S, Kramer JK. Receipt of recommended therapy by patients with advanced colorectal cancer. Am J Gastroenterol. 2006;101(6):1320–8.
20. Freeman RK, Van Woerkom JM, Vyverberg A, Ascioti AJ. The effect of a multidisciplinary thoracic malignancy conference on the treatment of patients with esophageal cancer. Ann Thorac Surg. 2011;92(4):1239–42. discussion 43

21. Menon M, Cunningham C, Kerr D. Addressing unwarranted variations in colorectal cancer outcomes: a conceptual approach. Nat Rev Clin Oncol. 2016; 13(11):706–12.

22. Burton S, Brown G, Daniels IR, Norman AR, Mason B, Cunningham D, et al. MRI directed multidisciplinary team preoperative treatment strategy: the way to eliminate positive circumferential margins? Br J Cancer. 2006;94(3):351–7.

23. Richardson B, Preskitt J, Lichliter W, Peschka S, Carmack S, de Prisco G, et al. The effect of multidisciplinary teams for rectal cancer on delivery of care and patient outcome: has the use of multidisciplinary teams for rectal cancer affected the utilization of available resources, proportion of patients meeting the standard of care, and does this translate into changes in patient outcome? Am J Surg. 2016;211(1):46–52.

24. Kontovounisios C, Tan E, Pawa N, Brown G, Tait D, Cunningham D, et al. Selection process can improve the outcome in locally advanced and recurrent colorectal cancer: activity and results of a dedicated multidisciplinary colorectal cancer centre. Color Dis. 2016; 19(4):331–8.

25. Wille-Jorgensen P, Sparre P, Glenthoj A, Holck S, Norgaard Petersen L, Harling H, et al. Result of the implementation of multidisciplinary teams in rectal cancer. Color Dis. 2013;15(4):410–3.

26. Frost M, Arvizu R, Jayakumar S, Schoonover A, Novotny P, Zahasky K. A multidisciplinary healthcare delivery model for women with breast cancer: patient satisfaction and physical and psychosocial adjustment. Oncol Nurs Forum. 1998;26(10):1673–80.

27. Walker MS, Ristvedt SL, Haughey BH. Patient care in multidisciplinary cancer clinics: does attention to psychosocial needs predict patient satisfaction? Psychooncology. 2003;12(3):291–300.

28. Yopp AC, Mansour JC, Beg MS, Arenas J, Trimmer C, Reddick M, et al. Establishment of a multidisciplinary hepatocellular carcinoma clinic is associated with improved clinical outcome. Ann Surg Oncol. 2014;21(4):1287–95.

29. Stephens MR, Lewis WG, Brewster AE, Lord I, Blackshaw GRJC, Hodzovic I, et al. Multidisciplinary team management is associated with improved outcomes after surgery for esophageal cancer. Dis Esophagus. 2006;19(3):164–71.

30. Junor EJ, Hole DJ, Gillis CR. Management of ovarian cancer: referral to a multidisciplinary team matters. Br J Cancer. 1994;70(2):363–70.

31. Houssami N, Sainsbury R. Breast cancer: multidisciplinary care and clinical outcomes. Eur J Cancer. 2006;42(15):2480–91.

32. Birchall M, Bailey D, King P, South West Cancer Intelligence Service H, Neck Tumour P. Effect of process standards on survival of patients with head and neck cancer in the south and west of England. Br J Cancer. 2004;91(8):1477–81.

33. Ye YJ, Shen ZL, Sun XT, Wang ZF, Shen DH, Liu HJ, et al. Impact of multidisciplinary team working on the management of colorectal cancer. Chin Med J. 2012;125(2):172–7.

34. Lan YT, Jiang JK, Chang SC, Yang SH, Lin CC, Lin HH, et al. Improved outcomes of colorectal cancer patients with liver metastases in the era of the multidisciplinary teams. Int J Color Dis. 2016;31(2):403–11.

35. Sidhom M, Poulsen M. Group decisions in oncology: doctors' perceptions of the legal responsibilities arising from multidisciplinary meetings. J Med Imaging Radiat Oncol. 2008;52(3):287–92.

36. Boyle FM, Robinson E, Heinrich P, Dunn SM. Cancer: communicating in the team game. ANZ J Surg. 2004;74(6):477–81.

37. Macaskill E, Thrush S, Walker E, Dixon J. Surgeons' views on multi-disciplinary breast meetings. Eur J Cancer. 2006;42(7):905–8.

38. Kim KH, Shin SJ, Cho MS, Ahn JB, Jung M, Kim TI, et al. A phase II study of preoperative mFOLFOX6 with short-course radiotherapy in patients with locally advanced rectal cancer and liver-only metastasis. Radiother Oncol. 2016;118(2):369–74.

39. Shin SJ, Yoon HI, Kim NK, Lee KY, Min BS, Ahn JB, et al. Upfront systemic chemotherapy and preoperative short-course radiotherapy with delayed surgery for locally advanced rectal cancer with distant metastases. Radiat Oncol. 2011;6(1):99.

40. Yoon HI, Koom WS, Kim TH, Ahn JB, Jung M, Kim TI, et al. Upfront systemic chemotherapy and short-course radiotherapy with delayed surgery for locally advanced rectal cancer with distant metastases: outcomes, compliance, and favorable prognostic factors. PLoS One. 2016;11(8):e0161475.

41. Hong NJL, Wright FC, Gagliardi AR, Paszat LF. Examining the potential relationship between multidisciplinary cancer care and patient survival: an international literature review. J Surg Oncol. 2010; 102(2):125–34.

42. Newman EA, Guest AB, Helvie MA, Roubidoux MA, Chang AE, Kleer CG, et al. Changes in surgical management resulting from case review at a breast cancer multidisciplinary tumor board. Cancer. 2006;107(10):2346–51.

43. Riedel RF, Wang X, McCormack M, Toloza E, Montana GS, Schreiber G, et al. Impact of a multidisciplinary thoracic oncology clinic on the timeliness of care. J Thorac Oncol. 2006;1(7):692–6.

44. Kelly SL, Jackson JE, Hickey BE, Szallasi FG, Bond CA. Multidisciplinary clinic care improves adherence to best practice in head and neck cancer. Am J Otolaryngol. 2013;34(1):57–60.

45. Friedland PL, Bozic B, Dewar J, Kuan R, Meyer C, Phillips M. Impact of multidisciplinary team management in head and neck cancer patients. Br J Cancer. 2011;104(8):1246–8.

46. Korman H, Lanni T Jr, Shah C, Parslow J, Tull J, Ghilezan M, et al. Impact of a prostate multidisciplinary clinic program on patient treatment decisions and on adherence to NCCN guidelines: the William Beaumont Hospital experience. Am J Clin Oncol. 2013;36(2):121–5.

47. Kidger J, Murdoch J, Donovan JL, Blazeby JM. Clinical decision-making in a multidisciplinary gynaecological cancer team: a qualitative study. BJOG. 2009;116(4):511–7.

48. Stalfors J, Lundberg C, Westin T. Quality assessment of a multidisciplinary tumour meeting for patients with head and neck cancer. Acta Otolaryngol. 2007; 127(1):82–7.

49. Delaney G, Jacob S, Iedema R, Winters M, Barton M. Comparison of face-to-face and videoconferenced multidisciplinary clinical meetings. Australas Radiol. 2004;48(4):487–92.

50. Blazeby JM, Wilson L, Metcalfe C, Nicklin J, English R, Donovan JL. Analysis of clinical decision-making in multi-disciplinary cancer teams. Ann Oncol. 2006; 17(3):457–60.

51. Wood J, Metcalfe C, Paes A, Sylvester P, Durdey P, Thomas M, et al. An evaluation of treatment decisions at a colorectal cancer multi-disciplinary team. Color Dis. 2008;10(8):769–72.

52. Leo F, Venissac N, Poudenx M, Otto J, Mouroux J. Multidisciplinary management of lung cancer: how to test its efficacy? J Thorac Oncol. 2007;2(1):69–72.

53. Bumm R, Feith M, Lordick F, Herschbach P, Siewert JR. Impact of multidisciplinary tumor boards on diagnosis and treatment of esophageal cancer. Eur Surg. 2007;39(3):136–40.

54. Lutterbach J, Pagenstecher A, Spreer J, Hetzel A, van Velthoven V, Nikkhah G, et al. The brain tumor board: lessons to be learned from an interdisciplinary conference. Onkologie. 2005;28(1):22–6.

55. Haward R, Amir Z, Borrill C, Dawson J, Scully J, West M, et al. Breast cancer teams: the impact of constitution, new cancer workload, and methods of operation on their effectiveness. Br J Cancer. 2003;89(1): 15–22.

56. Soukop M, Robinson A, Soukop D, Ingham-Clark CL, Kelly MJ. Results of a survey of the role of multidisciplinary team coordinators for colorectal cancer in England and Wales. Color Dis. 2007;9(2): 146–50.

57. Kunkler I, Fielding G, Macnab M, Swann S, Brebner J, Prescott R, et al. Group dynamics in telemedicine-delivered and standard multidisciplinary team meetings: results from the TELEMAM randomised trial. J Telemed Telecare. 2006;12(suppl 3):55–8.

58. Davison AG, Eraut CD, Haque AS, Doffman S, Tanqueray A, Trask CW, et al. Telemedicine for multidisciplinary lung cancer meetings. J Telemed Telecare. 2004;10(3):140–3.

59. Epstein RJ, Leung TW, Mak J, Cheung PS. Utility of a web-based breast cancer predictive algorithm for adjuvant chemotherapeutic decision making in a multidisciplinary oncology center. Cancer Investig. 2006;24(4):367–73.

60. Seroussi B, Bouaud J, Gligorov J, Uzan S. Supporting multidisciplinary staff meetings for guideline-based breast cancer management: a study with OncoDoc2. AMIA Annu Symp Proc. 2007;2007:656–60.

61. Harris J, Green JS, Sevdalis N, Taylor C. Using peer observers to assess the quality of cancer multidisciplinary team meetings: a qualitative proof of concept study. J Multidiscip Healthc. 2014;7:355.

62. Lamb BW, Wong HW, Vincent C, Green JS, Sevdalis N. Teamwork and team performance in multidisciplinary cancer teams: development and evaluation of an observational assessment tool. BMJ Qual Saf. 2011;20(10):849–56.

63. Pillay B, Wootten AC, Crowe H, Corcoran N, Tran B, Bowden P, et al. The impact of multidisciplinary team meetings on patient assessment, management and outcomes in oncology settings: a systematic review of the literature. Cancer Treat Rev. 2016;42: 56–72.

Molecular Basis of Colorectal Cancer: Tumor Biology

Zhao Ren and Zhang Tao

Abstract

Colorectal cancer is a heterogeneous disease entity in terms of both molecular carcinogenesis and morphologic multistep pathways. Three molecular carcinogenesis pathways have been identified: (1) chromosomal instability (CIN), (2) microsatellite instability (MSI), and (3) CpG island methylator phenotype (CIMP). The two morphologic multistep pathways are the classical pathway (the so-called adenoma–carcinoma sequence) and the serrated neoplasia pathway. CRC continues to be a significant public health problem, with a less than 10% of 5-year prognosis for metastatic CRC. Our increased understanding of the molecular events underlying CRC carcinogenesis will enable the development of new targeted therapies and the identification of clinical biomarkers that will inform their effective usage.

Keywords

Colorectal cancer · Tumor biology · Molecular carcinogenesis · MSI · CIN · CIMP · Serrated neoplasia

3.1 Introduction

Colorectal cancer (CRC) is now the third most common malignant disease in both men and women in Asia [1, 2]. While improvements in early detection have helped to reduce the incidence of CRC-related death over the past several decades, the overall frequency of the disease is likely to increase steadily due to its connection to western style diet and to obesity and chronic inflammation (i.e., inflammatory bowel disease). As a result, the search for new and effective therapies of CRC is incubated in the identification of the molecular etiology of the disease.

Over the last century, CRC genetics has emerged from an unrecognized field to a specialized one, encompassing all aspects of cancer care. The role of genetics in CRC has become critical to disease prevention, early detection, and effective treatment. As we enter the post-genomic era, it is possible that most of the genes that contribute to CRC in a meaningful way have been identified and consequently make CRC a preventable disease. Leveraging the extensive mutational information to establish new therapeutic strategies requires a combination of functional genomics, medical chemistry, and preclinical and clinical efforts.

Z. Ren (✉) • Z. Tao
Rui Jin Hospital, Shanghai Jiaotong University
School of Medicine, Shanghai, China

© Springer Nature Singapore Pte Ltd. 2018
N. K. Kim et al. (eds.), *Surgical Treatment of Colorectal Cancer*,
https://doi.org/10.1007/978-981-10-5143-2_3

3.2 Three Molecular Carcinogenesis Pathways and Two Morphologic Multistep Pathways

Colorectal cancer is a heterogeneous disease entity in terms of both molecular carcinogenesis and morphologic multistep pathways [3]. Three molecular carcinogenesis pathways have been identified [4]: (1) chromosomal instability (CIN), (2) microsatellite instability (MSI), and (3) CpG island methylator phenotype (CIMP). The two morphologic multistep pathways are the classical pathway (the so-called adenoma–carcinoma sequence) and the serrated neoplasia pathway (see in Fig. 3.1). The CIN pathway is characterized by alterations in the number and structure of chromosomes and accompanying genetic mutations of proto-oncogenes and tumor suppressor genes. The MSI pathway features alteration in the number of nucleotide repeats located in the exons and subsequent frame shift mutations in tumor suppressor genes or tumor-related genes. The CIMP pathway is characterized by widespread hypermethylation of numerous promoter CpG island loci and consequent inactivation of tumor suppressor genes or tumor-related genes. The classical pathway begins with premalignant lesions comprising conventional adenomas, including tubular or tubulovillous adenomas, whereas the serrated neoplasia pathway begins with hyperplastic polyps or sessile or traditional serrated adenomas. These two morphologic pathways are driven by different molecular pathways: the classical pathway is driven by either CIN or MSI, whereas the serrated neoplasia pathway has epigenetic instability as its initial driving force and MSI as an optional secondary force. Although Lynch syndrome CRCs and sporadic MSI-high (MSI-H) CRCs both have a high level of MSI, their premalignant lesions are different because they develop through different morphologic multistep pathways: Lynch syndrome tumors follow the classical pathway and manifest their premalignant lesions as tubular or tubulovillous adenoma [5, 6], whereas the premalignant lesions of sporadic MSI-H CRCs are sessile serrated adenomas that arise through the serrated neoplasia pathway and undergo further hypermethylation-associated inactivation of MLH1 and subsequent acquisition of high-level MSI [7]. The Cancer Genome Atlas study results demonstrate that the CIN and MSI pathways are mutually exclusive [8]. Whereas the CIMP pathway overlaps with the MSI pathway because of the presence of sporadic MSI-H CRCs, which are also usually CIMP high (CIMP-H), the CIMP pathway does not appear to be in an exclusive relationship with the

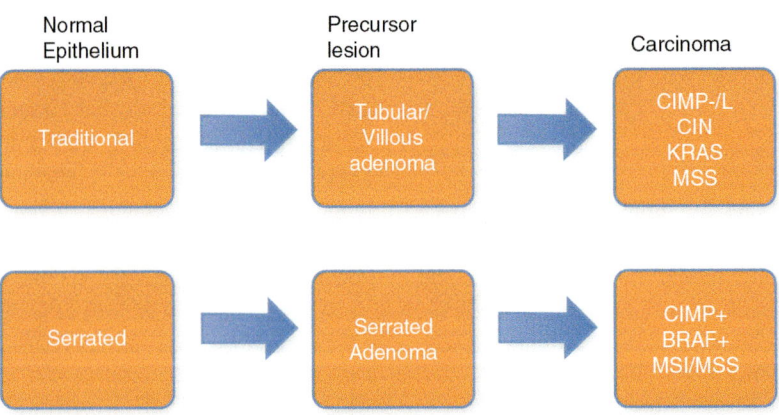

Fig. 3.1 Two morphologic multistep pathways: traditional pathway and serrated neoplasia pathway

CIN pathway. CIMP-H/non-MSI-H CRCs show some copy number variations across the genome, although the degree of CIN is less pronounced than that of CIMP-negative or CIMP-low (CIMP-0, CIMP-L)/non-MSI-H CRCs [9]. This finding suggests that the CIMP pathway itself may not be sufficient for the malignant transformation of serrated polyps and requires collaboration with either the CIN or MSI pathway to promote successful malignant transformation.

The phenotypes of serrated polyps vary considerably, and the entity mixed polyp reflects the considerable overlap among these lesions [10]. Sessile serrated adenoma/polyp (SSA/P) constitutes about 20% of all serrated polyps and is morphologically defined by the elongation of serrated crypts and distortion of the proliferative zone [11]. Progression of SSA/P is associated with the occurrence of cytological dysplasia and development of invasive adenocarcinoma. SSA/P and related adenocarcinomas are preferentially found in the right hemi-colon. Traditional serrated adenomas (TSA) are morphological variants of serrated adenomas and show considerable differences from SSA/P concerning mutation (*KRAS* mutation in about 25%), localization (left-sided), and methylation status (increased methylation, but not methylation of *MLH1*) [12].

Given the malignant potential of serrated polyps, two important serrated pathways of colorectal carcinogenesis were characterized: (1) sessile serrated pathway and (2) traditional serrated pathway. The resulting serrated adenocarcinoma has architectural similarity to a SSA/P that may be accompanied by additional morphological features including trabecular and mucinous areas. However, these CRCs can have *MSI-L* or *MSI-H*, *BRAF* or *KRAS* mutations, and CIMP [10, 13]. Given the molecular heterogeneity of serrated adenocarcinomas, a strong genotype-to-phenotype relation is not well established at present.

3.3 CIN

The molecular mechanisms underlying CIN include chromosomal segregation defects, centromere dysfunction, telomere dysfunction, loss of heterozygosity, and deficiency in DNA damage response.

3.3.1 Defects in Chromosomal Segregation

Chromosomal segregation defects include chromosome rearrangements, sequence changes, chromosomal number alterations, and chromosomal missegregation. The CIN phenotype can result from defects in pathways that regulate chromosomal segregation. The mitotic or spindle checkpoint ensures proper chromosome segregation by delaying the metaphase-to-anaphase transition until all pairs of duplicated chromatids are properly aligned on the spindle. Genes that encode proteins operating as spindle checkpoint regulators include *mitotic arrest-deficient* (*MAD1L1* and *MAD2L1*), *budding uninhibited by benzimidazoles 1* (*BUB1*), and *kinesin family member 11* (*KIF11*). Mutations in *BUB1* result in abnormal spindle checkpoint and CIN in chromosomally table cell lines [14]. Cells from dominant-negative mBub1 mutant mice demonstrate escape from apoptosis, continued cell cycle progression, and disrupted spindles [15]. Kinesin spindle protein, also known as Eg5, is a motor protein responsible for mitotic spindle formation and chromosomal separation during mitosis. Overexpression of *Eg5* in mice leads to spindle defects, CIN, and solid tumor formation [16]. Chromosomal missegregation due to defects in the mitotic checkpoint may lead to aneuploidy. After promoting chromosomal missegregation and aneuploidy, aneuploidy destabilizes the genome, gives rise to polyclonal mutations, and results in heterogeneous karyotypes [16, 17].

3.3.2 Centromere Dysfunction

Another proposed cause of CIN is abnormal centromere number and function. Centrosomes serve to anchor cytoplasmic microtubules as they are arranged into a mitotic spindle apparatus. Extra centrosomes in cancer cell lines may lead to the formation of multiple spindle poles during mitosis, resulting in unequal distribution of chromosomes and CIN [18]. Polo-like kinases (Plk) are serine/threonine kinases, which regulate centrosome duplication. Elevated expression of Plk1 has been observed in 73% of CRCs and correlated with tumor invasion, lymph node involvement, and staging [19]. The centrosome-associated Aurora A protein is amplified and positively associated with CIN in CRC, but metastatic CRC patients with increased Aurora A gene copy number have longer overall and progression-free survival, particularly in *KRAS* wild-type tumors [20, 21]. The related Aurora B protein regulates chromatid segregation, and its expression is correlated with advanced stages of CRC [22].

3.3.3 Telomere Dysfunction

CIN may also be driven by telomere dysfunction. Telomeres are hexameric DNA repeats (TTAGGG in humans) that protect the ends of eukaryotic chromosomes from fusing and breaking during segregation. A portion of telomeric DNA is lost after each round of DNA replication due the inability of DNA polymerase to completely synthesize the 3′ end of chromosomes. Cells with sufficiently shortened telomeres are targeted for senescence and apoptosis by DNA damage checkpoints. Cells that survive the checkpoint activate telomerase, which elongates telomeres.

3.3.4 Loss of Heterozygosity (LOH)

LOH is a key feature of CIN-positive tumors and distinguishes tumors arising from the CIN pathway from tumors arising from the MSI pathway. Approximately 25–30% of alleles are lost in tumors [23, 24]. Mitotic nondisjunction, recombination between homologous chromosomes, and chromosomal deletion are among the implicated mechanisms. One study found that the majority of losses on chromosome 18 involved the whole chromosome and were caused by mitotic nondisjunction. Losses that limited to a part of a chromosome were thought to be due to interchromosomal recombinations and deletions associated with DNA double-strand breaks [25].

3.3.5 Deficiencies in DNA Damage Response

Deficiencies in DNA damage response have been linked to human cancer. Inactivating mutations in ataxia telangiectasia-mutated (*ATM*) and ataxia telangiectasia and Rad3-related (*ATR*) protein kinases lead to the ataxia telangiectasia and Seckel syndromes, respectively [26]. Other syndromes linked to impaired DNA damage response include Li–Fraumeni syndrome (*TP53* mutations) and hereditary breast–ovarian cancer (*BRCA1* and *BRCA2* mutations). Of these genes, only TP53 has been directly implicated in human colorectal cancer. Haploinsufficiency of histone H2AX, an ATM and ATR substrate, leads to genomic instability and tumor susceptibility in a p53-deficient background, and mouse embryonic fibroblasts derived from ATM- and H2Ax-deficient mice show severe genomic instability [27–29]. Deficiency in *Chk1*, a DNA damage checkpoint protein, causes mitotic defects and disrupts Aurora B during mitosis, resulting in failure of cytokinesis and multinucleation [30].

3.3.6 Clinical Implications of CIN

Many of the genes identified by sequencing analysis were already well known to be somatically mutated in CRC (e.g., *APC*, *KRAS*, and *TP53*) (Table 3.1). Our insights into the genetic basis for CRC have allowed the identification of prognostic molecular markers. Patients with activating *KRAS* and *BRAF* mutations may experience worse overall survival outcomes compared to wild-type patients [31–33]. Patients with tumor harboring *KRAS* and *PIK3CA* mutations are more likely to develop liver metastases compared to wild-type patients [34]. *TP53* mutation may be associated with greater mortality, but this risk may be limited to patients with metastatic disease [35, 36]. There are contradictory reports on whether deletion of chromosome 18q is associated with poor outcomes; individual chromosomal deletions are currently used as molecular markers for CRC prognosis [37–39].

Table 3.1 Somatic mutations in oncogenes and tumor suppressor genes implicated in colorectal carcinogenesis

Gene	Chromosomal location	Type of mutation	Prevalence (%)	Function of gene product
Oncogenes				
KRAS	12q12	Point mutation (codons 12, 13 of exon 2)	40	Cell proliferation and survival
PIK3CA	3q26	Point mutations (E545K on exon 9, H1047R on exon 20)	15–30	Cell proliferation and survival
CDK8	13q12	Gene amplification	10–15	β-catenin activation
EGFR	7p12	Gene amplification	5–15	Cell proliferation and survival
BRAF	7q34	Point mutations activating kinase activity (most commonly V600E)	5–10	Cell proliferation and survival
CMYC	8q24	Gene amplification	5–10	Cell proliferation and survival
CCNE1	19q12	Gene amplification	5	
NRAS	1p13	Point mutation	<5	Cell proliferation and survival
CTNNB1	3p22	Stabilizing point mutations and in-frame deletions near N-terminus	<5	Regulation of Wnt pathway target genes that promote tumor growth and invasion
ERBB2 (HER2)	17q21	Gene amplification	<5	Cell proliferation and survival
MYB	6q22–q23	Gene amplification	<5	Stimulates growth of intestinal stem cells
Tumor suppressor genes				
APC	5q21	Frameshift, point mutation, deletion, allele loss leading to truncated protein	70–80	Inhibition of Wnt signaling
TP53	17q13	Point mutation (missense), allele loss	60–70	Cell cycle arrest, apoptosis, and autophagy induction
DCC	18q21	Point mutation	50	Cell surface receptor for netrin-1, triggers tumor cell apoptosis
TGFBR2	3p22	Frameshift, nonsense	25	Inhibition of cell growth
SMAD4	18q21	Nonsense, missense, allele loss	10–15	Intracellular mediator of the TGF-β pathway
PTEN	10q23	Nonsense, deletion	10	Inhibition of PI3K activity
ACVR2A	2q22	Frameshift	10	Cellular growth
SMAD2	18q21	Nonsense, deletion, allele loss	5–10	Intracellular mediator of the TGF-β pathway
FBXW7	4q31	Nonsense, missense, deletion	9	Targets oncoproteins for ubiquitin-mediated degradation
SMAD3	15q22	Nonsense, deletion	5	Intracellular mediator of the TGF-β pathway
TCF7L2	10q25	Frameshift, nonsense	5	Regulation of the Wnt signaling
BAX	19q13	Frameshift	5	Apoptotic activator
LKB1	19p13	Deletion	Rare	Regulation of cell polarity

Modified from Fearon ER. Molecular genetics of colorectal cancer. Annu Rev. Pathol 2011; 6:479–507

Years of research on the molecular mechanisms of CRC are slowly translating into the clinic. Patients with *KRAS* mutant tumors do not appreciably respond to inhibition of the EGFR; use of agents such as cetuximab is thus limited to patients with *KRAS* wild-type cancer [40]. A recent phase I clinical trial examined treatment of *BRAF* CRC with vemurafenib, a specific inhibitor of the *BRAF* protein, and demonstrated mixed results, which suggest the presence of primary resistance mechanisms [41]. Inhibition of the PI3K and downstream mTOR pathways has shown efficacy in a mouse model for *PIK3CA* wild-type CRC, and phase I clinical trials are planned [42]. Small molecule inhibitors of Aurora kinase, Plks, and the spindle motor protein Eg5 have shown promise in preclinical studies and have demonstrated safety and antitumor efficacy in phase I human trials [43–45].

CIN-related CRCs demonstrate no characteristic histomorphological pattern. They differ in tumor grading, occurrence of necrosis, and accumulation of extracellular mucin. The putative molecular founder event/mutation for the intestinal phenotype of CRCs has not been characterized up to now.

3.4   MSI

Microsatellite instability (*MSI*) is the condition of genetic hypermutability that results from impaired DNA mismatch repair (MMR). The presence of MSI represents phenotypic evidence that MMR is not functioning normally.

MMR corrects errors that spontaneously occur during DNA replication, such as single-base mismatches or short insertions and deletions. The proteins involved in MMR correct polymerase errors by forming a complex that binds to the mismatched section of DNA, excises the error, and inserts the correct sequence in its place [46]. Cells with abnormally functioning MMR are unable to correct errors that occur during DNA replication and consequently accumulate errors. This causes the creation of novel microsatellite fragments. PCR-based assays can reveal these novel microsatellites and provide evidence for the presence of MSI (Fig. 3.2).

Microsatellites are repeated sequences of DNA. These sequences can be made of repeating units of one to six base pairs in length. Although the length of these microsatellites is highly variable from person to person and contributes to the individual DNA "fingerprint," each individual has microsatellites of a set length. The most common microsatellite in humans is a dinucleotide repeat of the nucleotides C and A, which occurs tens of thousands of times across the genome.

MSI is found in up to 15% of sporadic CRCs and in almost all Lynch syndrome-associated CRCs due to either somatic inactivation of both alleles or an inherited germline mutation to one allele with additional somatic inactivation of the other [47]. A mismatch repair function usually corrects deletion/insertion errors during DNA replication. In MSI, sequence corrections resulting in alleles of varying lengths are not performed. The differences in length are diagnostic in PCR-based strategies using consensus primer panels. In standardized panels for MSI testing, two mononucleotides (BAT25 and BAT26) and three dinucleotide microsatellites (D5S346, D2S123, D17S250) were used [48]. MSI CRCs are not usually associated with mutations in *KRAS* or *TP53*. However, genes containing simple repeats such as *EGFR*, *BAX*, and *TGFbetaR*II are often mutated in these tumors. The *BRAF* status is another variable in MSI CRCs and a prognostic factor. Disease-free survival and overall survival are significantly improved in patients with MSI and nonmutated BRAF [49]. MSI CRCs do not have chromosomal abnormalities.

3.4.1   Clinical Implication of MSI

MSI is well recognized by its high frequency in stage II colon cancer, present in 15% of cases overall and around 25% of right-sided tumors, in comparison with a frequency of 14% in stage III colon cancer and 4% in metastatic disease [50]. Mismatch repair proteins are required for surveillance of the newly synthesized DNA strand following replication, where they serve to recognize mispaired bases, small insertions, and deletions incorporated by DNA polymerases [51]. Germline mutation of the mismatch repair genes *MLH1*, *MSH2*, *MSH6*, or *PMS2* causes Lynch syndrome (also known as hereditary nonpolyposis colorectal cancer—HNPCC), associated with early-onset colonic and endometrial cancer, in addition to tumors of the ovary, stomach,

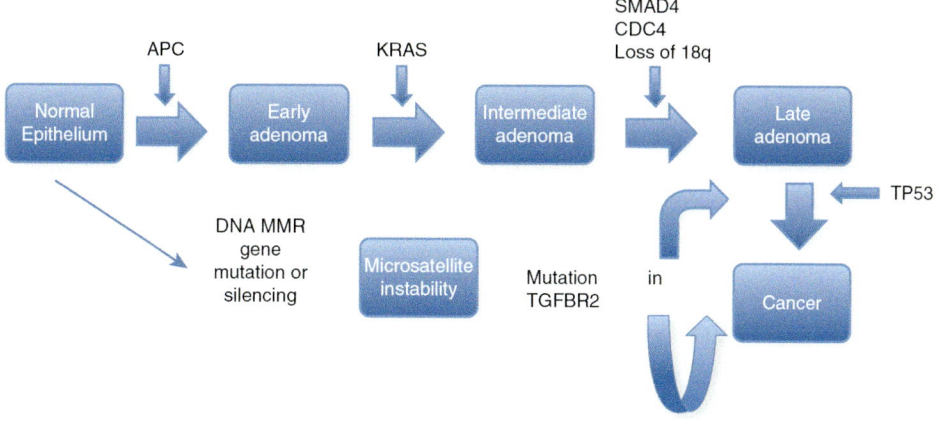

Fig. 3.2 Chromosomal instability and microsatellite instability

small bowel, pancreas, and other sites [52, 53]. Defective mismatch repair function in sporadic colonic cancer is commonly due to mutation of *MSH6* and *MSH2* or epigenetic silencing of MLH1 by promoter methylation [54]. In both hereditary and sporadic tumors, aberrant mismatch repair function leads to failure to repair defects caused by slippage of DNA polymerases at microsatellites—short tandem DNA repeats—and point mutations, resulting in a characteristic molecular phenotype of microsatellite instability (MSI) and mutation of the tumor suppressors *TGFβR2*, *IGF2R*, *BAX*, and *PTEN* and the oncogene *BRAF* [54–57]. MSI-high tumors are commonly proximal to the splenic flexure and poorly differentiated and demonstrate a prominent lymphocytic infiltrate [54]. Confirmation of tumor microsatellite instability can be performed either using PCR—by the demonstration of instability of at least two of five microsatellite markers examined—or by immunohistochemistry (IHC) for the mismatch repair proteins, as absent staining demonstrates excellent concordance with MSI-high status [58, 59]. Testing for MSI in stage II colonic cancer, and particularly in T3 tumors, is advised, as it has important prognostic and therapeutic implications, as discussed below.

3.5 CIMP

Unlike colorectal tumors from Lynch syndrome, sporadic CRC with MSI arises via a mechanism involving the CIMP. CIMP was originally grouped together with MSI tumors. The islands are CpG-rich regions within the genome and especially found in promoter sequences. DNA methylation of cytosines in the context of CpG dinucleotides is a central mechanism of epigenetic control, with essential roles in the maintenance of genome integrity, genomic imprinting, transcriptional regulation, and developmental processes [60, 61].

Genome-wide methylome analyses have highlighted extensive disruption of DNA methylation in CRC. Tumors are typically characterized by global loss of methylation (hypomethylation), predominantly in repetitive sequences, and focal gain in methylation (hypermethylation) in CpG islands, the latter often occurring simultaneously within defined megabase regions [62–64]. Hypermethylation within CpG islands is associated with transcriptional silencing of tumor suppressor genes, while hypomethylation within gene bodies can affect transcriptional elongation or alternative promoter usage and cause aberrant transcription of oncogenes [65–79]. Global loss of methylation may trigger cancer genomic instability and activation of transposons and genes within regions of repetitive sequence [69–71]. Both hypo- and hypermethylation occur early in tumorigenesis [72–79], and the average CRC genome carries thousands of methylation changes with marked impact on the cellular transcriptional program [80–82].

Genes that are frequently affected by this non-covalent epigenetic modification are *p16*, *MGMT*, and *hMLH1*. The presence and extent of CIMP have been used to classify CRC into three major subgroups, CIMP high (CIMP-H), CIMP low (CIMP-L) and non-CIMP (CIMP-0), with distinct clinical and molecular features (201, 202). CIMP-H is associated with proximal tumor location, female gender, BRAF mutation, *MLH1* methylation, and MSI; CIMP-L is characterized by proximal tumor location and *KRAS* mutation, while CIMP-0 is associated with distal tumor location, *TP53* mutation, and CIN [32, 83, 84].

3.5.1 Clinical Implications of CIMP

Clinically, CIMP CRCs are commonly found in a proximal location and often have methylation of the *hMLH1* mismatch repair gene. However, over 50% of the CIMP CRCs are microsatellite stable. In general, CIMP CRCs have a poor prognosis and are associated with mutations in *KRAS* and/or *BRAF*. The histological phenotype of CIMP CRCs is not well characterized or defined. In these carcinomas, a poor degree of histomorphological differentiation is frequently found reflecting some aspects of MSI. However, despite methylation of the *hMLH1* mismatch repair gene, histomorphological MSI-related histological features are not fully expressed in CIMP CRCs [85, 86].

Studies have identified a subset of CRCs that exhibit particularly widespread promoter hypermethylation, referred to as the CpG island methylator phenotype (CIMP) [85, 87]. CIMP is observed in ~30% of CRCs, and the presence and extent of CIMP have been used to classify CRC

into three major subgroups, CIMP high (CIMP-H), CIMP low (CIMP-L), and non-CIMP (CIMP-0), with distinct clinical and molecular features [82, 88]. CIMP-H is associated with proximal tumor location, female gender, BRAF mutation, *MLH1* methylation, and MSI; CIMP-L is characterized by proximal tumor location and *KRAS* mutation, while CIMP-0 is associated with distal tumor location, *TP53* mutation, and CIN [32, 82–84].

Aberrant DNA methylation patterns are attractive tumor biomarkers because of their high frequency in neoplasms, and the detection of methylation in DNA isolated from stool and/or blood has emerged as a promising approach for early diagnosis and surveillance of CRC [89, 90]. Microarray-based studies of hypermethylated CpG sites in CRC and benign adenomas have revealed a large number of tumor-specific candidate detection markers [91–93]. Translation of these candidates into blood- or stool-based diagnostic tests is actively being pursued by the academia and industry, involving method development, validation of specificity against normal tissues and other pathologies, and evaluation of performance against routine clinical assays (FOBT, CEA).

3.6 Consensus Molecular Subtypes

The CRC Subtyping Consortium (CRCSC) was formed to assess the presence or absence of core subtype patterns among existing gene expression-based CRC subtyping algorithms [94]. Four consensus molecular subtypes (CMS) with distinguishing features were concluded:

CMS1 (MSI immune, 14%), hypermutated, microsatellite unstable, strong immune activation, right-sided tumors, older age at diagnosis, females, hypermutation, *BRAF* mutation, and intermediate survival

CMS2 (canonical, 37%), epithelial, chromosomally unstable, marked WNT and MYC signaling activation, MSS, left-sided tumors, *TP53* mutation,

EGFR amplification/overexpression, and better survival

CMS3 (metabolic, 13%), epithelial, evident metabolic dysregulation, low CIN, moderate WNT/MYC pathway activation, *KRAS* mutation, *PIK3CA* mutation, IGFBP2 overexpression, and intermediate survival

CMS4 (mesenchymal, 23%), prominent transforming growth factor β activation, stromal invasion and angiogenesis, CIN/MSI heterogeneous, mesenchymal/TGF-β activation, younger age at diagnosis, NOTCH3/VEGFR2 overexpression, and worse survival.

These molecular subtypes of CRCs resolve inconsistencies among the reported gene expression-based CRC classifications and facilitate clinical translation.

Conclusions

CRC continues to be a significant public health burden. Whereas there have been significant advances in the development of targeted therapies, the 5-year prognosis for metastatic CRC still continues to be less than 10%. However, our increased understanding of the molecular events underlying CRC carcinogenesis will enable the development of new targeted therapies and the identification of clinical biomarkers that will inform their effective usage. This is an exciting time for cancer medicine, and we believe that the field is poised to make significant therapeutic breakthroughs.

The application of genomic approaches, in particular whole exome sequencing, presents issues beyond the assessment of molecular alterations related to the patient's original presentation of CRC. Given the comprehensive nature of these tests, incidental findings on clinically relevant variants in genes with no relationship to the primary diagnosis may be made. The revolutionary advances in genomic technologies are enabling the possibility of personalized medicine for CRC. Evolving platforms such as next generation sequencing (NGS) and high-density microarrays are starting to bring precision genomic profiling to the clinic at a reasonable cost. Ongoing innovations in existing applications and clinical informatics algorithms, as well as the many emerging technologies, will continue to advance translational cancer genomics and ultimately contribute to improving patients outcomes.

References

1. Sung JJ, Lau JY, Goh KL, et al. Increasing incidence of colorectal cancer in Asia: implications for screening. Lancet Oncol. 2005;6:871–6.
2. Jemal A, Bray F, Center MM, et al. Global cancer statistics. CA Cancer J Clin. 2011;61:69–90.
3. Bae JM, Kim JH, Kang GH. Molecular subtypes of colorectal cancer and their clinicopathologic features, with an emphasis on the serrated neoplasia pathway. Arch Pathol Lab Med. 2016;140:406–13.
4. Kanthan R, Senger JL, Kanthan SC. Molecular events in primary and metastatic colorectal carcinoma: a review. Pathol Res Int. 2012;2012:597497.
5. Walsh MD, Buchanan DD, Pearson SA, et al. Immunohistochemical testing of conventional adenomas for loss of expression of mismatch repair proteins in Lynch syndrome mutation carriers: a case series from the Australasian site of the colon cancer family registry. Mod Pathol. 2012;25(5):722–30.
6. Jass JR. Classification of colorectal cancer based on correlation of clinical, morphological and molecular features. Histopathology. 2007;50(1):113–30.
7. Goldstein NS. Small colonic microsatellite unstable adenocarcinomas and high-grade epithelial dysplasias in sessile serrated adenoma polypectomy specimens: a study of eight cases. Am J Clin Pathol. 2006;125(1):132–45.
8. Cancer Genome Atlas Network. Comprehensive molecular characterization of human colon and rectal cancer. Nature. 2012;487(7407):330–7.
9. Mo Q, Wang S, Seshan VE, et al. Pattern discovery and cancer gene identification in integrated cancer genomic data. Proc Natl Acad Sci U S A. 2013;110(11):4245–50.
10. Noffsinger AE. Serrated polyps and colorectal cancer: new pathway to malignancy. Annu Rev Pathol. 2009;4:343–64.
11. Torlakovic EE, Gomez JD, Driman DK, Parfitt JR, Wang C, Benerjee T, Snover DC. Sessile serrated adenoma (SSA) vs. traditional serrated adenoma (TSA). Am J Surg Pathol. 2008;32:21–9.
12. East JE, Saunders BP, Jass JR. Sporadic and syndromic hyperplastic polyps and serrated adenomas of the colon: classification, molecular genetics, natural history, and clinical management. Gastroenterol Clin N Am. 2008;37:25–46.

13. Leggett B, Whitehall V. Role of the serrated pathway in colorectal cancer pathogenesis. Gastroenterology. 2010;138:2088–100.

14. Bardelli A, Cahill DP, Lederer G, et al. Carcinogen-specific induction of genetic instability. Proc Natl Acad Sci U S A. 2001;98(10):5770–5.

15. Taylor SS, McKeon F. Kinetochore localization of murine Bub1 is required for normal mitotic timing and checkpoint response to spindle damage. Cell. 1997;89(5):727–35.

16. Castillo A, Morse HC III, Godfrey VL, Naeem R, Justice MJ. Overexpression of Eg5 causes genomic instability and tumor formation in mice. Cancer Res. 2007;67(21):10138–47.

17. Duesberg P, Fabarius A, Hehlmann R. Aneuploidy, the primary cause of the multilateral genomic instability of neoplastic and preneoplastic cells. IUBMB Life. 2004;56(2):65–81.

18. Ganem NJ, Godinho SA, Pellman D. A mechanism linking extra centrosomes to chromosomal instability. Nature. 2009;460(7252):278–82.

19. Takahashi T, Sano B, Nagata T, et al. Polo-like kinase 1 (PLK1) is overexpressed in primary colorectal cancers. Cancer Sci. 2003;94(2):148–52.

20. Dotan E, Meropol NJ, Zhu F, et al. Relationship of increased aurora kinase a gene copy number, prognosis and response to chemotherapy in patients with metastatic colorectal cancer. Br J Cancer. 2012; 106(4):748–55.

21. Herz C, Schlürmann F, Batarello D, et al. Occurrence of Aurora A positive multipolar mitoses in distinct molecular classes of colorectal carcinomas and effect of Aurora A inhibition. Mol Carcinog. 2011; 51(9):696–710.

22. Katayama H, Ota T, Jisaki F, et al. Mitotic kinase expression and colorectal cancer progression. J Natl Cancer Inst. 1999;91(13):1160–2.

23. Lengauer C, Kinzler KW, Vogelstein B. Genetic instability in colorectal cancers. Nature. 1997;386(6625): 623–7.

24. Lengauer C, Kinzler KW, Vogelstein B. Genetic instabilities in human cancers. Nature. 1998;396(6712): 643–9.

25. Thiagalingam S, Laken S, Willson JKV, et al. Mechanisms underlying losses of heterozygosity in human colorectal cancers. Proc Natl Acad Sci U S A 2001;98(5):2698–702.

26. Khanna KK, Jackson SP. DNA double-strand breaks: signaling, repair and the cancer connection. Nat Genet. 2001;27(3):247–54.

27. Bassing CH, Suh H, Ferguson DO, et al. Histone H2AX: a dosage-dependent suppressor of oncogenic translocations and tumors. Cell. 2003;114(3): 359–70.

28. Celeste A, Difilippantonio S, Difilippantonio MJ, et al. H2AX haploinsufficiency modifies genomic stability and tumor susceptibility. Cell. 2003;114(3): 371–83.

29. Zha S, Sekiguchi J, Brush JW, Bassing CH, Alt FW. Complementary functions of ATM and H2AX in development and suppression of genomic instability. Proc Natl Acad Sci U S A. 2008;105(27):9302–6.

30. Peddibhotla S, Lam MH, Gonzalez-Rimbau M, Rosen JM. The DNA-damage effector checkpoint kinase 1 is essential for chromosome segregation and cytokinesis. Proc Natl Acad Sci U S A. 2009;106(13):5159–64.

31. Van Cutsem E, Köhne C-H, Láng I, et al. Cetuximab plus irinotecan, fluorouracil, and leucovorin as first-line treatment for metastatic colorectal cancer: updated analysis of overall survival according to tumor KRAS and BRAF mutation status. J Clin Oncol. 2011;29(15):2011–9.

32. Ogino S, Nosho K, Kirkner GJ, et al. CpG island methylator phenotype, microsatellite instability, BRAF mutation and clinical outcome in colon cancer. Gut. 2009;58(1):90–6.

33. Ogino S, Shima K, Meyerhardt J, et al. Predictive and prognostic roles of BRAF mutation in stage III colon cancer: results from intergroup trial CALGB 89803. Clin Cancer Res. 2011;18(3):890–900.

34. Li H-T, Lu Y-Y, An Y-X, Wang X, Zhao Q-C. KRAS, BRAF and PIK3CA mutations in human colorectal cancer: relationship with metastatic colorectal cancer. Oncol Rep. 2011;25(6):1691–7.

35. Munro AJ, Lain S, Lane DP. P53 abnormalities and outcomes in colorectal cancer: a systematic review. Br J Cancer. 2005;92(3):434–44.

36. Russo A, Bazan V, Iacopetta B, Kerr D, Soussi T, Gebbia N. The TP53 colorectal cancer international collaborative study on the prognostic and predictive significance of p53 mutation: influence of tumor site, type of mutation, and adjuvant treatment. J Clin Oncol. 2005;23(30):7518–28.

37. Zhou W, Goodman SN, Galizia G, et al. Counting alleles to predict recurrence of early-stage colorectal cancers. Lancet. 2002;359(9302):219–25.

38. Diep CB, Thorstensen L, Meling GI, Skovlund E, Rognum TO, Lothe RA. Genetic tumor markers with prognostic impact in Dukes' stages B and C colorectal cancer patients. J Clin Oncol. 2003;21(5):820–9.

39. Ogino S, Nosho K, Irahara N, et al. Prognostic significance and molecular associations of 18q loss of heterozygosity: a cohort study of microsatellite stable colorectal cancers. J Clin Oncol. 2009;27(27): 4591–8.

40. Karapetis CS, Khambata-Ford S, Jonker DJ, et al. K-ras mutations and benefit from cetuximab in advanced colorectal cancer. N Engl J Med. 2008; 359(17):1757–65.

41. Tol J, Nagtegaal ID, Punt CJA. BRAF mutation in metastatic colorectal cancer. N Engl J Med. 2009; 361(1):98–9.

42. Roper J, Richardson MP, Wang WV, et al. The dual PI3K/mTOR inhibitor NVP-BEZ235 induces tumor regression in a genetically engineered mouse model of PIK3CA wild-type colorectal cancer. PLoS One. 2011;6(9):e25132.

43. Jani JP, Arcari J, Bernardo V, et al. PF-03814735, an orally bioavailable small molecule aurora kinase inhibitor for cancer therapy. Mol Cancer Ther. 2010; 9(4):883–94.

44. Schöffski P, Awada A, Dumez H, et al. A phase I, dose-escalation study of the novel Polo- like kinase inhibitor volasertib (BI 6727) in patients with advanced solid tumours. Eur J Cancer. 2012;48(2):179–86.

45. Infante JR, Kurzrock R, Spratlin J, et al. A phase I study to assess the safety, tolerability, and pharmacokinetics of AZD4877, an intravenous Eg5 inhibitor in patients with advanced solid tumors. Cancer Chemother Pharmacol. 2012;69(1):165–72.

46. Ehrlich M, editor. DNA alterations in cancer: genetic and epigenetic changes. Natick: Eaton; 2000. p. 178. ISBN 9781881299196. Retrieved 19 Feb 2015

47. Moreira L, Balaguer F, Lindor N, de la Chapelle A, Hampel H, Aaltonen LA, Hopper JL, Le Marchand L, Gallinger S, Newcomb PA, et al. Identification of Lynch syndrome among patients with colorectal cancer. JAMA. 2012;308:1555–65.

48. Zhang X, Li J. Era of universal testing of microsatellite instability in colorectal cancer. World J Gastrointest Oncol. 2013;5:12–9.

49. French AJ, Sargent DJ, Burgart LJ, Foster NR, Kabat BF, Goldberg R, Shepherd L, Windschitl HE, Thibodeau SN. Prognostic significance of defective mismatch repair and BRAF V600E in patients with colon cancer. Clin Cancer Res. 2008;14:3408–15.

50. Bertagnolli MM, Redston M, Compton CC, et al. Microsatellite instability and loss of heterozygosity at chromosomal location 18q: prospective evaluation of biomarkers for stages II and III colon cancer--a study of CALGB 9581 and 89803. J Clin Oncol. 2011;29:3153–62.

51. Kunkel TA, Erie DA. DNA mismatch repair. Annu Rev Biochem. 2005;74:681–710.

52. Lynch HT, Boland CR, Gong G, et al. Phenotypic and genotypic heterogeneity in the Lynch syndrome: diagnostic, surveillance and management implications. Eur J Hum Genet. 2006;14:390–402.

53. Boland CR, Goel A. Microsatellite instability in colorectal cancer. Gastroenterology. 2010;138:2073–2087.e3.

54. Ionov Y, Peinado MA, Malkhosyan S, et al. Ubiquitous somatic mutations in simple repeated sequences reveal a new mechanism for colonic carcinogenesis. Nature. 1993;363:558–61.

55. Rampino N, Yamamoto H, Ionov Y, et al. Somatic frameshift mutations in the BAX gene in colon cancers of the microsatellite mutator phenotype. Science. 1997;275:967–9.

56. Thibodeau SN, Bren G, Schaid D. Microsatellite instability in cancer of the proximal colon. Science. 1993;260:816–9.

57. Boland CR, Thibodeau SN, Hamilton SR, et al. A National Cancer Institute workshop on microsatellite instability for cancer detection and familial predisposition: development of international criteria for the determination of microsatellite instability in colorectal cancer. Cancer Res. 1998;58:5248–57.

58. Lindor NM, Burgart LJ, Leontovich O, et al. Immunohistochemistry versus microsatellite instability testing in phenotyping colorectal tumors. J Clin Oncol. 2002;20:1043–8.

59. Quasar Collaborative Group, Gray R, Barnwell J, et al. Adjuvant chemotherapy versus observation in patients with colorectal cancer: a randomised study. Lancet. 2007;370:2020–9.

60. Bock C, Tomazou EM, Brinkman AB, et al. Quantitative comparison of genome-wide DNA methylation mapping technologies. Nat Biotechnol. 2010;28:1106–14.

61. Laird PW. Principles and challenges of genome-wide DNA methylation analysis. Nat Rev Genet. 2010;11:191–203.

62. Feinberg AP, Vogelstein B. Hypomethylation distinguishes genes of some human cancers from their normal counterparts. Nature. 1983;89-92(180):301.

63. Berman BP, Weisenberger DJ, Aman JF, et al. Regions of focal DNA hypermethylation and long-range hypomethylation in colorectal cancer coincide with nuclear lamina-associated domains. Nat Genet. 2012;44:40–6.

64. Schweiger MR, Hussong M, Rohr C, et al. Genomics and epigenomics of colorectal cancer. Wiley Interdiscip Rev Syst Biol Med. 2013;5:205–19.

65. Baylin SB, Ohm JE. Epigenetic gene silencing in cancer - a mechanism for early oncogenic pathway addiction? Nat Rev Cancer. 2006;6:107–16.

66. Maunakea AK, Nagarajan RP, Bilenky M, et al. Conserved role of intragenic DNA methylation in regulating alternative promoters. Nature. 2010;466:253–7.

67. Hitchins MP, Rapkins RW, Kwok CT, et al. Dominantly inherited constitutional epigenetic silencing of MLH1 in a cancer-affected family is linked to a single nucleotide variant within the 5'UTR. Cancer Cell. 2011;20:200–13.

68. Shenker N, Flanagan JM. Intragenic DNA methylation: implications of this epigenetic mechanism for cancer research. Br J Cancer. 2012;106:248–53.

69. Eden A, Gaudet F, Waghmare A, et al. Chromosomal instability and tumors promoted by DNA hypomethylation. Science. 2003;300:455.

70. Rodriguez J, Frigola J, Vendrell E, et al. Chromosomal instability correlates with genome-wide DNA demethylation in human primary colorectal cancers. Cancer Res. 2006;66:8462–9468.

71. Howard G, Eiges R, Gaudet F, et al. Activation and transposition of endogenous retroviral elements in hypomethylation induced tumors in mice. Oncogene. 2008;27:404–8.

72. Oster B, Thorsen K, Lamy P, et al. Identification and validation of highly frequent CpG island hypermethylation in colorectal adenomas and carcinomas. Int J Cancer. 2011;129:2855–66.

73. Kibriya MG, Raza M, Jasmine F, et al. A genome-wide DNA methylation study in colorectal carcinoma. BMC Med Genet. 2011;4:50.

74. Kim YH, Lee HC, Kim SY, et al. Epigenomic analysis of aberrantly methylated genes in colorectal cancer identifies genes commonly affected by epigenetic alterations. Ann Surg Oncol. 2011;18:2338–47.

75. Spisák S, Kalmar A, Galamb O, et al. Genome-wide screening of genes regulated by DNA methylation in colon cancer development. PLoS One. 2012; 7:e46215.

76. Simmer F, Brinkman AB, Assenov Y, et al. Comparative genome-wide DNA methylation analysis of colorectal tumor and matched normal tissues. Epigenetics. 2012;7:1355–67.

77. Khamas A, Ishikawa T, Mogushi K, et al. Genome-wide screening for methylation-silenced genes in colorectal cancer. Int J Oncol. 2012;41:490–6.

78. Naumov VA, Generozov EV, Zaharjevskaya NB, et al. Genome-scale analysis of DNA methylation in colorectal cancer using Infinium HumanMethylation450 BeadChips. Epigenetics. 2013;8:921–34.

79. Hammoud SS, Cairns BR, Jones DA. Epigenetic regulation of colon cancer and intestinal stem cells. Curr Opin Cell Biol. 2013;25:177–83.

80. Suvà ML, Riggi N, Bernstein BE. Epigenetic reprogramming in cancer. Science. 2013;339:1567–70.

81. Luo Y, Wong CJ, Kaz AM, et al. Differences in DNA methylation signatures reveal multiple pathways of progression from adenoma to colorectal cancer. Gastroenterology. 2014;147:418–29.

82. Hinoue T, Weisenberger DJ, Lange CP, et al. Genome-scale analysis of aberrant DNA methylation in colorectal cancer. Genome Res. 2012;22:271–82.

83. Weisenberger DJ, Siegmund KD, Campan M, et al. CpG island methylator phenotype underlies sporadic microsatellite instability and is tightly associated with BRAF mutation in colorectal cancer. Nat Genet. 2006;38:787–93.

84. Ogino S, Odze RD, Kawasaki T, et al. Correlation of pathologic features with CpG island methylator phenotype (CIMP) by quantitative DNA methylation analysis in colorectal carcinoma. Am J Surg Pathol. 2006;30:1175–83.

85. Goel A, Nagasaka T, Arnold CN, Inoue T, Hamilton C, Niedzwiecki D, Compton C, Mayer RJ, Goldberg R, Bertagnolli MM, et al. The CpG island methylator phenotype and chromosomal instability are inversely correlated in sporadic colorectal cancer. Gastroenterology. 2007;132:127–38.

86. Suehiro Y, Wong CW, Chirieac LR, Kondo Y, Shen L, Webb CR, Chan YW, Chan AS, Chan TL, Wu TT, et al. Epigenetic-genetic interactions in the APC/WNT, RAS/RAF, and P53 pathways in colorectal carcinoma. Clin Cancer Res. 2008;14:2560–9.

87. Toyota M, Ahuja N, Ohe-Toyota M, et al. CpG island methylator phenotype in colorectal cancer. Proc Natl Acad Sci U S A. 1999;96:8681–6.

88. Shen L, Toyota M, Kondo Y, et al. Integrated genetic and epigenetic analysis identifies three different subclasses of colon cancer. Proc Natl Acad Sci U S A. 2007;104:18654–9.

89. Azuara D, Rodriguez-Moranta F, de Oca J, et al. Novel methylation panel for the early detection of colorectal tumors in stool DNA. Clin Colorectal Cancer. 2010;9:168–76.

90. Wang X, Kuang YY, Hu XT. Advances in epigenetic biomarker research in colorectal cancer. World J Gastroenterol. 2014;20:4276–87.

91. Schuebel KE, Chen W, Cope L, et al. Comparing the DNA hypermethylome with gene mutations in human colorectal cancer. PLoS Genet. 2007;3:1709–23.

92. Mori Y, Olaru AV, Cheng Y, et al. Novel candidate colorectal cancer biomarkers identified by methylation microarray-based scanning. Endocr Relat Cancer. 2011;18:465–78.

93. Yi JM, Dhir M, Guzzetta AA, et al. DNA methylation biomarker candidates for early detection of colon cancer. Tumour Biol. 2012;33:363–72.

94. Guinney J, et al. The consensus molecular subtypes of colorectal cancer. Nat Med. 2015;21(11):1350–6. https://doi.org/10.1038/nm.3967.

Part II

Anatomic Considerations in Rectal Cancer Surgery

Anatomical Basis of Rectal Cancer Surgery Focused on Pelvic Fascia

4

Jin-Tung Liang

Abstract

Fascial structures are the natural embryonic dissection plane for the precise surgery of rectal cancer. This chapter characterized the fascial structures implicated in the rectal cancer surgery, which include Toldt fascia, Denonvilliers' fascia, proper fascia of the rectum, endopelvic fascia (parietal layer of pelvic fascia), presacral fascia, rectosacral fascia, and Waldeyer's fascia. Toldt fascia is the extension of Gerota fascia and constitutes the natural dissection plane for the mobilization of left colon. The whole mesorectum was enclosed circumferentially by the thin layer of proper fascia of the rectum; the pelvic sacral bone was covered with the endopelvic fascia (parietal layer of pelvic fascia). Endopelvic fascia and proper fascia of the rectum fused at the level of sacral promontory, and the presacral space is entered after the fascial junction is incised.

Rectosacral fascia usually originated in the S4 level, and the retrorectal space is entered when this fascia is sharply incised. Waldeyer's fascia constitutes the fascia layer covering levator ani muscle. Denonvilliers' fascia is situated in front of proper fascia of the rectum. Usually, the anterior dissection for mobiliza-tion of the rectum is in front of Denonvilliers' fascia to ensure oncological efficacy; however, to enhance the preservation of sexual function, some surgeons suggest the dissection plane be back to the Denonvilliers' fascia. Full respect of the fascia structures is the basic principle for the precise implementation of total mesorectal excision for rectal cancer.

Keywords

Toldt fascia · Denonvilliers' fascia · Proper fascia of the rectum · Endopelvic fascia (parietal layer of pelvic fascia) · Presacral fascia · Rectosacral fascia · Waldeyer's fascia · Gerota fascia

4.1 Introduction

Total mesorectal excision (TME) has become the technical paradigm for the surgery of rectal cancer. The basic tenet of surgical oncology is to en bloc extirpate the cancer with its spreading lymphatic basin along the embryonic natural dissection plane. During the implementation of TME procedure, most colorectal surgeons adopted the following dissection sequences:

(1) Explore the duodeno-mesenteric fossa to find out the inferior mesenteric artery (IMV), and then ligate and transect IMV in the fashion of no-touch isolation technique.

J.-T. Liang
Department of Surgery, National Taiwan University Hospital, Taipei City, Taiwan
e-mail: jintung@ntu.edu.tw

(2) Medial-to lateral mobilization of the meso-colon belonging to the anatomic territory of descending-sigmoid colon along the Toldt fascial dissection plane.

(3) Isolate and transect the inferior mesenteric artery (IMA), in consideration of adequate lymph node clearance.

(4) Mobilize the rectosigmoid mesentery later-ally and downward to the junction of endo-pelvic and proper fascial of the rectum.

(5) Enter the presacral space along the holy plane posterior to the mesorectum, sharply incise the rectosacral fascia, and continue the dissection downward to the Waldeyer's fascia.

(6) Incise the Douglas pouch and dissect the anterior mesorectum downward to the pelvic floor along the Denonvilliers' fascia, prostate capsule in male, and rectovaginal septum in female, in consideration of the preservation of autonomic nerve supplies to genitourinary organs.

In order to ensure the quality surgery of rectal cancer and enhance the dissection efficiency, the importance of the respect for the fascial planes implicated in the TME procedure cannot be overemphasized.

4.2 Anatomic Concepts of Toldt Fascia

Dissection along the Toldt fascia is involved in the mobilization of descending colon to take down the colonic splenic flexure, which is an important procedure to facilitate a tension-free colorectal anastomosis following total mesorec-tal excision for the treatment of rectal cancer. Based on the "rotation and fusion" theory, during the developmental process of the embryonic dor-sal mesentery [1–4], the fascial layer, which anchors the ascending and descending colon to the retroperitoneum, should be sandwiched by two mesothelial layers belonging to the overlying mesocolon and the underlying retroperitoneum, respectively, as elegantly demonstrated by Culligan et al. [4]. It has been demonstrated that

the dissection plane for the mobilization of the ascending, descending, and sigmoid colon is within the Toldt fascial layer. The upper part of Toldt fascial layer fused closely with the meso-thelial layer of the overlying mesocolon; the low part of Toldt fascial layer fused closely with the mesothelial layer of the underlying retroperito-neum, and therefore, "mesofascial interface" and "retrofascial interface" were frequently utilized to label the transitions from the fascial layer to the mesothelial layer attached to the overlying mesocolon and the underlying retroperitoneum, respectively. In 1879, Carl Toldt identified a mes-entery associated with the ascending and descending colon and showed that, although these structures were flattened against the poste-rior abdominal wall, they remained separate from it, i.e., between them, there exists a fascial dis-section plane, which can be utilized to separate the mesocolon from the underlying retroperito-neum [1]. Given Toldt precise description, we proposed that Toldt fascia be an appropriate eponym for this fascial layer, within which a nat-ural embryonic dissection plane can be precisely developed for the mobilization of the whole col-orectum (Fig. 4.1).

Structurally, it has been found that the Toldt fascia was loose and even manifested as areolar tissues in texture. And, during the advancement of surgical dissection, we found minute vessels were present in this fascial plane and sometimes caused oozing of blood. Surfaces of the perirenal fat of bilateral kidneys are covered by the Gerota fascia, which consists of dense connective tissue fibers. On the anatomic territory of bilateral kid-neys, the floor of Toldt fascia fused securely with Gerota fascia and to separate the two layers was technically unfeasible. Sometimes, deliberate separation of Toldt and Gerota fascia might per-forate the Gerota fascia and overexpose the peri-renal fat.

From the kidney area, the fused Toldt and Gerota fascia, or the so-called retrofascial inter-face, extended in all directions. Upward, the fused fascia advanced into the dorsal surface of the duodenum, liver, and pancreas. Downward, the fused Toldt and Gerota fascia became a thin-ner layer of membrane-like structures covering

Fig. 4.1 (**a**) The correct dissection plane for the mobilization of descending-sigmoid mesocolon is within the Toldt fascia (gray area). (**b**) Recognition of the dissection plane along the Toldt fascia is just like identification of the junction between sky and blue sea, when you stand at the seven-miles' beach in Ishikawa Prefecture, Japan. Can you catch it? (**c**) Recognition of the dissection plane along the Toldt fascia is just like identification of the junction between gray sky and snowy peak, when you stand at the Hida Mountain in Hokuriku, Japan. Can you find it?

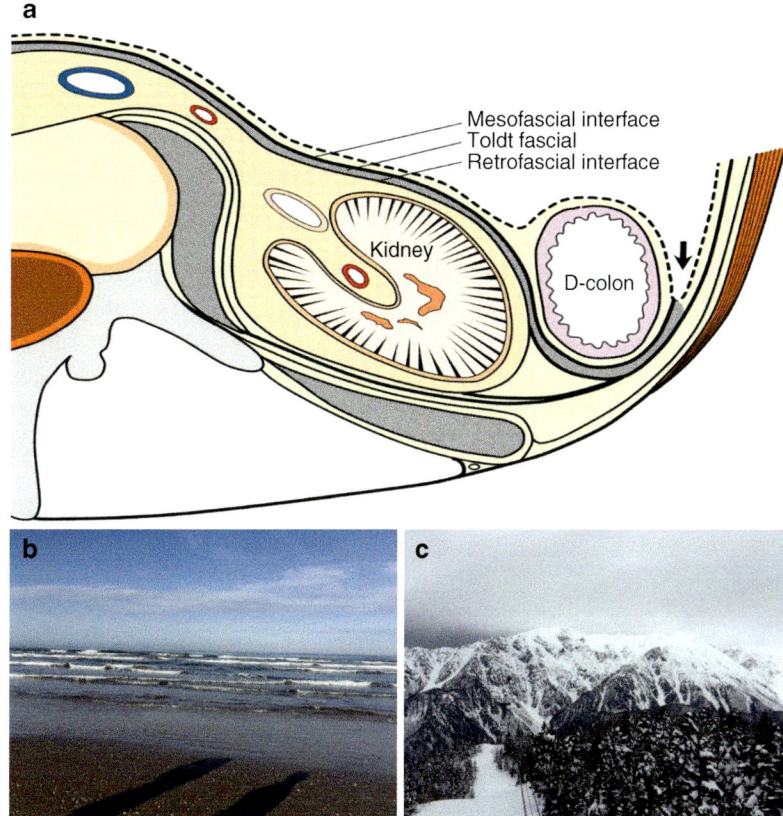

the gonadal vessels, bilateral ureters, and retroperitoneum structures. At this point we carefully preserved gonadal vessels and ureters and simultaneously kept the membrane intact. Any attempt to isolate the ureter might perforate this retrofascial interface and impair the continuity of the Toldt fascial plane.

Laterally, the Toldt fascia tapered at the area below the reflection of visceral and parietal peritoneum and then became sparse and continuous with the loose fibrous tissues surrounding the subperitoneal fatty tissues. Remarkably, Carl Toldt originally described the peritoneal reflection in the paracolic gutter, and later this structure is named as "white line of Toldt" in eponym. The white line of Toldt is formed due to the difference in the density of the connective tissues between the visceral and parietal peritoneum.

For patients with moderate body mass index (more than 24 kg/m²), the Toldt fascia was looser and areolar in nature, and therefore the dissection plane was fairly easy to develop. In contrast, for slim patients, especially the body mass index less than 18 kg/m², the Toldt fascia was nearly absent or invisible, and in such patients we could see Gerota fascia manifest as a whitish membrane and adhere closely to the thin mesocolon, and the development of a dissection plane between the two layers was very difficult and vulnerable to perforate the mesentery.

During the surgical dissection and by scrutiny of the surgical specimens, it has been demonstrated and reproduced that Toldt fascia was a contiguous anatomic structure for anchoring the mesentery to the retroperitoneum from ileocecal junction to the upper rectum, where the endopelvic fascia and proper fascia of the rectum met, as described in the previous cadaveric studies [1–4].

It needs to be further addressed that the misleading term "fascia of fusion" used to describe the Toldt fascia was first coined by Goligher [3].

Actually, Toldt fascia is composed of loose or even areolar fibrous tissues and contains lymphatics and minute blood vessels inside and can be dissected within. If Toldt fascia is a fused fascial structures in nature, it cannot be dissected within, just as we cannot make any dissection within the Denonvilliers' fascia [5], which is an obvious fused fascia overlying the anterior mesorectum. The fascia is developed from mesenchymal cells, whereas the peritoneum is from mesothelial cells. Recently, Culligan et al. have made an in-depth histologic study of Toldt fascia, pointing out that Toldt fascia is sandwiched by upper mesothelium attached to overlying mesocolon and retroperitoneal mesothelium [4]; therefore, it is conceivable that the mechanisms for the formation of Toldt fascia is through the "condensation theory" rather than "fusion theory," i.e., the mesenchymal cells were deposited in between when the visceral and parietal peritoneum of the dorsal mesentery began to fuse together during the embryonic stage [5]. Some authors suggested that the mobilization of the mesocolon of ascending and descending colon could be made along either the mesofascial interface or retrofascial interface; we feel that it is impractical for clinical surgery, and, otherwise, the best way for the development of correct dissection plane should be dissection within the Toldt fascia.

4.3 Rectosacral and Waldeyer's Fascia Revisited

During the clinical practice of total mesorectal excision for the treatment of middle and low rectal cancer, posterior mobilization of the rectum is along the holy plane, which consists of loose areolar connective tissues [6]. With further posterior downward mobilization, a thick tough fascia will be encountered, generally known as rectosacral fascia, and failure to recognize and divide the rectosacral fascia can perforate the mesorectum or lead to severe presacral hemorrhage. Division of the rectosacral fascia allows mobilization of the rectum as far as the anorectal junction and exposes the Waldeyer's fascia, conceptually known as the endopelvic fascia

covering the pelvic floor. However, there is significant confusion about what Waldeyer's fascia represents as the eponym has been used to describe the presacral fascia, the rectosacral fascia, or all fascia posterior to the rectum [7, 8]. This is because Wilhelm Waldeyer did not mention rectosacral fascia and just vaguely described the floor of retrorectal space as the fascia lying along the anococcygeal ligament [9, 10].

Based on the high-resolution images in robotic or laparoscopic surgery for patients with distal rectal cancer undergoing total mesorectal excision, the dissection of holy plane was vividly demonstrated and conceptualized. Briefly, the junction between proper rectal fascia and parietal layer of presacral fascia was incised, and the presacral space is easily entered and enlarged downward along the loose areolar tissue planes. At the level of the body of the fourth sacral vertebra (frequently) or the third sacral vertebra(less frequently), we might encounter the so-called rectosacral fascia, which varies in thickness from a thin transparent membrane to a thick, tough, opaque fascia, running from the periosteum overlying the vertebra body to insert into the proper fascia of the rectum about 3–5 cm above anorectal junction. However, rectosacral fascia was visualized in only 44% of patients undergoing laparoscopic surgery and 48% of patients undergoing robotic surgery. We think only a half minus of patients whose rectosacral fascia can be visualized is because the rectosacral fascia, most of the time, was too thin to be visualized under the strong sharp electrocautery during laparoscopic or robotic surgery or related to the quality of dissection, such as bleedings from bridging venules during dissection. After the rectosacral fascia is divided, a small space is entered inferior to the rectosacral fascia and the rectum, containing the rectococcygeus muscle and lying on the posterior attachment of levator ani to the coccyx and sacrum; this space maybe described as the infrarectal space, also known as the retrorectal space, since it is below the almost horizontal part of the rectum, in the upright position. The floor of retrorectal space consists of an extension of the parietal layer of presacral fascia enveloping the rectococcygeus muscle or its fibrous remnant, which blends with the medial edge of levator ani to form the upper part of the strong anococcygeal ligament. Based on the present study and with reference to the original description of Wilhelm Waldeyer [9–11], we strongly suggest that the fascia covering the floor of retrorectal space should mean Waldeyer's fascia. Remarkably, both rectosacral fascia and Waldeyer's fascia are more obvious in patients after concurrent chemoradiation therapy.

In summary, rectosacral fascia and Waldeyer's fascia are two distinct anatomical structures: The former traverses and separates the presacral space into superior compartment and inferior retrorectal space; the latter forms the floor of retrorectal space (Fig. 4.2). Further clarification of the rectosacral and Waldeyer's fascia would facili-

tate the precise and quality surgery for patients with distal rectal cancer. Sharp division of the condensed and thicker rectosacral fascia is preferred over blunt dissection in order to avoid inadvertent tearing of posterior mesorectal fascia and bleeding from presacral veins.

4.4 Dissection of Denonvilliers' Fascia Implicated in Total Mesorectal Excision

Ample imaging and surgical practices have suggested that the key to a successful anterior dissection in TME is based on the full appreciation of the Denonvilliers' fascia and its relationship to the anterior mesorectum [12–15]. The Denonvilliers'

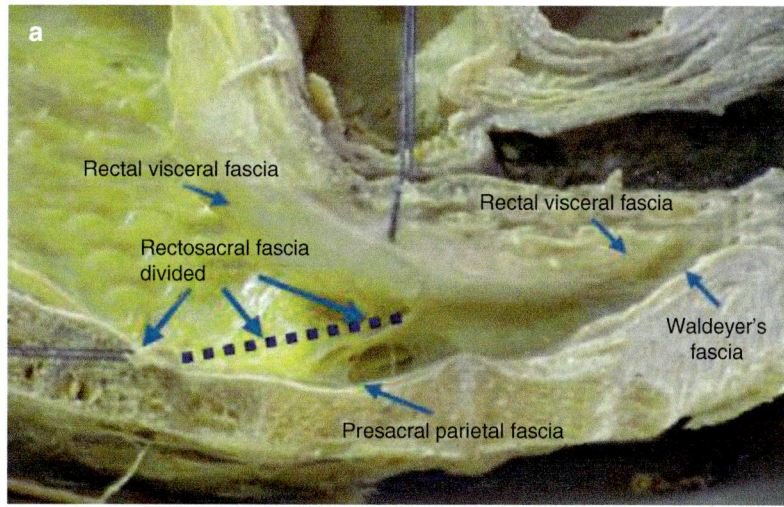

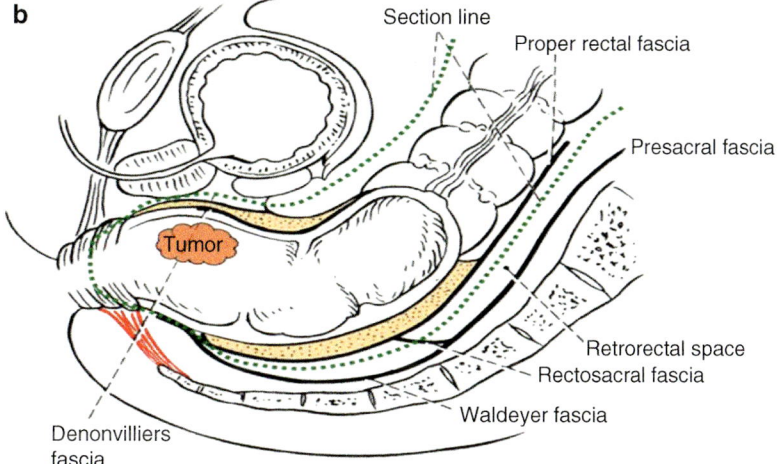

Fig. 4.2 (**a**) Retrorectal space after division of the rectosacral fascia (necessary to mobilize the rectum completely). Waldeyer's fascia denotes the thick endopelvic fascia covering the levator ani muscle. At the lower end (floor) of the retrorectal space, we can see presacral parietal fascia (endopelvic fascia) fuse with proper fascial of the rectum at the level of the anorectal junction. (**b**) Rectosacral fascia frequently originated from endopelvic fascia at S4 sacral level and less frequently from S3 level; Waldeyer's fascia is the endopelvic fascia covering the levator ani muscle. The green line is suggested dissection plane for a TME

fascia is generally considered macroscopically to be a one-layer fascia arising from the fusion of the two walls of the embryonic peritoneal cul-de-sac, and thus it histologically actually consists of two-layer fibromuscular tissues and extends from the peritoneal reflection cranially to the perineal body caudally [13]. Heald et al. advocated that there is usually no surgical plane behind the Denonvilliers' fascia and insisted that optimal TME for rectal cancer should be by dissection "in front of" this fascia [16, 17]. However, Lindsey et al., based on the histologic and embryologic evidences, pointed out that the fascia propria of the rectum and the Denonvilliers' fascia would be separable, and thus the correct natural dissection plane of TME should be "anterior" to the fascia propria of the rectum and "posterior" to the Denonvilliers' fascia [13, 14]. Moreover, Kinugasa et al. found that at the level of seminal vesicles, incision in front of the Denonvilliers' fascia was likely to injure superior parts of the pelvic nerve plexus and the left/right communication; and therefore to preserve all autonomic nerves for a normal genitourinary function, optimal TME for rectal cancer, in their opinion, required a dissection behind the Denonvilliers' fascia [15–18]. On the other hand, the concepts of Denonvilliers' fascia in female patients remain unclear for most colorectal surgeons. Actually, Denonvilliers' original description gave no account of the presence of such a fascia in the female, but gynecologists generally believe that the rectovaginal septum is the female counterpart and is a normal, constant structure [19, 20]. Heald et al. stated that the fascia is less obvious in women, but, importantly for the conduct of rectal dissection, it provides mobility for the rectum on the posterior vaginal wall [16].

For nearly all male patients (91%), the boundaries of Denonvilliers' fascia could be clearly recognized in laparoscopy [5]. Immediately after the peritoneum over the rectovesical pouch was incised, the bluish bubble-shaped seminal vesicles were exposed nakedly with little purposely dissection. Medially, the surface of seminal vesicles was generally covered with sparse areolar fibrous tissues, whereas, laterally, it was contiguous with some dense fibrous structures, which were postulated to contain the communicating nerve fibers from the nearby neurovascular bundle of Walsh.

Posterior to the seminal vesicles, we could see the Denonvilliers' fascia, varying in nature from a fragile translucent fibrous layer to a tough leathery membrane, manifesting itself as a trapezoidal "apron" covering the glistening fatty tissues of the anterior mesorectum (Fig. 4.3a). Although Lindsey et al. showed that the Denonvilliers' fascia and the anterior part of the fascia propria of the rectum proper rectal fascia were two separable layers in histology [12–14], it has been found that there was no natural dissection plane between the two layers in practice, because any attempt to dissect along this postulated surgical plane would have nearly resulted in the perforation of this fascial layer (Fig. 4.3b). This finding gave us the impression that the upper part of the Denonvilliers' fascia was more adherent to, or even fused with, the anterior part of the fascia propria of the rectum than to the seminal vesicles. Moreover, in laparoscopy, the Denonvilliers' fascia usually has clear left and right edges, which are fenced by the insertion of lateral ligaments at the anterolateral (2 and 10 o'clock) direction of the rectum. Remarkably, the Denonvilliers' fascia was even more prominent in male patients after preoperative concurrent chemoradiation therapy.

Technically, by pushing the seminal vesicles ventrally along the areolar tissue plane "in front of" the Denonvilliers' fascia, the anterior dissection in TME can be efficiently continued downward until the prostate is reached, where the Denonvilliers' fascia fuses with the prostate capsule and the natural surgical plane halts (Fig. 4.3c). Therefore, in order to continue the dissection, we had to incise the Denonvilliers' fascia at this site and shift the dissection plane to "behind" this fascia (Fig. 4.3d), and thereafter, by gentle pushing the very thin fatty tissues of the anterior mesorectum dorsally, the rectum could be completely separated from the prostate and mobilized to the pelvic floor. However, for tumors located at the anterior rectal wall with suspected invasion into the prostate capsule, we deliberately kept the dissection plane in front of the Denonvilliers' fascia and even into the pros-

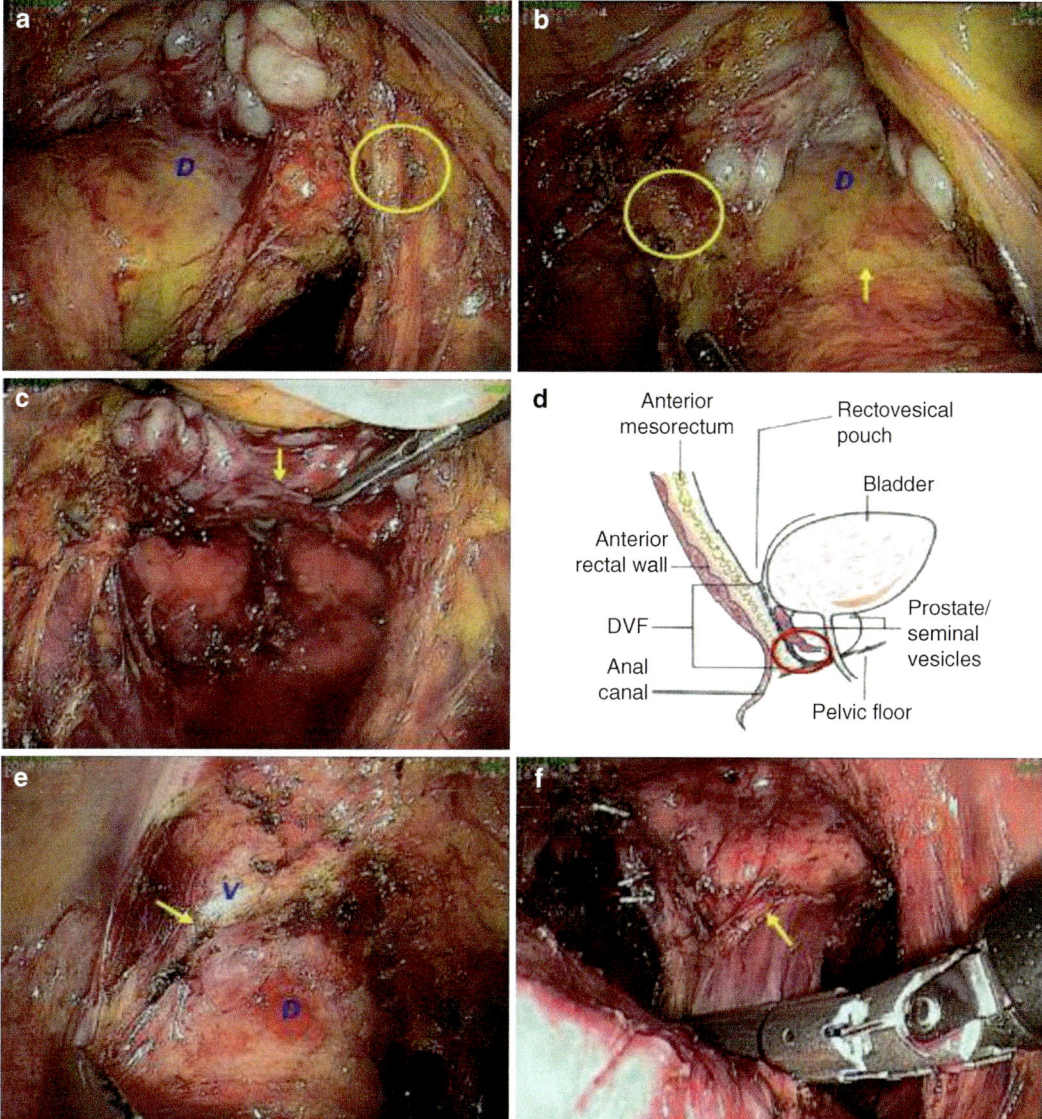

Fig. 4.3 (a) The Denonvilliers' fascia (*D*) is a fibrous layer in between seminal vesicles anteriorly and fatty mesorectum posteriorly. The left edge of Denonvilliers' fascia is at the insertion of the left lateral ligament. The left side of seminal vesicles is close to the neurovascular bundle of Walsh (yellow circle). (**b**) Attempt to dissect between the Denonvilliers' fascia and the fascia propria of the rectum resulted in perforation of this layer (arrow). (**c**) The tented structure (arrow) was the cutting end of the Denonvilliers' fascia, which was incised at the level of prostate so that the dissection could be continued downward. (**d**) The band of dotted lines indicates the Denonvilliers' fascia, whose lower part fuses with the posterior capsule of the prostate and could not be separated (red circle), modified from Lindsey et al. Br J Surg 2000;87:1288. (**e**) In some adipose females, there is still a scanty layer of fibrous tissue, which may be equivalent to Denonvilliers' fascia (*D*), covering the anterior mesorectum. In between the posterior vaginal wall (*V*) and anterior mesorectum, the rectovaginal septum is composed of intertwined fibrous tissues (arrow). (**f**) A laparoscopic view of the lower part of the rectovaginal septum (arrow), in which no distinct layer of the Denonvilliers' fascia could be found

tate parenchyma to ensure an adequate anterior resection margin for cancer. However, such dissection always resulted in more bleeding as well as postoperative sexual dysfunction, which was due to the unavoidable injury of the peri-prostate autonomic nerve plexus.

In contrast, the female Denonvilliers' fascia was found to be much less obvious as a distinct fibrous layer than in the male counterpart. Generally, the vagina and rectum are separated by a sheet of strong fibrous tissues, which have long been recognized by gynecologists as "rectovaginal septum." Under laparoscopy, after the peritoneum over cul-de-sac was excised, we could clearly identify the intertwined fibrous tissues in between the vaginal vault and the rectum. In more adipose women (body mass index $\geq$ 27 kg/m^2), posterior to this area of irregular fibrous tissues, we could still identify the shiny fatty tissues of the mesorectum, which tapered caudally (Fig. 4.3e). However, in thinner females, the anterior mesorectum is very scanty or actually not present, and therefore in this condition, it seems that the intervening fibrous tissue plate acts as the linking substances to anchor the posterior vaginal wall to the anterior rectal wall all the way from the level of cul-de-sac down to the perineal body [21].

Based on the observation in our previous study [5], we feel that there is no natural surgical plane between the rectum and vagina, and therefore, during surgical practice, we usually first clearly identify the whitish posterior vaginal wall and then push it ventrally and caudally against the backward-pulled rectum (Fig. 4.3f). By this sliding action, the vaginal wall can then be separated from the rectum, and simultaneously the anterior surface of the rectum can be kept attached by some fibrous tissues of the rectovaginal septum to ensure that the anterior resection margin was adequate during the whole dissection process. On the other hand, it has also been noted that in females after preoperative concurrent chemoradiation therapy, the so-called female Denonvilliers' fascia became more dense, unclear, and irregular and therefore more difficult to dissect.

4.5　In Conclusion

In assisting a resident in an operation, I frequently cited the ancient Chinese article entitled "Chinese Gastronomy," which was written by Chuangtse in the fourth century BC and emphasized the use of the cleaver (Fig. 4.4).

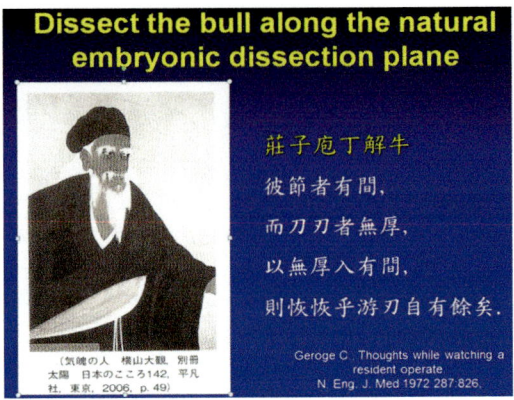

Fig. 4.4 The ancient Chinese Taoist Chungtse advocated if the dissection was performed along the natural dissection plane, the surgeons will meet the least resistance and greatly enhance the work efficiency, which is the core philosophy of the Chinese Taoism

Much of its wording seems applicable to our daily practice of colorectal cancer surgery, particularly the concept of working "with the mind, not the eye":

Prince Huei's cook was cutting up a bullock. Every blow of his hand, every heave of his shoulders, every trend of his foot, every thrust of his knee, every whshh of rent flesh, every chhk of the chopper, was in perfect rhythm-like the dancer of the Mulberry Grove, like the harmonious chords of Ching Shou.

"Well done!" cried the Prince. "Yours is skill indeed!"

"Sire," replied the cook laying down his chopper," I have always devoted myself to Tao, which is higher than mere skill. When I first began to cut up bullocks, I saw before me whole bullocks. After three years' practice, I no longer saw whole animals. And now I work with my mind and not with my eye. My mind works without control of the senses. Falling back on eternal principles, I glide through such great joints or cavities as there may be, according to the natural constitution of the animal. I do not even touch the convolution of muscle and tendon, still less attempt to cut through large bones.

"A good cook changes his chopper once a year because he cuts. An ordinary cook once a month because he hacks. But I have had this chopper for nineteen years, and although I have cut up many thousand bullocks, its edge is as if fresh from the whetstone. For at the joints there are always interstices, and the edge of chopper being without thickness, it remains only to insert that which is without thickness into such an interstice. Indeed there is plenty of room for the blade to move about. It is thus that I have kept my chopper for nineteen years as though fresh from the whetstone.

Nevertheless, where I come upon a knotty part which is difficult to tackle, I am all caution. Fixing my eye on it, I stay my hand, and gently apply my blade, until with a hivah the part yields like earth crumbling to the ground. Then I take out my chopper, stand up, and look around with an air of triumph.

"Bravo!" cried the Prince. "From the words of this cook I have learnt how to take care of my life." [22]

This quotation from the ancient manuscript is so self-explanatory that no comment is needed. It is stranger, however, that in books on surgical technique, much space is spent on advice on the gentle handling of tissues and the benefits of sharp dissection but little or none on how to find the natural tissue planes and separate them by a gentle traction and a minimum of dissection. Fully respecting the Toldt, Gerota, rectosacral, Waldeyer, Denonvilliers fascia, and its relation to the neighboring proper fascia of the rectum, endopelvic fascia, and rectal lateral ligament would ensure the quality surgery of rectal cancer, which can extrapolate to optimal oncological efficacy, even without the proof from randomized prospective clinical trials.

References

1. Coffey JC, O'Leary DP. The mesentery: structure, function, and role in disease. Lancet Gastroenterol Hepatol. 2016;1:238–47.
2. Coffey JC, Dillon M, Sehgal R, et al. Mesenteric-based surgery exploits gastrointestinal, peritoneal, mesenteric and fascial continuity from duodenojejunal flexure to the anorectal junction—a review. Dig Surg. 2015;32:291–300.
3. Culligan K, Coffey JC, Kiran RP, et al. The mesocolon: a prospective observational study. Color Dis. 2012;14:421–8.
4. Culligan K, Walsh S, Dunne C, et al. The mesocolon: a histological and electron microscopic characterization of the mesenteric attachment of the colon prior to and after surgical mobilization. Ann Surg. 2014;260:1048–56.
5. Liang JT, Cheng KW. Laparoscopic dissection of Denonvilliers' fascia implicated for total mesorectal excision for treatment of rectal cancer. Surg Endosc. 2011;25:935–40.
6. Liang JT, Cheng JC, Huang KC, Sun CT. Comparison of tumor recurrence between laparoscopic total meso-

rectal excision with sphincter preservation and laparoscopic abdominoperineal resection for low rectal cancer. Surg Endosc. 2013;27:3452–64.
7. Gordon PH, Nivatvongs S. Principles and practice of surgery for the colon, rectum, and anus. 3rd ed. New York: Informa Healthcare USA; 2007. p. 8–9.
8. Corman ML. Corman's colon and rectal surgery. 6th ed. Philadelphia: Lippincott Williams and Wilkins; 2013. p. 6.
9. Crapp AR, Cuthbertson AM. William Waldeyer and the rectosacral fascia. Surg Gynecol Obstet. 1974; 138(2):252–6.
10. Goligher J. Surgery of the anus rectum and colon. 5th ed. London: Bailliere Tindall; 1984. p. 5.
11. Skandalakis JE. Surgical anatomy: the embryologic and anatomic basis of modern surgery, vol. 2. Athens: PMP; 2004. p. 902–6.
12. Lindsey I, Guy RJ, Warren BF, Mortensen NJ. Anatomy of Denonvilliers' fascia and pelvic nerves, impotence, and implications for the colorectal surgeon. Br J Surg. 2000;87:1288–99.
13. Lindsey I, Warren B, Mortensen N. Optimal total mesorectal excision for rectal cancer is by dissection in front of Denonvilliers' fascia. Br J Surg. 2004; 91:121–3.
14. Lindsey I, Warren BF, Mortensen NJ. Denonvilliers' fascia lies anterior to the fascia propria and rectal dissection plane in total mesorectal excision. Dis Colon Rectum. 2005;48:37–42.
15. Kinugasa Y, Murakami G, Uchimoto K, Takenaka A, Yajima T, Sugihara K. Operating behind Denonvilliers' fascia for reliable preservation of urogenital autonomic nerves in total mesorectal excision: a histologic study using cadaveric specimens, including a surgical experiment using fresh cadaveric models. Dis Colon Rectum. 2006;49:1024–32.
16. Heald RJ, Moran BJ, Brown G, Daniels IR. Optimal total mesorectal excision for rectal cancer is by dissection in front of Denonvilliers' fascia. Br J Surg. 2004;91:121–3.
17. Liang JT, Chang KJ, Wang SM. Lateral ligaments contain important nerves. Br J Surg. 1998;85:1162.
18. Kinugasa Y, Murakami G, Suzuki D, Sugihara K. Histological identification of fascial structures posterolateral to the rectum. Br J Surg. 2007;94:620–6.
19. Richardson AC. The rectovaginal septum revisited: its relationship to rectocele and its importance in rectocele repair. Clin Obstet Gynecol. 1993;36:976–83.
20. Farrell SA, Dempsey T, Geldenhuys L. Histologic examination of 'fascia' used in colporrhaphy. Obstet Gynecol. 2001;98:794–8.
21. Nichols DH, Milley PS. Surgical significance of the rectovaginal septum. Am J Obstet Gynecol. 1970; 108:215–20.
22. Crile G. Thoughts while watching a resident operate. N Engl J Med. 1972;287:826.

The Lymphatic Spread of the Rectal Cancer

5

In Kyu Lee

Abstract

The lymph spread of the rectal cancer is various according to the tumor location. Pathways of lymphatic drainage are dived into three groups, the upper two thirds of the rectum, dentate line up to the lower third of the rectum, and the anal canal up to dentate line. Lymph node metastasis from rectal cancer usually occurs in regional rectal lymph nodes that consist of three groups: perirectal, intermediate and main lymph nodes, and lateral pelvic lymph nodes. The concept of total mesorectal excision is equally accepted in the West and East, but the role of lateral pelvic lymph node dissection is accepted differently. Therefore, recently selective pelvic lymph node dissection after preoperative chemoradiotherapy was proposed. Moreover, whole-mount sections or fat clearance techniques have been performed for the precise pathologic assessment after surgery. The lymph node metastasis of rectal cancer progresses differently under various conditions, so the management of rectal cancer should consider various aspects through multidisciplinary team approach.

Keywords

Rectal neoplasms · Lymphatic metastasis · Lymph node excision

I. K. Lee
Department of Surgery, College of Medicine,
Seoul St. Mary's Hospital, The Catholic University
of Korea, Seoul, South Korea
e-mail: cmcgslee@catholic.ac.kr

5.1 Introduction

The lymph node metastasis in rectal cancer surgery is more important than colon cancer for predicting prognosis. Unlike colon cancer, lymph node metastasis from rectal cancer occurs within the narrow pelvis with many nerves related to urination and sexual function and to the lateral pelvic lymph node outside the pelvic cavity. Therefore, several methods have been considered for the treatment of metastatic lymph nodes. Especially, the management of these lateral pelvic lymph nodes has many differences in treatment methods in the East and the West and will be discussed in this chapter.

5.2 The Pattern of the Lymphatic Drainage According to the Tumor Location

The lymphatic drainage begins as a network of intramural lymphatic plexuses under the mucosal layer of the rectum and flows into the lymph nodes along the arterial blood supply [1, 2]. Pathways of lymphatic drainage in the anus and rectum are dived into three groups, the upper two thirds of the rectum, dentate line up to the lower third of the rectum, and the anal canal up to dentate line [1–3]. There is a difference in the lymphatic spread method depending on the location of the tumor according to the groups (Fig. 5.1).

© Springer Nature Singapore Pte Ltd. 2018
N. K. Kim et al. (eds.), *Surgical Treatment of Colorectal Cancer*,
https://doi.org/10.1007/978-981-10-5143-2_5

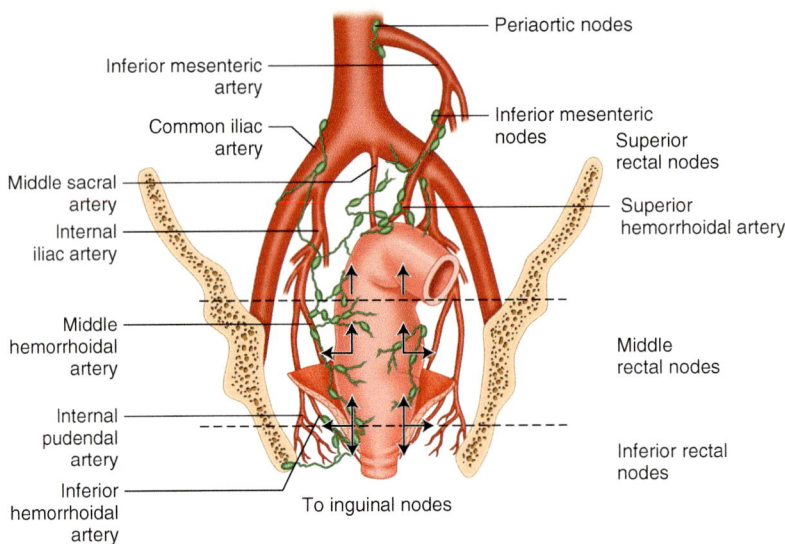

Fig. 5.1 The pattern of the lymphatic drainage according to the tumor location

1. In the first group, lymphatics in the upper two thirds of the rectum drain into the perirectal lymph node along the superior rectal vessels and then toward the origin of the inferior mesenteric artery [1–3]. These perirectal lymph nodes are located in the mesorectum within holy plane which Heald et al. introduced as the concept of total mesorectal excision [2, 4].

2. In the second group, lymphatics in the lower third of the rectum primarily drain cephalad but laterally along the middle rectal vessels to the internal iliac nodes [1, 2, 5]. Rectal endoscopic lymphoscintigraphy study showed no lateral drainage to internal iliac nodes among healthy volunteers whose rectums had been injected both above and below the peritoneal reflection, but lateral drainage occurred in all control subjects whose anal canal had been injected above the dentate line [6, 7]. Lateral drainage pathways were variable and inconsistent, and lateral spread occurs in neoplasms of the anal canal or in rectal cancer when there is obstruction of the cranial drainage path [1–3, 7]. Above the dentate line, the drainage is primarily to the inferior mesenteric nodes and laterally into the internal iliac

nodes as some secondary through the inferior and middle rectal lymphatics like the lower third rectum [1].

3. In the third group, lymphatics between the dentate line and anal verge drain into inguinal lymph nodes which are main drainage site and internal iliac lymph nodes through the middle rectal nodes [1, 3]. The anal canal from the levator ani to the anal verge is composed of two parts, endodermal origin above the dentate line and ectodermal origin below the dentate line, which have different innervations, vasculature and lymphatics [1]. Therefore, lymphatics did not communicate across the dentate line and did not perforate the levator ani muscles in infant cadavers study [1, 2]. However, there is possibility of downward spread of cancer over mucocutaneous junction, especially when superior pathways were obstructed by cancer, and spread of carcinoma of the rectum to inguinal nodes rarely occurs and then usually in late cases [3, 8].

Intramural spread extension beyond 2 cm from visible edge of the tumor and positive nodes distal to the tumor are rare, but these cases occur in advanced and high-grade tumors or proximal nodal metastasis, respectively [2, 9, 10]. The majority of mesorectal lymph nodes are located in the posterior section; a great proportion are within the upper mesorectum, and a few are in the distal mesorectum [11]. Metastasis of lymph nodes was most likely to occur in the bowel segment affected by the tumor and in the segments 1 cm distal or proximal to the tumor [12].

5.3 Lymph Node Groups

Regional rectal lymph nodes consist of three groups: perirectal, intermediate (inferior mesenteric trunk nodes) and main lymph nodes (inferior mesenteric nodes), and lateral pelvic lymph nodes are included as a fourth group in the rectum [13] (Fig. 5.2). The lateral lymph nodes include the common iliac lymph nodes, the proximal and distal internal iliac lymph nodes, the obturator lymph nodes, and the external iliac lymph nodes [13]. Nakamura et al. defined the anatomical location of the lateral lymph node as follows [5]. The common iliac lymph nodes are located in the region surrounded by the left and right common iliac arteries. The caudal border extends to the obturator foramen. The internal iliac lymph nodes are surrounded by the internal iliac artery, the superior vesical artery, and the region extending from the left and right hypogastric nerves to the pelvic nerve plexus. The caudal margin of this group of lymph nodes extends to Alcock's canal. The internal iliac lymph nodes are subclassified into the central internal iliac nodes and the peripheral internal iliac nodes; the border is defined by the superior vesical artery. The lateral border of the obturator lymph nodes is defined by the external iliac artery and the pelvic wall. The dorsal border of this group of nodes is defined by the sciatic nerve and the piriformis muscle. The medial border is defined by the internal iliac artery and the superior vesical artery. The caudal border extends to the obturator foramen. Para-aortic nodes are proximal to the main lymph nodes, and other lymph nodes include lateral and median sacral nodes, aortic bifurcation nodes, and inguinal nodes [13].

5.4 Concept of Lymphadenectomy

Lymph node dissection other than lymph nodes included in total mesorectal excision has several views. For suspicious lymph node metastasis beyond the TME, removal of lymph node metastasis or histologic biopsy in many guidelines was performed, and for lymph nodes not clinically suspicious, extensive lymph node dissection is not recommended for preventive purposes [14]. The incidence of lateral pelvic lymph node (LPLN) metastasis has been reported to be approximately 15–20% in patients with locally advanced rectal cancer who underwent lateral pelvic lymph node dissection (LPLND) [15–19]. In Western countries, surgeons do not perform LPLN regularly because preoperative CRT without surgery can provide acceptable local control and LPLN metastasis is generally considered a metastatic disease [16, 20]. Therefore, preoperative chemotherapy is the widely accepted standard treatment for patients with stage II, III rectal cancer.

In about 1950, LPLND was attempted and then Japanese considered LPLND a standard procedure for the surgical treatment of advanced lower rectal cancer [5, 21]. Therefore, the Western TME is described as a limited resection [22].

A standard resection of LPLN involves dissection along the parietal pelvic fascia and the internal iliac artery [2, 22]. The lateral, medical, cranial, caudal, and dorsal anatomical borders of LPLND are the external iliac artery, pelvic plexus, bifurcation of the common iliac artery, levator ani muscle, and sciatic nerve, respectively [16]. Whereas an extended resection also includes excision of the internal iliac vessels preserving the superior vesical artery and obturator nerve by Japanese surgeons [2, 22].

5.5 Debated About Lateral Pelvic Lymph Node Dissection (West vs. East)

As a basis for the controversy of the East and the West on lateral pelvic lymph node dissection, the West insist that a meta-analysis comparing

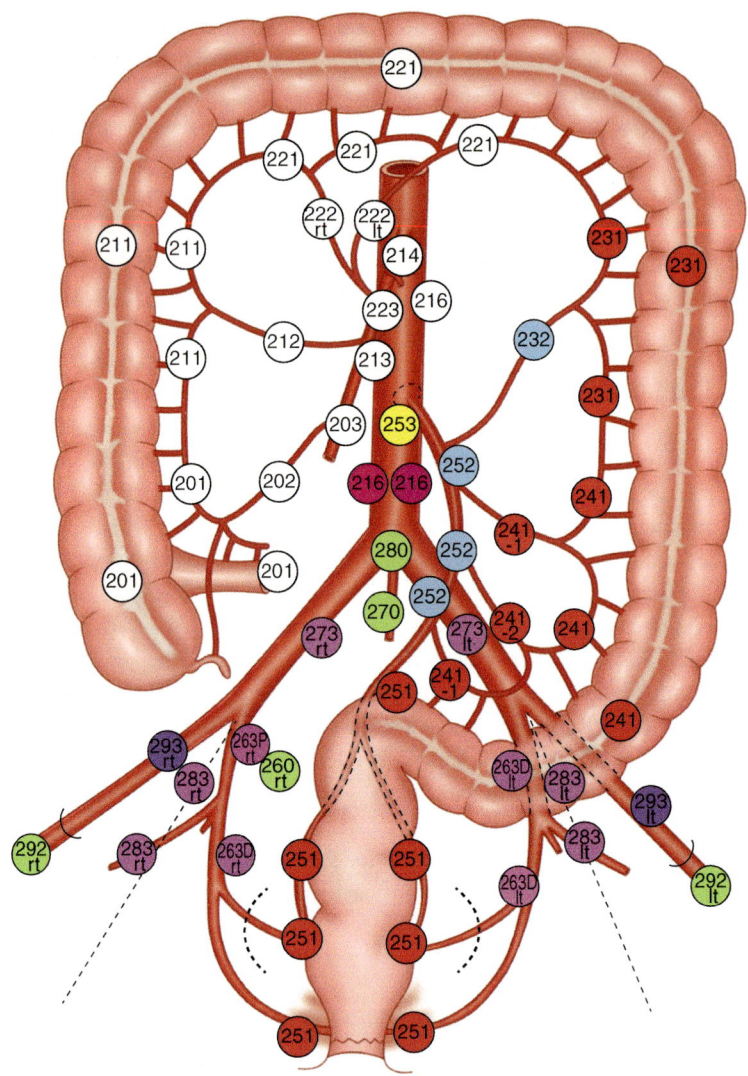

Fig. 5.2 Lymph node groups

extended and non-extended lymphadenectomy of LPLN in patients with rectal cancer showed no significant difference in overall cancer-specific advantage [23]. Furthermore, LPLND increases operating time, intraoperative blood loss, and rates of autonomic nerve dysfunction, such as urination dysfunction and male sexual dysfunction in this meta-analysis [23]. However, the Japan Clinical Oncology Group compared TME only with TME with LPLND for clinical stage II or stage III lower rectal cancer without LPLN enlargement [24–26]. In this randomized controlled trial, LPLND with autonomic nerve preservation may not increase the incidence of sexual dysfunction in men and also did not increase any grade 3–4 postoperative complications including anastomotic leakage of all grades in spite of longer operation time and greater blood loss [24, 25]. Moreover, TME with LPLND group had lower local recurrence than TME alone groups [26]. In other study, patients with stage T3, T4 tumors who underwent preoperative CRT and TME alone had LPLN metastasis as a major cause of local recurrence [27]. Therefore, the East, especially Japan, has advocated LPLND.

5.6 Selective Pelvic Lymph Node Dissection After Preoperative Chemoradiotherapy

With high prevalence of preoperative CRT for rectal cancer, some of the studies showed the major local recurrence was pelvic lymph node area. Recently, the need of selective LPLND has been reported for rectal cancer based on pre- or posttreatment imaging after preoperative CRT [15, 16, 28, 29].

In the studies that emphasized the importance of LPLN status before CRT, pathological LPLN metastasis was reported as 66% in advanced low rectal cancer and 51.6% in advanced rectal cancer when LPLND was performed in patients with suspected LPLN metastasis based on MDCT or MRI before CRT [15, 16]. Moreover, none developed local recurrence in these patients with LPLND [15, 16]. The incidence of lateral pelvic lymph node metastasis after chemoradiotherapy was estimated to be 22% in low rectal cancer and 8.1%

in rectal cancer [15, 16]. They suggested that incidence of LPLN metastasis is high even after preoperative CRT, and LPLND might improve local control and survival of patients with LPLN metastasis in advanced low rectal cancer treated with preoperative CRT [15, 16]. Moreover, there is increasing opinions that LPLN short-axis diameter after CRT was significantly associated with LPLN recurrence, the 5-year overall survival and 5-year disease-free survival rates [28, 29]. They recommended that the decision to perform LPLND should be based on the LPLN response to preoperative CRT [28, 29]. Therefore, if selective LPLND is performed on the base of pre- or posttreatment imaging after preoperative CRT, the LPLN metastasis itself is not a poor prognostic indicator after preoperative CRT and LPLND, and LPLN metastasis can be a regional disease that is amenable to curative resection [15, 16, 28, 29].

5.7 Pathologic Assessment of Rectal Lymph Node

LN involvement is one of the most significant prognostic factors. Many guidelines recommend a minimum of 12 lymph nodes retrieval. However, harvest of 12 LNs is difficult to achieve especially in rectal cancer. One limitation of the current N-stage system is that it cannot provide a precise prognosis for patients who did not have over 12 lymph nodes dissected. The number of metastatic lymph nodes, total number of lymph nodes examined, number of negative metastatic lymph nodes, lymph node ratio, and the number of apical lymph nodes were examined to complement the N-stage system. Lymph node ratio and apical lymph nodes are complementary in rectal cancer [30]. Most pathologists believe that LNs measuring ≥5 mm can be identified by routine methods, but LN <5 mm are difficult to recognize [31]. However, fat clearance techniques show LN harvesting including 70–92% small LNs, with some reporting a small lymph node ratio as high as 45–78% [11]. Therefore, small LN evaluation through fat clearance techniques increase the accuracy of staging, and also, whole-mount sections facilitate the precise and effective assessment of rectal cancer.

Conclusion

According to extent of disease, adequate lymphadenectomy is the most important treatment for rectal cancer. With the understanding of lymphatic spread of the rectal cancer, the lymph node metastasis of rectal cancer happened by various methods under different conditions, so there is a limit to only either treatment of radical resection or CRT. Therefore, the management of rectal cancer should be approached under accurate diagnosis and various treatment methods through a multidisciplinary team approach.

References

1. Dujovny N, Quiros RM, Saclarides TJ. Anorectal anatomy and embryology. Surg Oncol Clin N Am. 2014;13:277–93.
2. Bell S, Sasaki J, Sinclair G, Chapuis PH, Bokey EL. Understanding the anatomy of lymphatic drainage and the use of blue-dye mapping to determine the extent of lymphadenectomy in rectal cancer surgery: unresolved issues. Color Dis. 2009;11:443–9.
3. Blair JB, Holyoke A. A note on the lymphatics of the middle and lower rectum and anus. Anat Rec. 1950; 108:635–43.
4. Heald RJ, Husband EM, Ryall RD. The mesorectum in rectal cancer surgery-the clue to pelvic recurrence? Br J Surg. 1982;69:613–6.
5. Nakamura T, Watanabe M. Lateral lymph node dissection for lower rectal cancer. World J Surg. 2013;37:1808–13.
6. Montori A, Miscusi G, Saracca L, et al. Transrectal sonography and endoscopic lymphoscintigraphy in the preoperative staging of rectal cancer. Dig Surg. 1984;1:200–4.
7. Arnaud JP, Bergamaschi R, Schloegel M, Ollier JC, Haegele P, Grob JC, Adloff M. Progress in the assessment of lymphatic spread in rectal cancer. Rectal endoscopic lymphoscintigraphy. Dis Colon Rectum. 1990; 33:398–401.
8. Grinnell RS. The lymphatic and venous spread of carcinoma of rectum. Ann Surg. 1942;116:200–16.
9. Hida J, Yasutomi M, Maruyama T. Lymph node metastases detected in the mesorectum distal to carcinoma of the rectum by the clearing method: justification of total mesorectal excision. J Am Coll Surg. 1997;184:584–8.
10. Williams NS, Dixon MF, Johnston D. Reappraisal of the 5 centimetre rule of distal excision for carcinoma of the rectum: a study of distal intramural spread and of patients' survival. Br J Surg. 1987;70:150–4.
11. Yao Y-F, Wang L, Liu Y-Q, Li J-Y, Gu J. Lympn node distribution and pattern of metastases in the mesorectum following total mesorectal excision using the modified fat clearing technique. J Clin Pathol. 2011; 64:1073–7.
12. Cserni G, Tarjan M, Bori R. Distance of lymph nodes from the tumor, an important feature in colorectal cancer specimens. Arch Pathol Lab Med. 2001;125:246–9.
13. Japanese Society for Cancer of the Colon and Rectum. Japanese classification of colorectal carcinoma, 2nd ed. (English). Tokyo: Kanehara; 2009.
14. Korean Clinical Practice Guideline for Colon and Rectal Cancer v.1.0. Ivy Plan, Korean Medical Association, Seoul; 2012.
15. Ishihara S, Kawai K, Tanaka T, Kiyomatsu T, Hata K, Nozawa H, Morikawa T, Watanabe T. Oncological outcomes of lateral pelvic lymph node metastasis in rectal cancer treated with preoperative chemoradiotherapy. Dis Colon Rectum. 2017;60:469–76.
16. Akiyoshi T, Ueno M, Matsueda K, Konishi T, Fujimoto Y, et al. Selective lateral pelvic lymph node dissection in patients with advanced low rectal cancer treated with preoperative chemoradiotherapy based on pretreatment imaging. Ann Surg Oncol. 2014;21:189–96.
17. Mori T, Takahashi K, Yasuno M. Radical resection with autonomic nerve preservation and lymph node dissection techniques in lower rectal cancer surgery and its results: the impact of lateral lymph node dissection. Langenbeck's Arch Surg. 1998;383: 409–15.
18. Moriya Y, Sugihara K, Akasu T, Fujita S. Importance of extended lymphadenectomy with lateral node dissection for advanced lower rectal cancer. World J Surg. 1997;21:728–32.
19. Ueno M, Oya M, Azekuru K, Yamaguchi T, Muto T. Incidence and prognostic significance of lateral lymph node metastasis in patients with advanced low rectal cancer. Br J Surg. 2005;92:756–63.
20. Kusters M, Beets GL, van de Velde CJ, et al. A comparison between the treatment of low rectal cancer in Japan and the Netherlands, focusing on the patterns of local recurrence. Ann Surg. 2009;10:1053–62.
21. Sauer I, Bacon HE. A new approach of excision of carcinoma of the lower portion of the rectum and anal canal. Surg Gynecol Obstet. 1952;95:229–42.
22. Takahashi T, Ueno M, Azekura K, Ota H. The lymphatic spread of rectal cancer and the effect of dissection: Japanese contribution and experience. In: des Soreide O, Norstein J, editors. Rectal Cancer surgery. Optimisation standardisation documentation. Berlin: Springer-Verlag; 1997. p. 165–80.
23. Georgiou P, Tan E, Gouvas N, Antoniou A, Brown G, Nicholls RJ, Tekkis P. Extended lymphadenectomy versus conventional surgery for rectal cancer: a meta-analysis. Lancet Oncol. 2009;10:1053–62.
24. Fujita S, Akasu T, Mizusawa J, Saito N, et al. Postoperative morbidity and mortality after mesorectal excision with and without lateral lymph node dissection for clinical stage II or stage III lower rectal

cancer (JCOG0212): results from a multicentre, randomized controlled, non-inferiority trial. Lancet Oncol. 2012;13:616–21.

25. Saito S, Fujita S, Mizusawa J, Kanemitsu Y, Saito N, et al. Male sexual dysfunction after rectal cancer surgery: results of a randomized trial comparing mesorectal excision with and without lateral lymph node dissection for patients with lower rectal cancer: Japan Clinical Oncology Group Study JCOG0212. Eur J Surg Oncol. 2016;42:1851–8.

26. Fujita S, Mizusawa J, Kanemitsu Y, Ito M, et al. Mesorectal excision with or without lateral lymph node dissection for clinical stage II/III lower rectal cancer (JCOG0212): a multicenter, randomized controlled, noninferiority trial. Ann Surg. 2017;266:201–7.

27. Kim TH, Jeong SY, CHoi DH, et al. Lateral lymph node metastasis is a mjor cause of locoregional recurrence in rectal cancer treated with preoperative chemoradiotherapy and curative resection. Ann Surg Oncol. 2008;15:729–37.

28. Oh HK, Kang SB, Lee SM, Lee SY, Ihn MH, Kim DW, Park JH, Kim YH, Lee KH, Kim JS, Kim JW, Kim JH, Chang TY, Park SC, Sohn DK, Oh JH, Park JW, Ryoo SB, Jeong SY, Park KJ. Neoadjuvant chemoradiotherapy affects the indications for lateral pelvic node dissection in mid/low rectal cancer with clinically suspected lateral node involvement: a multicenter retrospective cohort study. Ann Surg Oncol. 2014;21:2280–7.

29. Kim MJ, Kim TH, Kim DY, Kim SY, Baek JY, Chang HJ, Park SC, Park JW, Oh JH. Can chemoradiation allow for omission of lateral pelvic node dissection for locally advanced rectal cancer? J Surg Oncol. 2015;111:459–64.

30. Kwon TS, Choi SB, Lee YS, Kim J-G, Oh ST, Lee IK. Novel methods of lymph node evaluation for predicting the prognosis of colorectal cancer patients with inadequate lymph node harvest. Cancer Res Treat. 2016;48:216–24.

31. Herrera-Ornelas L, Justiniano J, Castillo N, et al. Metastases in small lymph nodes from colon cancer. Arch Surg. 1987;122:1253–6.

Anal Sphincter Complex Preservation

6

Ji Won Park and Seung-Yong Jeong

Abstract

To save the sphincter, understanding the anatomy of anal sphincter complex is essential. The anal canal extends from the level of the levator ani muscle to the anal verge. The muscularis propria of the rectum is consisted of the inner circular and outer longitudinal smooth muscle layer. The internal and external sphincters together can maintain anal continence. Intersphincteric groove lies between the subcutaneous external anal sphincter and the internal anal sphincter. This is one of the landmarks for intersphincteric resection. In the middle and low rectal cancer, total mesorectal excision should be performed. For distal rectal cancer, a 1-cm distal margin may be acceptable. To avoid positive circumferential resection margin, the surgeons should follow the principles of total mesorectal excision and perform en bloc resection of contiguous tissues when clinically indicated.

Keywords

Anatomy · Rectum · Anal canal · Peritoneal reflection · Anal sphincter complex · Resection margin

6.1 Introduction

Treatment of patients with low-lying rectal cancer requires achieving the incompatible goals. For oncologic outcomes, wider resection is needed to get safer margin. For functional outcomes, rectal preservation is required to maintain bowel function. Recently, sphincter-saving surgery has been more frequently applied than abdominoperineal resection for the treatment of rectal cancer [1, 2].

To save the sphincter, understanding the anatomy of anal sphincter complex is essential. This anatomy includes anorectal sphincter muscle, pelvic nerve plexus, and perirectal vessels. In addition, colorectal surgeons should be familiar with tumor spreading of rectal cancer and surgical technique for sphincter saving. The purpose of this chapter is to provide a review of the anatomy of rectum and anal sphincter complex and adequate tumor resection margin in sphincter preservation.

J. W. Park · S.-Y. Jeong (✉)
Department of Surgery, Seoul National University College of Medicine, Seoul, South Korea

Colorectal Cancer Center, Seoul National University Cancer Hospital, Seoul, South Korea

Cancer Research Institute,
Seoul National University, Seoul, South Korea
e-mail: syjeong@snu.ac.kr

6.2   Anatomy

6.2.1   Rectum

The large intestine is consisted of the colon and rectum. The rectum is the distal part of the large bowel, not covered by the peritoneum. The definition of the rectum is varied. Anatomists defined the rectum as the bowel between the third sacral vertebra S3 and dentate line. Surgeons usually consider the rectum as the bowel between the sacral promontory and anal verge. However, these definitions cannot be precisely applied before surgery. Practically, the distance from the anal verge, measured by the rigid scope, has been widely used. Based on the results of local recurrence, the National Cancer Institute Rectal Cancer Focus Group suggested 12 cm from the anal verge for the definition of the rectum [3]. The proximal tumor above 12 cm from the anal verge behaves like sigmoid colon cancer in terms of recurrence pattern and prognosis.

6.2.2   Peritoneal Reflection

Another anatomical landmark for the rectum is the peritoneal reflection. The peritoneal reflection can be used for application of transanal endoscopic microsurgery. If the tumor is located above the peritoneal reflection, free perforation can occur with the opening of peritoneum during transanal endoscopic microsurgery. The rectum below the peritoneal reflection has a distinctive lateral lymphatic and hematogenous drainage system, compared with intraperitoneal rectum. Extraperitoneal rectum is invested with the adjacent pelvic wall, which could be the foci of recurrences. Survival rate can be poorer in the tumor below the peritoneal reflection than in the tumor above the peritoneal reflection [4]. Yun et al. investigated the location of the peritoneal reflection in Korean live human [5]. The distance of the peritoneal reflection was about 8–14 cm from the anal verge. The taeniae coli have coalesced into outer longitudinal muscle below the peritoneal reflection.

The rectum contains typically left superior, right middle, and left inferior folds, created by submucosal curves called the valves of Houston. The folds are located at approximately 4–5 cm, 6–8 cm, and 9–10 cm from the anal verge, respectively. The peritoneal reflection is located at the level of the second valve of Houston.

6.2.3   Anal Sphincter Complex

The anal canal extends from the level of the levator ani muscle to the anal verge. The length of the anal canal is approximately 2.5–4 cm. The muscularis propria of the rectum is consisted of the inner circular and outer longitudinal smooth muscle layer (Fig. 6.1). The inner circular smooth muscle layer of the rectum continues as the internal anal sphincter. The outer longitudinal muscle conjoins with fibers from the levator ani muscle. Surrounded by the levator ani muscle, the anal canal passes through the pelvic diaphragm. The levator ani is formed by the pubococcygeus, puborectalis, and iliococcygeus. The outer layer of anal sphincter complex is formed by the puborectalis muscle superiorly and the external anal sphincter inferiorly. The puborectalis muscle and the upper part of the internal sphincter form the anorectal ring. This ring can be palpated and should be identified and saved during surgery since injury of this ring can produce incontinence. The external sphincter has three separate parts: subcutaneous, superficial, and deep part (Figs. 6.1 and 6.2). These three parts together can maintain anal continence. The subcutaneous external anal sphincter attaches to the perianal skin anteriorly, encircling the anus. The superficial external anal sphincter continues with the anococcygeal ligament and surrounds the anus canal. The deep external anal sphincter also surrounds the anus canal without attachments. The internal anal sphincter is under control of the autonomic nervous system. However, the external anal sphincter is under voluntary control. The external anal sphincter has a high resting tone, which can be influenced by voluntary efforts. Intersphincteric groove lies between the subcutaneous external anal sphincter and the internal anal sphincter. This is one of the landmarks for intersphincteric resection.

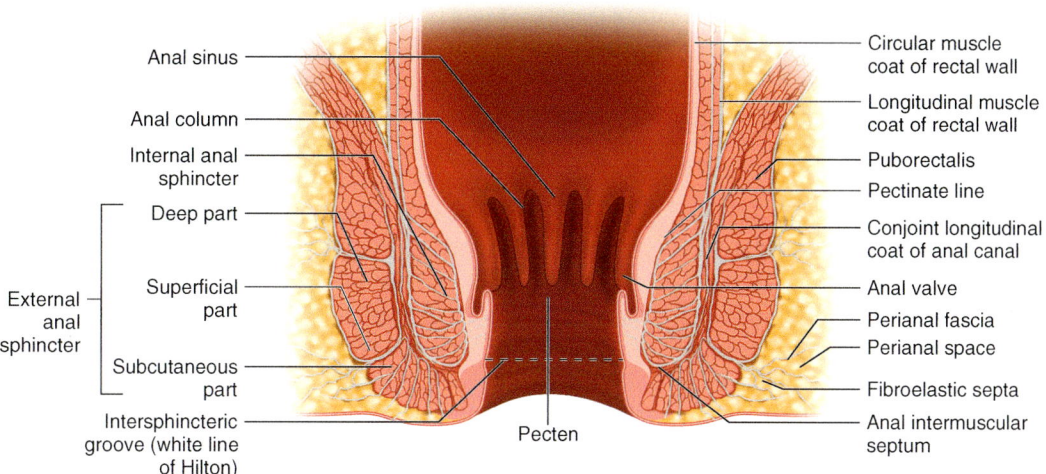

Fig. 6.1 Anal sphincter muscle

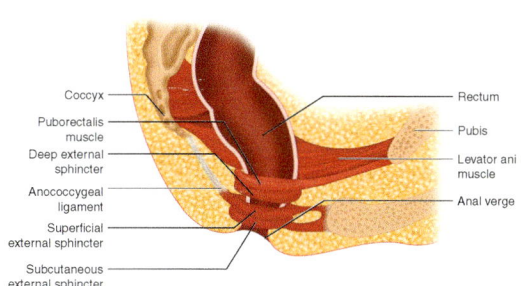

Fig. 6.2 Extrinsic muscles of the anal canal. (1) Coccyx; (2) pubis; (3) levator ani muscle; (4) puborectalis muscle; (5) deep external sphincter; (6) superficial external sphincter; (7) subcutaneous external sphincter; (8) anococcygeal ligament; (9) anal verge; (10) rectum (By permission of JE Skandalakis, SW Gray, and JR Rowe. Anatomical Complications in General Surgery. New York: McGraw-Hill, 1983)

6.2.4 Epithelium of the Anal Canal

The interior part of the anal canal is formed by three histologic regions. Outside of the anal verge, the cutaneous region is covered by the squamous epithelium of the external anoderm. Above the anal verge to the dentate line, the transitional region is composed of columnar, transitional, or stratified squamous epithelium.

Above the dentate line, the mucosal region contains columnar epithelium. The columns of Morgagni are folds of the mucosa above the dentate line. These columns extend upward from the dentate line to the level of the puborectalis sling. The anal crypts are located between the columns of Morgagni. The dentate line marks the transition between the visceral region above and the somatic region below.

6.2.5 Artery Supply

The superior rectal artery, as the terminal branch of the inferior mesenteric artery, supplies the rectum and the upper anal canal. At the upper rectum, the superior rectal artery bifurcates into two vessels: the larger right branch and the smaller left branch [6]. These branches finally penetrate the muscle layer to reach the submucosa. The middle rectal artery, arising from the internal iliac artery, supplies distal rectum and the middle anal canal. The middle rectal artery reaches the rectal wall in the lateral ligament. In a study with 32 cadaver dissections, the middle rectal artery was observed in only 28.1% as the component of the lateral ligament [7]. The inferior rectal artery, originating from the internal pudendal artery, supplies the distal anal canal and the sphincter muscle. The inferior rectal artery reaches the submucosa and subcutaneous tissue of the anal canal. These terminal branches communicate with the branches of the middle and superior rectal artery through intramural collaterals [8].

6.2.6 Venous Drainage

Blood from the rectum and anal canal drains into either the systemic or portal venous system. The upper and middle portion of the rectum drains into the portal venous system via the superior rectal vein. Blood from the lower portion of the rectum and the anal canal drains into systemic venous system via the middle and inferior rectal vein.

6.2.7 Lymphatic Drainage

Most lymphatic drainage of the rectum and the anal canal follows the pathway of the artery (Fig. 6.3). One lymphatic pathway is superior direction. Mesorectal nodes drain to nodes on the superior rectal artery. They subsequently drain to clustered nodes around the inferior mesenteric artery [9]. This pattern of lymphatic drainage is different from that suggested by Ernest Miles, who had the concept of the lymphatic drainage into nodes above and below the pelvic floor in the rectum. Another lymphatic pathway is lateral direction. The middle and low rectum drains to the iliac nodes along the middle and inferior rectal vessels. For removal of metastatic lymph nodes in this area, lateral pelvic lymph node dissection must be applied. The anal canal below the dentate line drains the inguinal nodes.

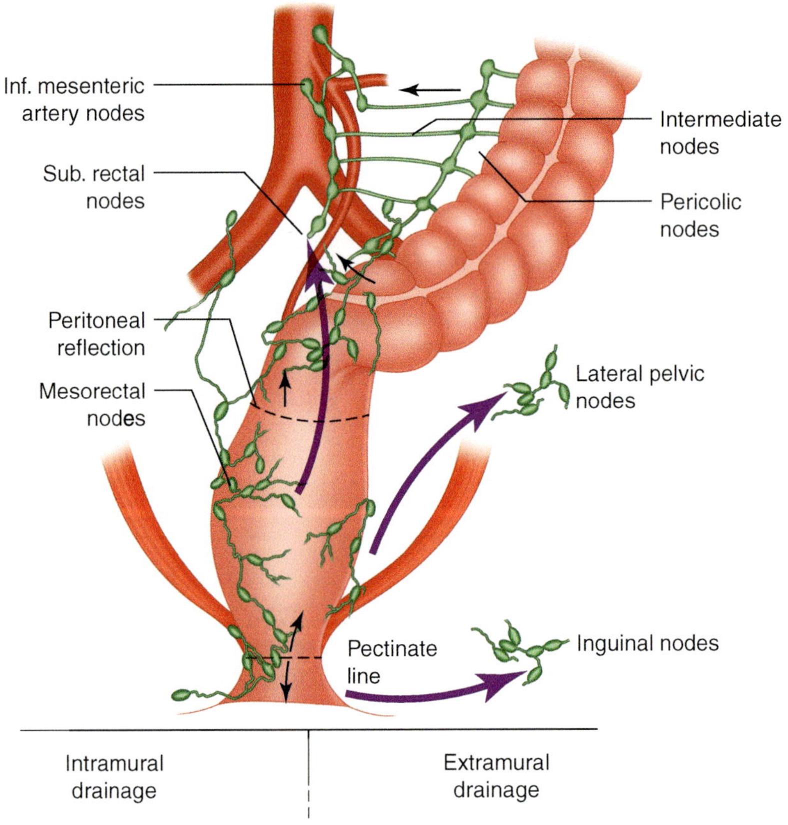

Fig. 6.3 Lymphatic drainage of the rectum and the anal canal. (By permission of JE Skandalakis, SW Gray, and JR Rowe. Anatomical Complications in General Surgery. New York: McGraw-Hill, 1983)

6.2.8 Innervation

The sympathetic supply of the rectum arises from L1, L2, and L3. The parasympathetic supply of the rectum and the anal canal arises from S2, S3, and S4 though sacral foramen. The sympathetic nerve via the hypogastric plexus and the parasympathetic nerve join and form the pelvic plexus at the level of the lower third of the rectum, around the lateral ligament. The pelvic plexus regulates sexual and urinary function. Injury of the pelvic plexus during rectal dissection can induce impotence, ejaculatory dysfunction, and bladder paresis [10, 11] (Fig. 6.4).

Lumbar sympathetic nerves (L5) that cause contraction and sacral parasympathetic nerves (S2, S3, and S4) that inhibit contraction supply motor innervation of the internal anal sphincter via the pelvic plexus ganglia. The external anal sphincter is innervated by the rectal branch of the pudendal nerve (S2 and S3) and by the perineal branch of S4. The puborectalis muscle is innervated by the pudendal nerve. Sensation of the anal canal comes from the inferior rectal branch of the pudendal nerve. This sensation has a key role to maintain anal continence through detecting rectal fullness and discriminating the compound of rectal content. Nerve supply in the anal canal is extensive below the dentate line.

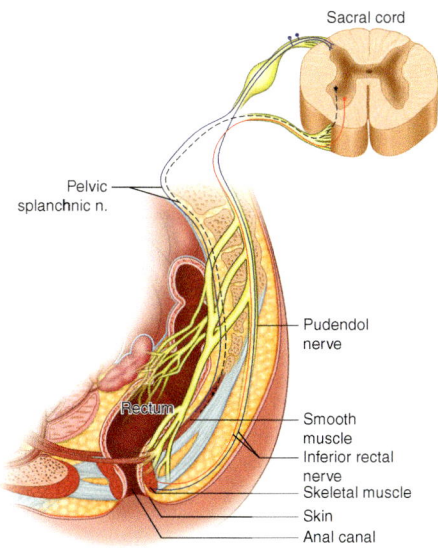

Fig. 6.4 Innervation of the rectum and the anal canal (motor fibers are shown in red, parasympathetic fibers as interrupted lines, and sensory fibers in blue. The fibers in the pelvic splanchnic nerves reach the intestine by way of plexuses)

6.3 Tumor Margin in Rectal Cancer

6.3.1 Distal Resection Margin

Several histologic studies found that tumor spread in the distal mesorectum, as the extramural spread, was up to 5 cm beyond the lower margin of the tumor [12]. In the upper rectal cancer, distal resection with 5-cm margin can be oncologically safe instead of total resection of mesorectum. In the middle and low rectal cancer, total mesorectal excision should be performed.

Because the amount of mesorectum diminishes close to the pelvic floor, intramural spread should be considered than extramural spread for distal resection of low rectal cancer. According to the length of intramural spread, adequate distal resection can be determined in low rectal cancer. In non-irradiated tumor, distal intramural spread of tumor rarely exceeds 1.5 cm [13, 14]. A 2-cm distal margin may be adequate because of not being compromised by shorter distal margins [14–17]. In early stage, distal spread is rarely found beyond 1 cm. In patients with preoperative chemoradiotherapy, distal intramural spread is limited to less than 1 cm [18]. Currently, preoperative radiotherapy is recommended for locally advanced middle or low rectal cancer. Therefore, a 1-cm distal margin may be acceptable for distal rectal cancer [17, 19].

6.3.2 Circumferential Resection Margin

Circumferential resection margin (CRM) is one of the main prognostic factors in rectal cancer. CRM positivity is associated with high local recurrence and poor survival [20]. In well-performed total mesorectal excision, the rate of

CRM involvement is less than 10% [21, 22]. The definition of CRM involvement has an ongoing debate. Most studies used ≤1 mm as the CRM positive. On the base of local recurrence, 2 mm has also been used as a cutoff value [23]. In patients with preoperative chemoradiotherapy, CRM was a prognostic factor for both local recurrence and survival [24]. To avoid positive CRM, the surgeons should follow the principles of TME and perform en bloc resection of contiguous tissues when clinically indicated.

References

1. Park SJ, Lee KY, Lee SH. Laparoscopic surgery for colorectal cancer in Korea: Nationwide data from 2008~2013. J Minim Invasive Surg. 2015;18(2): 39–43.
2. Warschkow R, Ebinger SM, Brunner W, Schmied BM, Marti L. Survival after abdominoperineal and sphincter-preserving resection in nonmetastatic rectal cancer: a population-based time-trend and propensity score-matched SEER analysis. Gastroenterol Res Pract. 2017;2017:6058907.
3. Nelson H, Petrelli N, Carlin A, Couture J, Fleshman J, Guillem J, et al. Guidelines 2000 for colon and rectal cancer surgery. J Natl Cancer Inst. 2001;93(8):583–96.
4. Hwang MR, Park JW, Kim DY, Chang HJ, Hong YS, Kim SY, et al. Prognostic impact of peritonealisation in rectal cancer treated with preoperative chemoradiotherapy: extraperitoneal versus intraperitoneal rectal cancer. Radiother Oncol. 2010;94(3):353–8.
5. Yun HR, Chun HK, Lee WS, Cho YB, Yun SH, Lee WY. Intra-operative measurement of surgical lengths of the rectum and the peritoneal reflection in Korean. J Korean Med Sci. 2008;23(6):999–1004.
6. Goligher JC. In: Duthie HL, Nixon HH, editors. Surgery of the anus, rectum and colon, vol. x. 2nd ed. London: Baillière; 1967. p. 1110.
7. Lin M, Chen W, Huang L, Ni J, Yin L. The anatomy of lateral ligament of the rectum and its role in total mesorectal excision. World J Surg. 2010;34(3):594–8.
8. Vogel P, Klosterhalfen B. The surgical anatomy of the rectal and anal blood vessels. Langenbecks Arch Chir. 1988;373(5):264–9.
9. Heald RJ, Moran BJ. Embryology and anatomy of the rectum. Semin Surg Oncol. 1998;15(2):66–71.
10. Beck DE, Wexner SD. Fundamentals of anorectal surgery, vol. xiii. New York: Health Professions Division, McGraw-Hill; 1992. p. 509.
11. Gerstenberg TC, Nielsen ML, Clausen S, Blaabjerg J, Lindenberg J. Bladder function after abdominoperineal resection of the rectum for anorectal cancer. Urodynamic investigation before and after operative in a consecutive series. Ann Surg. 1980;191(1):81–6.
12. Lopez-Kostner F, Lavery IC, Hool GR, Rybicki LA, Fazio VW. Total mesorectal excision is not necessary for cancers of the upper rectum. Surgery. 1998;124(4):612–7. discussion 7-8
13. Lazorthes F, Voigt JJ, Roques J, Chiotasso P, Chevreau P. Distal intramural spread of carcinoma of the rectum correlated with lymph nodal involvement. Surg Gynecol Obstet. 1990;170(1):45–8.
14. Shirouzu K, Isomoto H, Kakegawa T. Distal spread of rectal cancer and optimal distal margin of resection for sphincter-preserving surgery. Cancer. 1995;76(3): 388–92.
15. Williams NS, Dixon MF, Johnston D. Reappraisal of the 5 centimetre rule of distal excision for carcinoma of the rectum: a study of distal intramural spread and of patients' survival. Br J Surg. 1983;70(3):150–4.
16. Kwok SP, Lau WY, Leung KL, Liew CT, Li AK. Prospective analysis of the distal margin of clearance in anterior resection for rectal carcinoma. Br J Surg. 1996;83(7):969–72.
17. Andreola S, Leo E, Belli F, Lavarino C, Bufalino R, Tomasic G, et al. Distal intramural spread in adenocarcinoma of the lower third of the rectum treated with total rectal resection and coloanal anastomosis. Dis Colon Rectum. 1997;40(1):25–9.
18. Moore HG, Riedel E, Minsky BD, Saltz L, Paty P, Wong D, et al. Adequacy of 1-cm distal margin after restorative rectal cancer resection with sharp mesorectal excision and preoperative combined-modality therapy. Ann Surg Oncol. 2003;10(1):80–5.
19. Vernava AM 3rd, Moran M, Rothenberger DA, Wong WD. A prospective evaluation of distal margins in carcinoma of the rectum. Surg Gynecol Obstet. 1992; 175(4):333–6.
20. Nagtegaal ID, Quirke P. What is the role for the circumferential margin in the modern treatment of rectal cancer? J Clin Oncol. 2008;26(2):303–12.
21. Nagtegaal ID, van de Velde CJ, van der Worp E, Kapiteijn E, Quirke P, van Krieken JH, et al. Macroscopic evaluation of rectal cancer resection specimen: clinical significance of the pathologist in quality control. J Clin Oncol. 2002;20(7):1729–34.
22. Quirke P, Steele R, Monson J, Grieve R, Khanna S, Couture J, et al. Effect of the plane of surgery achieved on local recurrence in patients with operable rectal cancer: a prospective study using data from the MRC CR07 and NCIC-CTG CO16 randomised clinical trial. Lancet. 2009;373(9666):821–8.
23. Nagtegaal ID, Marijnen CA, Kranenbarg EK, van de Velde CJ, van Krieken JH, Pathology Review Committee, et al. Circumferential margin involvement is still an important predictor of local recurrence in rectal carcinoma: not one millimeter but two millimeters is the limit. Am J Surg Pathol. 2002;26(3):350–7.
24. Hwang MR, Park JW, Park S, Yoon H, Kim DY, Chang HJ, et al. Prognostic impact of circumferential resection margin in rectal cancer treated with preoperative chemoradiotherapy. Ann Surg Oncol. 2014;21(4):1345–51.

Part III

Optimized Treatment for Locally Advanced Rectal Cancer

Risk Factors for Recurrence and Tumor Response Evaluation After Neoadjuvant Therapy-Based Radiological Study

7

Joon Seok Lim, Honsoul Kim, and Nieun Seo

Abstract

This chapter describes pretreatment MR imaging features to enable the risk stratification for selecting high-risk rectal cancer patients. These features include mrCRM (mr-circumferential resection margin), extramural tumor spread, clinical nodal status, extramural vessel invasion, low positioning of cancer, and lateral pelvic lymph node metastases. Tumor response evaluation on MR imaging after neoadjuvant treatment is also described in terms of MR volumetry, MR tumor regression grade (mrTRG), and diffusion-weighted imaging.

Keywords

Rectal cancer · Risk stratification · MRI · Tumor response evaluation

7.1 Introduction

The main imaging modality for local staging of rectal cancer is magnetic resonance imaging (MRI), as it defines the tumor and relevant anatomy providing the most detail on the important prognostic factors that influence treatment choice. The preoperative prognostic stratification based on MR imaging enables patient selection according to risk of both local and systemic tumor recurrence. This stratification is very important for managing rectal cancer, avoiding the morbidity associated potential overtreatment and allowing aggressive treatment for high-risk patients. These high-risk patients should undergo neoadjuvant therapy before total mesorectal excision. This chapter describes MR imaging features to enable the stratification. These features include mrCRM (mr-circumferential resection margin), extramural tumor spread, clinical nodal status, extramural vessel invasion, low positioning of cancer, and lateral pelvic lymph node metastases.

7.2 High-Risk Factors on MRI Findings

7.2.1 mrCRM

The circumferential resection margin (CRM) is a powerful prognostic factor for rectal cancer patients. Many studies have established that pathologic CRM (pCRM) is important not only for local recurrence but also for the distant metastasis and patient survival [1]. As the pCRM is obtained after surgical resection, preoperative assessment of CRM involvement is critical for selecting patients for preoperative intensive treatment and predicting patient prognosis.

J. S. Lim (✉) · H. Kim · N. Seo
Department of Radiology, Yonsei Cancer Center,
Yonsei University College of Medicine,
Seoul, South Korea
e-mail: JSLIM1@yuhs.ac

© Springer Nature Singapore Pte Ltd. 2018
N. K. Kim et al. (eds.), *Surgical Treatment of Colorectal Cancer*,
https://doi.org/10.1007/978-981-10-5143-2_7

Among various preoperative imaging modalities, magnetic resonance imaging (MRI) is the most widely accepted preoperative imaging in rectal cancer. High-resolution MRI can accurately delineate the local tumor extent and its relation to the mesorectal fascia [2, 3]. As with pCRM, a positive CRM on MRI (mrCRM) is defined as tumor within 1 mm from the mesorectal fascia [4]. For lower-third rectal tumors, mrCRM involvement is regarded as tumor within 1 mm of the levator muscle [5]. CRM can be positive due to tumor deposits, extramural vascular invasion, or suspicious metastatic lymph nodes as well as main tumor extension [4]. As the mesorectal fat in the anterior direction can be relatively thinner than that in other directions, the rectum can be close to anterior CRM. To discuss anterior CRM involvement, the tumor should be at least a T3 tumor [4].

MRI can predict pCRM with a high degree of certainty [2, 6]. According to a systematic review and meta-analysis, the mean sensitivity and specificity of MRI for predicting CRM were 76.3% and 85.9%, respectively [2]. Both pCRM and mrCRM are significant predictors for local tumor recurrence [5, 7] (Fig. 7.1). According to a previous study by MERCURY study group, involvement of mrCRM is also significantly associated with distant metastatic disease [7]. Furthermore, preoperative assessment of CRM on MRI is superior to preoperative American Joint Committee on Cancer (AJCC) TNM-based criteria for predicting risk of local recurrence, disease-free survival, and overall survival [7]. Another study by the same group assessed MRI after neoadjuvant therapy for rectal cancer [5]. In this study, preoperative mrCRM independently predicted local recurrence, whereas MRI-assessed tumor regression grade (TRG) was significant factor for overall survival and disease-free survival [5].

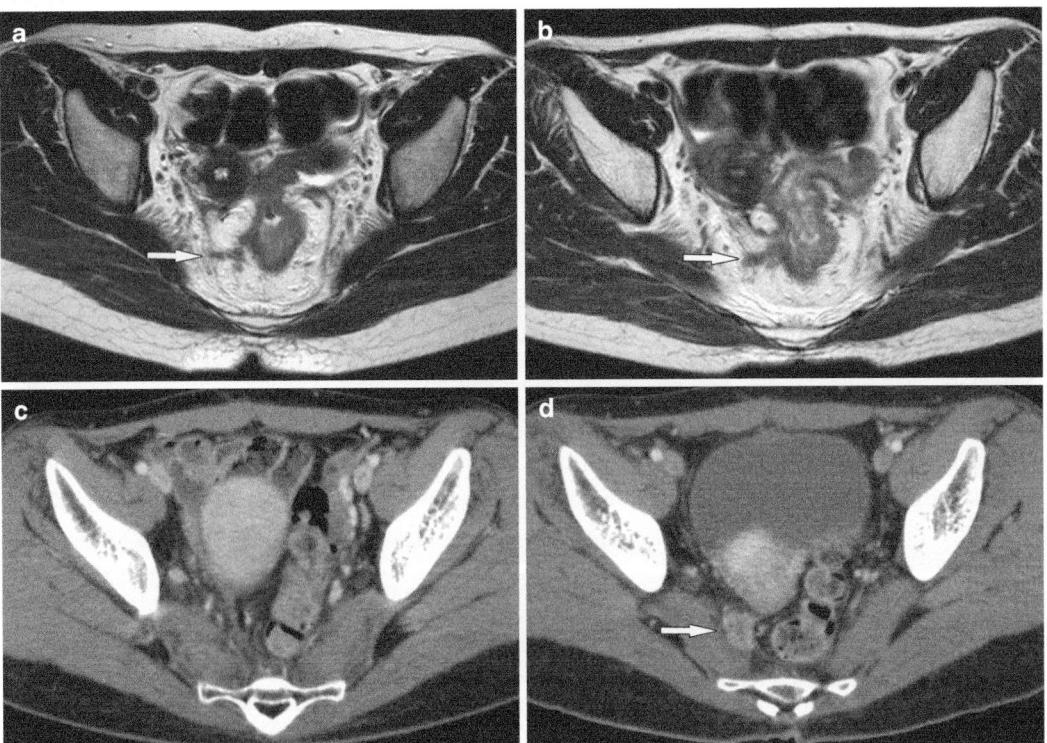

Fig. 7.1 Axial T2-weighted MR images of a 28-year-old woman with rectal cancer obtained before (**a**) and after (**b**) neoadjuvant chemoradiotherapy showed persistent mesorectal fascial involvement (arrows) at 9 o'clock by tumor extension. (**c**) A portal phase axial CT image obtained a year after surgery demonstrated no local tumor recurrence. (**d**) However, a portal phase axial CT image taken 2 years after surgery revealed enhancing soft tissue lesion in right pelvic wall (arrow), suggestive of local recurrence

7.2.2 Extramural Tumor Spread

Tumor staging using T component of TNM system is a traditional method for stratification of patient prognosis, but T staging has limitations in rectal cancer. The major limitation of T staging is that T3 tumors which account for the majority of rectal cancers at the time of presentation have heterogeneous clinical outcome according to the depth of extramural tumor spread [8]. In a previous histopathologic study published by a University of Erlangen group, T3 tumors with extramural spread of more than 5 mm have a cancer-specific 5-year survival rate of 54%. On the other hand, for T3 tumors with extramural tumor spread of 5 mm or less, the cancer-specific survival rate was greater than 85% [9]. Therefore, the depth of extramural spread is an essential factor in determining patient prognosis [4].

In this context, preoperative stratification of T3 tumors on the radiological study is important for optimal selection of patients who may benefit from preoperative therapy. The Union for International Cancer Control (UICC) criteria have been widely used for subclassification of T3 rectal cancer (T3a, <1 mm; T3b, 1–5 mm; T3c, >5–15 mm; and T3d, >15 mm) [10] (Fig. 7.2). Other criteria by the Radiologic Society of North America (RSNA)

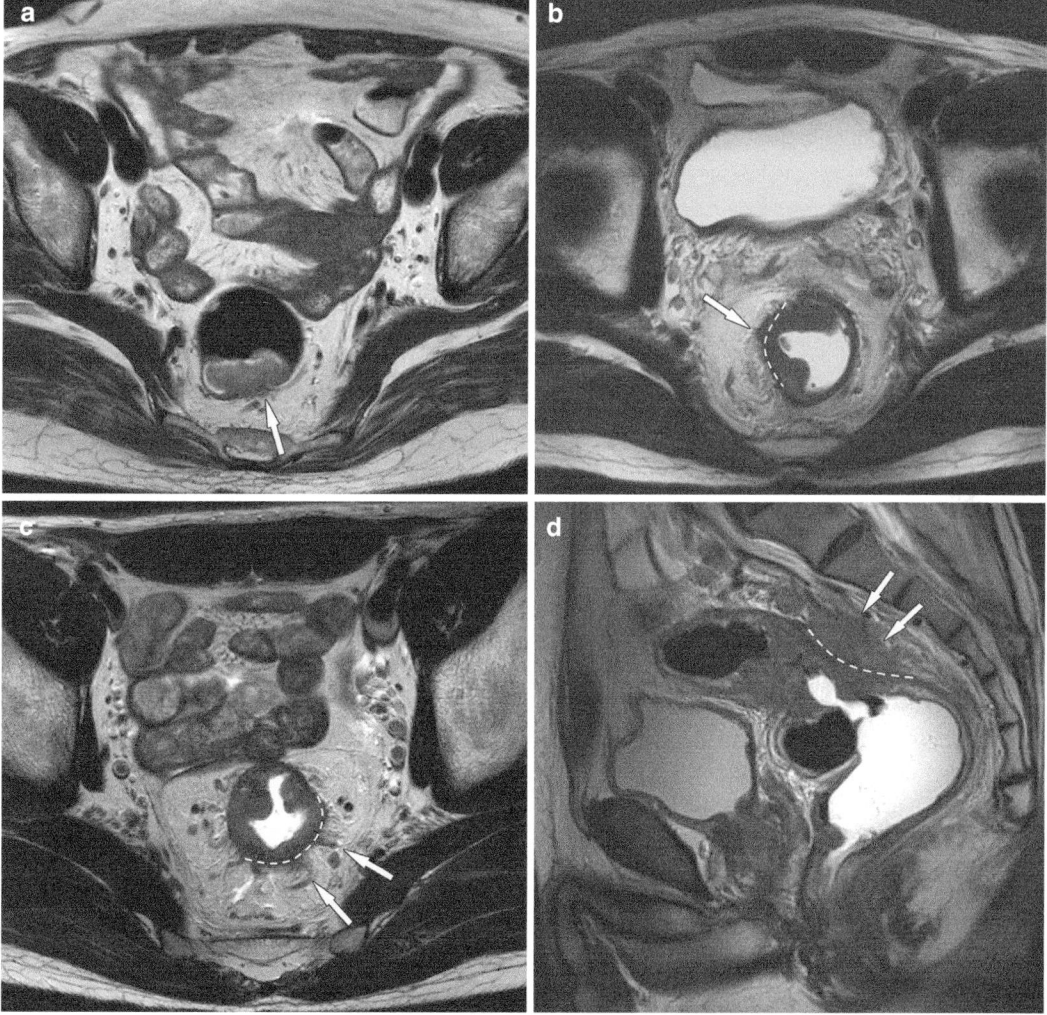

Fig. 7.2 Axial (**a–c**) and sagittal (**d**) T2-weighted MR images of subclassification of T3 tumor extramural spread by the Union for International Cancer Control (UICC) criteria. (**a**) T3a (<1 mm), (**b**) T3b (1–5 mm), (**c**) T3c (>5–15 mm), and (**d**) T3d (>15 mm). Arrow = extramural tumor spread, dashed line = expected border of the muscularis propria

stratified extramural depth of tumor invasion into three groups (T3a, <5 mm; T3b, 5–10 mm; and T3c, >10 mm) [11]. MRI is known to be accurate for stratifying T3 tumors compared with histopathologic extramural tumor spread [8, 12]. In addition, MRI assessment of extramural tumor spread using either UICC criteria or RSNA proposal is significantly associated with patient survival [12, 13]. In particular, the cutoff extramural tumor spread of 5 mm is radiologically reliable and clinically meaningful criteria for predicting prognosis and selecting optimal treatment strategy.

7.2.3 Clinical Nodal Status

Nodal staging in rectal cancer is important because the number of lymph node metastases is associated with prognosis. Nodal involvement on MRI has traditionally determined with size criteria. However, there is substantial overlap in size between normal, reactive, and metastatic lymph nodes [4, 14]. Moreover, micrometastasis is not rare in normal-sized lymph nodes. Therefore, size-based criteria do not seem to be a reliable method to assess lymph node metastasis in rectal cancer. Instead, criteria based on the shape, border, and signal intensity of lymph nodes have been shown to be more reliable [14, 15]. According to these criteria, suspicious lymph nodes are defined as lymph nodes with irregular, spiculated, or indistinct borders or mixed heterogeneous signal intensity [14, 15] (Fig. 7.3). By using these criteria, some investigators argued that the diagnostic accuracy of MRI to determine lymph node metastasis is up to 85% [14, 15]. Recently, the relative unimportance of nodal status in predicting the local recurrence has been highlighted because lymph node status is less influential than other poor prognostic factors in total mesorectal excision era. Some investigators insisted that preoperative nodal status may not be an independent risk factor for local recurrence because MRI does not have sufficient diagnostic nodal accuracy and even pathologic N1 disease does not show any difference compared with node positive patients in term of local recurrence, if good quality of TME is performed [16, 17].

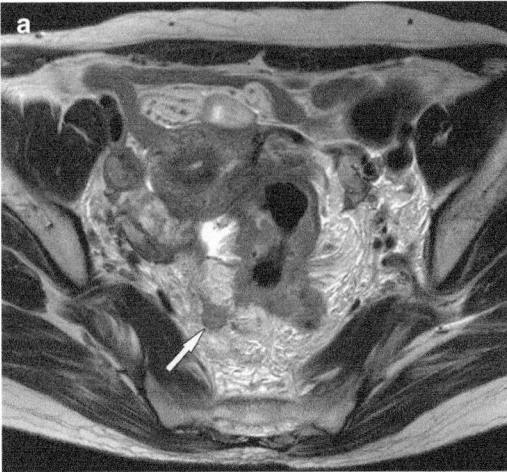

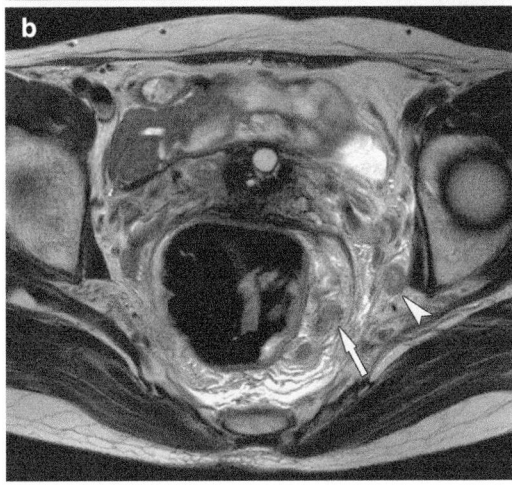

Fig. 7.3 Axial T2-weighted MR images at the level of upper (**a**) and middle (**b**) portion of the rectum. (**a**) A lymph node with spiculated and irregular borders (arrow) is noted at the right lateral aspect of mesorectum, which suggests metastasis. (**b**) Several lymph nodes in indistinct borders and mixed signal intensity are located in left side of mesorectum (arrow) and left pelvic side wall (arrowhead), which suggest metastases

7.2.4 Extramural Vessel Invasion

Extramural vessel invasion (EMVI) is defined as the presence of tumor cells within blood vessels beyond the muscularis propria nearby the primary malignancy and is more frequently observed in locally advanced lesions [18]. Histological EMVI is related to poor prognosis, high local recurrence, and distant metastasis [19]. Similarly, EMVI detected on preoperative MRI is known as a risk factor associated with a higher risk of pathological CRM involvement as well as increased tumor relapse after treatment [20–23].

To document a positive EMVI on MRI, it is important to identify the presence of an intravascular tumor component showing intermediate signal intensity [19]. The lesion may be associated with an irregular contour and/or nodular expansion (Fig. 7.4) in more obvious cases but could also merely demonstrate slight vascular expansion. Meanwhile, findings such as minimal extramural stranding or nodular extension that is apart from a vascular structure usually are not considered to represent EMVI [18]. EMVI should be recognized as a potential source of malignant embolic shower-promoting systemic metastasis, and it has been reported that the presence of EMVI revealed on preoperative MRI is an independent risk factor for promoting distant metastasis, especially when identified in larger vessels (≥3 mm) [18, 24].

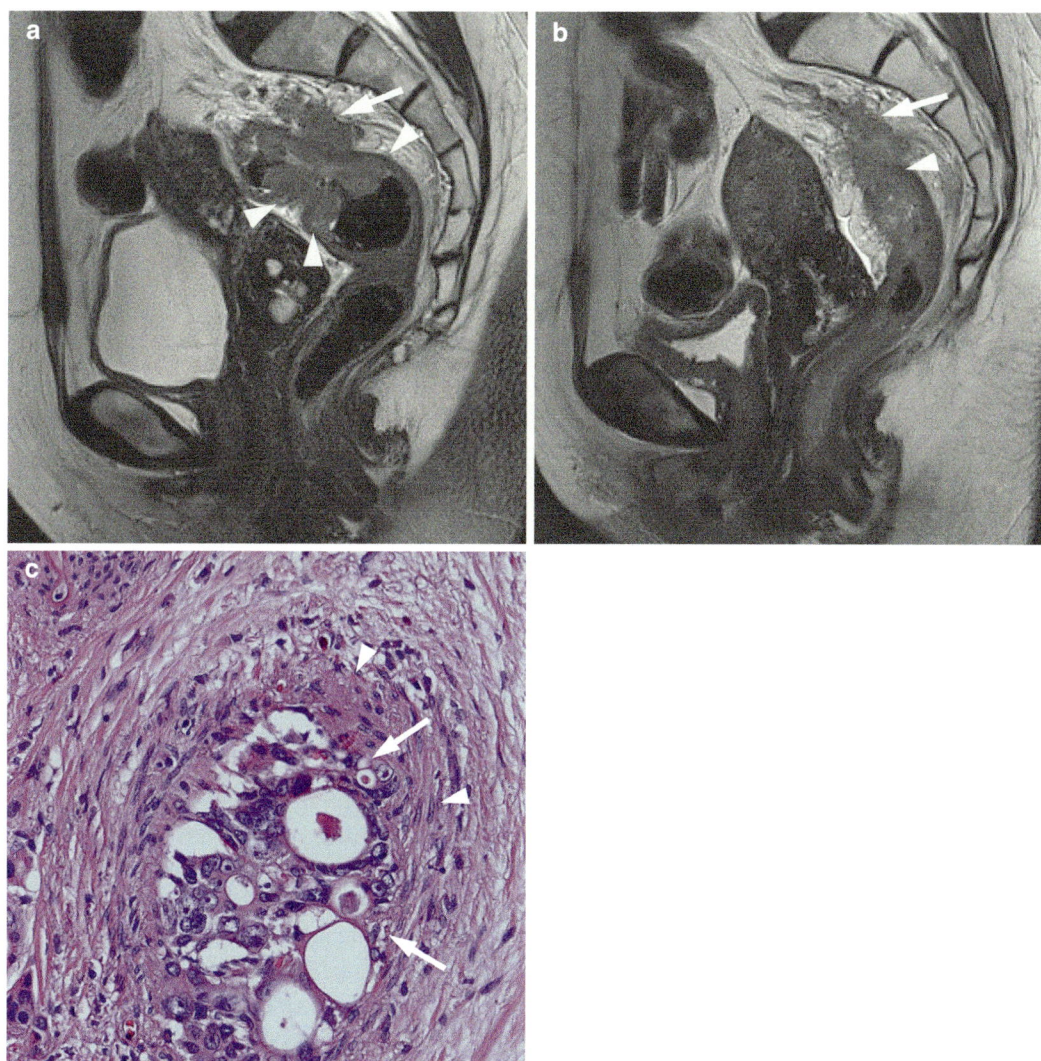

Fig. 7.4 (**a**) Pre-CCRT and (**b**) post-CCRT T2-weighed sagittal MR image of a 52-year-old woman with rectal cancer demonstrating the main mass (arrowhead) and adjacent extramural vessel invasion (arrow). (**c**) Microscopic examination of the surgical specimen (hematoxylin-eosin stain, X 40) revealed a vessel (arrowhead) containing tumor cells (arrows) documenting the presence of extramural vessel invasion

7.2.5 Low Positioning of Tumoral Distal Margin

Lower rectal cancer (defined as adenocarcinoma less than 6 cm from the anal verge) is known to have a significantly worse prognosis when compared with those of mid and upper rectal cancers [25]. The mesorectal fascia tapers below the origin of the levator muscles at the far distal rectal area, and consequently there is no mesorectum which serves as a protective barrier to contain tumor spread below the level of puborectalis sling [4, 26]. It has been reported that lower rectal cancers located at this level are associated with higher rate of pathological CRM involvement and poor oncological outcome [3, 23, 27, 28]. In similar lines, the overall risk of pathological CRM involvement has been reported to increase if the lower rectal cancer invades the anterior quadrant, probably because relatively less volume is removed anteriorly than in other quadrants even if extra-levator abdominoperineal excision is conducted [23].

Conventionally low rectal cancers are treated by abdominoperineal resection. Because of the oncologic rule of a 1-cm distal resection margin, lower rectal cancers that are at least 1 cm apart from the puborectal junction are considered suitable for classical sphincter preservation surgery [29, 30]. As result, whether or not lower rectal cancers extend within 1 cm distance from the anorectal junction has substantial significance and in order to accomplish successful resection of a cancer at this area both the mesorectal fascia plane and the intersphincteric plane must be clear of tumor. The MERCURY II study has prospectively validated that MRI can reliably evaluate the extent of lower rectal cancer invasion in regard with the lower rectal plane (Fig. 7.5) and therefore predict the risk of pathological CRM involvement, of which information aids to select the correct plane of surgery and guide the proper selection of preoperative therapy [23].

7.2.6 Lateral Pelvic LN Metastases

Rectal cancer patients of whom the lower margin extends at or below the peritoneal reflection occa-

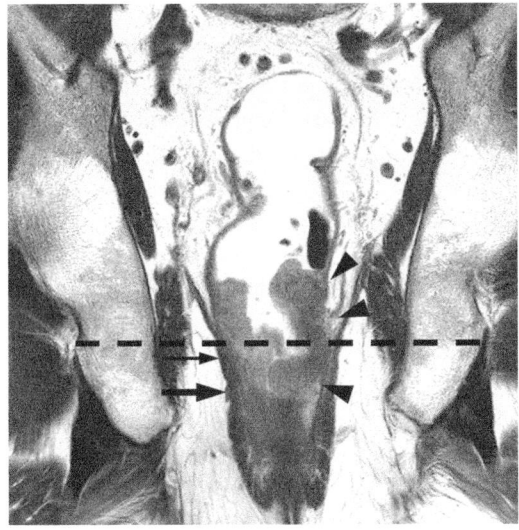

Fig. 7.5 T2-weighed oblique coronal MR image of a 63-year-old male with rectal cancer (arrowheads) extending below the imaginary line (dotted line) 1 cm above the puborectalis muscle (large arrow) and directly invading the right levator ani muscle (small arrow). The patient underwent CCRT and curative resection; however positive pathologic CRM was reported

sionally develop metastasis at the lateral pelvic LNs (common iliac, internal iliac, external iliac, and obturator nodes) which are located outside the surgical field of TME [31]. A retrospective study in Japan reported that T3 or T4 lower rectal cancer patients developed lateral pelvic LN metastasis in 18.1% [32].

Ongoing debate exists on the optimal strategy to treat a potential, but not obvious lateral pelvic LN metastasis. One study reported the incidence of local tumor recurrence in patients who had undergone TME or ME with lateral LN dissection (LLND) to be similar with those who had undergone TME or ME alone without adjuvant radiotherapy [33]. Meanwhile, a recent multicenter randomized controlled trial combining LLND in addition to ME in rectal cancer patients located below the peritoneal reflection of whom lacked clinical evidence of enlarged lateral pelvic LN reported a reduced incidence of local tumor recurrence (especially in the lateral pelvis): the incidence of local recurrence were 7% and 13% in the ME with LLND and ME alone groups, respectively [31]. However, when preoperative radiological studies demon-

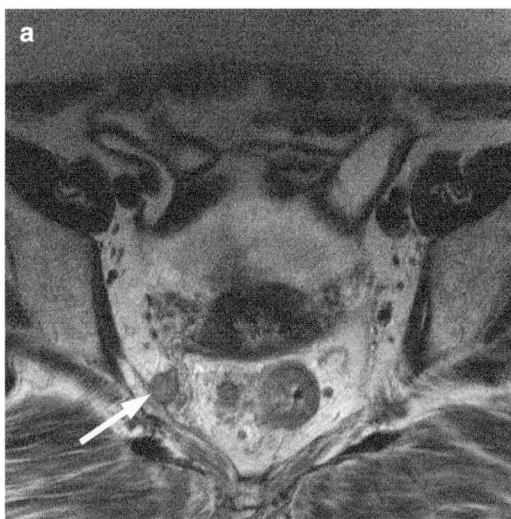

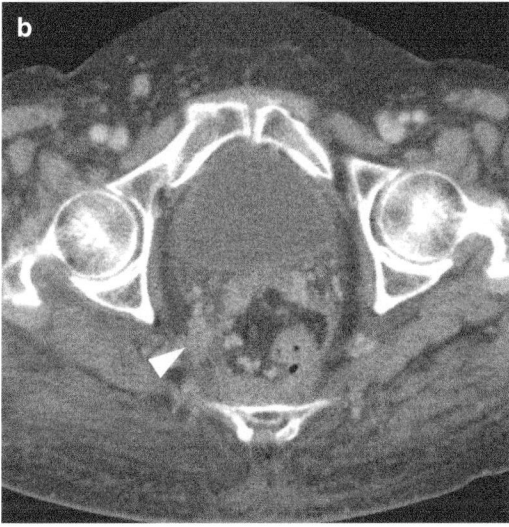

Fig. 7.6 A 73-year-old female patient with rectal cancer who underwent curative resection and lateral pelvic LN dissection. (**a**) The preoperative T2-weighed oblique axial MR image revealed an enlarged lymph node (arrow) of which the short diameter measured 1 cm along the right internal iliac chain, highly suggestive of nodal metastasis. (**b**) The occurrence of right pelvic tumor recurrence (arrowhead) was detected by CT 7 months after surgery

strated a lateral pelvic LN (Fig. 7.6), the size of the LN positively correlated with the risk for lateral pelvic tumor recurrence after preoperative CCRT and curative resection [34]. Collectively, lateral pelvic LN metastasis is a valid risk factor influencing the clinical outcome that should be considered while establishing the treatment strategies. A few studies have suggested that radiological assessment

of the lateral pelvic LN is relatively reliable and that if lateral pelvic LN is not detected on CT or MRI, then lateral pelvic LN metastasis is a relatively uncommon event to occur [35–37]. However, in general, imaging studies are considered not reliable in predicting the absence of nodal metastasis, and therefore further evidence on the diagnostic performance of radiological studies in regard with lateral pelvic LN assessment seems necessary.

7.3 Tumor Response Evaluation After Neoadjuvant Therapy

Preoperative concurrent chemotherapy and radiation therapy (CRT) results in a decreased rate of local recurrence and in preservation of the anal sphincter. As a result, CCRT is widely used in the treatment of rectal cancer (1). Pre-CRT MR imaging has undeniable role for selecting high-risk patients for the neoadjuvant treatment. However, post-CRT MR imaging has controversial role for a change in the surgical plan and prediction of the prognosis. This debate has been caused by the low accuracy of post-CRT MRI in diagnosing CRM status and pathologic TN status. The factors related to these issues include fibrosis, desmoplastic reaction, edema, inflammation, and viable tumor nets at a fibrotic scar from a previous tumor (2). In spite of such difficult situation, post-CRT MRI has been regarded as important tool for predicting prognosis including pathologic complete remission. MR volumetry, MR tumor regression grade (mrTRG), and diffusion-weighted imaging may be helpful in prediction and assessment of tumor response and patients' prognosis. In this section, we will discuss and illustrate post-CRT MR imaging findings after CRT for rectal cancer and the roles of MR volumetry, MR tumor regression grade (mrTRG), and diffusion-weighted imaging.

7.3.1 MR Volumetry

Traditionally assessment of CRT response on post-CRT MR imaging is performed with two-dimensional measurements of orthogonal tumor

Fig. 7.7 A 56-year-old man with locally advanced rectal cancer. The segmentation of the lesion is manually drawn along the tumor margin (green arrow). The 3D volume of the rectal tumor is automatically calculated. The mean tumor volumes were 52.6 cm³ at pre-CRT phase (right column). After CRT, the measured volume is prominently decreased (18.1 cm³) (left column)

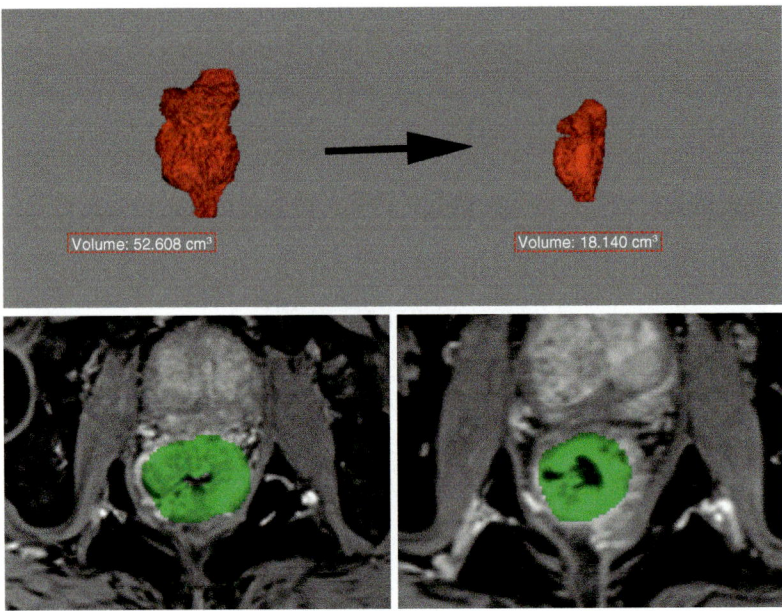

diameters. This measurement may be inaccurate owing to the irregular configuration of the tumor. However, MR volumetry provides three dimensionally reconstructed tumor volume by summing each of the crossly sectional volumes of the entire tumor lesion by using software (Fig. 7.7). It has been reported that higher tumor volume reduction ratios following CRT were significantly associated with a high rate of pathological complete response in patients with rectal cancer. Kang et al. reported that more than 75% of the tumor volume reduction ratios after CRT was completed were significantly associated with a high pathologic complete response rate [38]. Early tumor volume reduction during CRT (second week after CRT initiation) may also be a good indicator for predicting CRT treatment outcome [38]. However, MR volumetry has intrinsic limitation for predicting complete remission and down-staging after CRT, because it does not reflect the microscopic tumor status.

7.3.2 mrTRG

Dworak or Mandard tumor regression systems describe the varying degree of replacement of tumor with fibrous or fibroinflammatory tissue [39, 40]. Improved disease-free survival in patients with complete or partial pathologic tumor regression grades has been known, compared with minimal pathologic tumor regression. MERCURY group suggested an MRI-based tumor regression grading based on the results with pathologic tumor regression grade (G1, complete response, no evidence of treated tumor; G2, good response, dense fibrosis or mucin, no obvious residual tumor; G3, moderate response, significant residual tumor signal but there is >50% fibrosis or mucin; G4, slight response, mainly tumor with small areas of low-intensity fibrosis or mucin; G5, no response, tumor is unchanged from baseline) (Fig. 7.8) [5, 41]. In their study, there was a significant difference in disease-free survival and overall survival between mrTRG 1–3 (good responder) and mrTRG 4/5 (poor responder)); the 5-year DFS was 72% and 27%, respectively. Yu et al. found a similar significant difference in DFS and OS: mrTRG 1/2 (good responder), mrTRG 3 (intermediate responder), and mrTRG 4/5 (poor responder) had a 3-year DFS of 82%, 72%, and 61%, respectively [42]. Therefore, mrTRG is emerging as promising imaging biomarker for stratifying rectal cancer patients with regard to future management. Organ-saving surgery or deferral surgery with intensive follow-up is applying in good responders on mrTRG in several clinical trials.

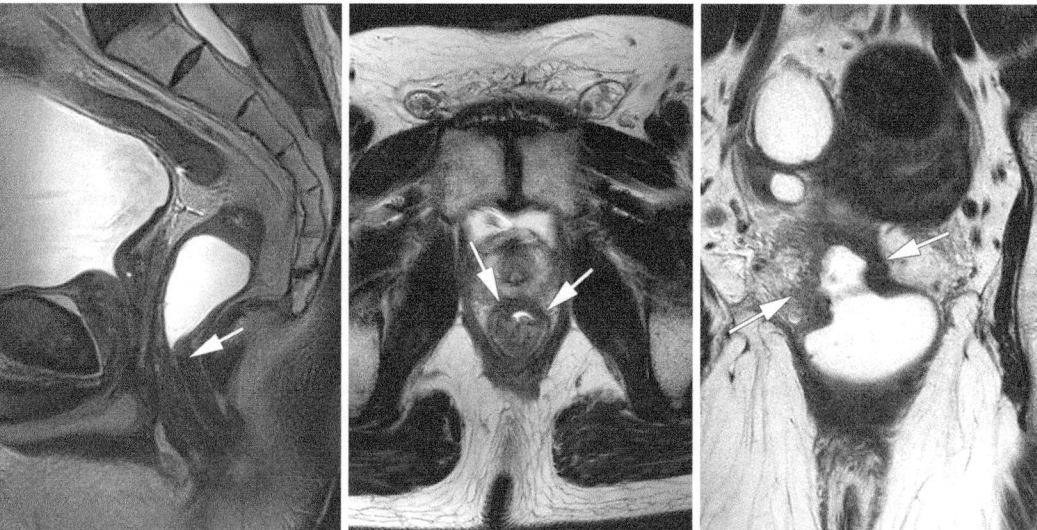

Fig. 7.8 mrTRG. Post-CRT MR image shows mrTRG G1 (right: non-visualization of the treated tumor), G2 (middle: dense fibrotic change only), and G3 (left: tumoral fibrotic low signal intensity portions exceed 50% of overall tumor volume) cases

7.3.3   Diffusion-Weighted Magnetic Resonance Imaging

Diffusion-weighted magnetic resonance imaging (DWI) has shown to be a promising modality to identify good treatment responders after CRT. DWI is based upon the motion of water molecules in intracellular and extracellular spaces. In case of tumors, there is an increased cellular environment and more restriction of water diffusion. Apparent diffusion coefficient (ADC) values are calculated to quantify the diffusion restriction. Low pre-CRT ADC values and a large increase of ADC values after CRT were correlated with pathological good response [43–47] (Fig. 7.9). Park et al. reported that DWI to T2-weighted imaging could improve the prediction of negative CRM after CRT compared with T2-weighted imaging alone [46]. Sun et al. reported that the mean percentage of tumor ADC change in the responder group was significantly higher than that of the non-responder group after 1 and 2 weeks of CRT [47]. However, there is considerable variability in reported ADCs for differentiating responders and non-responders. It is unclear whether these results will be reproducible in other centers. In addition, manually drawing ROIs along the rectal cancer margin for ADC values measurement

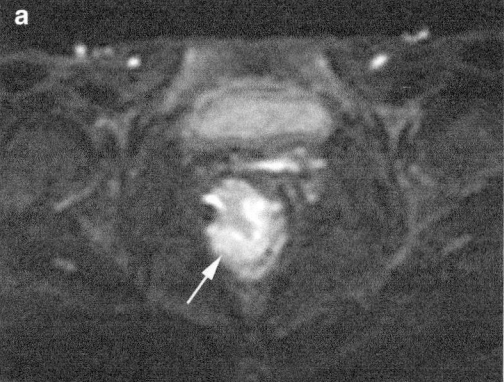

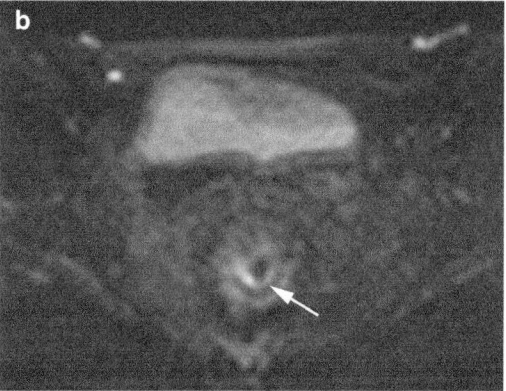

Fig. 7.9 Diffusion-weighted imaging for monitoring tumor response. (**a**) Diffusion-weighted axial image obtained with a b value of 1000 s/mm^2 before CRT shows high-signal-intensity (diffusion restriction) tumoral lesion in the rectum. (**b**) Post-CRT diffusion-weighted image shows near disappearance of the high-signal-intensity lesions in the rectum

may cause inter- or intraobserver variations. Distortion due to imaging artifacts on DWI is not also rare findings, particularly around air-tissue interfaces.

References

1. Nagtegaal ID, Quirke P. What is the role for the circumferential margin in the modern treatment of rectal cancer? J Clin Oncol. 2008;26(2):303–12.

2. van der Paardt MP, Zagers MB, Beets-Tan RG, Stoker J, Bipat S. Patients who undergo preoperative chemoradiotherapy for locally advanced rectal cancer restaged by using diagnostic MR imaging: a systematic review and meta-analysis. Radiology. 2013;269(1):101–12.

3. MERCURY Study Group. Diagnostic accuracy of preoperative magnetic resonance imaging in predicting curative resection of rectal cancer: prospective observational study. BMJ. 2006;333(7572):779.

4. Nougaret S, Reinhold C, Mikhael HW, Rouanet P, Bibeau F, Brown G. The use of MR imaging in treatment planning for patients with rectal carcinoma: have you checked the "DISTANCE". Radiology. 2013;268(2):330–44.

5. Patel UB, Taylor F, Blomqvist L, George C, Evans H, Tekkis P, et al. Magnetic resonance imaging-detected tumor response for locally advanced rectal cancer predicts survival outcomes: MERCURY experience. J Clin Oncol. 2011;29(28):3753–60.

6. Beets-Tan RG, Beets GL, Vliegen RF, Kessels AG, Van Boven H, De Bruine A, et al. Accuracy of magnetic resonance imaging in prediction of tumour-free resection margin in rectal cancer surgery. Lancet. 2001;357(9255):497–504.

7. Taylor FG, Quirke P, Heald RJ, Moran BJ, Blomqvist L, Swift IR, et al. Preoperative magnetic resonance imaging assessment of circumferential resection margin predicts disease-free survival and local recurrence: 5-year follow-up results of the MERCURY study. J Clin Oncol. 2014;32(1):34–43.

8. MERCURY Study Group. Extramural depth of tumor invasion at thin-section MR in patients with rectal cancer: results of the MERCURY study. Radiology. 2007;243(1):132–9.

9. Merkel S, Mansmann U, Siassi M, Papadopoulos T, Hohenberger W, Hermanek P. The prognostic inhomogeneity in pT3 rectal carcinomas. Int J Color Dis. 2001;16(5):298–304.

10. Hermanek P, Henson DE, Hutter RV, Sobin LH. UICC TNM supplement 1993: a commentary on uniform use. Berlin: Springer; 1993.

11. Kaur H, Choi H, You YN, Rauch GM, Jensen CT, Hou P, et al. MR imaging for preoperative evaluation of primary rectal cancer: practical considerations. Radiographics. 2012;32(2):389–409.

12. Cho SH, Kim SH, Bae JH, Jang YJ, Kim HJ, Lee D, et al. Prognostic stratification by extramural depth of tumor invasion of primary rectal cancer based on the Radiological Society of North America proposal. AJR Am J Roentgenol. 2014;202(6):1238–44.

13. Shin R, Jeong SY, Yoo HY, Park KJ, Heo SC, Kang GH, et al. Depth of mesorectal extension has prognostic significance in patients with T3 rectal cancer. Dis Colon Rectum. 2012;55(12):1220–8.

14. Brown G, Richards CJ, Bourne MW, Newcombe RG, Radcliffe AG, Dallimore NS, et al. Morphologic predictors of lymph node status in rectal cancer with use of high-spatial-resolution MR imaging with histopathologic comparison. Radiology. 2003;227(2):371–7.

15. Kim JH, Beets GL, Kim MJ, Kessels AG, Beets-Tan RG. High-resolution MR imaging for nodal staging in rectal cancer: are there any criteria in addition to the size? Eur J Radiol. 2004;52(1):78–83.

16. Hunter CJ, Garant A, Vuong T, Artho G, Lisbona R, Tekkis P, et al. Adverse features on rectal MRI identify a high-risk group that may benefit from more intensive preoperative staging and treatment. Ann Surg Oncol. 2012;19(4):1199–205.

17. Chand M, Moran BJ, Jones RG, Heald RJ, Brown G. Lymph node status does not predict local recurrence in the total mesorectal excision era. Dis Colon Rectum. 2014;57(1):127–9.

18. Smith NJ, Barbachano Y, Norman AR, Swift RI, Abulafi AM, Brown G. Prognostic significance of magnetic resonance imaging-detected extramural vascular invasion in rectal cancer. Br J Surg. 2008;95(2):229–36.

19. Talbot IC, Ritchie S, Leighton MH, Hughes AO, Bussey HJ, Morson BC. The clinical significance of invasion of veins by rectal cancer. Br J Surg. 1980;67(6):439–42.

20. Chand M, Evans J, Swift RI, Tekkis PP, West NP, Stamp G, et al. The prognostic significance of post-chemoradiotherapy high-resolution MRI and histopathology detected extramural venous invasion in rectal cancer. Ann Surg. 2015;261(3):473–9.

21. Mantke R, Schmidt U, Wolff S, Kube R, Lippert H. Incidence of synchronous liver metastases in patients with colorectal cancer in relationship to clinico-pathologic characteristics. Results of a German prospective multicentre observational study. Eur J Surg Oncol. 2012;38(3):259–65.

22. Kim H, Myoung S, Koom WS, Kim NK, Kim MJ, Ahn JB, et al. MRI risk stratification for tumor relapse in rectal cancer achieving pathological complete remission after neoadjuvant chemoradiation therapy and curative resection. PLoS One. 2016;11(1):e0146235.

23. Battersby NJ, How P, Moran B, Stelzner S, West NP, Branagan G, et al. Prospective validation of a low rectal cancer magnetic resonance imaging staging system and development of a local recurrence risk stratification model: the MERCURY II study. Ann Surg. 2016;263(4):751–60.

24. Sohn B, Lim JS, Kim H, Myoung S, Choi J, Kim NK, et al. MRI-detected extramural vascular invasion is an independent prognostic factor for synchronous metastasis in patients with rectal cancer. Eur Radiol. 2015;25(5):1347–55.
25. Moran BJ, Holm T, Brannagan G, Chave H, Quirke P, West N, et al. The English national low rectal cancer development programme: key messages and future perspectives. Colorectal Dis. 2014;16(3):173–8.
26. Shihab OC, Heald RJ, Rullier E, Brown G, Holm T, Quirke P, et al. Defining the surgical planes on MRI improves surgery for cancer of the low rectum. Lancet Oncol. 2009;10(12):1207–11.
27. Nagtegaal ID, van de Velde CJ, Marijnen CA, van Krieken JH, Quirke P, Dutch Colorectal Cancer Group, et al. Low rectal cancer: a call for a change of approach in abdominoperineal resection. J Clin Oncol. 2005;23(36):9257–64.
28. Marr R, Birbeck K, Garvican J, Macklin CP, Tiffin NJ, Parsons WJ, et al. The modern abdominoperineal excision: the next challenge after total mesorectal excision. Ann Surg. 2005;242(1):74–82.
29. Shirouzu K, Isomoto H, Kakegawa T. Distal spread of rectal cancer and optimal distal margin of resection for sphincter-preserving surgery. Cancer. 1995;76(3):388–92.
30. Rullier E, Denost Q, Vendrely V, Rullier A, Laurent C. Low rectal cancer: classification and standardization of surgery. Dis Colon Rectum. 2013;56(5):560–7.
31. Fujita S, Mizusawa J, Kanemitsu Y, Ito M, Kinugasa Y, Komori K, et al. Mesorectal excision with or without lateral lymph node dissection for clinical stage II/III lower rectal cancer (JCOG0212): a multicenter, randomized controlled, noninferiority trial. Ann Surg. 2017;266:201.
32. Sugihara K, Kobayashi H, Kato T, Mori T, Mochizuki H, Kameoka S, et al. Indication and benefit of pelvic sidewall dissection for rectal cancer. Dis Colon Rectum. 2006;49(11):1663–72.
33. Moriya Y, Sugihara K, Akasu T, Fujita S. Importance of extended lymphadenectomy with lateral node dissection for advanced lower rectal cancer. World J Surg. 1997;21(7):728–32.
34. Kim TH, Jeong SY, Choi DH, Kim DY, Jung KH, Moon SH, et al. Lateral lymph node metastasis is a major cause of locoregional recurrence in rectal cancer treated with preoperative chemoradiotherapy and curative resection. Ann Surg Oncol. 2008;15(3):729–37.
35. Yano H, Saito Y, Takeshita E, Miyake O, Ishizuka N. Prediction of lateral pelvic node involvement in low rectal cancer by conventional computed tomography. Br J Surg. 2007;94(8):1014–9.
36. Fujita S, Yamamoto S, Akasu T, Moriya Y. Risk factors of lateral pelvic lymph node metastasis in advanced rectal cancer. Int J Color Dis. 2009;24(9):1085–90.
37. Akasu T, Iinuma G, Takawa M, Yamamoto S, Muramatsu Y, Moriyama N. Accuracy of high-resolution magnetic resonance imaging in preoperative staging of rectal cancer. Ann Surg Oncol. 2009;16(10):2787–94.
38. Kang JH, Kim YC, Kim H, Kim YW, Hur H, Kim JS, et al. Tumor volume changes assessed by three-dimensional magnetic resonance volumetry in rectal cancer patients after preoperative chemoradiation: the impact of the volume reduction ratio on the prediction of pathologic complete response. Int J Radiat Oncol Biol Phys. 2010;76(4):1018–25.
39. Dworak O, Keilholz L, Hoffmann A. Pathological features of rectal cancer after preoperative radiochemotherapy. Int J Color Dis. 1997;12(1):19–23.
40. Mandard AM, Dalibard F, Mandard JC, Marnay J, Henry-Amar M, Petiot JF, et al. Pathologic assessment of tumor regression after preoperative chemoradiotherapy of esophageal carcinoma. Clinicopathologic correlations. Cancer. 1994;73(11):2680–6.
41. Jhaveri KS, Hosseini-Nik H. MRI of rectal cancer: an overview and update on recent advances. AJR Am J Roentgenol. 2015;205(1):W42–55.
42. Battersby NJ, Moran B, Yu S, Tekkis P, Brown G. MR imaging for rectal cancer: the role in staging the primary and response to neoadjuvant therapy. Expert Rev Gastroenterol Hepatol. 2014;8(6):703–19.
43. Jacobs L, Intven M, van Lelyveld N, Philippens M, Burbach M, Seldenrijk K, et al. Diffusion-weighted MRI for early prediction of treatment response on preoperative chemoradiotherapy for patients with locally advanced rectal cancer: a feasibility study. Ann Surg. 2016;263:522.
44. Lambrecht M, Vandecaveye V, De Keyzer F, Roels S, Penninckx F, Van Cutsem E, et al. Value of diffusion-weighted magnetic resonance imaging for prediction and early assessment of response to neoadjuvant radiochemotherapy in rectal cancer: preliminary results. Int J Radiat Oncol Biol Phys. 2012;82(2):863–70.
45. Jung SH, Heo SH, Kim JW, Jeong YY, Shin SS, Soung MG, et al. Predicting response to neoadjuvant chemoradiation therapy in locally advanced rectal cancer: diffusion-weighted 3 Tesla MR imaging. J Magn Reson Imaging. 2012;35(1):110–6.
46. Park MJ, Kim SH, Lee SJ, Jang KM, Rhim H. Locally advanced rectal cancer: added value of diffusion-weighted MR imaging for predicting tumor clearance of the mesorectal fascia after neoadjuvant chemotherapy and radiation therapy. Radiology. 2011;260(3):771–80.
47. Sun YS, Zhang XP, Tang L, Ji JF, Gu J, Cai Y, et al. Locally advanced rectal carcinoma treated with preoperative chemotherapy and radiation therapy: preliminary analysis of diffusion-weighted MR imaging for early detection of tumor histopathologic downstaging. Radiology. 2010;254(1):170–8.

Neoadjuvant Therapy for Locally Advanced Rectal Cancer

8

Jin Gu

Abstracts

Worldwide, colorectal cancer is the third most commonly occurring cancer. Local recurrence and distance metastasis, especially in patients with low rectal cancers, present the main problems for surgeons. Even after undergoing total mesorectal excision (TME), the local recurrence rate for stage III patients is 20–30%. The available treatments of rectal cancers are far from satisfactory; the 5- and 10-year surgical rates are 35% and 22%, respectively. To improve the local control and long-term survival rates, it is necessary for patients with resectable stage II–III cancers to receive neoadjuvant therapy before undergoing surgery. Per the evidence, preoperative chemoradiotherapy (CRT) can significantly reduce the local recurrence of locally advanced rectal cancers and increase the rates of anus preservation. Hence, most guidelines, such as those of the National Comprehensive Cancer Network (NCCN), the European Society for Medical Oncology (ESMO), and the American Cancer Society (ACS), have strongly recommended the implementation of presurgery CRT as standard neoadjuvant therapy for locally advanced rectal cancers.

Keywords

Neoadjuvant therapy · Rectal cancer · Locally advanced · Surgery · Chemoradiotherapy

8.1 Introduction

Worldwide, rectal cancer is the third most commonly occurring cancer [1]. Surgery remains the mainstay of therapy for patients with rectal cancers [2]. However, local recurrence and distance metastasis, especially in patients with low rectal cancers, present the main problems for surgeons [3]. Even after undergoing total mesorectal excision (TME), the local recurrence rate for stage III patients is 20–30% [4]. The available treatments of rectal cancers are far from satisfactory; the 5- and 10-year surgical rates are 35% and 22%, respectively [5, 6].

To improve the local control and long-term survival rates, it is necessary for patients with resectable stage II–III cancers to receive neoadjuvant therapy before undergoing surgery [2]. Therefore, surgery combined with adjuvant therapy, including radiotherapy (RT) and chemoradiotherapy (CRT), with postoperative adjuvant chemotherapy (CT), for locally advanced rectal cancers has formed the basis of several reports published in the early 1990s [7, 8]. Postoperative CRT has been established as a standard treatment in the United States [6, 7]. Since then, physicians

J. Gu
Department of Colorectal Surgery, Peking University Cancer Hospital, Beijing, People's Republic of China
e-mail: zlguj@hsc.pku.edu.cn

have compared the advantages of preoperative and postoperative RT, more attentively [9]. RT for rectal cancers, whether or not combined with CT based on 5-fluorouracil (5-FU) or in combination with oxaliplatin, presents an important concern of treatment [4]. Additionally, 2 schedules of treatments with RT have been explored: short-term treatment that delivers 25 Gy of radiation in 5 fractions during 1 week, followed immediately by surgery, and conventional schedules that deliver 40–50 Gy in 20–25 fractions during 4–5 weeks, followed by surgery 3–6 weeks later [6]. Physicians have started to explore other regimens of RT or CRT. Clinical research has emphasized the use of either single-agent CT or combined CT [4]. Researchers have also aimed to improve the efficacy of RT, including the reduction of radiation toxicity before surgery [4, 10]. By the end of the last century, many studies had reported the course of RT, including long- and short-term regimens, and evidence-based medicine had optimized the regimens of CT, using quantitative random samples in control studies [8].

In the twenty-first century, science and technology have greatly advanced, and the equipment for RT has been upgraded. The advancements in RT techniques, such as precise RT, the application of three-dimensional (3D) conformal therapy, and intensity-modulated RT, have further improved its therapeutic accuracy and effects [11]. Furthermore, the selection of appropriate indications for CRT has been standardized. Clinical research has shown that RT has extended the waiting times for surgery, which significantly demonstrates its therapeutic effectiveness [12].

During this period, the renewal and the development of various ideas and surgical techniques, such as TME, represented milestones in the field of rectal cancer surgery [13]. TME significantly decreased local recurrence rates and improved survivals in patients with locally advanced rectal cancers [14]. Meanwhile, standardizing surgical pathological evaluation, utilizing the concept of circumferential resection margins (CRMs), and developing neoadjuvant therapy have enabled significant progress in the combined treatments for rectal cancers [15]. Per the evidence, preoperative CRT can significantly reduce the local recurrence of locally advanced rectal cancers and increase the rates of anus preservation [16]. Hence, most guidelines, such as those of the National Comprehensive Cancer Network (NCCN), the European Society for Medical Oncology (ESMO), and the American Cancer Society (ACS), have strongly recommended the implementation of presurgery CRT as standard neoadjuvant therapy for locally advanced rectal cancers.

8.2 Pretreatment Staging with Magnetic Resonance Imaging (MRI) and Endoscopic Ultrasound (EUS)

For patients with rectal cancers, pretreatment staging is vital. Treatment planning requires defining the depths of tumor invasions in relation to the bowel wall, the presence of metastatic regional lymph nodes, and the precise relationship of the tumors to other pelvic structures, such as the mesorectal fascia (MRF), levator muscle, anal sphincters, and other adjacent organs [17, 18]. Additionally, the assessments of pelvic nodal basins outside the MRF and retroperitoneal nodes, liver, and lungs can provide useful information that may influence treatment strategies [19]. The Magnetic Resonance Imaging and Rectal Cancer European Equivalence (MERCURY) study group has recently published a prospective observational study on the diagnostic accuracy of MRI in predicting curative resections of rectal cancers [20, 21]. This multicenter study, comprising 11 units in Europe, analyzed 408 patients with rectal cancers who underwent MRIs before TMEs [21]. The MRI findings were compared to the results of standardized pathological examinations of the specimens [21]. The conclusions from the MERCURY study indicated that tagged MRI is currently the best technique for predicting CRM status and clinical outcomes of rectal cancers; it allows staging and planning of individualized treatments by a multidisciplinary team before surgery is performed [21]. Additionally, EUS demonstrated superior evaluations of tumor invasions [22]. Therefore, MRI and EUS are strongly recommended by the NCCN and ESMO guidelines as golden standards of evaluation for patients with rectal cancers.

8.3   The Indications of Pre- or Postoperative CRT for Locally Advanced Rectal Cancer

Evidence suggests that surgery with neoadjuvant therapy, including neoadjuvant CRT or RT, has improved local control of tumors and that some patients could benefit from such treatment [23]. However, the selection of appropriate patients is critical because not all patients with rectal cancers benefit from neoadjuvant therapy [24, 25]. Unfortunately, there are no relative accurate ways to select patients who can benefit from preoperative neoadjuvant therapy [26, 27]. Therefore, the NCCN guidelines can only specify the indications for patients with rectal cancers who can undergo neoadjuvant therapy, based on limited clinical evidence [22]. In fact, it is generally recognized that upper rectal cancers that are 11–15 cm from the anal verge do not require neoadjuvant therapy because of their biological behavior as colon cancers [20, 27]. A phase III randomized study in the Netherlands showed that tumor location was a prognostic factor for treatment efficacy [24, 25]. Middle and lower rectal cancers can benefit more from neoadjuvant CRT than upper rectal cancers [9, 26–31]. The NCCN guidelines have recommended that patients with rectal cancers that are 12 cm from the anal verge are eligible to accept neoadjuvant CRT before undergoing surgery [22]. Among these patients, the postoperative local recurrence rate for stage T1 rectal cancers is approximately 5%; hence, CRT is not necessary [4, 29]. For patients with low-risk rectal cancers (classified as T1-T2/N1, T3/N0, per tumor-node-metastasis classification), their postoperative local recurrence rates are significantly different from patients with mid- (T1-T2/N2, T3/N1, T4/N0) and high-risk (T3/N2, T4/N1, T4/N2) rectal carcinomas [28, 30]. Patients with low-risk rectal cancers may not benefit by treatment

with combined CRT with surgery but may experience increasing toxicities from RT and CT [25, 31]. Thus, most patients with T1-2N0M0 rectal cancers can be cured by surgery [27]. In contrast, 22% of pathological diagnoses have indicated the presence of positive nodal metastases in mid-risk patients with stratified T3N0 rectal cancers, using EUS or MRI [4]. Therefore, the prognoses of stratifications among this subtype of patients may be underestimated. Patient groups treated with established preoperative neoadjuvant RT and CRT should include patients with rectal tumors that are located within 12 cm of the anus, stratification stage (c/pT3-4b), or mesentery and pelvic nodal metastases (c/pN1-2), but without distant metastases (M0).

8.3.1   Neoadjuvant CRT: Preoperative CRT Versus Preoperative RT

Neoadjuvant CRT uses preoperative RT and preoperative CT [22]. Preoperative CRT can be further divided into 5-FU-based CRT and RT combined with CT [6, 7]. RT is then divided into long-term RT (45.0–50.4 Gy), which is more popular in North America, and short-term RT, 25.0 Gy (5 × 5 Gy), which is more popular in Europe [6]. An increasing number of studies show that the combination of CT with neoadjuvant RT could effectively improve local remission rates and synergistic sensitization; the most frequently used CT agent is 5-FU; other combined chemotherapeutic and molecular-targeted drugs are still being tested in ongoing clinical studies [3, 6].

8.3.1.1 Preoperative Versus Postoperative CRT for Rectal Cancer

In the early 1990s, postoperative CRT was established as standard treatment in the United States [6]. A study from the Duluth Community Clinical Oncology Program designed a combination regimen to optimize the contributions of CT, decrease recurrences, and improve survivals, in contrast to treatments with adjuvant RT alone [5]. They concluded that the combination of postoperative local therapy, with radiation and FU, and systemic therapy, with an FU-based regimen, significantly and substantively improved the results of therapy for rectal carcinomas with poor prognoses, compared with treatments with postoperative RT alone [5]. From the end of the twentieth century, encouraging results of treatments with preoperative RT have been reported. One such representative study from the German Rectal Cancer Study Group randomly assigned 401 patients with clinical stage T3 or T4 node-positive disease to receive preoperative CRT and 402 such patients to receive postoperative CRT [32]. The overall 5-year survival rates in these groups of patients were 76% and 74%, respectively, and the 5-year cumulative incidences of local relapses were 6% and 13% [32]. They concluded that preoperative CRT improved local control and was associated with reduced toxicities, but did not improve overall survivals (OS), compared with postoperative CRT [32]. Based on this study and other evidence from literature, we believe that preoperative CRT showed the superiority of postoperative therapy as standard therapy for locally advanced rectal cancers.

8.3.1.2 CT with Preoperative RT for Rectal Cancer

Preoperative CRT is recommended for selected patients with rectal cancers. Because of the relatively high rates of observed side effects with preoperative RT, especially as part of CRT, some studies focused on determining whether adjuvant postoperative CT should be appropriate for patients with rectal cancers. In 2006, the European Organization for Research and Treatment of Cancer (EORTC) Radiotherapy Group Trial 22921 published their study on CT with preoperative RT for the treatment of rectal cancers [33]. They randomly assigned patients with clinical stage T3 or T4 resectable rectal cancers to receive preoperative RT, preoperative CRT, preoperative RT and postoperative CT, or preoperative CRT and postoperative CT [33]. After a median follow-up of 5.4 years, they concluded that in patients with rectal cancers who received preoperative RT, the addition of preoperative or postoperative FU-based CT had no significant effects on survivals [34, 35]. Regardless

of whether it is administered before or after surgery, CT confers significant benefits with respect to local control [6, 33, 35].

8.3.1.3 TME with or Without Preoperative RT for Rectal Cancer

Local recurrence following surgery for rectal cancer remained a serious problem. Heald first reported TME in 1982, but decreasing the local recurrence rates and improving patient survivals, regional recurrences, and distant metastases, including liver and lung involvement, remained challenging for surgeons [36]. RT was administered to improve local control and survival after conventional surgery [37]. Two well-known trials using preoperative RT with surgery to improve local control have been published. In 1997, the Swedish Rectal Cancer Trial reported that a short-course regimen of high-dose preoperative RT reduces local recurrence rates and improves survivals among patients with resectable rectal cancers [37]. Another study from the Dutch Colorectal Cancer Group randomly assigned 1861 patients with resectable rectal cancers, to groups treated with either preoperative RT followed by TME, or TME alone [38]. The results indicated that short-term preoperative RT reduced the risk of local recurrence in patients with rectal cancers who undergo standardized TME [38]. A few meta-analyses concluded that the combination of preoperative RT and surgery, compared with surgery alone, significantly improved overall and cancer-specific survivals [3, 38].

8.3.1.4 Short-Course RT Versus Long-Course RT

Currently, preoperative CRT is widely used as standardized treatment for locally advanced rectal cancers. There are two treatment regimens: one delivers 25 Gy in 5 fractions during 1 week, followed immediately by surgery, and the other conventional regimen delivers 40–50 Gy in 20–25 fractions during 4–5 weeks, followed by surgery 6–8 weeks later [15]. Till date, many northern European countries have developed a treatment regimen that includes short-course RT following surgery, which has significantly controlled local recurrence after surgery and prolonged survival times [32]. However, because of the relatively high dose administered per fraction (5 Gy), the occurrence of adverse events, such as severe diarrhea, led patients to refuse adjuvant RT in China [39]. To reduce the incidence of these side effects, we investigated a modified short-course regimen that could potentially decrease the fractional dose from 5 Gy to 3 Gy and the total dose to 30 Gy (10 × 3 Gy) [40]. Our results indicated that the modified short-course regimen of 30 Gy (10 × 3 Gy) can significantly reduce local recurrence and improve survivals in patients who show downstaging, and the rates of occurrence of complications in these cases are acceptable [40]. Long-course RT is usually incorporated with preoperative CT. The results of the CAO/ARO/AIO-94 (Working Group of Surgical Oncology/Working Group of Radiation Oncology/Working Group of Medical Oncology of the Germany Cancer Society) trial have indicated that this could increase the rates of anus preservation and 5-year local control and could also limit the occurrence of toxic reactions to 3–4° (including acute and late-stage reactions) and anastomotic stricture [32]. Comparison of the two neoadjuvant therapies revealed that preoperative long-course RT could improve the tumor downstaging rates and lower the rates of CRM positivity; however, there were no differences between the two with respect to the rates of anus preservation, OS, or local control. This difference may be related to the waiting times for surgeries after RT; yet both regimens should be considered comprehensively, according to the tolerance of patients and the waiting times. Although preoperative CRT has been used as standard treatment for locally advanced rectal cancers, limited evidence from clinical trials indicates that it could also improve long-term survivals and the rates of anal sphincter retention.

8.3.2   Preoperative RT Versus Preoperative RT for Rectal Cancer

As previously mentioned, patients with rectal cancers could benefit from preoperative CRT. The European Organization for Research and Treatment of Cancer (EORTC) 22921 trial has illustrated that patients with rectal cancers who received preoperative RT with FU-based CT reap significant benefits with respect to local control [6]. Additionally, a recent meta-analysis from China concluded that capecitabine was more efficient than 5-FU, in terms of tumor responses, during neoadjuvant treatments for patients with locally advanced rectal cancers, with favorably low toxicities, except for the occurrence of the hand-foot syndrome [41].

8.3.2.1   5-FU Combined with Oxaliplatin

Neoadjuvant CRT, including RT and single-agent CT with 5-FU, is the standard treatment for locally advanced rectal cancers. Many clinical studies have evaluated the effect of combination therapies, namely, 5-FU plus oxaliplatin with neoadjuvant CRT. The clinical trials including ACCORD 12/80405, STAR-01, and National Surgical Adjuvant Breast and Bowel Project (NSABP) R-04 have verified that the combinations of 5-FU or capecitabine with oxaliplatin do not improve the rates of pathologic complete responses (pCR), operative downstaging, anus preservation, or positive lymph node harvest [42–44]. Aschele et al. found that adding oxaliplatin to FU-based preoperative CRT significantly increases the toxicity of treatments, without affecting the primary tumor responses [43]. The occurrence rates of adverse reactions (mainly diarrhea) increased correspondingly [43]. In contrast, the Chinese **FORWARC** study divided patients with locally advanced rectal cancers into different groups corresponding to the administered neoadjuvant therapy, namely, CRT combined with 5-FU and mFOLFOX6 (modified folinic acid, FU, and oxaliplatin-6), respectively, and CT with mFOLFOX6 [4]. Preliminary results show that the pCR rates for each group were 14.3%, 28.0%, and 6.1%, respectively [4]. This may also indicate the differences in oxaliplatin sensitization between patients in the Eastern and Western countries. Thus, treatment of Eastern patients with the combined oxaliplatin regimen still requires further validation.

8.3.3 Molecular-Targeted Agents in Neoadjuvant Therapy for Rectal Cancer

Till date, few intensive studies have been conducted on molecular-targeted agents for neoadjuvant therapy for rectal cancers. There is some research on the anti-epidermal growth factor receptors (EGFR) antibodies, e.g., cetuximab and panitumumab; small molecular tyrosine kinase inhibitors of the EGFR, such as gefitinib and erlotinib; and anti-angiogenesis drugs (e.g., bevacizumab); however, no consensus has been established yet.

The binding of cetuximab, an anti-EGFR monoclonal antibody [45], prevents the activation of signal transduction pathways and interrupts downstream phosphorylation reactions [46], which prevents further tumor growth [47]. Studies have shown that the administration of cetuximab during neoadjuvant therapy for rectal cancers with wild-type V-Ki-ras2 Kirsten rat sarcoma viral oncogene homolog (KRAS) results in pCR rates of 0–25% (Table 8.1).

These studies include patients who exhibit immunologic tolerance and in whom the pathologic downstaging rates have increased without raising the pCR rates, which may be explained by the following reasons: (1) molecular-targeted drugs are not toxic to cells. Adding cetuximab to CRT may not reduce tumor sizes in the short term, but it may shrink the tumors steadily in the long term. (2) The pCR rate can be used for the assessment of preoperative combined therapy; however, it cannot replace OS times, local recurrence rates, or other classical standards. (3) The prospective reveals small sample sizes. They may be biased during case selection and treatment, due to the lack of randomized controlled trials. (4) Studies were conducted several years ago and thus do not consider the status of the KRAS or neuroblastoma RAS viral oncogene homolog (NRAS) genes.

Table 8.1 Trials integrating cetuximab into neoadjuvant chemoradiotherapy for resectable rectal cancers

Study	Evaluable patients (n)	pCR rate	Concomitant chemoradiotherapy regimen	Patients with KRAS mutations (%)	Grade 3 or 4 (CTCAE v.3) toxicities
Machiels et al. [45]	38	2/38 (5%)	Capecitabine 650–825 mg/m² b.i.d., 7 days a week Radiotherapy 45.0 Gy	12/39 (31%)	Neutropenia: 3% Vomiting: 2.5% Diarrhea: 15% Rash: 0%
Bertolini et al. [46]	38	3/38 (8%)	5-FU 225 mg/m²/day continuous infusion over 7 days a week Radiotherapy 50–50.4 Gy	9/40 (22.5%)	Febrile neutropenia: 2.5% Nausea/vomiting: 0% Diarrhea: 7.5% Rash: 7.5%
Rodel et al. [47]	45	4/45 (9%)	Capecitabine 500–825 mg/m² b.i.d., days 1–14 and 22–35 Oxaliplatin 50 mg/m², days 1, 8, 22, and 29	NA	Leukopenia: 6% Nausea/vomiting: 4% Diarrhea: 19% Skin rash: 2%
Horisberger et al. [48]	50	4/50 (8%)	Capecitabine 500 mg/m² b.i.d. Irinotecan 40 mg/m², 5 days a week Radiotherapy 50.4 Gy	NA	Leukopenia: 4% Nausea/vomiting: 2% Diarrhea: 30% Skin rash: 6%
Kim [49]	39	9/39 (23%)	Capecitabine 825 mg/m² b.i.d., 5 days a week Irinotecan 40 mg/m², 5 days a week Radiotherapy 50.4 Gy	5/38 (13%)	Neutropenia: 5.1% Vomiting: 0% Diarrhea: 5.1% Skin rash: 2.6%

pCR pathologic complete response, *CTCAE* common terminology criteria for adverse events, *NA* not available, *b.i.d* twice a day, *5-FU* 5-fluorouracil

This could also be a possible reason why the pCR rates are low. In a more recent multicenter random stage II clinical trial, EXPERT-C, 165 patients with high-risk rectal cancers, divided into simple cetuximab (+) and cetuximab (−) subgroups randomly, underwent a 4-week regimen, consisting of capecitabine combined with oxaliplatin (CAPOX), followed by capecitabine-based concurrent CRT after CT induction [50]. The data indicate that 90 patients with wild-type KRAS/v-raf murine sarcoma viral oncogene homolog B (BRAF) showed similar pCR rates (11–7%, $p = 0.71$), either with or without the addition of capecitabine [50]. In summary, there are no significant differences in OS or progression-free survival between the two subgroups, whereas an

increase in adverse reactions has been reported in those patients who added cetuximab to their treatment regimens.

8.3.3.1 Bevacizumab

The vascular endothelial growth factor (VEGF) plays an essential role in tumor angiogenesis. Inhibiting VEGF by bevacizumab can block oxygen supply to the tumor cells and increase their sensitivities to RT [51]. Other functions of bevacizumab have been studied, especially in patients with rectal cancers that harbored KRAS mutations. The pCR rates for locally advanced rectal carcinomas are 13.3–32%, with administration of bevacizumab during neoadjuvant therapy (Table 8.2).

Table 8.2 Bevacizumab with conventional chemoradiotherapy: an overview of the discussed studies

Study	Evaluable patients (n)	pCR rate	Concomitant chemoradiotherapy regimen	Stage	Postoperative complications (n)
Willett et al. [51]	32	16%	BV 5 or 10 mg/kg, 5-FU 225 mg/m² daily, RT 50.4 Gy in 28 fr	II–III	Anastomotic leak with presacral abscess (1) Vaginal tear with presacral hematoma and abscess (1) Pelvic hematoma (1) Delayed healing of perineal incision (2) Ileus (2) Neurogenic bladder (1) Perforated ileostomy (1) Pulmonary embolus (1) Wound infection (3)
Crane et al. [52]	25	32%	BV 5 mg/kg, CAPE 900 mg/m² b.i.d., RT 50.4 Gy in 28 fr	II–III	Wound complications requiring surgical intervention (3) 32% Minor complications (5)
Velenik et al. [53]	61	13.3%	BV 5 mg/kg, CAPE 825 mg/m² b.i.d., RT 50.4 Gy in 28 fr	II–III	Delayed wound healing (18) infection/abscess (12) Anastomotic leakage (7) Pneumothorax (1)
Salazar et al. [54]	90	16% vs. 11%	Arm A: BV 5 mg/kg, CAPE 825 mg/m² b.i.d., RT 45 Gy in 25 fr Arm B: CAPE 825 mg/m² b.i.d., RT 45 Gy in 25 fr	II–III	16% vs. 13% (not specified)
Gasparini et al. [55]	43	14%	BV 5 mg/kg, CAPE 825 mg/m² b.i.d., RT 50.4 Gy in 28 fr	II–III	Bowel perforation (1) 14% Anastomosis failure (1) Abscess (1)
Landry et al. [56]	49	17%	BV 5 mg /kg, CAPE 825 mg/m² b.i.d., RT 50 Gy in 25 fr	II–III	29 patients (53%) with worst grade 3 toxicities 8 patients (15%) with worst grade 4 toxicities

BV bevacizumab, *RT* radiotherapy, *5-FU* 5-fluorouracil, *CAPE* capecitabine, *fr* fractions, *pCR* pathological complete response

Nonetheless, the effects of treatment with bevacizumab during neoadjuvant CRT for locally advanced rectal cancers remain unclear. Many studies have demonstrated moderate increases in the pCR rates with bevacizumab combined with CRT; however, other related adverse reactions should be considered at the same time.

8.3.4 Total Neoadjuvant Therapy for Rectal Cancer

Although adjuvant CT was implemented for pT3-4 or pT1-2N+ rectal cancers, and is recommended by the NCCN guidelines, its role in rectal cancers remains less clear, and its inclusion in treatment regimens is at least partially extrapolated from colon cancer trials [5, 22, 57, 58]. Recently, multiple trials have reported promising outcomes using a "total neoadjuvant therapy" (TNT) approach, in which all RT and CT were delivered in the preoperative setting [57]. Compared with neoadjuvant treatment, the adjuvant treatment has relatively low compliance and tolerability. These may be the reasons why the distant metastasis rates and the local recurrences for rectal cancers remain high. Although preoperative RT could improve the local recurrence, the OS rates are rarely affected. Thus, whether simple adjuvant CT can control the local recurrence and the metastasis of tumors, while preventing other side effects caused by CT or RT, is still one of the most popular fields for research. In theory, on the one hand, neoadjuvant therapy has evident advantages. Systematic administration has more effective whole body control than using neoadjuvant RT or CRT, and it can kill mic-

rosatellites to lower the distal metastasis risk. On the other hand, primary tumor regression, resulting from neoadjuvant CT, can also theoretically lower the risks for local recurrence. The first study that proposed the concept of neoadjuvant CT and validated its effectiveness prospectively, MSKCC, administrated FOLFOX (6 cycles), bevacizumab (4 cycles), or both, to 32 patients with "low- to mid-risk" locally advanced rectal cancers [59]. The results indicate that 25% of the pathology in these patients was completely relieved. After a 4-year follow-up, no local occurrence has been seen. The 4-year disease-free survival rate is 84%, and the OS rate is 91% [59]. Comprehensively, neoadjuvant CT can compare favorably with the conventional CRT. This study has also stimulated a series of randomized controlled studies of neoadjuvant therapy for locally advanced rectal cancers (Table 8.3).

These results suggest that single-agent neoadjuvant CT could lower the local recurrence rates to some extent. Although it can potentially prolong patient survival times and rates, the CT regimens and the assessment standards are different in the reported studies; therefore the conclusion needs more support of persuasive evidence. Additionally, the effects of neoadjuvant therapy cannot be evaluated objectively because of the lack of cases, long-term follow ups, or other control studies. Therefore, there are other ongoing clinical trials, such as PROSPECT (NCT01515787, Preoperative Radiation or Selective Preoperative Radiation and Evaluation before Chemotherapy and TME) and BACCHUS (NCT01650428, Bevacizumab and Combination Chemotherapy in rectal cancer Until Surgery), which might change the outcomes from the current studies.

Table 8.3 Studies on treatment of rectal cancers with neoadjuvant chemotherapy alone

Study	Year	n	Regimen	pCR rate (%)	Outcomes
Ishii et al. [60]	2010	26	CPT-11 + 5-FU + leucovorin, 8 weeks	3.8	5-year DFS: 74%, 5-year OS: 84%
Uehara et al. [61]	2013	32	CAPOX + Bev, 12 weeks	13.3	R0 resection rate: 90%
Hasegawa et al. [62]	2014	25	CAPOX + Bev, 12 weeks	4.3	R0 resection rate: 93%
Schrag et al. [63]	2014	32	FOLFOX + Bev, 8 weeks	25.0	4-year DFS: 84%, 5-year DFS: 91%

pCR pathological complete response, *FU* fluorouracil, *CAPOX* capecitabine + oxaliplatin, *FOLFOX* fluorouracil + leucovorin + oxaliplatin, *DFS* disease-free survival, *OS* overall survival, *Bev* bevacizumab, *CPT-11* Irinotecan

8.3.5   The Necessity of Undergoing Neoadjuvant Therapy for Upper Rectal Cancers and MRI-Diagnosed T3a and T3b Carcinomas

The main goals of neoadjuvant therapy for locally advanced rectal cancers are reducing the local recurrence rates and increasing the sphincter preservation. However, the need for this therapy in T3N0 locally advanced rectal carcinomas is still debatable. Some studies have reported that postoperative local recurrence rates of under 8% can be achieved for patients with T3N0 rectal cancers [14]. These patients may not need neoadjuvant therapy before undergoing surgery. Tumor location, CRM, and nerve involvements can determine tumor recurrence [64]. Due to the limitations of pretreatment evaluations, discrepancies exist in the staging of locally advanced rectal cancers. The pathological data validates that 22–28% patients with cT3N0 cancers show lymph nodal metastasis after surgery; therefore, the NCCN guidelines recommend neoadjuvant therapy for such patients [21]. The ESMO guidelines use MRIs to assess tumor staging, the extent of spread to the lymph nodes (N staging), and the location of the tumors to the anal verge, the invasion of the MRF, and extramural vascular invasions (EMVI) [22]. This assessment can categorize the recurrence risks for the extreme-low-risk, the low-risk, the mid-risk, and the high-risk groups [65]. Within these groups, the patients diagnosed as extreme-low-risk and low-risk for tumor recurrence can directly undergo surgical operations without neoadjuvant therapy [65]. Similarly, the presence of cT3N0 carcinomas, invasion depths lesser than 5 mm without MRF invasion or EMVI, and surgical intervention should be considered first if the tumor is located above the anal sphincter [66]. The MERCURY study indicates that without a prognosis of high-risk tumor recurrence by MRI assessment (tumor infiltrations cannot be found in the mesenteric space or tumor thrombi cannot be found in the vessels if the tumor invasions remain less than 5 mm), the local recurrence rate after surgery is only 1.7% [67]. Therefore, even though neo-

adjuvant therapy is recommended as standard treatment, we suggest further analysis of cT3 carcinoma staging, thus avoiding the unnecessary side effects of administering neoadjuvant therapy to those who may not benefit from it.

8.4   The Efficacy of Neoadjuvant Therapy

The results of worldwide randomized trials of adjuvant RT for rectal cancer indicated that some patients could benefit from neoadjuvant RT, obtaining downstaging or clinical complete responses. After CRT and surgery, 15–27% of the patients have no residual viable tumors during pathological examinations; this constitutes achieving pCR [68]. Recent studies have shown that patients with pCRs had favorable outcomes with regard to local control, distant recurrence, disease-free survival, and OS [38, 41, 68]. Unfortunately, objective methods to predict the efficacy of neoadjuvant therapy do not exist. Many patients demonstrated no responses to neoadjuvant therapy but experienced the side effects of RT.

A study from the Peking University Cancer Hospital showed that approximately 20–30% of the patients with rectal cancers achieved complete remissions after undergoing preoperative CRT, irrespective of MRI scanning or clinical pathology [69]. Additionally, some patients experienced tumor progressions during the course of CRT, and a few presented with distant metastasis before surgery [69].

Several studies have attempted to define patients who may benefit from CRT, to omit further adjuvant treatments, and to intensify treatments for those who show no responses.

8.4.1   Complete Clinical Remission

8.4.1.1   Defining Complete Clinical Remission

The tumor is deemed to be in complete clinical remission if the following conditions are satisfied [70]: (1) only fibrosis is found by MRI scanning, without any clear indications of tumor residuals; (2) no suspicious lymph nodes are found by MRI scanning; (3) only scars or ulcers are found by endoscopic examination; (4) only scars or ulcers can be discovered from the pathologic tests of the multiple punch biopsies of the original tumor site; and (5) no clear tumor residues are found by digital rectal examination.

8.4.1.2 Patients with Restaged cCR (Clinical Complete Response) (yT0N0) Cancers Either Underwent Surgery or Adopted a "Wait-and-See" Approach

Approximately 15–27% of the patients appear to achieve complete clinical remission after neoadjuvant therapy [20]. After the pathology validates the complete remission, clinicians need to determine whether the patient can avoid surgery, which can further preclude surgical complications, such as infections, hemorrhage, pelvic nerve injury, and anterior resection syndrome. Furthermore, without undergoing surgery, some patients can avoid ostomy and retaining their anal function, which can improve their quality of living. Accordingly, increasing research has confirmed that appropriately selected patients can manage the tumor regrowth rates in acceptable ranges [70].

The first study of the "wait-and-see" approach, which entails observational management of patients with rectal cancers who had cCR after neoadjuvant CRT, was reported by Habr-Gama et al. [71]. Forty-five patients with locally advanced rectal cancers who achieved cCRs following neoadjuvant therapy were enrolled in a study from the Peking University Cancer Hospital; of these, 32 were assigned to the "wait-and-see" group, and the remaining 13 were assigned to the surgery group (intent-to-treat). The median follow-up time was 24 months (range, 3–51). Of the patients who were followed up for more than 12 months ($n = 37$), eight developed tumor progression (seven from the wait-and-see group and one from the surgery group, respectively). In the "wait-and-see" group, the local regrowth was 23.1% (6/26), while the distant metastasis

rate was 3.8% (1/26). We concluded that the "wait-and-see" approach has acceptable safety and efficiency, and it may become an alternative treatment for the patients who achieved cCR following neoadjuvant therapy. A recent publication has raised a debate on whether some patients who get to achieve cCR could undertake a "wait-and-see" approach, to avoid mutilating surgeries, although it is true that the criteria of a cCR, with or without the excision of the residual scar, have not been validated yet [72]. Therefore, choosing the "wait-and-see" approach cautiously can be one of the possible measures to achieve the same survival rates as with surgery. Additionally, patients with diagnosed distant metastasis and local recurrence can also undertake further treatments. Habr-Gama et al. also proposed that the "wait-and-see" period after neoadjuvant therapy did not mean that surgical treatments would never be necessary [72]. In addition to careful follow-ups, the condition of individual patients should be considered to determine their personal therapy, based on their consent.

8.4.2 The Effect of Neoadjuvant Therapy on the Surgical Strategy

8.4.2.1 Timing of Surgery After Neoadjuvant Therapy

Research has shown that prolonged interval time between RT and surgery may lead to increases in the cCR or pCR rates within a certain period. Several data support the fact that the tumor pCR rates increase after 5 weeks of neoadjuvant therapy but decrease after 10–11 weeks [73]. Current research showed that the period between 7 and 10 weeks (usually between 6 and 8 weeks) after neoadjuvant therapy is optimal for surgery. This period can not only relieve the acute toxic side effects of neoadjuvant therapy, but it can also repress tumor growth [3, 74]. While there are no observed decreases in surgical difficulties or the postsurgical complications after this time (10 weeks), the long-term toxic effects may increase.

8.4.2.2 Radical or Local Resection for yT1N0 Cancers

According to the preexisting guidelines, the suggested treatment for yT1N0 rectal cancers remains radical resection, to obtain more precise R0 resections [22]. Previous research indicates that 42% of cases with cN+ cancers have positive lymph nodes in their dissected specimens, after neoadjuvant therapy [75]. In some patients with ypT0 carcinomas, 16% show positive lymph node involvement; in contrast, cases with cT3-T4N0 cancers can maintain 3-year local non-recurrence rates of 96.9%, if neoadjuvant therapy could reveal their downstaging to ypT0-1 [75]. Meanwhile, another study suggested that local resections should excise at least 1 cm of margins and the full-thickness resections. If patients experience tumor regrowth or distant metastasis, salvage surgery would be needed [76].

Conclusion

Preoperative neoadjuvant therapy is the standard treatment for mid-to-low locally advanced rectal cancers. The method of treatment may vary, but the overall effects are undoubted. Numerous clinical practices and other evidence suggest that preoperative CRT can improve the rates of local control and increase the opportunities for patients with low-third rectal cancers to preserve their anal sphincters, but only a few studies provide limited evidence that demonstrates the benefit in OS rates from CRT. Till date, based on the NCCN guidelines, standard neoadjuvant CRT uses single 5-FU-based chemotherapy. The applications of neoadjuvant CT are yet being studied in clinical trials, whereas CRT for rectal cancers has been refined further. The future directions of CRT include achieving higher local control rates, more refined treatments, and smaller side effects. Although more clinical evidence is required to evaluate the effects of preoperative or molecular-targeted combined CT, we believe that with the rapid developments in molecular biology, the era of precise treatments for rectal cancer is approaching.

References

1. Ferlay J, Soerjomataram I, Dikshit R, Eser S, Mathers C, Rebelo M, et al. Cancer incidence and mortality worldwide: sources, methods and major patterns in GLOBOCAN 2012. Int J Cancer. 2015;136(5):E359–86. https://doi.org/10.1002/ijc.29210.
2. Dbeis R, Smart NJ, Daniels IR. Focusing the management of rectal cancer. Ann Transl Med. 2016;4(24):521. https://doi.org/10.21037/atm.2016.11.80.
3. Trakarnsanga A, Ithimakin S, Weiser MR. Treatment of locally advanced rectal cancer: controversies and questions. World J Gastroenterol. 2012;18(39):5521–32. https://doi.org/10.3748/wjg.v18.i39.5521.
4. Li Y, Wang J, Ma X, Tan L, Yan Y, Xue C, Hui B, Liu R, Ma H, Ren J. A review of neoadjuvant chemoradiotherapy for locally advanced rectal cancer. Int J Biol Sci. 2016;12(8):1022–31. https://doi.org/10.7150/ijbs.15438.
5. Krook JE, Moertel CG, Gunderson LL, et al. Effective surgical adjuvant therapy for high-risk rectal carcinoma. N Engl J Med. 1991;324:709–15.
6. Mineur L, Maingon P, Radosevic-Jelic L, Daban A, Bardet E, Beny A. Chemotherapy with preoperative radiotherapy in rectal cancer. N Engl J Med. 2006;355(11):1114–23.
7. NIH consensus conference: adjuvant therapy for patients with colon and rectal cancer. JAMA. 1990;264:1444–50.
8. Madoff RD. Chemoradiotherapy for rectal cancer—when, why, and how? N Engl J Med. 2004;351(17):1790–2.
9. Sauer R, Becker H, Hohenberger W, Rödel C, Wittekind C, Fietkau R, Martus P, Tschmelitsch J, Hager E, Hess CF, Karstens JH, Liersch T, Schmidberger H, Raab R, German Rectal Cancer Study Group. Preoperative versus postoperative chemoradiotherapy for rectal cancer. N Engl J Med. 2004;351:1731–40.
10. Belluco C, Forlin M, Olivieri M, Cannizzaro R, Canzonieri V, Buonadonna A, Bidoli E, Matrone F, Bertola G, De Paoli A. Long-term outcome of rectal cancer with clinically (EUS/MRI) metastatic mesorectal lymph nodes treated by neoadjuvant chemoradiation: role of organ preservation strategies in relation to pathologic response. Ann Surg Oncol. 2016;23:4302–9. https://doi.org/10.1245/s10434-016-5451-5.
11. Arbea L, Ramos LI, Martínez-Monge R, Moreno M, Aristu J. Intensity-modulated radiation therapy (IMRT) vs. 3D conformal radiotherapy (3DCRT) in locally advanced rectal cancer (LARC): dosimetric comparison and clinical implications. Radiat Oncol. 2010;5:1–9.
12. Petrelli F, Sgroi G, Sarti E, Barni S. Increasing the interval between neoadjuvant chemoradiotherapy and surgery in rectal cancer. Ann Surg. 2013;263(3):458–64. https://doi.org/10.1097/SLA.0000000000000368.

13. Heald RJ. The 'Holy Plane' of rectal surgery. J R Soc Med. 1988;81(9):503–8.

14. Frasson M, Garcia-Granero E, Roda D, Flor-lorente B. Preoperative chemoradiation may not always be needed for patients with T3 and T2N+ rectal cancer. Cancer. 2011;117:3118–25. https://doi.org/10.1002/cncr.25866.

15. Weiser MR, Zhang Z, Schrag D. Locally advanced rectal cancer: time for precision therapeutics. Am Soc Clin Oncol Educ Book. 2015;35:e192–6.

16. Hong TS, Kachnic LA. Preoperative chemoradiotherapy in the management of localized rectal cancer: the new standard. Gastrointest Cancer Res. 2007;1:49–56.

17. Kouyama Y, Kudo S-E, Miyachi H, Ichimasa K, Hisayuki T, Oikawa H, Matsudaira S, Kimura YJ, Misawa M, Mori Y, Kodama K, Kudo T, Hayashi T, Wakamura K, Katagiri A, Hidaka E, Ishida F, Hamatani S. Practical problems of measuring depth of submucosal invasion in T1 colorectal carcinomas. Int J Color Dis. 2016;31:137–46.

18. Ong MLH, Schofield JB. Assessment of lymph node involvement in colorectal cancer. World J Gastrointest Surg. 2016;8:179–92.

19. Samdani T, Garcia-Aguilar J. Imaging in rectal cancer: magnetic resonance imaging versus endorectal ultrasonography. Surg Oncol Clin N Am. 2014;23:59–77.

20. Ferrari L, Fichera A. Neoadjuvant chemoradiation therapy and pathological complete response in rectal cancer. Gastroenterol Rep. 2015;3(4):277–88. https://doi.org/10.1093/gastro/gov039.

21. Lombardi R, Cuicchi D, Pinto C, Di Fabio F, Iacopino B, Neri S, Tardio ML, Ceccarelli C, Lecce F, Ugolini G, Pini S, Di Tullio P, Taffurelli M, Minni F, Martoni A, Cola B. Clinically-staged T3N0 rectal cancer: is preoperative chemoradiotherapy the optimal treatment? Ann Surg Oncol. 2010;17:838–45. https://doi.org/10.1245/s10434-009-0796-7.

22. Cedars Sinai. Rectal cancer. NCCN Clinical Practice Guidelines in Oncology, versuib 2. 2017. Retrieved from http://www.cedars-sinai.edu/Patients/Programs-and-Services/Colorectal-Cancer-Center/Services-and-Treatments/Rectal-Cancer.aspx

23. Jo P, Nietert M, Gusky L, Kitz J, Conradi LC, Müller-Dornieden A, Schüler P, Wolff HA, Rüschoff J, Ströbel P, Grade M, Liersch T, Beißbarth T, Ghadimi MB, Sax U, Gaedcke J. Neoadjuvant therapy in rectal cancer - biobanking of preoperative tumor biopsies. Sci Rep. 2016;6:35589. https://doi.org/10.1038/srep35589.

24. Snijders HS, Leersum NJ, Van Henneman D, Vries AC, De Tollenaar RAEM, Stiggelbout AM, Wouters MW, Dekker JWT. Optimal treatment strategy in rectal cancer surgery: should we be cowboys or chickens? Ann Surg Oncol. 2015;22(11):3582–9. https://doi.org/10.1245/s10434-015-4385-7.

25. Brændengen M, Tveit KM, Berglund Å, Birkemeyer E, Gunilla Frykholm LP, Wiig JN, Byström P, Bujko K, Glimelius B. Randomized phase III study comparing preoperative radiotherapy with chemoradiotherapy in nonresectable rectal cancer. J Clin Oncol. 2008;26(22):3687–94. https://doi.org/10.1200/JCO.2007.15.3858.A.

26. Gunderson LL, Sosin H. Areas of failure found at reoperation (secondor symptomatic look) following curative surgery for adenocarcinoma ofthe rectum: clinicopathologic correlation and implications foradjuvant therapy. Cancer. 1974;34:1278–92.

27. Higgins GA, Humphrey EW, Dwight RW, et al. Preoperative radiation and surgery for cancer of the rectum. Veterans administration surgical oncology group trial II. Cancer. 1986;58(2):352–9.

28. Izar F, Fourtanier G, Pradere B, et al. Pre-operative radiotherapy as adjuvant treatment in rectal cancer. Cancer. 1992;16(1):106–11. Discussion 111–2.

29. Hyams DM, Mamounas EP, Petrelli N, et al. A clinical trial to evaluate the worth of preoperative multimodality therapy in patients with operable carcinoma of the rectum: a progress report of National Surgical Breast and Bowel Project Protocol R-03. Dis Colon Rectum. 1997;40(2):131.

30. Aklilu M, Eng C. The current landscape of locally advanced rectal cancer. Nat Rev Clin Oncol. 2011;8(11):649–59.

31. Lai LL, Fuller CD, Kachnic LA, et al. Can pelvic radiotherapy be omitted in select patients with rectal cancer? Semin Oncol. 2006;33(11):70–4.

32. Sauer R, Liersch T, Merkel S, Fietkau R, Hohenberger W, Hess C. Preoperative versus postoperative chemoradiotherapy for locally advanced rectal cancer: results of the German CAO/ARO/AIO-94 randomized phase III trial after a median follow-up of 11 years. J Clin Oncol. 2012;30(16):1926–33. https://doi.org/10.1200/JCO.2011.40.1836.

33. Bosset JF, Pavy JJ, Hamers HP, et al. Determination of the optimal dose of 5-fluorouracil when combined with low dose D,L-leucovorin and irradiation in rectal cancer: results of three consecutive phase II studies. Eur J Cancer. 1993;29A:1406–10.

34. Bosset JF, Calais G, Mineur L, et al. Enhanced tumoricidal effect of chemotherapy with preoperative radiotherapy for rectal cancer: preliminary results—EORTC 22921. J Clin Oncol. 2005;23:5620–7.

35. Bosset JF, Calais G, Daban A, et al. Pre-operative chemoradiotherapy versus preoperative radiotherapy in rectal cancer patients: assessment of acute toxicity and treatment compliance—report of the 22921 randomised trial conducted by the EORTC Radiotherapy Group. Eur J Cancer. 2004;40:219–24.

36. Heald RJ, Husband EM, Ryall RD. The mesorectum in rectal cancer surgery: the clue to pelvic recurrence? Br J Surg. 1982;82:613–6.

37. Swedish Rectal Cancer Trial. Improved survival with preoperative radiotherapy in resectable rectal cancer. N Engl J Med. 1997;336:980–7.

38. Kapiteijn E, Marijnen CA, Nagtegaal ID, Putter H, Steup WH, Wiggers T, Rutten HJ, Pahlman L, Glimelius B, van Krieken JH, Leer JW, van de Velde CJ. Preoperative radiotherapy combined with total mesorectal excision for resectable rectal cancer. N Engl J Med. 2001;345:638–46.

39. Shi C, Zhou H, Li X, Cai Y. A retrospective analysis on two-week short-course pre-operative radiotherapy in elderly patients with resectable locally advanced rectal cancer. Sci Rep. 2016;6:37866. https://doi.org/10.1038/srep37866.

40. Wang L, Li YH, Cai Y, Zhan TC, Gu J. Intermediate neoadjuvant radiotherapy combined with total mesorectal excision for locally advancd rectal cancer: outcomes after a median follow-up of 5 years. Clin Colorectal Cancer. 2016;15(2):152–7.

41. Liu G, Yan J, He Q, An X, Pan Z, Ding P. Effect of neoadjuvant chemoradiotherapy with capecitabine versus fluorouracil for locally advanced rectal cancer: a meta-analysis. Gastroenterol Res Pract. 2016;2016:1–10. https://doi.org/10.1155/2016/1798285.

42. Allegra CJ, Yothers G, O'Connell MJ, Beart RW, Wozniak TF, Pitot HC, Shields AF, Landry JC, Ryan DP, Arora A, Evans LS, Bahary N, Soori G, Eakle JF, Robertson JM, Moore DF, Mullane MR, Marchello BT, Ward PJ, Sharif S, Roh MS, Wolmark N. Neoadjuvant 5-FU or capecitabine plus radiation with or without oxaliplatin in rectal cancer patients: a phase III randomized clinical trial. J Natl Cancer Inst. 2015;107:djv248.

43. Aschele C, Cionini L, Lonardi S, Pinto C, Cordio S, Rosati G, Artale S, Tagliagambe A, Ambrosini G, Rosetti P, Bonetti A, Negru ME, Tronconi MC, Luppi G, Silvano G, Corsi DC, Bochicchio AM, Chiaulon G, Gallo M, Boni L. Primary tumor response to preoperative chemoradiation with or without oxaliplatin in locally advanced rectal cancer: pathologic results of the STAR-01 randomized phase III trial. J Clin Oncol. 2011;29:2773–80.

44. Gérard J-P, Azria D, Gourgou-Bourgade S, Martel-Lafay I, Hennequin C, Etienne P-L, Vendrely V, François E, de La Roche G, Bouché O, Mirabel X, Denis B, Mineur L, Berdah J-F, Mahé M-A, Bécouarn Y, Dupuis O, Lledo G, Seitz J-F, Bedenne L, Juzyna B, Conroy T. Clinical outcome of the ACCORD 12/0405 PRODIGE 2 randomized trial in rectal cancer. J Clin Oncol. 2012;30:4558–65.

45. Machiels JP, Sempoux C, Scalliet P, et al. Phase I/II study of preoperative cetuximab, capecitabine, and external beam radiotherapy in patients with rectal cancer. Ann Oncol. 2007;18:738–44.

46. Bertolini F, Chiara S, Bengala C, et al. Neoadjuvant treatment with single-agent cetuximab followed by 5-FU, cetuximab,and pelvic radiotherapy: a phase II study in locally advanced rectal cancer. Int J Radiat Oncol Biol Phys. 2009;73:466–72.

47. Rodel C, Arnold D, Hipp M, et al. Phase I-II trial of cetuximab,capecitabine, oxaliplatin, and radiotherapy as preoperative treatment in rectal cancer. Int J Radiat Oncol Biol Phys. 2008;70:1081–6.

48. Horisberger K, Treschl A, Mai S, et al. Cetuximab in combination with capecitabine, irinotecan, and radiotherapy for patients with locally advanced rectal cancer: results of a phase II MARGIT trial. Int J Radiat Oncol Biol Phys. 2009;74:1487–93.

49. Kim SY, Hong YS, Kim DY, et al. Preoperative chemoradiation with cetuximab, irinotecan, and capecitabine in patients with locally advanced resectable rectal cancer: a multicenter phase II study. Int J Radiat Oncol Biol Phys. 2011;81(3):677–83.

50. Dewdney A, Cunningham D, Tabernero J, et al. Multicenter randomized phase II clinical trial comparing neoadjuvant oxaliplatin, capecitabine, and preoperative radiotherapy with or without cetuximab followed by total mesorectal excision in patients with high-risk rectal cancer (EXPERT-C). J Clin Oncol. 2012;30(14):1620–7.

51. Willett CG, Duda DG, di Tomaso E, Boucher Y, Ancukiewicz M, Sahani DV, Lahdenranta J, Chung DC, Fischman AJ, Lauwers GY, Shellito P, Czito BG, Wong TZ, Paulson E, Poleski M, Vujaskovic Z, Bentley R, Chen HX, Clark JW, Jain RK. Efficacy, safety, and biomarkers of neoadjuvant bevacizumab, radiation therapy, and fluorouracil in rectal cancer: a multidisciplinary phase II study. J Clin Oncol. 2009;27:3020–6.

52. Crane CH, Eng C, Feig BW, Das P, Skibber JM, Chang GJ, Wolff RA, Krishnan S, Hamilton S, Janjan NA, Maru DM, Ellis LM, Rodriguez-Bigas MA. Phase II trial of neoadjuvant bevacizumab, capecitabine, and radiotherapy for locally advanced rectal cancer. Int J Radiat Oncol Biol Phys. 2010;76:824–30.

53. Velenik V, Ocvirk J, Music M, Bracko M, Anderluh F, Oblak I, Edhemovic I, Brecelj E, Kropivnik M, Omejc M. Neoadjuvant capecitabine, radiotherapy, and bevacizumab (CRAB) in locally advanced rectal cancer: results of an open-label phase II study. Radiat Oncol. 2011;6:105.

54. Salazar R, Capdevila J, Laquente B. A randomized phase II study of capecitabine-based chemoradiation with or without bevacizumab in resectable locally advanced rectal cancer: clinical and biological features. BMC Cancer. 2015;15:60.

55. Gasparini G, Torino F, Ueno T, Cascinu S, Troiani T, Ballestrero A, Berardi R, Shishido J, Yoshizawa A, Mori Y, Nagayama S, Morosini P, Toi M. A phase II study of neoadjuvant bevacizumab plus capecitabine and concomitant radiotherapy in patients with locally advanced rectal cancer. Angiogenesis. 2012;15:141–50.

56. Landry JC, Feng Y, Cohen SJ, Staley CA. Phase 2 study of preoperative radiation with concurrent capecitabine, oxaliplatin, and bevacizumab followed by surgery and postoperative 5-fluorouracil, leucovorin, oxaliplatin (FOLFOX), and bevacizumab in patients with locally advanced rectal cancer: ECOG 3204. Cancer. 2013;119(8):1521–7.

57. Ludmir EB, Palta M, Willett CG, Czito BG. Total neoadjuvant therapy for rectal cancer: an emerging option. Cancer. 2017;123:1497–506.

58. Sclafani F, Cunningham D. Neoadjuvant chemotherapy without radiotherapy for locally advanced rectal cancer. Future Oncol. 2014;10(14):2243–57.

59. Fernandez-Martos C, Pericay C, Aparicio J, et al. Phase II, randomized study of concomitant chemoradiother-

apy followed by surgery and adjuvant capecitabine plus oxaliplatin (CAPOX) compared with induction CAPOX followed by concomitant hemoradiotherapy and surgery in magnetic resonance imaging-defined, locally advanced rectal cancer: Grupo cancer de recto 3 study. J Clin Oncol. 2010;28(5):859–65.

60. Ishii Y, Hasegawa H, Endo T, et al. Medium-term results of neoadjuvant systemic chemotherapy using irinotecan, 5-fluorouracil,and leucovorin in patients with locally advanced rectal cancer. Eur J Surg Oncol. 2010;36:1061–5.

61. Uehara K, Hiramatsu K, Maeda A, et al. Neoadjuvant oxaliplatin and capecitabine and bevacizumab without radiotherapyfor poor-risk rectal cancer: N-SOG 03 phase II trial. Jpn J Clin Oncol. 2013;43:964–71.

62. Hasegawa J, Nishimura J, Mizushima T, et al. Neoadjuvant capecitabine and oxaliplatin (XELOX) combined with bevacizumab for high-risk localized rectal cancer. Cancer Chemother Pharmacol. 2014; 73:1079–87.

63. Schrag D, Weiser MR, Goodman KA, et al. Neoadjuvant chemotherapy without routine use of radiation therapy for patients with locally advanced rectal cancer: a pilot trial. J Clin Oncol. 2014;32:513–8.

64. Trakarnsanga A, Gonen M, Shia J, et al. What is the significance of the circumferential margin in locally advanced rectal cancer after neoadjuvant chemoradiotherapy? Ann Surg Oncol. 2013;20:1179–84.

65. Glimelius B, Tiret E, Cervantes A, et al. Rectal cancer: ESMO clinical practice guidelines for diagnosis, treatment and follow-up. Ann Oncol. 2013;24(6):81–8.

66. Wang Q-X, Li S-H, Zhang X, Xie L, Cai P-Q, An X, et al. Identification of locally advanced rectal cancer with low risk of local recurrence. PLoS One. 2015; 10(1):e0117141.

67. MERCURY Study Group. Extramural depth of tumor invasion at thin-section MR in patients with rectal cancer: results of the MERCURY study. Radiology. 2007;243(1): 132–9.

68. Mass M, Nelemans PJ, Valentini V, et al. Long-term outcome in patients with a pathological complete response after chemoradiation for rectal cancer: a pooled analysis of individual patient data. Lancet Oncol. 2010;11:835–44.

69. Sun YS, Zhang XP, Tang L, Ji JF, Gu J, Cai Y, Zhang XY. Locally advanced rectal carcinoma treated with preoperative chemotherapy and radiation therapy: preliminary analysis of difussion-weighted MR imaging for early detection of tumor histopathologic downstaging. Radiology. 2009;254:170–8.

70. Maas M, Beets-Tan RG, Lambregts DM, et al. Wait-and-see policy for clinical complete responders after chemoradiation for rectal cancer. J Clin Oncol. 2011;29(35):4633.

71. Habr-Gama A, Perez RO, Nadalin W, Sabbaga J, Ribeiro U Jr, Silva e Sousa AH Jr, Campos FG, Kiss DR, Gama- Rodrigues J. Operative versus nonoperative treatment for stage 0 distal rectal cancer following chemoradiation therapy: long term results. Ann Surg. 2004;240:711–7.

72. Hernandez-Carcia I, Viudez A, Suarez J, et al. Clinical complete response in locally advanced rectal cancer: can we offer a wait-and-see policy? Ann Oncol. 2013;24(3):853.

73. Kwak YK, Kim K, Lee JH, et al. Timely tumor response analysis after preoperative chemoradiotherapy and curative surgery in locally advanced rectal cancer: a multi-institutional study for optimal surical timing in rectal cancer. Radiother Oncol. 2016;119(3):512–8.

74. Lefevre JH, Mineur L, Kotti S, et al. Effect of interval (7 or 11 weeks) between neoaduavant radiochemotherapy and surgery on complete pathologic response in rectal cancer: a multicenter, randomized, controlled trial (GRECCAR-6). J Clin Oncol. 2016;34:3773.

75. Bujko K, Nowacki MP, Michalski W, Bebenek M, Kryj M. Long-term results of a randomized trial comparing preoperative short-course radiotherapy with preoperative conventionally fractionated chemoradiation for rectal cancer. Br J Surg. 2006;93:1215–23. https://doi.org/10.1002/bjs.5506.

76. Trotti A, Barthel JS, Kim CJ, Yeatman TJ, Coppola D, Trotti A, Williams B. Local excision of T2 and T3 rectal cancers after downstaging chemoradiation. Ann Surg. 2001;234(3):352–9. https://doi.org/10.1097/00000658-200109000-00009.

Tailored Surgical Treatment Based on Response to Neoadjuvant Therapy

9

In Ja Park and Chang Sik Yu

Abstract

Introduction of neoadjuvant chemoradiotherapy for rectal cancer results in diversity of surgical treatment. It is based on the variable response to neoadjuvant therapy. Favorable oncologic outcomes of patients with good response to neoadjuvant therapy have been reported, and organ-preserving strategies have extended its application for these patients. However, definition of good response to neoadjuvant therapy has not clearly defined, and different categorization has been used in many researches. Usually pathologic regression grade is used for identification of good responder, but the pathologic grading system is diverse. Recently MRI is increasing in use to define response to neoadjuvant therapy because pathologic assessment is not available before surgical treatment. MRI is more useful to set plan to surgical strategies. But, the accuracy of MRI is not satisfactory as well as other imaging modalities. Therefore, we have to determine the definition of response level and standard method of assessment.

There are ongoing active studies regarding surgical or observational strategies for good responders to neoadjuvant therapy.

Functional preservation was the most attractive aspect of these strategies, but the long-term functional and oncological outcomes are not well established. In addition, the surveillance strategies are not yet established and have no consensus. Before extension of organ-preserving strategies, indication, and surveillance have to be preconditioned.

Although researches focused on good responder to neoadjuvant therapy is increasing, poor responders is not interested in surgical field. Considerate approach to poor responder to neoadjuvant therapy is needed in surgical as well as medical treatment.

Keywords

Neoadjuvant therapy · Rectal cancer · Organ-preserving strategy · Response level

9.1 Introduction

Neoadjuvant therapy was initiated as an attempt to improve oncologic outcome and provided a chance to introduce changes in the surgical treatment environment. Although there are different views on whether neoadjuvant therapy improves survival rate, numerous studies have reported a decrease in local recurrence in patients treated with neoadjuvant therapy, and it has been established as a standard treatment for locally advanced rectal cancer,

I. J. Park (✉) · C. S. Yu
Department of Colon and Rectal Surgery,
University of Ulsan College of Medicine and Asan
Medical Center, Seoul, South Korea
e-mail: ipark@amc.seoul.kr; csyu007@gmail.com

© Springer Nature Singapore Pte Ltd. 2018
N. K. Kim et al. (eds.), *Surgical Treatment of Colorectal Cancer*,
https://doi.org/10.1007/978-981-10-5143-2_9

alongside TME [1–3]. However, there is a wide range of tumor regression after neoadjuvant therapy, and oncologic outcome differs by degree of regression, which led to the pursuit of diversity in surgical treatment [4–6]. Recently, in addition to interest in quality of life and realization of the need for individualized treatment, there has been an increase in the need for various surgical treatments according to the response to neoadjuvant therapy. In this chapter, we review such various types of surgical treatments, their outcomes, and problems from evaluation of response after neoadjuvant therapy.

9.2   Evaluation of Tumor Response After Neoadjuvant Therapy

When pursuing diversity of treatment according to oncologic response after neoadjuvant therapy, the fundamental standard criterion is needed to evaluate the level of response before determination of adequate treatment among diverse options. The evaluation of response after neoadjuvant therapy follows various degrees of pathologic tumor regression grade (TRG), which is based on the percentage of fibrosis and residual tumor (Fig. 9.1) [7, 8]. However, as studies have been published showing that ypT stage better reflects prognosis than degree of tumor regression, whether to use the degree of pathological regression as an evaluation standard for the level of response and to what extent tumors should be classified as good responders have not been established. Regardless, degree of pathological regression or ypT stage is determined after the primary lesion is completely resected and therefore cannot be used for determining surgical treatment after neoadjuvant therapy. Hence, the level of response from neoadjuvant therapy is evaluated through various radiological and physical examinations prior to determining the direction of surgical treatment.

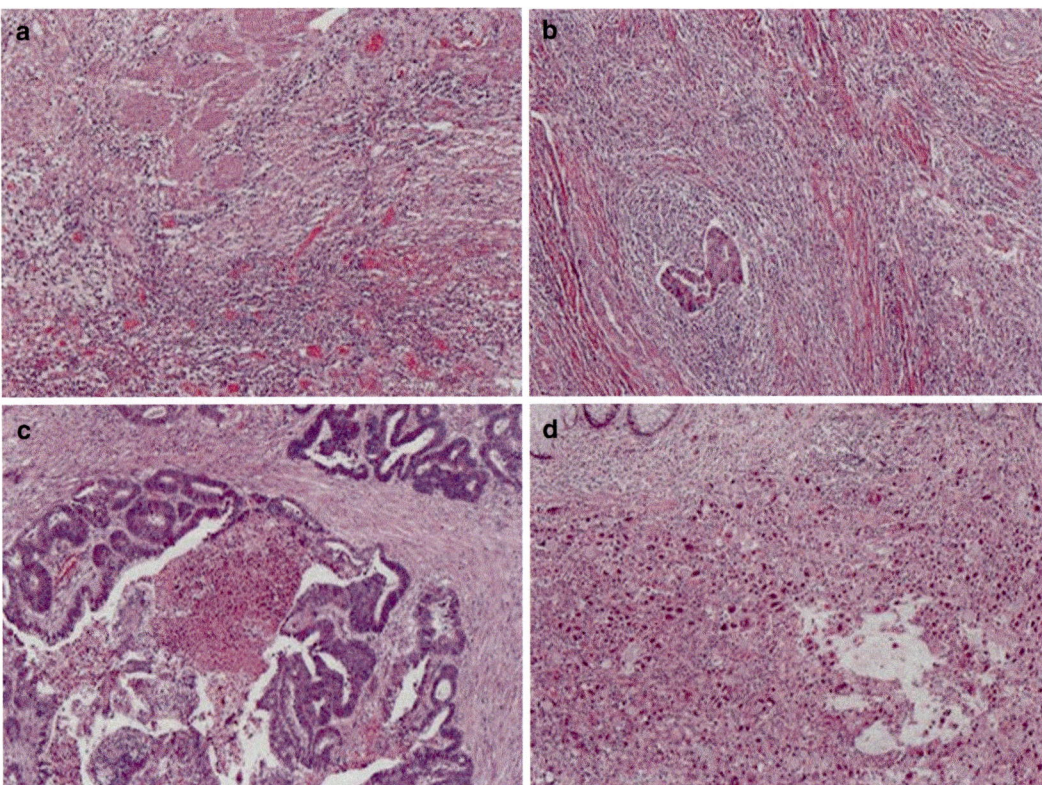

Fig. 9.1 Pathologic tumor regression grade (TRG). (**a**) Total regression. No viable tumor cells are identified. (**b**) Near total regression. Fibrosis and scattered tumor cells. (**c**) Moderate regression. Predominantly fibrosis with scattered tumor cells. (**d**) Minimal regression. Predominantly tumor with significant fibrosis

The most widely used and consistently studied evaluation method is magnetic resonance imaging (MRI). As the indication for neoadjuvant therapy is determined through MRI, the response can be also evaluated through MRI, which is an advantage of this technique. However, the accuracy of restaging evaluation after neoadjuvant therapy is not satisfactory. Numerous studies and metastasis analyses currently report that the accuracy of the T stage is 34–82%, and the accuracy of the N stage is 60–88% [9–13]. There have been attempts to improve the accuracy of MRI using various auxiliary methods. The addition of diffusion-weighted imaging improves the accuracy of assessment of complete responders up to 82–88% [14, 15]. However, evaluating the depth of tumor invasion is still limited, and the accuracy of predicting total regression also varies, according to reports.

In order to assess the response to treatment, Brown G group [16], who continuously studied the evaluation of stage based on MRI, proposed MRI-based tumor regression grade (mrTRG) to classify the degree of response, taking into account the percentage of fibrosis and residual tumor by MRI, similarly to the evaluation of pathological regression (Fig. 9.2). It has been shown that prognosis can be sufficiently predicted from tumor classification using mrTRG [16, 17]. Studies on the evaluation of tumor response after neoadjuvant therapy are focused on the T stage, and this is true of both pathological and MRI evaluations. There is no consensus standard for the degree of pathological regression

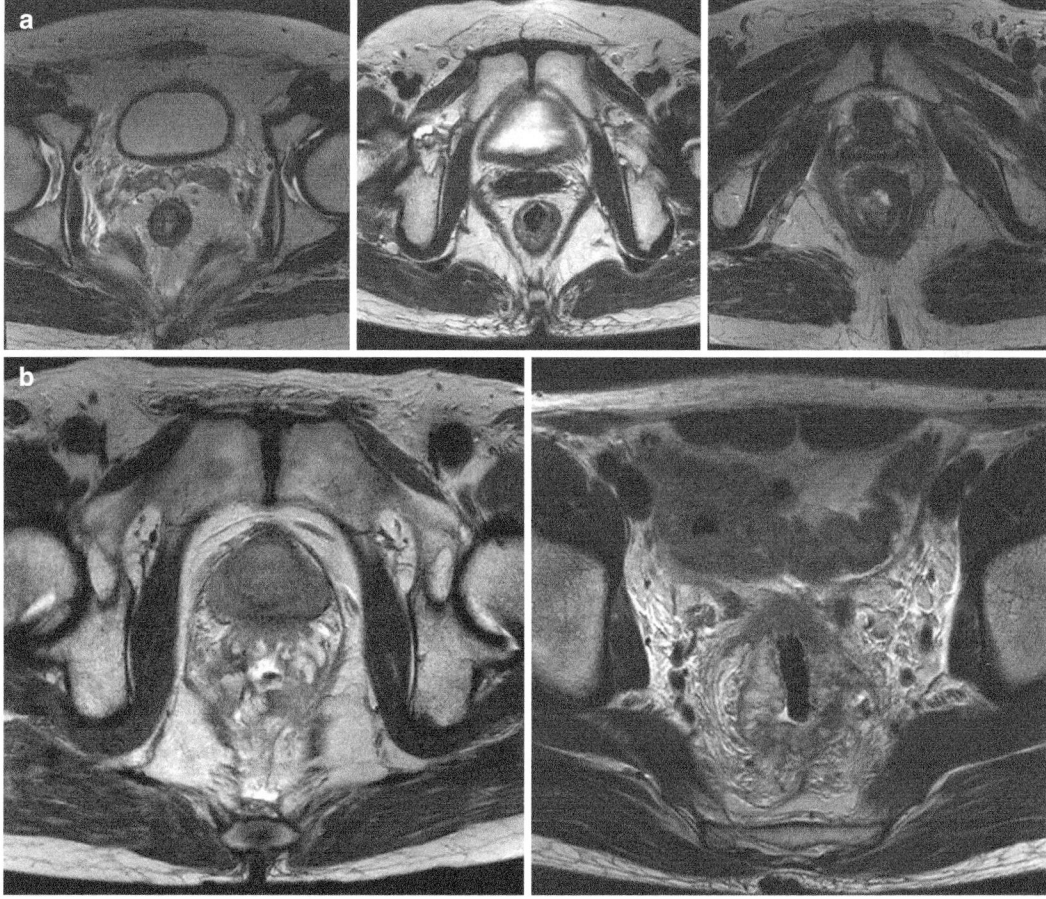

Fig. 9.2 Tumor regression grade by MRI imaging (mrTRG). (**a**) Good MRI tumor regression with mrTRG (grades 1, 2, 3): complete remission, fibrosis or more fibrosis than tumor in the residual lesion. (**b**) Poor MRI tumor regression with mrTRG (grades 4 and 5): more tumor than fibrosis in the residual lesion or unchanged/increased tumor

for the N stage, and very few studies have been conducted in this area. Although there have been numerous studies on diagnosing lymph node (LN) metastasis by MRI, the standard for metastasis varies between studies, and the accuracy is below the desired standards [11–13]. The mrTRG also does not take into account LN metastasis. However, LN metastasis is one of the most important factors affecting prognosis. It is generally known that the frequency of LN metastasis varies according to progression as assessed by T stage [18]. Previous studies have attempted to indirectly assess and predict LN metastasis through the T stage; however, we believe that the evaluation of the N stage requires more attention when examining LN metastasis.

In addition to MRI, there have been attempts to evaluate the depth of invasion using computed tomography (CT) and endorectal ultrasound (ERUS), but the results were disappointing, and these techniques are not usually independently used in the clinic. As the metabolic activity of the actual tumor is evaluated, there have been approaches examining the use of positron-emission tomography (PET). Based on the results of previous studies, PET/CT seems to be a useful addition to the current repertoire of imaging modalities in assessing rectal cancer and treatment response [19]. However, availability and validation means are lacking for PET, and it appears to be a more useful tool for specific situations, when additional information is needed. It would provide information about systemic metastatic or accompanying lesions. There have been many efforts to try various surgical treatments on good responders after neoadjuvant therapy and to differentially apply adjuvant treatment according to the level of response. However, there is no consensus on the method, evaluation standard, or accuracy for evaluating response. In particular, noninvasive diagnostic methods and prognosis evaluation of metastatic LNs are not sufficiently reflected in the evaluation of response after neoadjuvant therapy.

Currently, the implementation of tailored treatment according to the level of response after neoadjuvant therapy and establishing the standard of response level are ongoing. Therefore, it is vital that we maintain constant interest and make efforts for the application of tailored treatment, as well as the establishment of the standard that will be its basis. This will be the most important factor for the proper application of tailored treatment.

9.3 Organ-Preserving Strategies for Patients with Good Response After Neoadjuvant Therapy

Organ-preserving strategies are used to avoid rectal excision in patients who are likely to have no residual tumor, as clear tumor shrinkage was observed after neoadjuvant therapy. Such strategies are largely divided into local excision and "wait and watch" strategies. Both strategies require proper surveillance to ensure the best patient outcome.

9.3.1 Local Excision

The most appealing advantage of local excision is that the degree of pathological regression can be directly evaluated. Therefore, it can be considered as the method that allows for final confirmation and complementation of the limitations of physical, radiological, and endoscopic examinations. However, LNs cannot be evaluated, as only the primary tumor is excised. The LN metastasis rate increases along with the progression of the primary tumor; however, a number of reports have shown that local excision alone can yield favorable long-term prognosis in cases of total regression, in which LN metastasis is reported as below 2–17% after neoadjuvant therapy [6, 20–22]. Studies have reported acceptable oncologic outcome after local excision in patients with clinically good response to neoadjuvant therapy (Table 9.1).

There are conflicting views on the relationship between the extent of progression and the range of local excision. Some studies reported acceptable oncologic outcome after local excision, even for ypT2 lesions. However, up to 20% of ypT2

Table 9.1 Oncologic outcomes after excision for rectal cancer patients treated with neoadjuvant therapy

Author	Year	No.	Chemotherapeutic agent	Radiation dose, Gy	cCR, %	Interval, weeks[a]	pCR, %	Radical surgery, %[b]	Median F/U, mon	Local recurrence, %	Disease-free survival, %	Overall survival, %
Kim	2001	26	5FU/45	45	84.6	–	65.4	22.2	19	4.2	–	–
Ruo	2002	10	5FU/5FU-LV	36–50.4	–	4–6	30	0	28.5	10	–	78
Hershman	2003	33	5FU	39–45	–	6–8	21.2	0	45	15.4	CSS 94	78
Nair	2008	44	5FU	45	70.5	–	56.8	41.7	64	7.7	–	–
Callender	2010	47	5FU	45–52.5	–	–	48.9	0	63	10.6	–	–
Belluco	2011	29	5FU 5FU/LV Xeloda XELOX	45–50.4			58.6					
Kenelly	2012	10	5FU Xeloda	50	50	8	60	0	24	0	–	–
Issa	2012	31	5FU-LV	45	–	5–18	74.2	8	87	0	–	86.7
Perez	2013	27	5-FU/LV	50.4–54	–	7.9 (4.7–15.4)[c]	64	30.8	24	5.3	–	–
Bujko	2013	89	No CTx	50.4 or 25	–	6.4 (3.6–17.4)[c]	35.9	–	–	21.5		
Marks	2013	49	Xeloda	45 ± 10.8	–	12 (7–46)[c]	22.4	–	36.3	6.1	–	88
Puciarelli	2013	63	Xeloda XELOX	45, 56	30.2	9.3 (5.9–20.1)[c]	66.7	55	–	3.2		
Lee	2014	27	5FU/FOLFOX	44–50.4	–	4–8	55.6	–	81.9	11.1	–	–
Noh	2014	17	FU Xeloda S1	44–54	–	7.6 (5.7–10.7)[c]	58.8	–	75	11.8	82	–
Guerrieri	2014	305	5FU	50.4	80 (26.2)	5.7–7.1	–	–	52	11.1	–	–
Stipa	2014	43	5FU/Xeloda	50.4	–	–	30.2	–	81	39.5	–	–
Verseveld	2015	55	Xeloda	50–50.4	–	8–10	44.7	47.1	17	10.3	–	–
Jung	2016	43	5FU/Xeloda	50–50.4	–	6–8	61.9	–	56	4.8	95.2	96.6
ACOSOG Z6041	2016	79	FOLFOX	50.4	–	4–8	49	–	56	4	79.3	80.3

FU fluorouracil, *LV* leucovorin, *FOLFOX* fluorouracil and oxaliplatin, *XELOX* Xeloda and oxaliplatin, *cCR* clinical complete remission, *pCR* pathologic complete remission, *CSS* cancer-specific survival, *CTX* chemotherapy, *TS-1* tegafur/gimeracil/oteracil, *AOSOG* American College of Surgeons Oncology Group
[a]Interval, weeks from completion of neoadjuvant therapy and surgery
[b]Percentage of patients who receive radical resection among patients showing pathologic risk factors on local excision
[c]Mean (range)

lesions are known to have LN metastasis, and patient prognosis is poor when LN metastasis is present, even when radical resection is performed. This makes it difficult to generalize the application of local excision in ypT2 lesions. Hence, radical resection is currently recommended when the lesion is ypT2 or higher after local excision or when there are pathological risk factors, such as margin involvement. However, less than 70% of patients in whom radical resection is recommended after local excision actually undergo the procedure [23–25]. Long-term follow-up of these patients suggests extremely poor prognosis. Therefore, interest in the compliance of immediate salvage surgery in patients who are to receive radical resection after local excision, as well as efforts to improve compliance, is required.

Surgical complications that can occur after local excision are also an important matter. In the ACOSOG Z6041 trial [23], a recently published phase II study examining local excision after neoadjuvant therapy reported that 23% of patients experienced surgery-related grade 3–4 complications. Such local excision-related problems raise the interests in nonsurgical treatment.

9.3.2 Wait and Watch

This strategy gained attention when Habr-Gama et al. first published the long-term oncologic outcome of patients who received nonsurgical treatment for rectal cancer after neoadjuvant therapy in 2004 [20]. Their group observed excellent outcome in terms of local recurrence and disease-free survival, which was of great interest in the field (Table 9.2). However, they faced criticism, as their results could not be reproduced in follow-up studies by other groups (Table 9.3). The Habr-Gama group used colonoscopy, MRI, and CT as standards for evaluating response, but these methods lacked accuracy in evaluating local lesions, and the group was criticized for not adequately assessing patient outcome. In the wait and watch method, detection of tumor regrowth is vital for surveillance. Luminal regrowth is reported to occur in 6–60% of patients, and the timing of its occurrence and detection varies [26–28].

Upon early detection, salvage surgery can increase favorable outcome. However, detection is difficult under submucosal growth or when the lesion is accompanied, and performing salvage surgery on patients with tumor regrowth already

Table 9.2 Series from Habr-Gama group regarding wait and watch strategies for rectal cancer treated with neoadjuvant therapy

Year	No.	cCR, %	Follow-up duration, months	Local recurrence, %	Disease-free survival, %	Overall survival, %
2004	265	26.8	57.3	3	100	92
2005	260	27.3	57	0	–	92
2006	361	27.4	60	5	93	85
2006	360	27.5	NS	6	–	NS
2011	173	38.7	65	4.6	96	72

Table 9.3 Studies regarding wait and watch strategies for rectal cancer after neoadjuvant therapy

Author	Year	No	Follow-up duration, months	Local regrowth, %	Disease-free survival, %
Lim	2007	27	49	41	–
Hughes	2010	10	–	60	–
Dalton	2012	12	25.5	50	–
Maas	2011	21	25	5	2Y 89
Smith	2012	32	28	19	2Y 88
Appelt	2015	40	23.9	15.5	–
OnCoRe	2016	129	33	34	3Y 83

in progress leads to poor prognosis and is impossible in some cases. Wait and watch strategies, which have received criticism in the past, are regaining attention owing to problems that occur after local excision, as described above. Studies have been conducted on the subjects of nonsurgical treatment and their outcome, and these will continue to be examined. However, as no solid results have been presented, precaution should be taken in the application of wait and watch, and the ongoing study results must be monitored.

9.3.3   Surveillance and Indication

The method and period of surveillance are important factors to consider when performing organ-preserving treatment, such as the local excision and wait and watch strategies. Most experts agree that surveillance should be conducted more frequently in these cases than in radical resections, and surveillance is generally conducted fairly often. However, there is no consensus as to appropriate testing methods, intervals, and endpoints. Tailored surveillance must be considered when tailored treatment is applied, and it should be continuously improved.

The indication for neoadjuvant therapy is being extended, and patients who did not receive radical resection are increasing. It is increasing patients with early lesions who received neoadjuvant therapy as well as locally advanced rectal cancer. This is because organ-preserving treatment can be performed in good responders, contributing to better prognoses regardless of pretreatment clinical stage. Unlike the actual treatment, there are cases in which the indication becomes extended unintentionally, such as decreasing compliance for radical resection after local excision. Sometimes, patients are reluctant to surgical resection after completion of neoadjuvant therapy. Prognosis after neoadjuvant therapy is not clearly defined yet. In addition, oncological fate of patients who did not receive radical resection after neoadjuvant therapy has been reported in small cohorts. Indeed, in this case, the long-term effects of radiation therapy on urination and bowel functions have not been

considered, and indications that do not include the consideration of treatment for recurrence can be extended. Hence, precaution is needed to not excessively extend the indication.

9.4   Treatment for Lateral Pelvic Node Enlargement After Neoadjuvant Therapy

The current radiological diagnostic method has low accuracy for diagnosing LN metastasis. Additionally, MRI, the standard method for determining local clinical stage, also has low accuracy for diagnosing LN metastasis [29–31]. This weakness of diagnostic methods is one of the limitations of lateral node treatment. Unlike diagnosis, the oncologic effects of the lesion itself can be a factor influencing the determination of the optimal treatment method. Typically, in Western society, lateral node metastasis is assessed as distant disease and treated accordingly. In Eastern society, lateral node dissection has been strongly supported and is performed frequently. However, there have been conflicting views on its therapeutic effects [30, 32]. As shown in the study comparing cases with neoadjuvant therapy and lateral node dissection, it is known that these two methods yield similar treatment outcomes [30, 31]. Thus, treatment of lateral node metastasis should be different in patients who receive neoadjuvant therapy and those who do not.

If lateral node enlargement still exists after neoadjuvant therapy in patients who had lateral node enlargement prior to neoadjuvant therapy, there should be no disagreement from a diagnostic viewpoint for performing lateral node dissection or sampling [29–34]. However, there have been studies showing that it is unclear whether the diagnostic criterion for LN metastasis is identical after neoadjuvant therapy and whether the metastasis was diagnosed, regardless of the size. Hence, the optimal treatment when the LN size decreased after neoadjuvant therapy has not been determined. Some researchers presented LN size as a standard, and others reported that lateral wall recurrence is the most common local recurrence after neoadjuvant therapy and recommended lateral node component surgery. However, diagnostic criteria and comparison of treatment outcomes are still lacking. Therefore, additional studies for determining the optimal standard for radiological diagnosis, as well as prospective studies attempting to establish the need for surgery in the lateral lymph node and standards for the operation range, are needed. Furthermore, the oncological meaning of lateral LN metastasis in poor responders to neoadjuvant therapy and the proposition of treatment beyond surgery should also be examined.

References

1. Sauer R, Becker H, Hohenberger W, Rödel C, Wittekind C, Fietkau R, Martus P, Tschmelitsch J, Hager E, Hess CF, Karstens JH, Liersch T, Schmidberger H, Raab R, German Rectal Cancer Study Group. Preoperative versus postoperative chemoradiotherapy for rectal cancer. N Engl J Med. 2004;351:1731–40.
2. Gérard JP, Conroy T, Bonnetain F, Bouché O, Chapet O, Closon-Dejardin MT, Untereiner M, Leduc B, Francois E, Maurel J, Seitz JF, Buecher B, Mackiewicz R, Ducreux M, Bedenne L. Preoperative radiotherapy with or without concurrent fluorouracil and leucovorin in T3-4 rectal cancers: results of FFCD 9203. J Clin Oncol. 2006;24:4620–5.
3. Bosset JF, Collette L, Calais G, Mineur L, Maingon P, Radosevic-Jelic L, Daban A, Bardet E, Beny A, Ollier JC, EORTC Radiotherapy Group Trial 22921. Chemotherapy with preoperative radiotherapy in rectal cancer. N Engl J Med. 2006;355:1114–23.
4. Rödel C, Martus P, Papadoupolos T, Füzesi L, Klimpfinger M, Fietkau R, Liersch T, Hohenberger W, Raab R, Sauer R, Wittekind C. Prognostic significance of tumor regression after preoperative chemoradiotherapy for rectal cancer. J Clin Oncol. 2005; 23:8688–96.
5. Fokas E, Liersch T, Fietkau R, Hohenberger W, Beissbarth T, Hess C, Becker H, Ghadimi M, Mrak K, Merkel S, Raab HR, Sauer R, Wittekind C, Rödel C. Tumor regression grading after preoperative chemoradiotherapy for locally advanced rectal carcinoma revisited: updated results of the CAO/ARO/AIO-94 trial. J Clin Oncol. 2014;32:1554–62.
6. Park IJ, You YN, Agarwal A, Skibber JM, Rodriguez-Bigas MA, Eng C, Feig BW, Das P, Krishnan S, Crane CH, Hu CY, Chang GJ. Neoadjuvant treatment response as an early response indicator for patients with rectal cancer. J Clin Oncol. 2012;30:1770–6.
7. Trakarnsanga A, Gönen M, Shia J, Nash GM, Temple LK, Guillem JG, Paty PB, Goodman KA, Wu A, Gollub M, Segal N, Saltz L, Garcia-Aguilar J, Weiser MR. Comparison of tumor regression grade systems

for locally advanced rectal cancer after multimodality treatment. J Natl Cancer Inst. 2014;106(10):dju248.
8. Rullier A, Laurent C, Capdepont M, Vendrely V, Bioulac-Sage P, Rullier E. Impact of tumor response on survival after radiochemotherapy in locally advanced rectal carcinoma. Am J Surg Pathol. 2010; 34:562–8.
9. Pomerri F, Pucciarelli S, Maretto I, et al. Prospective assessment of imaging after preoperative chemoradiotherapy for rectal cancer. Surgery. 2011;149:56–64.
10. Johnston DF, Lawrence KM, Sizer BF, et al. Locally advanced rectal cancer: histopathological correlation and predictive accuracy of serial MRI after neoadjuvant chemotherapy. Br J Radiol. 2009;82:332–6.
11. Memon S, Lynch AC, Bressel M, Wise AG, Heriot AG. Systematic review and meta-analysis of the accuracy of MRI and endorectal ultrasound in the restaging and response assessment of rectal cancer following neoadjuvant therapy. Color Dis. 2015;17:748–61.
12. Larsen SG, Wiig JN, Emblemsvaag HL, et al. Extended total mesorectal excision in locally advanced rectal cancer (T4a) and the clinical role of MRI-evaluated neo-adjuvant downstaging. Color Dis. 2009; 11:759–67.
13. Koh DM, Chau I, Tait D, Wotherspoon A, Cunningham D, Brown G. Evaluating mesorectal lymph nodes in rectal cancer before and after neoadjuvant chemoradiation using thin-section T2-weighted magnetic resonance imaging. Int J Radiat Oncol Biol Phys. 2008;71:456–61.
14. Kim SH, Lee JM, Hong SH, et al. Locally advanced rectal cancer: added value of diffusion-weighted MR imaging in the evaluation of tumor response to neoadjuvant chemo- and radiation therapy. Radiology. 2009;253:116.
15. Ha HI, Kim AY, Yu CS, Park SH, Ha HK. Locally advanced rectal cancer: diffusion-weighted MR tumour volumetry and the apparent diffusion coefficient for evaluating complete remission after preoperative chemoradiation therapy. Eur Radiol. 2013; 23:3345–53.
16. Patel UB, Taylor F, Blomqvist L, George C, Evans H, Tekkis P, Quirke P, Sebag-Montefiore D, Moran B, Heald R, Guthrie A, Bees N, Swift I, Pennert K, Brown G. Magnetic resonance imaging-detected tumor response for locally advanced rectal cancer predicts survival outcomes: MERCURY experience. J Clin Oncol. 2011;29:3753–60.
17. Kim H, Myoung S, Koom WS, Kim NK, Kim MJ, Ahn JB, Hur H, Lim JS. MRI risk stratification for tumor relapse in rectal cancer achieving pathological complete remission after neoadjuvant chemoradiation therapy and curative resection. PLoS One. 2016; 11:e0146235.
18. Sprenger T, Rothe H, Conradi LC, Beissbarth T, Kauffels A, Kitz J, Homayounfar K, Wolff H, Ströbel P, Ghadimi M, Wittekind C, Sauer R, Rödel C, Liersch T. Stage-dependent frequency of lymph node metastases in patients with rectal carcinoma after preoperative chemoradiation: results from the CAO/ARO/AIO-94 trial and from a comparative prospective evaluation

with extensive pathological workup. Dis Colon Rectum. 2016;59:377–85.

19. Rymer B, Curtis NJ, Siddiqui MR, Chand M. FDG PET/CT can assess the response of locally advanced rectal cancer to neoadjuvant chemoradiotherapy: evidence from meta-analysis and systematic review. Clin Nucl Med. 2016;41(5):371.

20. Habr-Gama A, Perez RO, Nadalin W, et al. Operative versus nonoperative treatment for stage 0 distal rectal cancer following chemoradiation therapy: long-term results. Ann Surg. 2004;240:711–8.

21. Jang TY, Yu CS, Yoon YS, Lim SB, Hong SM, Kim TW, Kim JH, Kim JC. Oncologic outcome after preoperative chemoradiotherapy in patients with pathologic T0 (ypT0) rectal cancer. Dis Colon Rectum. 2012;55:1024–31.

22. Hughes R, Glynne-Jones R, Grainger J, et al. Can pathological complete response in the primary tumour following pre-operative pelvic chemoradiotherapy for T3-T4 rectal cancer predict for sterilisation of pelvic lymph nodes, a low risk of local recurrence and the appropriateness of local excision? Int J Color Dis. 2006;21:11–7.

23. Garcia-Aguilar J, Renfro LA, Chow OS, Shi Q, Carrero XW, Lynn PB, Thomas CR Jr, Chan E, Cataldo PA, Marcet JE, Medich DS, Johnson CS, Oommen SC, Wolff BG, Pigazzi A, McNevin SM, Pons RK, Bleday R. Organ preservation for clinical T2N0 distal rectal cancer using neoadjuvant chemoradiotherapy and local excision (ACOSOG Z6041): results of an open-label, single-arm, multi-institutional, phase 2 trial. Lancet Oncol. 2015;16:1537–46.

24. Stipa F, Picchio M, Burza A, Soricelli E, Vitelli CE. Long-term outcome of local excision after preoperative chemoradiation for ypT0 rectal cancer. Dis Colon Rectum. 2014;57:1245–52.

25. Pucciarelli S, De Paoli A, Guerrieri M, La Torre G, Maretto I, De Marchi Mantello G, Gambacorta MA, Canzonieri V, Nitti D, Valentini V, Coco C. Local excision after preoperative chemoradiotherapy for rectal cancer: results of a multicenter phase II clinical trial. Dis Colon Rectum. 2013;56:1349–56.

26. Renehan AG, Malcomson L, Emsley R, Gollins S, Maw A, Myint AS, Rooney PS, Susnerwala S, Blower A, Saunders MP, Wilson MS, Scott N, O'Dwyer ST. Watch-and-wait approach versus surgical resection after chemoradiotherapy for patients with rectal cancer (the OnCoRe project): a propensity-score matched cohort analysis. Lancet Oncol. 2016;17:174–83.

27. Habr-Gama A, Perez RO, Proscurshim I, Campos FG, Nadalin W, Kiss D, Gama-Rodrigues J. Patterns of fail-

ure and survival for nonoperative treatment of stage c0 distal rectal cancer following neoadjuvant chemoradiation therapy. J Gastrointest Surg. 2006;10:1319–28.

28. Hughes R, Harrison M, Glynne-Jones R. Could a wait and see policy be justified in T3/4 rectal cancers after chemo-radiotherapy? Acta Oncol. 2010;4:378–81.

29. Ogawa S, Hida J, Ike H, Kinugasa T, Ota M, Shinto E, Itabashi M, Kameoka S, Sugihara K. Selection of lymph node-positive cases based on perirectal and lateral pelvic lymph nodes using magnetic resonance imaging: study of the Japanese Society for Cancer of the colon and Rectum. Ann Surg Oncol. 2016;23:1187–94.

30. Akiyoshi T, Matsueda K, Hiratsuka M, Unno T, Nagata J, Nagasaki T, Konishi T, Fujimoto Y, Nagayama S, Fukunaga Y, Ueno M. Indications for lateral pelvic lymph node dissection based on magnetic resonance imaging before and after preoperative chemoradiotherapy in patients with advanced low-rectal cancer. Ann Surg Oncol. 2015;22(Suppl 3):S614–20.

31. Lim SB, Yu CS, Kim CW, Yoon YS, Park SH, Kim TW, Kim JH, Kim JC. Clinical implication of additional selective lateral lymph node excision in patients with locally advanced rectal cancer who underwent preoperative chemoradiotherapy. Int J Color Dis. 2013;28:1667–74.

32. Fujita S, Mizusawa J, Kanemitsu Y, Ito M, Kinugasa Y, Komori K, Ohue M, Ota M, Akazai Y, Shiozawa M, Yamaguchi T, Bandou H, Katsumata K, Murata K, Akagi Y, Takiguchi N, Saida Y, Nakamura K, Fukuda H, Akasu T, Moriya Y, Colorectal Cancer Study Group of Japan Clinical Oncology Group. Mesorectal excision with or without lateral lymph node dissection for clinical stage II/III lower rectal cancer (JCOG0212). Ann Surg. 2017;266:201. https://doi.org/10.1097/SLA.0000000000002212. [Epub ahead of print].

33. Ishihara S, Kawai K, Tanaka T, Kiyomatsu T, Hata K, Nozawa H, Morikawa T, Watanabe T. Oncological outcomes of lateral pelvic lymph node metastasis in rectal cancer treated with preoperative chemoradiotherapy. Dis Colon Rectum. 2017;60:469–76.

34. Oh HK, Kang SB, Lee SM, Lee SY, Ihn MH, Kim DW, et al. Neoadjuvant chemoradiotherapy affects the indications for lateral pelvic node dissection in mid/low rectal cancer with clinically suspected lateral node involvement: a multicenter retrospective cohort study. Ann Surg Oncol. 2014;21:2280.

Pathologic Assessment and Specimen Quality After Total Mesorectal Excision of Rectal Cancer

Hoguen Kim

Abstract

After introduction of total mesorectal excision in rectal cancer surgery and effective neoadjuvant therapy, a considerable improvement of clinical outcome had occurred in rectal cancer patients. The pathologic reports of resected rectal cancers provide valuable information for the adequacy of the surgical treatment and predictive factors for future therapy. The evaluation of completeness of resection, preparation of adequate specimen, and evaluation of prognostic and predictive factors through microscopic evaluation and molecular analysis should be included for the proper management of rectal cancer patients.

Keywords

Rectal cancer · Total mesorectal excision · Pathology report · Circumferential resection margin · Predictive factors

10.1 Introduction

Pathologic evaluation of rectal cancer provides information regarding the adequacy of prior treatment, risk stratification for follow-up, and prognostic

H. Kim
Department of Pathology,
Yonsei University College of Medicine,
Seoul, South Korea
e-mail: hkyonsei@yuhs.ac

and predictive factors for subsequent systemic treatment. Remarkable improvements in the clinical outcomes of rectal cancers have resulted from the use of effective neoadjuvant therapies and improved surgical methods. Resected rectal cancer specimens are generally obtained using one of three surgery methods: total mesorectal excision (TME), tumor-specific mesorectal excision (TSME), and abdominoperineal resection [1, 2]. Following its introduction [3], the proven efficacy of TME has led to its worldwide designation as a standard surgical treatment for rectal cancer. TME requires a precise perpendicular and circumferential excision of the visceral mesorectal tissue down to the level of the levator muscles. The distinction between TME and TSME is based on the extent of mesorectal excision. Therefore, the application of rectal surgery depends on both the tumor location and invasion depth. TME is recommended for distal rectal cancers, whereas TSME, which comprises a precisely perpendicular and circumferential excision of the mesorectum to an appropriate resection margin level, is recommended for proximal rectal tumors located more than 5 cm from the distal extent of the mesorectum.

The pathology reports of resected rectal cancers contain several unique points: first, a macroscopic evaluation of surgical completeness; second, a measurement of the distance between the deepest invasion point and radial resection margin; and third, an evaluation of the effects of neoadjuvant therapy. This chapter will describe the approach to a surgical pathology report for a resected rectal cancer, together with the relevant microscopic evaluation and prognostic/predictive factors. Special requirements for a pathology report after neoadjuvant therapy will also be described.

10.2 Completeness of TME

Although TME made a considerable contribution toward reducing the local recurrence, a subset of rectal cancer cases experience postoperative recurrence. These local recurrences in rectal cancer cases are largely attributed to isolated metastases within the mesorectum, distal to the primary tumor [3]. The mesorectum is surrounded by a thin fascia, which is considered the outer layer during TME excision; complete separation of the mesorectum and fascia is a known predictor of a rare intrapelvic recurrence, and incomplete separation may increase the rate of local recurrence [1]. Therefore, a macroscopic evaluation of the surgical plane reflects the completeness of TME excision and is an important indicator of surgical quality and prognostic factor for rectal cancer outcomes [4]. The current College of American Pathologists (CAP) guidelines for the macroscopic evaluation of excision completeness comprise the presence of mesorectal defects, coning, and the circumferential resection margin (CRM) status as shown in Table 10.1 [5].

Table 10.1 Guidelines for the macroscopic evaluation of a TME specimen

Complete	Nearly complete	Incomplete
Intact bulky mesorectum with a smooth surface	Moderate bulk to the mesorectum	Little bulk to the mesorectum
Only minor irregularities of the mesorectal surface	Irregularity of the mesorectal surface with defects greater than 5 mm, but none extending to the muscularis propria	Defects in the mesorectum down to the muscularis propria
No surface defects greater than 5 mm in depth No coning toward the distal margin of the specimen After transverse sectioning, the circumferential margin appears smooth	No areas where the muscularis propria is visible except at the insertion site of the levator ani muscles	After transverse sectioning, the circumferential margin appears very irregular

invasion. Next, we divide this slice into four blocks according to the anatomical position. Subsequently, we process the other perpendicular tumor-containing slices using the same method. Whole-mount slide production is not routinely performed.

10.3 Adequate Specimen Preparation

Optimal tissue sampling is essential for an adequate microscopic analysis. For primary tumors, the area of deepest invasion should be identified before fixation. We usually sample at least five tissue blocks to identify the deepest layer of tumor invasion and measure the CRM. The recommended protocols include fixation of the entire specimen, marking of the radial resection margin with ink, and crosscutting of the entire encircled area. Routinely, we cut the fixed specimen perpendicularly at 1-cm intervals and select one slice that contains the area of deepest

10.4 Evaluation of CRM

The statuses of the distal and lateral (i.e., radial or mesorectal) resection margins are well-known predictive factors of local recurrence [1]. In brief, recurrence is inevitable if residual tumor remains at the distal or radial margin. The CRM is defined as the distance in millimeters between the deepest invasion point of a rectal cancer and the margin of resection in the retroperitoneum or mesentery [1]. The CRM is produced by the surgical resection of pericolic or perirectal fibroadipose tissues or pelvic structures [1]. During TME, complete mesorectal excisions are subsequently performed in the planar fascia surrounding the mesorectum, and a large fat column separates the tumor and involved lymph nodes from the CRM.

A large CRM is an important prognostic factor related to a low risk of local recurrence [1]. The internationally accepted cutoff value for a positive CRM is 1 mm [1]. Tumors with a CRM distance of <1 mm are considered high risk for recurrence. By contrast, a CRM distance exceeding 1 cm is associated with a significantly reduced risk of local recurrence and improved survival prognosis [6, 7]. An optimal macroscopic evaluation and sufficient sampling are necessary for an adequate CRM evaluation. We recommend an analysis of the resected surgical specimen according to the CAP guidelines. Furthermore, adequate fixation of the specimen and marking of the radial margin are essential to ensure that the distance between the leading edge of the tumor and the radial resection margin is accurately measured. We routinely fix the whole specimen, cut it perpendicularly, and mark the external surface with four different colors according to the anatomical

positions (ventral, dorsal, right, and left). Either a paraffin block in f pieces according to anatomical position (Fig. 10.1) or a whole-mount block (Fig. 10.2) of perpendicularly cut specimens can be used for an adequate CRM measurement.

10.5   Evaluation of Distal Resection Margin

A local recurrence may arise from an incomplete distal mesorectal excision, although the importance of this factor is less clear than that of incomplete radial resection. Tumor involvement in the distal resection margin might result from continuous intraluminal and/or intramural tumor growth and/or discontinuous growth [8]. The resection margins should be carefully evaluated for the presence of extramural vascular invasion, lymph node metastasis, or tumor deposits. The distance between the tumor and its resection margin is also important. The internationally accepted cutoff

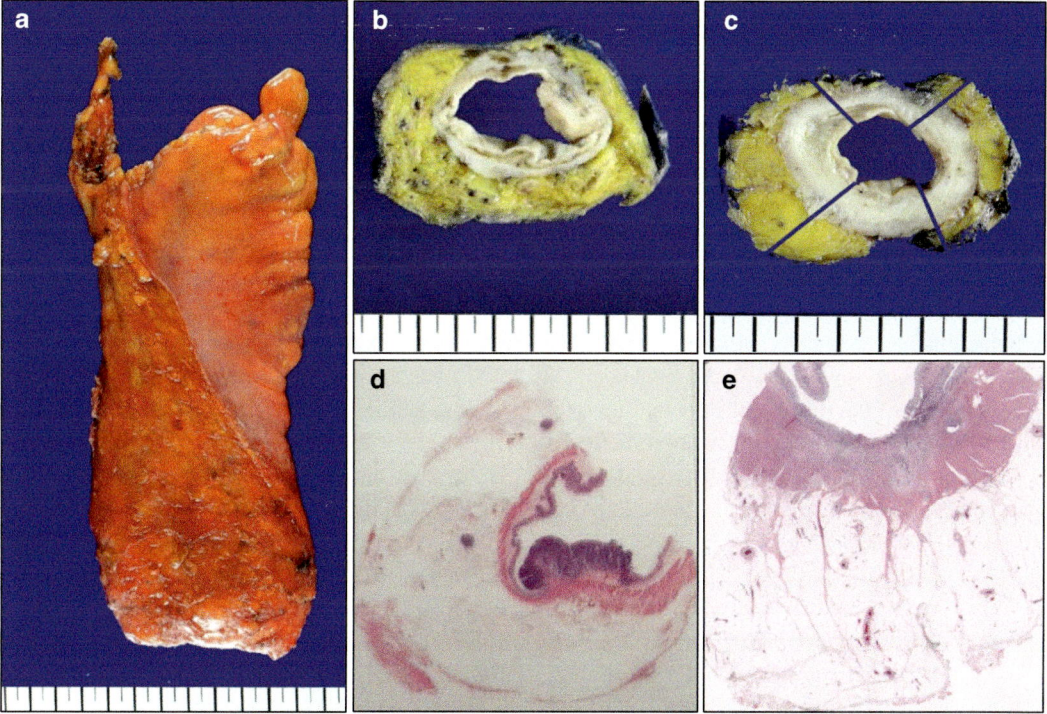

Fig. 10.1 Specimen preparation for the pathologic evaluation of a rectal cancer. After a gross evaluation of the TME specimen, the whole sample is fixed (**a**) and cut perpendicularly (**b**). The cut specimen is then divided into four parts (**c**) according to the anatomical position, and the CRM is evaluated on each slide (**d**, **e**)

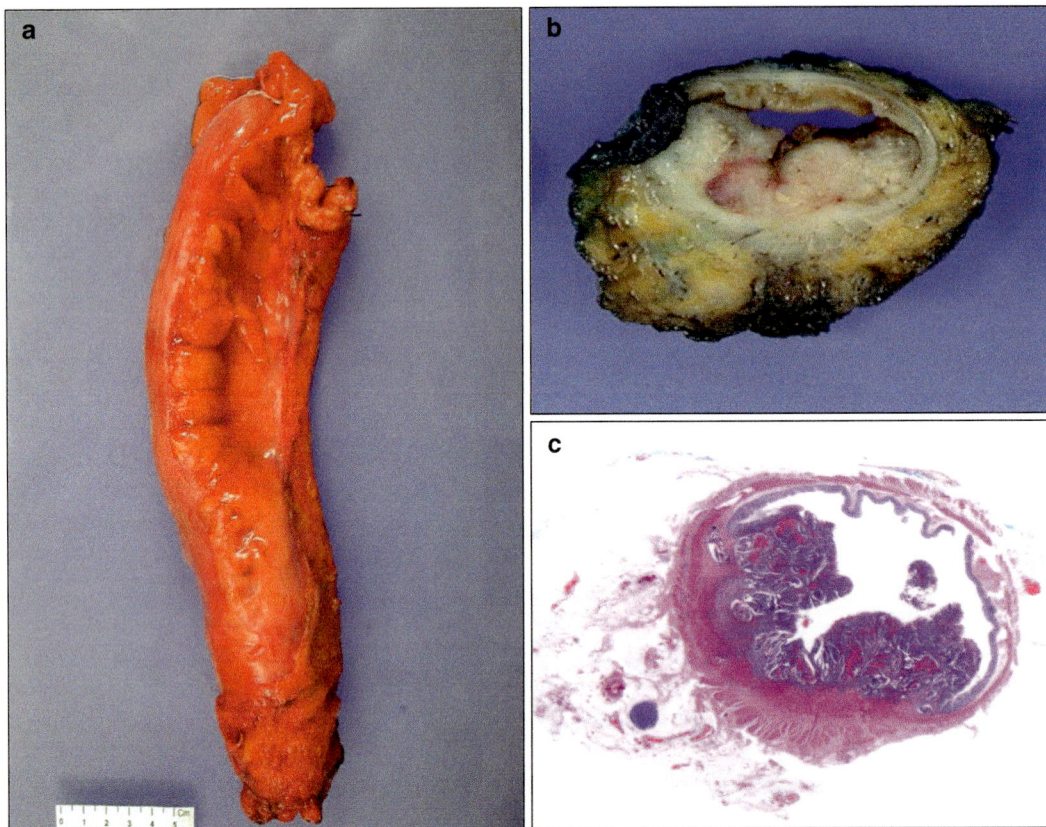

Fig. 10.2 Preparation of a whole-mount section from a surgically resected rectal cancer. After a gross evaluation of the TME specimen, the whole sample is fixed (**a**) and cut perpendicularly (**b**). The representative cut specimen is used to form one block (**c**) for CRM evaluation

value for a safe distal margin distance is 1 cm [6]. However, an increased distal resection margin will also contain sufficient regional lymph nodes and will facilitate an adequate evaluation of the lymph node metastasis status. To ensure an adequate measurement of the distal and proximal margins, an adequate length-preserving fixation method is required to avoid fixation-induced shrinkage. In particular, an unfixed colorectal specimen can shrink by up to 50% after formalin fixation.

10.6 Evaluation of Tumor Regression After Neoadjuvant Therapy

Neoadjuvant chemotherapy is applied to most locally advanced rectal cancers. An accurate pathology report requires information about systematic earlier treatments because rectal cancers treated with neoadjuvant therapy might exhibit significant histopathological effects. The effects of neoadjuvant therapy can be described in two ways: tumor down-staging and tumor regression. Tumor down-staging can be interpreted as tumor shrinkage [9, 10]. Down-staging and regression grades may overlap in some tumors. Tumor down-staging, in which the tumor infiltration depth is reduced because of tumor shrinkage, is associated with a good patient prognosis [11]. By contrast, the association of tumor regression with improved prognosis is less clear. This latter ambiguity is partly attributable to the ability of tumor regression to leave residual tumors in deep tissue areas, a phenomenon associated with an unfavorable prognosis. The presence of tumor cells in deep serial tumor sections has been reported in the context of complete regression [12], and the distinction between partial regression and rare regression is impossible for low-density tumors. These findings will require more detailed investigations in the future.

Although the impact of a good prognostic prediction remains unclear, the tumor regression grade (TRG) is an important factor for rectal cancers [1]. According to the CAP guidelines, tumor regression must be evaluated in the resected specimens and recorded. The primary tumor site, regional lymph nodes, peritumoral tumor satellite nodules, and/or tumor deposits should be subjected to a careful analysis, and the report should include the prefix "y" before pT and pN. Acellular mucin pools may be recognized in rectal cancers treated with neoadjuvant therapy. This finding is considered to indicate complete tumor eradication and is not used in the assignment of ypT and ypN categories. Currently, many protocols involve a tumor regression score evaluation [13–15], and the American Joint Committee on Cancer (AJCC) introduced modified Ryan scheme [15] for tumor regression scoring as shown in Table 10.2 and Fig. 10.3.

10.7 Pathology Reports for Rectal Cancer Resection

Pathology reports for resected rectal cancers provide valuable information about the adequacy of prior treatments and facilitate decisions regarding future therapy. This information about the tumor stage and prognostic and predictive factors is essential for optimal patient care. In addition to the pathologic, prognostic, and/or predictive factors, some molecular characteristics of the tumors may be included. The specific requirements for rectal cancer pathology reporting include a macroscopic evaluation of the surgical quality according to different surgical approaches, the CRM, and tumor regression grading in response to neoadjuvant therapy. Additionally, a microscopic evaluation for tumor staging, histologic subtype, and molecular results may facilitate precise predictions regarding future therapies.

The system used for pathological tumor staging (pTNM) after a microscopic examination is identical to the system used for other colon cancers, except that T4a is not applicable to rectal cancers. Tis, T1, T2, and T3 are assigned to intramucosal rectal cancers, cancers involving the submucosa, cancers that have penetrated to but not through the muscularis propria, and cancers that have penetrated through the muscularis propria, respectively. Colon cancers that involve the visceral peritoneum are classified as T4a, whereas those that directly invade an adjacent organ or structure are classified as T4b. However, the distal rectum is not peritonealized, and therefore T4a is not applicable to distal rectal cancers.

Table 10.2 Comparison of rectal cancer tumor regression grading/scoring systems

Ryan scheme [15]		Mandard grade [13]		Dworak et al [14]	
Description	Tumor regression grade	Description	Mandard grade	Description	Tumor regression grade
No viable cancer cells	0 (Complete response)	No residual tumor	1	No vital tumor cells detectable	4
Single cells or small groups of cancer cells	1 (Moderate response)	Rare residual cancer cells	2	Only scattered tumor cells in the space of fibrosis with/without acellular mucin	3
Residual cancer outgrown by fibrosis	2 (Minimal response)	Fibrosis outgrowing residual cancer	3	Predominantly fibrosis with scattered tumor cells (slightly recognizable histologically)	2
Minimal or no tumor death; extensive residual cancer	3 (Poor response)	Residual cancer outgrowing fibrosis	4	Predominantly tumor with significant fibrosis and/or vasculopathy	1
		Absence of regressive changes	5	No regression	0

Fig. 10.3 Representative images of tumor regression grades

Description	Ryan Scheme	
No viable cancer cells	0	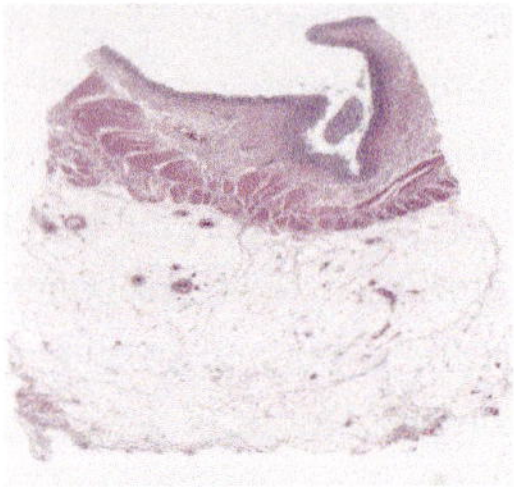
Single cells or small groups of cancer cells	1	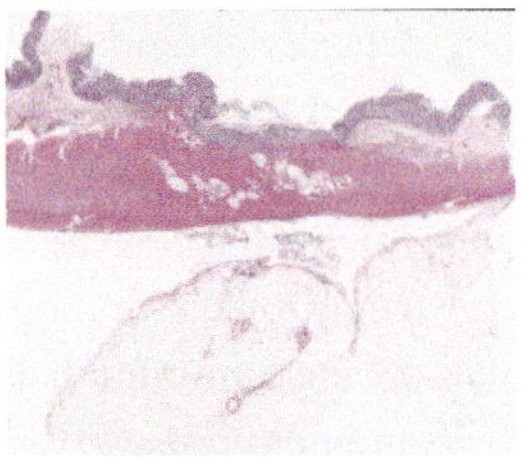
Residual cancer outgrown by fibrosis	2	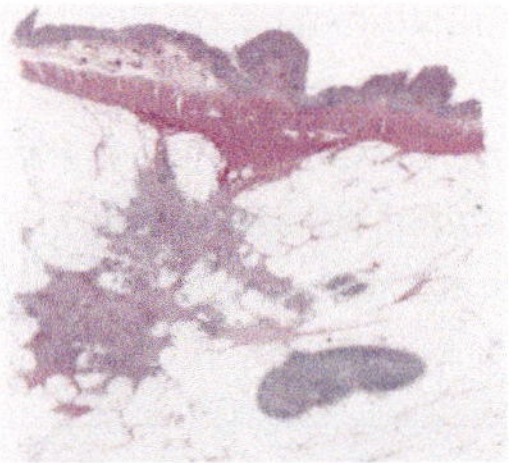
Minimal or no tumor death; extensive residual cancer	3	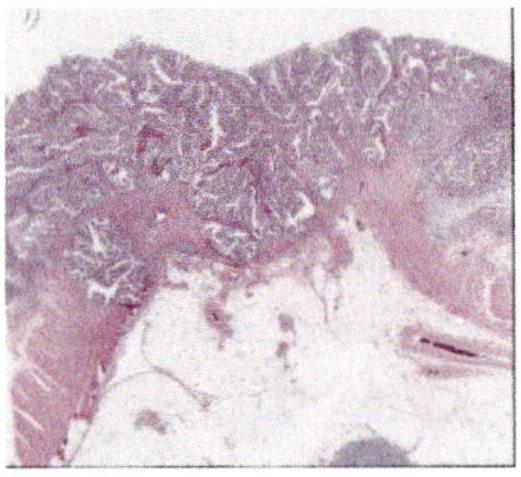

The histologic subtype is usually assigned according to the World Health Organization (WHO) classification [16]; however, most cases are classified as adenocarcinoma not otherwise specified. A subset of a specific subtype, such as signet ring cell carcinoma, is associated with a poor prognosis [17].

Other microscopic findings associated with a poor prognosis include lymphovascular and perineural invasion. Tumor deposits may result from the complete replacement of a lymph node metastasis or from lymphovascular and/or perineural invasion. In the 8th edition of the AJCC manual, tumor deposits are defined as discrete tumor nodules within the lymph node drainage area of a primary carcinoma, without identifiable lymph node tissue or an identifiable vascular or neural structure. The N1c category encompasses all colorectal cancers in which a tumor deposit is present without an identified lymph node metastasis, and this comprises level II evidence.

10.8 Molecular Markers Facilitating Subsequent Treatment Decisions for Rectal Cancers

Currently, the molecular markers recommended to support decisions regarding future therapy include the microsatellite instability (MSI) test and K-ras, N-ras, and BRAF mutation analyses.

Although prognosis is based predominantly upon the pathological disease stage, it is difficult to predict the outcomes of patients with Stage II and III cancers because they tend to have intermediate survival rates and it is currently impossible to predict responses to adjuvant chemotherapy. Among the listed molecular markers, the MSI test has been recommended as a prognostic predictor for colorectal cancers [1], and K-ras and N-ras mutation analyses were introduced as predictive markers of cetuximab therapy outcomes among colorectal carcinomas in the 8th edition of the AJCC manual [18].

Two major molecular pathways, the chromosomal instability pathway and microsatellite instability pathway, are known to be involved in these cancers. The microsatellite instability pathway begins with the inactivation of one of several genes responsibility for DNA nucleotide mismatch repair, leading to extensive mutations in repetitive DNA sequences. Tumors with high microsatellite instability (MSI-H) comprise approximately 15% of colorectal carcinomas. Most MSI-H tumors are sporadic and result from *MLH1* hypermethylation. Sporadic MSI-H tumors often harbor *BRAF* mutations, whereas *KRAS* mutations are distinctly less frequent [19, 20]. Compared with other types of colorectal carcinomas, MSI-H tumors are associated with a better prognosis, reduced responsiveness to FOLFOX therapy, and better responsiveness to immunotherapy [21]. MSI-H tumors are associated with a right-side preponderance, a high proportion of mucinous and signet ring cell-type histology, and high peritumoral lymphoid reactivity [22]. Therefore, the MSI-H test has only limited value among rectal cancers, as the incidence of MSI-H carcinoma in the rectum is less than 3%. The incidence of *KRAS* or *NRAS* mutation among rectal cancers is similar to that of colorectal cancers at other sites.

The use of markers predictive of therapeutic response or resistance is important for the individualization of chemoradiation for patients with advanced disease or the determination of candidacy for adjuvant therapy. Investigations of predictive markers, including key biomarkers for the identification of molecular subtypes, are ongoing. Additionally, large-scale clinical evaluations of molecular markers are currently in progress.

References

1. Amin MB, et al; AJCC cancer staging manual. 8th edn. New York: Springer; 2016. 251–269.
2. Monson JR, et al. Practice parameters for the management of rectal cancer (revised). Dis Colon Rectum. 2013;56(5):535–50.
3. Heald RJ, et al. The mesorectum in rectal cancer surgery–the clue to pelvic recurrence? Br J Surg. 1982;69(10):613–6.
4. Nagtegaal ID. Current concepts of colorectal cancer resection pathology. Histopathology. 2015;66(1):102–11.
5. Washington MK, et al. Protocol for the examination of specimens from patients with primary carcinoma of the colon and rectum. Arch Pathol Lab Med. 2009;133(10):1539–51.
6. Bujko K, et al. Is the 1-cm rule of distal bowel resection margin in rectal cancer based on clinical evidence? A systematic review. Ann Surg Oncol. 2012; 19(3):801–8.
7. Nagtegaal ID, Quirke P. What is the role for the circumferential margin in the modern treatment of rectal cancer? J Clin Oncol Off J Am Soc Clin Oncol. 2008;26(2):303–12.
8. Williams NS, et al. Reappraisal of the 5 cm rule of distal excision for carcinoma of the rectum: a study of distal intramural spread and of patients' survival. Br J Surg. 1983;70(3):150–4.
9. Gosens MJ, et al. Circumferential margin involvement is the crucial prognostic factor after multimodality treatment in patients with locally advanced rectal carcinoma. Clin Cancer Res Off J Am Assoc Cancer Res. 2007;13(22 Pt. 1):6617–23.
10. Perez RO, et al. Fragmented pattern of tumor regression and lateral intramural spread may influence margin appropriateness after TEM for rectal cancer following neoadjuvant CRT. J Surg Oncol. 2014;109(8):853–8.
11. Vironen J, et al. Tumour regression grading in the evaluation of tumour response after different preoperative radiotherapy treatments for rectal carcinoma. Int J Color Dis. 2005;20(5):440–5.
12. Park SY, et al. Is step section necessary for determination of complete pathological response in rectal cancer patients treated with preoperative chemoradiotherapy? Histopathology. 2011;59(4):650–9.
13. Mandard A-M, et al. Pathologic assessment of tumor regression after perspective chemotherapy of esophageal carcinoma. Cancer. 1994;73(6):2680–6.
14. Dworak O, Keilholz L, Hoffmann A. Pathological features of rectal cancer after preoperative radiochemotherapy. Int J Color Dis. 1997;12(1):19–23.
15. Ryan R, et al. Pathological response following long-course neoadjuvant chemoradiotherapy for locally advanced rectal cancer. Histopathology. 2005;47(2): 141–6.
16. Bosman FT, World Health Organization, International Agency for Research on Cancer. WHO classification of tumours of the digestive system. Lyon: International Agency for Research on Cancer; 2010. p. 417.

17. Hugen N, et al. Colorectal signet-ring cell carcinoma: benefit from adjuvant chemotherapy but a poor prognostic factor. Int J Cancer. 2015;136(2):333–9.
18. Karapetis CS, et al. K-ras mutations and benefit from cetuximab in advanced colorectal cancer. N Engl J Med. 2008;359:1757–65.
19. Cancer Genome Atlas Network. Comprehensive molecular characterization of human colon and rectal cancer. Nature. 2012;487:330–7.
20. Woerner SN, et al. Microsatellite instability in the development of DNA mismatch repair deficient tumors. Cancer Biomark. 2006;2:69–86.
21. Le DT, et al. PD-1 blockade in tumors with mismatch-repair deficiency. N Engl J Med. 2015;372:2509–20.
22. Kim H, et al. Clinical and pathological characteristics of sporadic colorectal carcinomas with DNA replication errors in microsatellite sequences. Am J Pathol. 1994;145(1):148–56.

Part IV

Standard Surgical Techniques in Rectal Cancer Surgery

Total Mesorectal Excision: History and Surgical Outcomes

11

Wai Lun Law

Abstract

Colorectal cancer is a common malignancy globally, and management of rectal cancer is particularly challenging. Not only should the treatment achieve good local disease control and favorable survival; but the body functions should also be preserved. Since the introduction of abdominoperineal resection by Sir Ernest Miles for rectal cancer resection more than a century ago, the operation had been the gold standard treatment for rectal cancer until the recent 2–3 decades. However, both the oncologic and functional outcomes of conventional abdominoperineal resection have been far from satisfactory.

The introduction of total mesorectal excision by Sir Richard Heald revolutionized the surgical treatment for rectal cancer. He postulated that most of the local recurrence was due to the incomplete excision of the mesorectum. He introduced sharp mesorectal excision along the embryonic plane in rectal resection. Sphincter preservation was achieved by close shave anterior resection. In addition, identification and preservation of the pelvic autonomic nerves could be facilitated with sharp dissection in the relatively bloodless operating field. A very low local recurrence rate and a favorable survival were demonstrated in Heald's early reports. The technique could be learned and attained by training through workshops and live demonstrations.

Currently total mesorectal excision is regarded as the gold standard surgical technique for rectal cancer. The principles of the operation also form the basis of minimally invasive techniques such as laparoscopic, robotic, and transanal approaches.

Keywords

Total mesorectal excision · History · Outcomes

11.1 History of Rectal Cancer Surgery to the Era of Total Mesorectal Excision

Colorectal cancer is the third most common cancer in the world, and in 2012, nearly 1.4 million new cases were diagnosed, and 700,000 patients died of the disease [1, 2]. Rectal cancer contributes 30–40% of all colorectal cancer [3, 4], and the management is more complex and challenging than colon cancer. The optimal management often involves multimodality treatment strategy,

W. L. Law
Department of Surgery, The Univeristy of Hong Kong, Queen Mary Hospital, Hong Kong, People's Republic of China
e-mail: lawwl@hku.hk

© Springer Nature Singapore Pte Ltd. 2018
N. K. Kim et al. (eds.), *Surgical Treatment of Colorectal Cancer*,
https://doi.org/10.1007/978-981-10-5143-2_11

sophisticated and radical surgery, and good peri-operative care. In addition to achieving a favorable oncologic outcome, attention should also be paid to the impact of the disease and treatment on the quality of life.

The objectives of treatment of rectal cancer can be summarized by Charles Mayo's "Evolution in the Treatment of Cancer of the Rectum" in which he stated that "Certain definite results are desired in operations on cancer of the rectum, namely, permanent cure, low operative mortality and a controllable anus, or its better substitute" [5]. After more than a century, these objectives still apply nowadays to the management of rectal cancer.

Historically, rectal cancer was described in ancient time and was considered incurable until the recent two centuries. The first successful resection of rectal tumor was performed in 1826 by Jacques Lisfranc, who excised a few centimeters of distal rectum after everting the rectum and dissecting below the peritoneal reflection [6, 7]. The exposure of this perineal approach, which was originally performed without anesthesia and hemostasis, was limited to the upper rectum and was associated with a high recurrence rate. In the latter half of the nineteenth century, with the introduction of anesthesia and asepsis, more radical techniques using the perineal and posterior approach for resection of rectal cancer developed. However, the posterior or perineal approach was associated with a high mortality as well as a high recurrence rate. Vogel reviewed 1500 cases from 12 prominent surgeons prior to 1900. The operative mortality was 20.9% and the recurrence rate was 80% [6].

The gold standard treatment of rectal cancer in most part of the twentieth century was abdominoperineal resection, described by Sir Ernest Miles in England. He recognized the issue of local recurrence after perineal/posterior resection for rectal cancer. After postmortem dissection of patients with perineal resections, Miles found recurrences occurred in the pelvic peritoneum, the mesorectum, and the lymph nodes over the bifurcation of the left common iliac artery, and he realized that a more radical resection, to address the upward, lateral, and downward spread of the disease, was needed to reduce the recurrence.

Miles developed the en bloc resection of rectal cancer with the combined abdominal and perineal operations to allow more radical lymphadenectomy. Miles principles included (1) the necessity of an abdominal anus, (2) resection of the rectum and the sigmoid, (3) resection of the mesorectum, (4) removal of the group of lymph nodes situated over the bifurcation of the common iliac artery, and (5) wide perineal part of the operation with resection of the levator ani so that the lateral and downward spread could be extirpated. He reported his 12 procedures in in 1908 [8]. The mortality rate was 42% and the survivors were disease-free for 1 year.

The abdominoperineal resection had been the gold standard treatment for rectal cancer for many decades in the last century, and in the late half of the century, attempt was made for sphincter preservation in proximal rectal cancer. Dukes demonstrated that the downward and lateral spread of rectal cancer emphasized by Miles was overestimated [9]. The downward and lateral spread was found to be unusual unless the tumor was advanced or the upward draining lymphatics were blocked by tumor deposit. The feasibility of sphincter preservation was demonstrated by Dixon, the then surgical chair at the Mayo Clinic, who reported in 1948 the results of anterior resection of 426 patients with cancer from 6 to 20 cm from the anal verge with a low mortality rate of 5.9% [10]. Sphincter preservation was further facilitated with the development of circular stapling devices and surgical techniques such as pull-through procedure with coloanal anastomosis, described by Alan Parks [11]. However, the morbidity and mortality associated with anastomotic leak limited the wide application of sphincter-saving operation.

Despite all these advances, rectal cancer surgery remained a major undertaking with significant mortality and morbidity. The majority of patients with mid and distal rectal cancer required a permanent colostomy. The local recurrence rate remained high and the survival was not favorable. In the 1970s and 1980s, the high local recurrence rates were recognized, and the adjuvant therapy for rectal cancer was considered to reduce the local recurrence after surgery. In randomized trials comparing surgical with or without chemoradiation/radiation, the local recurrence rates in the surgery-alone arms were in the range of 20–30% [12, 13], and reduction of local recurrence could be achieved with adjuvant radiation/chemoradiation therapy. In the National Cancer Institute Consensus Conference in 1990, postoperative chemoradiation was recommended for patients with stage II and stage III rectal cancer.

11.2 Development of Total Mesorectal Excision

Conventional pelvic dissection was performed with blunt presacral dissection. This was still described in textbook in 1998 [14]. The blunt dissection easily torn the fascial propria to enter the mesorectum and left the mesorectal disease, leading to an increased chance of positive lateral margins. Havenga et al. proposed the mechanism of local recurrence caused by blunt dissection [15]. At the level of S3, the thick rectosacral fascia would be encountered, and by avoiding tearing the presacral fascia, which would lead to severe hemorrhage, the surgeon's fingers would follow the less resistant plane and break the fascia propria to enter the meorectum. A portion of the mesorectum would be sheared off, and the presence of tumor in the mesorectum would become the source of tumor recurrence.

Up till 1970s, the local recurrence rate for rectal cancer after surgery was 20–30%. The functional outcomes were also poor after conventional surgery using blunt dissection. The urogenital dysfunction was reported to occur in up to 50% of patients, as the damage to the pelvic autonomic nerves was usually considered inevitable during the blunt pelvic dissection. Thus, a more optimal surgical technique to reduce the operative mortality and morbidity, to increase the sphincter-saving rate, to reduce the local recurrence, to improve the survival, as well as to improve the functional outcomes was very much needed.

In the 1980s the importance of the circumferential margin was recognized. In 1986, Phil Quirke reported that in 52 patients with rectal cancer with whole-mount section, a positive lateral resection margin was found in 27% and local recurrence occurred in 83% of patients with circumferential margin involvement [16]. In our institution, similar findings were observed, and local recurrence occurred in 53% of patients with a positive lateral margin, which was identified as an independent prognostic factor for tumor recurrence [17].

Richard Heald realized that better technique could improve the outcome of rectal cancer surgery in the majority of patients with rectal cancer. He developed a technique of dissection based on the embryonic bloodless plane, which he called the holy plane. Sharp dissection was used for en bloc excision of the rectum together with the intact mesorectum to the level of the levator muscles. He termed this technique total mesorectal excision. He believed that rectal cancer was a supralevator disease and the patient could be cured with preservation of the anal sphincter, using meticulous dissection. In 1982, he reported that tumor deposits were found in the mesorectum distal to the primary cancer and proposed that in the situation of rectal cancer, which was considered a slow-growing disease, if the rectum and the mesorectum surrounded by mesorectal fascia could be removed en bloc, better local control of the disease could be achieved [18].

The fundamental principles of TME involve sharp dissection under direct vision of the rectum with the mesorectum under the cover of the fascia propria, and a clear circumferential margin could be achieved. The sharp dissection was performed down to levator muscles with the rectum and mesorectum excised at this level. By performing sharp dissection, the excessive blood loss, which occurred commonly with blunt dissection and tearing the presacral venous plexus, was avoided. Regarding the autonomic nerve preservation, sharp dissection enabled identification and preservation of the hypogastric nerves as well as the sacral nerves in the bloodless operating field. Thus, the bladder and sexual functions have been significantly improved with this technique.

The rationale of total mesorectal excision and the need to completely remove the mesorectum for mid and distal rectum was proven by histology studies. Reynolds et al. found that in 39% of 44 patients with T3 cancer, non-nodal tumor foci were found within the mesorectum [19]. Distal spread actually occurred in 70% of patients with mesorectal tumor foci, and spread beyond 2 cm was not uncommon. As the distal mesorectal spread is at most 3–4 cm from the distal border, it is now commonly accepted that total mesorectal excision is not necessary for proximal rectal cancer, provided the mesorectum is removed 4–5 cm distal to the cancer. In our study on patients with anterior resection for rectal cancer, we found that the application of partial mesorectal excision for proximal cancer with a 4–5 cm mesorectal margin could achieve similar oncologic outcome as total mesorectal excision with fewer complications, especially anastomotic leakage [20]. Now tumor-specific mesorectal excision according to the level of the tumor is commonly accepted.

Heald reported his original series of 115 patients in 1986 [21] with a local recurrence rate of 3.7%, and the cumulative probability of survival at 5 years was 87%. The abdominoperineal rate was 11%.

There was significant skepticism on the original report by Heald. The patients treated in Basingstoke were independently reviewed by Professor MacFarlane who took a sabbatical from Vancouver. He followed up the 13-year data of Basingstoke and found that after curative anterior resection for rectal cancer, the actuarial local recurrence rate was 4% at 5 years and the overall recurrence rate is 18%. MacFarlane also identified a group of 135 high-risk patients with Dukes' B (B2) and Dukes' C cancer operations. When compared with the reports from conventional surgery plus radiation or combined chemoradiation from the NCCTG study, results from total mesorectal excision alone were substantially superior, and the concept of total mesorectal excision was confirmed and validated [22]. Heald later popularized his technique in different countries and took part in workshops and training programs. It was shown that the technique of total mesorectal excision could be acquired by training program and workshops with live surgery [23]. The improvement in outcome with the adoption of total mesorectal excision was also demonstrated in national audit, which compared the outcomes before and after adoption of the

technique [24]. Total mesorectal excision thus became the gold standard technique for rectal cancer surgery.

11.3 Outcomes of Total Mesorectal Excision

The application of total mesorectal excision has improved the outcomes of rectal cancer surgery in many aspects. The anal sphincter can be preserved in most of the patients, and the number of abdominoperineal resections has dropped significantly in recent decades. With meticulous sharp dissection under direct vision along the embryonic plane, the blood loss can also be reduced, and the autonomic nerves can be better identified and preserved. This will reduce the postoperative sexual and bladder dysfunction. The most important impact is the improvement in the oncologic outcomes. Most series showed a reduction of local recurrence and an improvement in survival with the adoption of total mesorectal excision.

11.3.1 Sphincter Preservation

Heald postulated that with total mesorectal excision, a narrow distal mural margin was oncologically acceptable and safe. The conventional "5-cm rule" of distal margin in rectal cancer surgery was reappraised. Williams et al. examined the distal mural spread in patients with rectal cancer [25]. In the 50 patients studied, distal mural spread for more than 1 cm occurred in only 10% of the specimens, and all these patients had poorly differentiated Dukes' C cancer. The authors also did not find any difference in the survival of patients who had distal margin more and less than 5 cm. The acceptance of a short distal margin allowed more patients to be treated with a sphincter-saving operation.

Heald proved that a short distal margin was oncologically safe provided total mesorectal excision was performed. In the study, which compared patients with distal margin of greater than 1 cm with those less than 1 cm, Karanjia and colleagues did not find any difference in the local recurrence rate or the survival rate between the two groups [26]. With the application of close shave anterior resection, Heald and colleagues reported that abdominoperineal resection was only performed in 37 out of the 517 patients with rectal cancer up to 15 cm from the anal verge [27]. In a study comparing the rates of abdomino-perineal resection before and after the adoption of TME, Arbman and colleagues found the reduction of abdominoperineal resections from 48% to 14% [28].

11.3.2 Perioperative Mortality and Morbidity

Rectal cancer surgery was regarded as a major undertaking associated with significant morbidity and mortality. The blood loss and sepsis were the two most common causes leading to significant morbidity. Total mesorectal excision is in fact a complex operation with multiple steps including splenic flexure mobilization, high ligation of inferior mesenteric vessels, meticulous pelvic dissection, and creation of a distal rectal or anal anastomosis. The operating time was longer than conventional blunt procedure, and Heald reported that the operation time for total mesorectal excision with sphincter preservation was about 4 h [29]. However, the sharp pelvic dissection in total mesorectal dissection allowed clear separation of the visceral layer of the pelvic fascia from the presacral fascia, and the chance of tearing the presacral venous plexus was reduced. The troublesome bleeding from the presacral venous plexus is not common in total mesorectal excision, and the blood loss is usually less than conventional rectal excision. Murty [30] reported blood loss of one unit and transfusion was needed in 15% of patients. In our study on total mesorectal resection with low anastomosis, the median blood loss was 400 ml [20]. With the application of minimally invasive surgery, the blood loss was further reduced [31]. The mortality of the operation was also low, ranging from 0% to 4% [27, 28, 32].

Anastomotic leak is a dreadful complication after colorectal surgery. An extraperitoneal anastomosis after resection for mid and distal rectal can-

cer is associated with a high risk of anastomotic leak, likely due to tension, poor blood supply, and difficult access. In total mesorectal excision with sphincter preservation, the transection of the bowel is invariably at the distal rectum or the anal canal, and the anastomosis is usually located at or below the pelvic floor; thus the leakage rate is particularly high. Karanjia et al. [33] reported Heald's series of 219 patients with low anterior resection with total mesorectal excision; the clinical and radiological leakage rates were 11.0% and 6.4%, respectively. A diversion stoma was suggested in view of the high leakage rate. Rullier et al. showed similar results with the leakage rate of 12% in patients after total mesorectal excision [34]. They also showed that the leakage rate for anastomoses below 5 cm from the anal verge was 6.5 times when compared to that of anastomosis [34]. In our study on 196 patients who underwent low anterior resection with TME and all the anastomoses were below 5 cm from the anal verge, the anastomotic leakage rate was 10.5% [35]. The male gender and the absence of diversion stoma were risk factors for a high anastomotic leakage rate. Thus, in cases of low anterior resection with total mesorectal excision, a proximal diversion is suggested to reduce the leakage rate and the septic consequence of the anastomotic leak. Whether a colostomy or an ileostomy provides better diversion and fewer complications is controversial in randomized trials [36, 37]. Recent meta-analysis showed that the ileostomy had the advantages of a lower incidence of prolapse and a lower wound infection rate after closure [38]. However, other studies did not showed clear advantages of either option of diversion [39].

11.3.3 Bladder and Sexual Functions

Sharp dissection in total mesorectal excision also enables better identification and preservation of the pelvic autonomic nerves. Conventional rectal cancer surgery has been associated with a high incidence of autonomic nerve injury, leading to postoperative bladder and sexual dysfunction. Preservation of the autonomic nerves is an integral part of total mesorectal excision, and this is made possible by sharp dissection in the holy plane in a bloodless field. In terms of the male sexual function, Havenga et al. [40] reported that in male patients younger than 60 years, 86% could engage in intercourse and 87% could achieve orgasm after surgery. Total mesorectal excision has also significantly improved the recovery of bladder function after surgery. In Nesbakken et al.'s study, bladder dysfunction occurred in 2 patients out of the 35 patients after TME [41]. The identification and preservation of the pelvic autonomic nerves was demonstrated to be an important factor for good outcome after surgery. Junginger et al. reported that the complete identification of the nerves was associated with a lower incidence of bladder dysfunction and that the experience was important in the identification of the pelvic nerves [42]. Despite the meticulous dissection and tedious identification of the pelvic autonomic nerves, the bladder and sexual dysfunction still contributes to the morbidity after total mesorectal excision. The application of laparoscopy was not found to improve the bladder and sexual function [43]. However, recent reports on total mesorectal excision using surgical robotic system, which enabled better identification of the pelvic autonomic nerves, demonstrated better recovery of the bladder and sexual functions [44, 45].

11.3.4 Oncologic Outcomes

The technique of total mesorectal excision revolutionized the rectal cancer surgery and is now regarded as the gold standard treatment. The technique began as an open approach, and in the recent two decades of rapid development of minimally invasive surgery, using laparoscopic, robotic, or transanal approaches, the basic principles of total mesorectal excision remain when applied to these approaches.

The impact on the oncologic outcomes is the most important aspect of total mesorectal excision. Local recurrence after rectal cancer surgery was a common occurrence in the pre-total mesorectal excision era, and in most cases the patients did not suffer from distal metastasis. The sufferings inflicted by local recurrence were tremendous and treatment using involves radical exenterative surgery, which adversely affected the quality of life. The reduction in the local recurrence is the most significant outcome brought by total mesorectal excision. Heald reported in 519 patients with total mesorectal excision, the local recurrence rate was 6% in 5 years and 8% in 10 years [27]. The local control in sphincter-saving operation was even better, and the local recurrence rate was 2% at 5 years. Enker et al. also reported a local recurrence of 7.3% in 246 high-risk patients, who suffered from Dukes' B and Dukes' C cancer [32]. The local recurrence rates and survivals in early series of TME are shown in Table 11.1. Most of them reported a local recurrence rate of less than 10%, and most of the patients did not undergo any adjuvant radiation therapy.

With the reduction in local recurrence, the survival of patients has also been improved with the adoption of total mesorectal excision. Heald et al. reported [27] a 5-year disease-free survival of 80% in those who underwent curative anterior

Table 11.1 Oncologic outcomes of early series of total mesorectal excision

Study (Year)	N	Patients' characteristics	Follow-up	Local recurrence	Overall survival
Enker et al. (1995) [32]	246	B and C	72 months	7%	Node −: 87%
					Node +: 64%
Heald el al. (1998) [27]	519	All stages	99 months	3%	80%
Zaheer et al. (1998) [62]	514	All stages	5.6 years	7%	78%
Martling et al. (2000) [23]	381	All stages	24 months	6%	79%
Nesbakken et al. (2002) [63]	134	A, B, and C	38 months	9%	66%
Wibe et al. (2002) [24]	686	A, B, and C	29 months	7%	
Piso et al. (2004) [64]	337	All stages	5 years	8.6%	69.3%

resection. Enker et al. also showed that the survival of patients with stage II and stage III disease was 74.2% [32].

The learning and the adoption of total mesorectal excision were demonstrated to improve the outcomes significantly. Martling showed that with program and workshops to train TME surgeons, significant improvement in the outcome could be achieved [23]. The outcomes of the patients with abdominal surgery for rectal cancer after the TME project in Stockholm County were compared to those recruited in the Stockholm I and Stockholm II trials (pre-TME era) [23]. The local recurrence was significantly reduced (6% vs. 15% and 14%), and the cancer-related death showed similar findings (9% vs. 15% and 16%). Thus the technique of TME could be trained and applied widely after training.

11.4 Evolution of Approach of Total Mesorectal Excision

Total mesorectal excision was regarded as a complex operation and was originally performed with the open technique. It involved multiple steps including high ligation of the inferior mesentery vessels, full mobilization of splenic flexure, meticulous pelvic dissection to the pelvic floor, and fashion of a distal rectal or anal anastomosis. In the era of minimally invasive surgery, which began in the late 1980s, there was enthusiasm on applying laparoscopy in colorectal surgery. However, because of the complexity of the procedure and the need to deal with cancer, the application of laparoscopy in rectal cancer was considered not fast, when compared to other procedures. However, Milsom demonstrated that all the steps of total mesorectal excision including colorectal anastomosis with intracorporeal application of stapler could be performed in a cadaveric model [46]. Laparoscopic total mesorectal excision with abdominoperineal resection was initially attempted, and the abdominal incision could be avoided [47, 48].

With improvement of techniques and instruments, laparoscopic pelvic dissection can be performed under the direct vision with magnified view. The development of laparoscopic stapler devices enabled intracorporeal rectal transection and anastomosis. The safety and feasibility of laparoscopic anterior resection with TME for rectal cancer were reported by different skillful laparoscopic surgeons [49–51]. Randomized trials started in the late 1990s even when the technique was not mature [52]. Despite a high conversion rate [53–55], the oncologic outcome of the laparoscopic group in terms of the local recurrence and survival rates were comparable to open surgery. Whether the quality of the TME specimen by laparoscopic resection is equivalent to open surgery is still controversial. The recently published ALaCart and ACOSOG Z6051 trials failed to prove that the specimens resected by laparoscopic surgery were not inferior to those removed with open operations [56, 57].

The use of surgical robotic system can overcome some of the limitations of conventional laparoscopy, and robotic surgery has been widely applied to other fields of pelvic surgery, such as prostate resection and gynecological operations. The surgical robot enables an ergonomic and stable platform for the surgeon to operate with versatile instruments on a magnified and 3-dimension view. This facilitates precise dissection in the pelvis under direct vision, which is the main concept of total mesorectal excision. Early results showed a lower conversion rate and better recovery of the bladder and sexual functions [44, 58]. The quality of the TME specimens was similar to those removed by laparoscopic or open resection. Available comparative data demonstrated similar long-term oncologic outcomes as laparoscopic resection [59, 60]. However, the cost and availability of the robot limit its wide application, and long-term survival data from randomized trials are still lacking.

Based on the concept of total mesorectal excision, the transanal approach was developed to perform the dissection proximally from the distal rectum or the anal canal. The distal margin can be well defined in the beginning of the procedure, and the difficulty of distal rectal transection with endoscopic staplers in laparoscopic or robotic surgery can be avoided. Encouraging initial results have been reported [61]. However, the long-term results comparing with other approaches of total mesorectal excision are still pending.

Conclusion

Total mesorectal excision has revolutionized the surgical technique in treatment of rectal cancer and has become the gold standard technique. The technique has significantly affected the outcome of surgery in terms of the perioperative blood loss, the incidence of sphincter preservation, the oncologic outcomes, as well as the recovery of bladder and sexual functions. With the development of different minimally invasive approaches, the principles of total mesorectal excision form the foundation of these developments with the objectives to further improve the postoperative as well as the functional outcome without compromising the oncologic results.

References

1. Arnold M, Sierra MS, Laversanne M, Soerjomataram I, Jemal A, Bray F. Global patterns and trends in colorectal cancer incidence and mortality. Gut. 2017;66(4):683–91.
2. Ferlay J, Soerjomataram I, Ervik M. GLOBOCAN 2012 v1.0, cancer incidence and mortality worldwide: IARC cancer base no. 11. Lyon: International Agency for Research on Cancer; 2013.
3. Devesa SS, Chow WH. Variation in colorectal cancer incidence in the United States by subsite of origin. Cancer. 1993;71(12):3819–26.
4. Jensen OM. Different age and sex relationship for cancer of subsites of the large bowel. Br J Cancer. 1984;50(6):825–9.
5. Mayo CH. Evolution in the treatment of cancer of the rectum. J Am Med Assoc. 1903;XL(17):1127–9.
6. Graney MJ, Graney CM. Colorectal surgery from antiquity to the modern era. Dis Colon Rectum. 1980;23(6):432–41.
7. Lisfranc J. Memoire sur l'excision de la partie inferieure du rectum devenue carcinomateuse. Mem Ac R Chir. 1833;3:291–302.
8. Miles WE. A method of performing abdominoperineal excision for carcinoma of the rectum and the terminal portion of the pelvic colon. Lancet. 1908;ii:1812–3.
9. Dukes CE. The spread of cancer of the rectum. Br J Surg. 1930;17:643–8.
10. Dixon CF. Anterior resection for malignant lesions of the upper part of the rectum and lower part of the sigmoid. Ann Surg. 1948;128:425–42.
11. Parks AG, Percy JP. Resection and sutured colo-anal anastomosis for rectal carcinoma. Br J Surg. 1982;69(6):301–4.
12. Krook JE, Moertel CG, Gunderson LL, Wieand HS, Collins RT, Beart RW, et al. Effective surgical adjuvant therapy for high-risk rectal carcinoma. N Engl J Med. 1991;324(11):709–15.
13. Gastrointestinal Tumor Study G. Prolongation of the disease-free interval in surgically treated rectal carcinoma. N Engl J Med. 1985;312(23):1465–72.
14. Corman MC. Carcinoma of rectum. In: Corman MC, editor. Colon and rectal surgery, vol. IV. Philadelphia: Lippincot-Raven; 1998. p. 733–862.
15. Havenga K, DeRuiter MC, Enker WE, Welvaart K. Anatomical basis of autonomic nerve-preserving total mesorectal excision for rectal cancer. Br J Surg. 1996;83(3):384–8.
16. Quirke P, Durdey P, Dixon MF, Williams NS. Local recurrence of rectal adenocarcinoma due to inadequate surgical resection. Histopathological study of lateral tumour spread and surgical excision. Lancet. 1986;2(8514):996–9.
17. Ng IO, Luk IS, Yuen ST, Lau PW, Pritchett CJ, Ng M, et al. Surgical lateral clearance in resected rectal carcinomas. A multivariate analysis of clinicopathologic features. Cancer. 1993;71(6):1972–6.
18. Heald RJ, Husband EM, Ryall RD. The mesorectum in rectal cancer surgery–the clue to pelvic recurrence? Br J Surg. 1982;69(10):613–6.
19. Reynolds JV, Joyce WP, Dolan J, Sheahan K, Hyland JM. Pathological evidence in support of total mesorectal excision in the management of rectal cancer. Br J Surg. 1996;83(8):1112–5.
20. Law WL, Chu KW. Anterior resection for rectal cancer with mesorectal excision: a prospective evaluation of 622 patients. Ann Surg. 2004;240(2):260–8.
21. Heald RJ, Ryall RD. Recurrence and survival after total mesorectal excision for rectal cancer. Lancet. 1986;1(8496):1479–82.
22. MacFarlane JK, Ryall RD, Heald RJ. Mesorectal excision for rectal cancer. Lancet. 1993;341(8843):457–60.
23. Martling AL, Holm T, Rutqvist LE, Moran BJ, Heald RJ, Cedemark B. Effect of a surgical training programme on outcome of rectal cancer in the County of Stockholm. Stockholm colorectal cancer study group, Basingstoke bowel cancer research project. Lancet. 2000;356(9224):93–6.
24. Wibe A, Moller B, Norstein J, Carlsen E, Wiig JN, Heald RJ, et al. A national strategic change in treatment policy for rectal cancer–implementation of total mesorectal excision as routine treatment in Norway. A national audit. Dis Colon Rectum. 2002;45(7):857–66.
25. Williams NS, Dixon MF, Johnston D. Reappraisal of the 5 centimetre rule of distal excision for carcinoma of the rectum: a study of distal intramural spread and of patients' survival. Br J Surg. 1983;70(3):150–4.
26. Karanjia ND, Schache DJ, North WR, Heald RJ. 'Close shave' in anterior resection. Br J Surg. 1990;77(5):510–2.
27. Heald RJ, Moran BJ, Ryall RD, Sexton R, MacFarlane JK. Rectal cancer: the Basingstoke experience of

total mesorectal excision, 1978–1997. Arch Surg. 1998;133(8):894–9.

28. Arbman G, Nilsson E, Hallbook O, Sjodahl R. Local recurrence following total mesorectal excision for rectal cancer. Br J Surg. 1996;83(3):375–9.

29. Heald RJ, Karanjia ND. Results of radical surgery for rectal cancer. World J Surg. 1992;16(5):848–57.

30. Murty M, Enker WE, Martz J. Current status of total mesorectal excision and autonomic nerve preservation in rectal cancer. Semin Surg Oncol. 2000;19(4):321–8.

31. Mohamed ZK, Law WL. Outcome of tumor-specific mesorectal excision for rectal cancer: the impact of laparoscopic resection. World J Surg. 2014;38(8): 2168–74.

32. Enker WE, Thaler HT, Cranor ML, Polyak T. Total mesorectal excision in the operative treatment of carcinoma of the rectum. J Am Coll Surg. 1995;181(4): 335–46.

33. Karanjia ND, Corder AP, Holdsworth PJ, Heald RJ. Risk of peritonitis and fatal septicaemia and the need to defunction the low anastomosis. Br J Surg. 1991;78(2):196–8.

34. Rullier E, Laurent C, Garrelon JL, Michel P, Saric J, Parneix M. Risk factors for anastomotic leakage after resection of rectal cancer. Br J Surg. 1998;85(3):355–8.

35. Law WI, Chu KW, Ho JW, Chan CW. Risk factors for anastomotic leakage after low anterior resection with total mesorectal excision. Am J Surg. 2000;179(2):92–6.

36. Law WL, Chu KW, Choi HK. Randomized clinical trial comparing loop ileostomy and loop transverse colostomy for faecal diversion following total mesorectal excision. Br J Surg. 2002;89(6):704–8.

37. Edwards DP, Leppington-Clarke A, Sexton R, Heald RJ, Moran BJ. Stoma-related complications are more frequent after transverse colostomy than loop ileostomy: a prospective randomized clinical trial. Br J Surg. 2001;88(3):360–3.

38. Chen J, Zhang Y, Jiang C, Yu H, Zhang K, Zhang M, et al. Temporary ileostomy versus colostomy for colorectal anastomosis: evidence from 12 studies. Scand J Gastroenterol. 2013;48(5):556–62.

39. Guenaga KF, Lustosa SA, Saad SS, Saconato H, Matos D. Ileostomy or colostomy for temporary decompression of colorectal anastomosis. Cochrane Database Syst Rev. 2007;24(1):CD004647.

40. Havenga K, Enker WE, McDermott K, Cohen AM, Minsky BD, Guillem J. Male and female sexual and urinary function after total mesorectal excision with autonomic nerve preservation for carcinoma of the rectum. J Am Coll Surg. 1996;182(6):495–502.

41. Nesbakken A, Nygaard K, Bull-Njaa T, Carlsen E, Eri LM. Bladder and sexual dysfunction after mesorectal excision for rectal cancer. Br J Surg. 2000;87(2):206–10.

42. Junginger T, Kneist W, Heintz A. Influence of identification and preservation of pelvic autonomic nerves in rectal cancer surgery on bladder dysfunction after total mesorectal excision. Dis Colon Rectum. 2003;46(5):621–8.

43. Jayne DG, Brown JM, Thorpe H, Walker J, Quirke P, Guillou PJ. Bladder and sexual function following resection for rectal cancer in a randomized clinical trial of laparoscopic versus open technique. Br J Surg. 2005;92(9):1124–32.

44. Kim JY, Kim NK, Lee KY, Hur H, Min BS, Kim JH. A comparative study of voiding and sexual function after total mesorectal excision with autonomic nerve preservation for rectal cancer: laparoscopic versus robotic surgery. Ann Surg Oncol. 2012;19(8):2485–93.

45. Broholm M, Pommergaard HC, Gogenur I. Possible benefits of robot-assisted rectal cancer surgery regarding urological and sexual dysfunction: a systematic review and meta-analysis. Color Dis. 2015;17(5):375–81.

46. Milsom JW, Bohm B, Decanini C, Fazio VW. Laparoscopic oncologic proctosigmoidectomy with low colorectal anastomosis in a cadaver model. Surg Endosc. 1994;8(9):1117–23.

47. Fleshman JW, Wexner SD, Anvari M, LaTulippe JF, Birnbaum EH, Kodner IJ, et al. Laparoscopic vs. open abdominoperineal resection for cancer. Dis Colon Rectum. 1999;42(7):930–9.

48. Darzi A, Lewis C, Menzies-Gow N, Guillou PJ, Monson JR. Laparoscopic abdominoperineal excision of the rectum. Surg Endosc. 1995;9(4):414–7.

49. Law WL, Lee YM, Choi HK, Seto CL, Ho JW. Laparoscopic and open anterior resection for upper and mid rectal cancer: an evaluation of outcomes. Dis Colon Rectum. 2006;49(8):1108–15.

50. Kim SH, Park IJ, Joh YG, Hahn KY. Laparoscopic resection for rectal cancer: a prospective analysis of thirty-month follow-up outcomes in 312 patients. Surg Endosc. 2006;20(8):1197–202.

51. Leroy J, Jamali F, Forbes L, Smith M, Rubino F, Mutter D, et al. Laparoscopic total mesorectal excision (TME) for rectal cancer surgery: long-term outcomes. Surg Endosc. 2004;18(2):281–9.

52. Guillou PJ, Quirke P, Thorpe H, Walker J, Jayne DG, Smith AM, et al. Short-term endpoints of conventional versus laparoscopic-assisted surgery in patients with colorectal cancer (MRC CLASICC trial): multicentre, randomised controlled trial. Lancet. 2005;365(9472): 1718–26.

53. Jayne DG, Guillou PJ, Thorpe H, Quirke P, Copeland J, Smith AM, et al. Randomized trial of laparoscopic-assisted resection of colorectal carcinoma: 3-year results of the UK MRC CLASICC trial group. J Clin Oncol. 2007;25(21):3061–8.

54. Jayne DG, Thorpe HC, Copeland J, Quirke P, Brown JM, Guillou PJ. Five-year follow-up of the Medical Research Council CLASICC trial of laparoscopically assisted versus open surgery for colorectal cancer. Br J Surg. 2010;97(11):1638–45.

55. Bonjer HJ, Deijen CL, Haglind E, Group CIS. A randomized trial of laparoscopic versus open surgery for rectal cancer. N Engl J Med. 2015;373(2):194.

56. Stevenson AR, Solomon MJ, Lumley JW, Hewett P, Clouston AD, Gebski VJ, et al. Effect of laparoscopic-assisted resection vs open resection on pathological outcomes in rectal cancer: the ALaCaRT randomized clinical trial. JAMA. 2015;314(13):1356–63.

57. Fleshman J, Branda M, Sargent DJ, Boller AM, George V, Abbas M, et al. Effect of laparoscopic-assisted resection vs open resection of stage II or III rectal cancer on pathologic outcomes: the ACOSOG Z6051 randomized clinical trial. JAMA. 2015;314(13):1346–55.

58. Xiong B, Ma L, Huang W, Zhao Q, Cheng Y, Liu J. Robotic versus laparoscopic total mesorectal excision for rectal cancer: a meta-analysis of eight studies. J Gastrointest Surg. 2015;19(3):516–26.

59. Law WL, Foo DCC. Comparison of short-term and oncologic outcomes of robotic and laparoscopic resection for mid- and distal rectal cancer. Surg Endosc. 2017;31(7):2798–807.

60. Lim DR, Bae SU, Hur H, Min BS, Baik SH, Lee KY, et al. Long-term oncological outcomes of robotic versus laparoscopic total mesorectal excision of mid-low rectal cancer following neoadjuvant chemoradiation therapy. Surg Endosc. 2017;31(4):1728–37.

61. Fernandez-Hevia M, Delgado S, Castells A, Tasende M, Momblan D, Diaz del Gobbo G, et al. Transanal total mesorectal excision in rectal cancer: short-term outcomes in comparison with laparoscopic surgery. Ann Surg. 2015;261(2):221–7.

62. Zaheer S, Pemberton JH, Farouk R, Dozois RR, Wolff BG, Ilstrup D. Surgical treatment of adenocarcinoma of the rectum. Ann Surg. 1998;227(6):800–11.

63. Nesbakken A, Nygaard K, Westerheim O, Mala T, Lunde OC. Local recurrence after mesorectal excision for rectal cancer. Eur J Surg Oncol. 2002;28(2):126–34.

64. Piso P, Dahlke MH, Mirena P, Schmidt U, Aselmann H, Schlitt HJ, et al. Total mesorectal excision for middle and lower rectal cancer: a single institution experience with 337 consecutive patients. J Surg Oncol. 2004;86(3):115–21.

Total Mesorectal Excision and Preservation of the Pelvic Autonomic Nerves: Technical Tips and Pitfall

12

Nam Kyu Kim

Abstract

To obtain relevant oncologic outcome and good functional outcome after rectal cancer surgery, total mesorectal excision (TME) with pelvic autonomic nerve (PAN) preservation is essential. Adequate TME with intact mesorectal fascia is very important to achieve clearance of lymphatics; also, avoiding nerve injuries including superior and inferior hypogastric nerves and neurovascular bundles in the pelvis is essential for good postoperative voiding and sexual function. In this context, this chapter is highlighting on fascial anatomy for TME and autonomic nerve structures. On the basis of the anatomy, technical tips for TME with PAN preservation are introduced by the author. This review of anatomy for TME and technical issues for preserving PAN will provide you an insight of desirable TME.

Keywords

Colorectal cancer · Low anterior resection · Total mesorectal excision · Pelvic autonomic nerve

The incidence of colorectal cancer has increased rapidly during the last 20 years in Korea and now ranks as the third most common cancer and fourth most common cause of cancer mortality [1]. Considering the recent annual trend of cases of colorectal cancer in Korea, the proportion of rectal cancer cases has decreased, but distal colon cancer has shown a rapid increase [2]. In this context, it is important for the colorectal surgeon to determine how to remove these tumors with curative intent and without any complications. With the adoption of the concept of total mesorectal excision (TME), proposed by Dr. Heald [3], the local recurrence rates have decreased dramatically, and promising results have been shown in terms of functional preservation and operative safety [4, 5]. We continue to improve the technique to gain enhanced oncologic outcomes in locally advanced rectal cancer. Additionally, the complete mesocolic excision (CME) and central vessel ligation (CVL) concepts, proposed by Dr. Hohenberg [6], which involve planned anatomical dissection and apical lymph node dissection, are becoming more emphasized, subsequently improving oncologic outcomes. The fascial anatomy of the rectum and its lymphatic spread pattern should be understood for a successful operation.

12.1 Basic Anatomy

The rectum is located in the pelvic cavity; the lower third of the anterior portion is extraperitoneally located, while the posterior part is fully

N. K. Kim
Department of Surgery, Yonsei University College of Medicine, Seoul, South Korea
e-mail: namkyuk@yuhs.ac

© Springer Nature Singapore Pte Ltd. 2018
N. K. Kim et al. (eds.), *Surgical Treatment of Colorectal Cancer*,
https://doi.org/10.1007/978-981-10-5143-2_12

extraperitoneal (Fig. 12.1). The length of the rectum is 12–15 cm. The rectal muscle wall is surrounded by a fatty layer known as the mesorectum, which contains blood vessels, lymphatics, and lymph nodes. The rectum, including the mesorectum, is enveloped by the endopelvic fascia. This structure contacts with the adjacent pelvic organs such as the prostate, seminal vesicles, posterior vaginal wall, and cervix of the uterus [7–9].

Additionally, the rectum passes through the pelvic floor and becomes the anus. At this level, a funnel-shaped muscular sheet structure is present, called the pelvic diaphragm. The pelvic floor muscles consist of three named muscles, the puborectalis, pubococcygeus, and iliococcygeus muscles. The puborectalis muscle wraps around the rectum and makes a sharp anorectal angle, which aids in fecal continence [7–9].

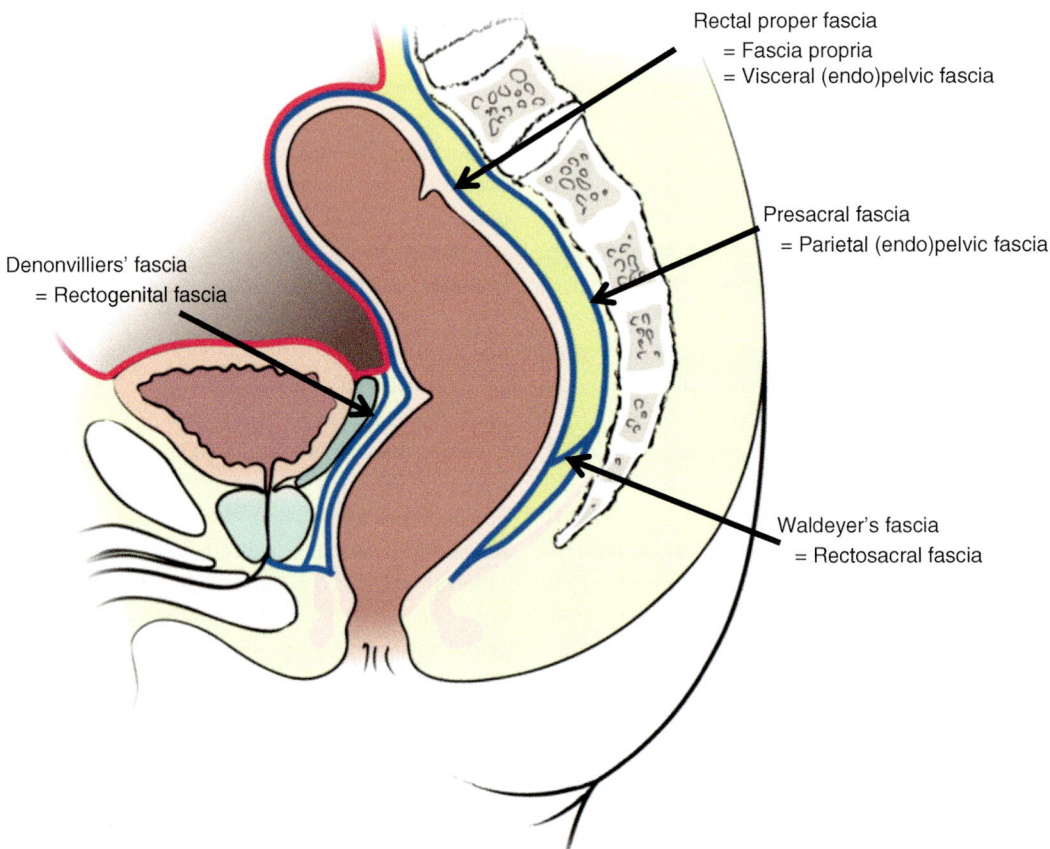

Rectal proper fascia
= Fascia propria
= Visceral (endo)pelvic fascia

Denonvilliers' fascia
= Rectogenital fascia

Presacral fascia
= Parietal (endo)pelvic fascia

Waldeyer's fascia
= Rectosacral fascia

Fig. 12.1 Location of the rectum in the pelvic cavity and nomina of the fascia structures around the rectum. Rectal proper fascia, the fascia covering mesorectum, also called visceral endopelvic fascia; presacral fascia, the fascia covering the sacrum, also called parietal endopelvic fascia; Denonvilliers' fascia, a dense membrane between the rectum and the seminal vesicles, also called rectogenital fascia; Waldeyer's fascia, a dense connective tissue layer between the posterior part of the rectal proper fascia and the presacral fascia at the level of S3 and S4

12.2   The Fascial Anatomy

It is important to understand the fascial planes around the rectum and the adjacent organs to obtain a sharp pelvic dissection along the embryologic planes. If pelvic dissection proceeds along the correct fascial plane, the operation can be finished without bleeding. Bisset et al. described a fibrous envelope surrounding the perirectal fat, called the mesorectum, and named it the fascia propria [8]. It corresponds to the visceral pelvic fascia. Histological studies of gross specimens and cadavers have revealed a variable thickness of the fascia propria [8]. Unless the fascia covering bony structures and muscles is open, the nerve structures cannot usually be seen (Fig. 12.2) [7]. At the S4 level, relatively dense connective tissue between the presacral fascia and the rectal proper fascia is encountered [7, 10, 11]. This fascia is known as the rectosacral fascia, or Waldeyer's fascia. Crapp and Cuthbertson pointed out its clinical significance because failure to recognize and divide it may result in hemorrhage from the presacral venous plexus [12]. The thickness of this fascia varies between individuals. In thick case, blunt dissection by hand may result in avulsion injury of the presacral venous system [12].

Sharp division of the rectosacral fascia enables pelvic dissection reaching down to the coccyx level; the pelvic plexus can then be visualized at the posterolateral side of the pelvic wall. In males, at the level of the seminal vesicles, pelvic dissection is extended to Denonvilliers' fascia, a dense connective tissue layer at the anterior part of the rectum. By incising this membrane, the rectum is dissected from the seminal vesicles (Fig. 12.3). Denonvilliers first described this as a membrane behind the seminal vesicles and in front of the rectum [13]. The consistency varies from a thin, transparent layer to a tough, thick membrane. It seems to be more prominent in young male patients, and it is composed of dense collagen fibers and coarse elastic fibers. The Denonvilliers' fascia should be opened on the lower part of the anterior aspect of the rectum, and one should dissect down along its posterior aspect to avoid injury to the neurovascular bundles running to the genitalia [13, 14]. Detailed surgical techniques used to preserve pelvic autonomic nerves will be discussed further on.

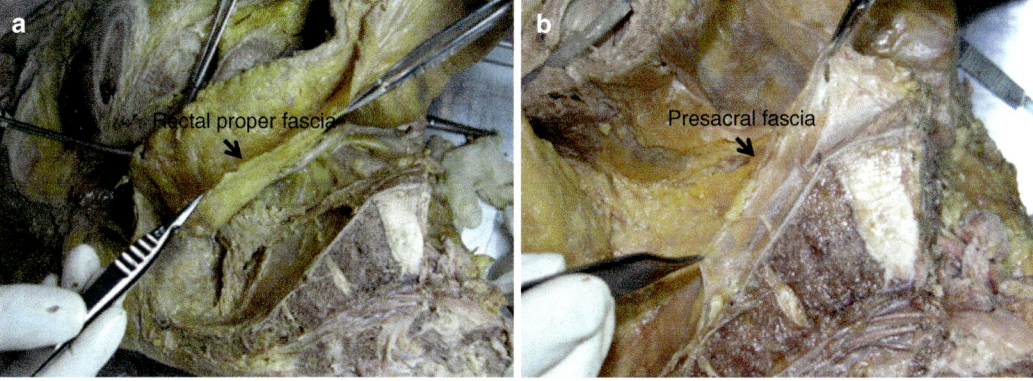

Fig. 12.2 Hemipelvis specimen in a cadaveric dissection. (**a**) The structure being picked up is the thickened rectal proper fascia. (**b**) The structure being picked up is the presacral fascia covering the sacrum

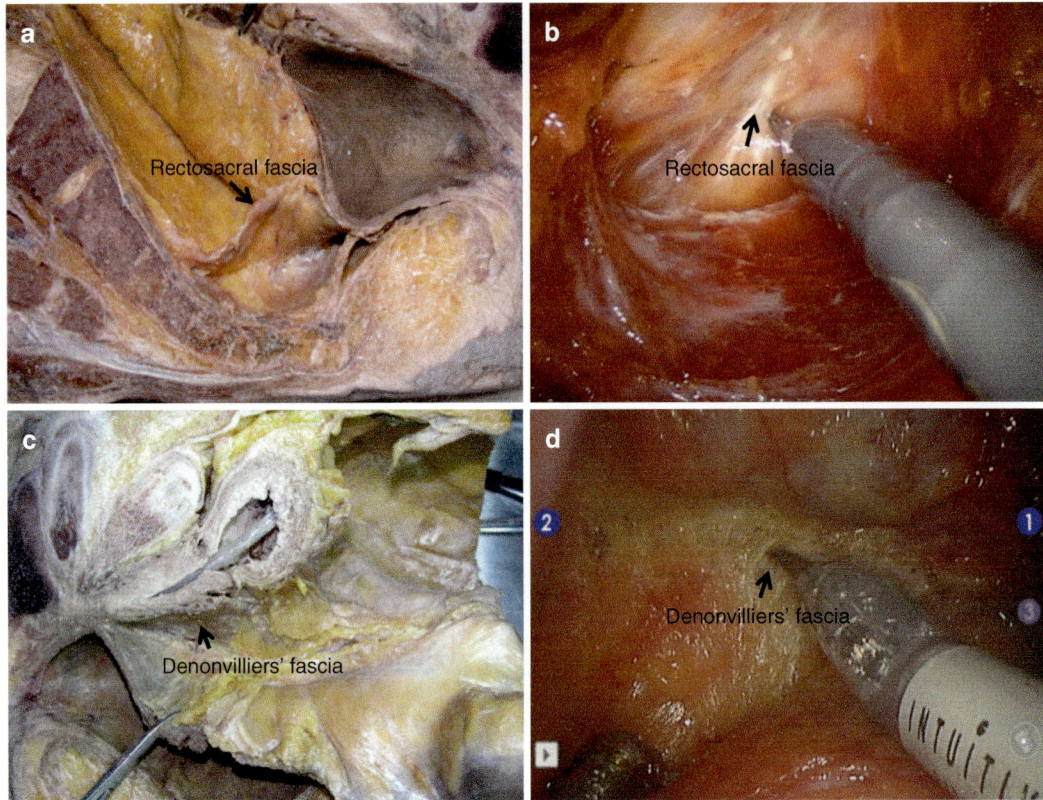

Fig. 12.3 Anatomy of fascia. (**a**) Rectosacral fascia connecting the presacral fascia at the level of S3 and the rectal proper fascia in a cadaveric hemipelvis dissection. (**b**) Rectosacral fascia encountered during robotic surgery. (**c**) Denonvilliers' fascia in a cadaveric hemipelvic dissection. (**d**) Denonvilliers' fascia encountered during robotic surgery

12.3 The Anatomy of the Mesorectum

The rectum is surrounded by a layer of fat tissue; this layer is called the mesorectum [3]. Some important knowledge about the mesorectum exists. First, the mesorectum contains blood vessels, lymphatics, and lymph nodes. It is enveloped by the thin mesorectal fascia, which has a shiny appearance and consists of collagen fibers, as proven by histological examination. Secondly, the posterolateral part of the mesorectum has the thickest appearance, whereas the anterior part has the thinnest structure [7]. Thirdly, the mesorectum is almost absent approximately 2 cm above the levator ani muscles [3]. At this point, only the rectal wall remains (Fig. 12.4). In other words, the meso-

rectum starts to taper down from the attachment of the rectosacral fascia. Hence, in surgery for middle and lower rectal cancer, removal of nearly the entire mesorectum has become standard.

12.4 The Anatomy of the Pelvic Floor

The levator ani forms the pelvic floor. It consists of the pubococcygeus, puborectalis, and iliococcygeus muscles. These muscles actually insert into the pelvic sidewall, which is like a membranous sheet and adheres to the rectal proper fascia. According to sex and body mass index (BMI), various types of pelvic floor can be observed based on the coronal axial views of rectal magnetic resonance imaging (MRI) (Fig. 12.5).

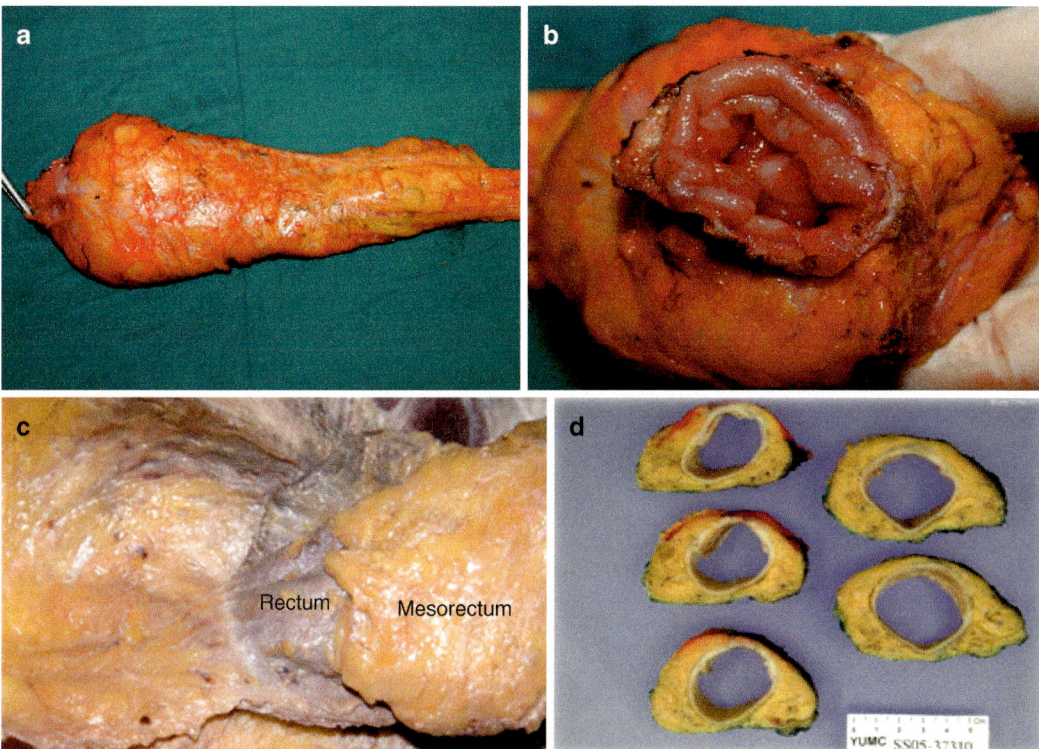

Fig. 12.4 Anatomy of the mesorectum. (**a**) Specimen of a total mesorectal excision, showing a shiny intact meso-rectal fascia appearance. (**b**) The mesorectum is well developed around the rectal wall. (**c**) Mesorectum tapered down from the attachment of the rectosacral fascia in a cadaveric dissection. (**d**) Prominent thickness of the pos-terolateral part of the mesorectum viewed in whole mount sections

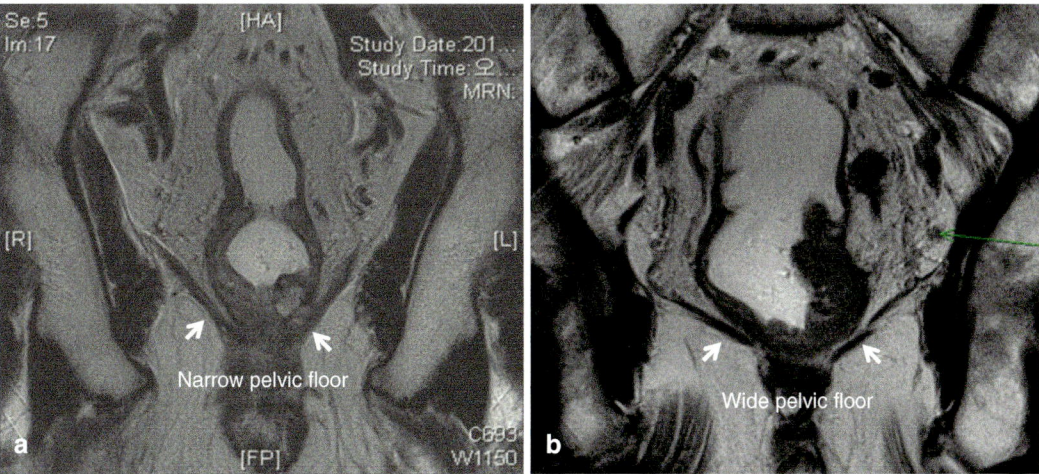

Fig. 12.5 Pelvic floor images on the coronal axial view of a magnetic resonance image (MRI). (**a**) Steep coning down of the pelvic floor with a narrow angle. (**b**) Gradual coning down of the pelvic floor with a wide angle

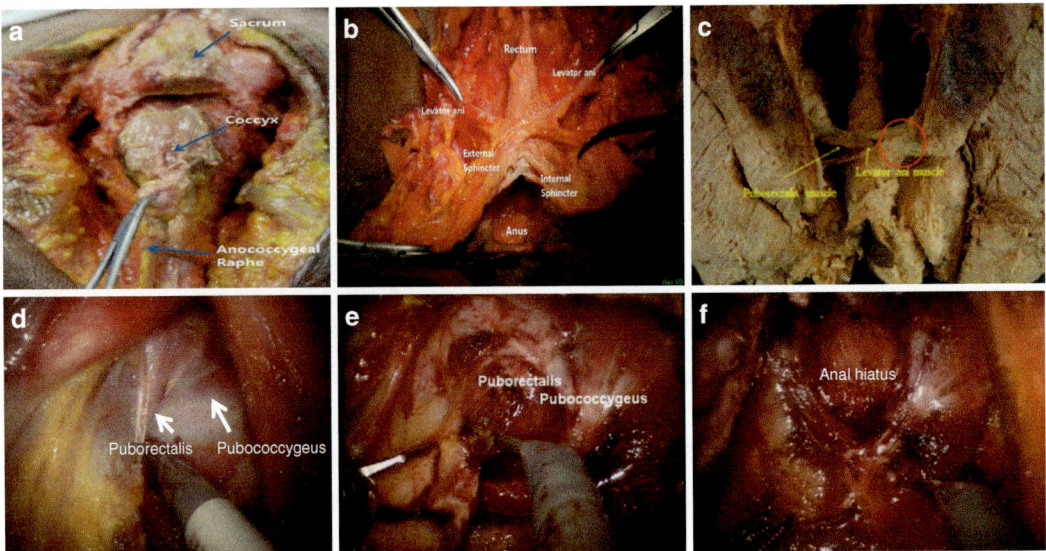

Fig. 12.6 Anatomy of the pelvic floor muscles. (**a**) Posterior aspect of the pelvis after division of the sacrum. (**b**) After removal of the sacrum, the funnel-shaped pelvic floor is shown with the sphincter complex. (**c**) Fixed cadaveric specimen showing the pelvic floor and puborectalis muscle. (**d**, **e**) With deep pelvic dissection, the pelvic floor muscles (puborectalis and pubococcygeus) are exposed. (**f**) Anal hiatus (triangular opening) with the anococcygeal ligament formed from the pelvic floor muscles, through which the rectum passes

The U-shaped puborectalis muscle can be clearly seen during dissection and has a role in preventing fecal incontinence by making a sharp anorectal angle. This funnel-shaped structure is usually attached to the mesorectum and its enveloping fascia. If the attached mesorectum is completely mobilized from the pelvic floor, we can then see the anococcygeal raphe and anal hiatus. In operative findings, the rectal muscle layer seems to be intermingled with the surrounding external anal sphincter complex (Fig. 12.6). Around this area, the anorectal ring can be identified, which is usually present 4 cm from the anal verge.

12.5 Pelvic Autonomic Nerve Structure

The superior hypogastric nerve descends and forms a plexus in the vicinity of the origin of the inferior mesenteric artery. This plexus forms a dense network around the inferior mesenteric artery. Therefore, during dissection of the lymph nodes around the origin of the inferior mesenteric artery or ligation of the inferior mesenteric artery, the superior hypogastric nerve may be injured. If this occurs, retrograde ejaculation can develop. The inferior hypogastric nerve descends to the pelvis by crossing the left common iliac artery at the level of the first sacrum and descends further into the pelvic cavity along the pelvic sidewall. Therefore, during the separation of the mesosigmoid colon from the gonadal vessels and the ureters, the superior and inferior hypogastric nerve plexus must be preserved [15, 16].

Pelvic dissection must be kept along the plane between the inferior hypogastric nerve fibers and rectal proper fascia in the pelvic cavity. Occasionally, fine branches to the rectal proper fascia are noted, which are vulnerable to cutting during dissection.

The inferior hypogastric nerve forms the pelvic nerve plexus at the lateral pelvic wall by encountering the parasympathetic sacral nerve originating from the second, third, and fourth sacral foramens. Numerous small neurovascular bundles running from the pelvic plexus to the genitalia cross the seminal vesicles in the 10 and 2 o'clock directions (Fig. 12.7) [7, 13, 16].

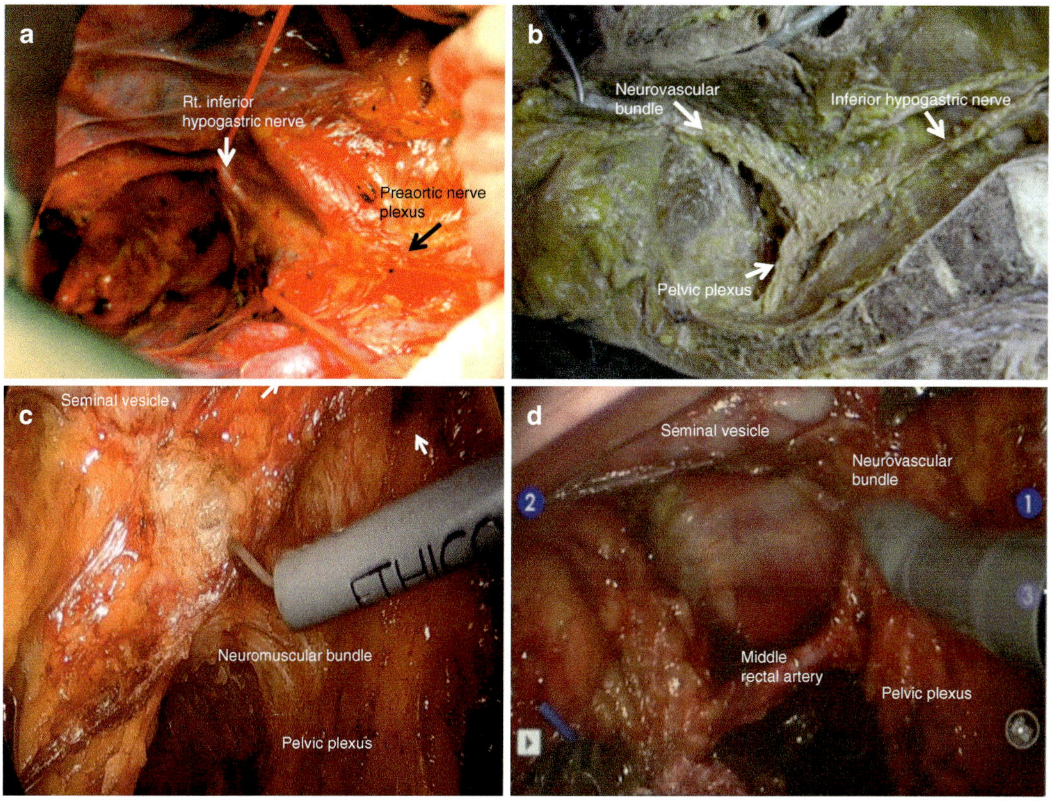

Fig. 12.7 Pelvic autonomic nerve structures. (**a**) Both inferior hypogastric nerves at sides of the pelvic wall, going down to the deep pelvis, merging with the sacral parasympathetic nerves from S2–4, and finally forming the pelvic plexus with a mesh-like structure. (**b**) Y-shaped pelvic autonomic nerve structures seen in the hemipelvis of a cadaveric section, showing that the inferior hypogastric nerve descends along each side of the pelvic wall and merges with the sacral parasympathetic nerves to become the pelvic plexus. This is densely attached to the lateral part of the mesorectal fascia, and the neurovascular bundle extends to the genitalia. (**c**) Laparoscopic view of the pelvic plexus and neurovascular bundles. (**d**) It shows a robotic view of the middle rectal artery arising near the pelvic plexus and piercing pelvic plexus. Denonvilliers' fascia continues with the right-side neurovascular bundles, which arise from the pelvic plexus. These structures can be seen after full mobilization of the rectum from the underlying pelvic floor muscles

Y-shaped pelvic autonomic nerve structures are clearly seen at the hemipelvis during cadaveric dissection [7]. The inferior hypogastric nerves descend along each side of the pelvic wall, and well mesh-like structures are densely attached to the lateral part of the mesorectal fascia, previously called the lateral ligament. The middle rectal artery has been reported to be present at approximately 20% of cases and mostly unilaterally [17]. The mean diameter of this vessel is 1.6 mm [17]; therefore, meticulous dissection with cauterization by monopolar or bipolar devices is sufficient to dissect this area. It usually pierces the pelvic plexus; thus, nerve preservation techniques are important for preserving sexual and voiding functions. To achieve these goals, it is important to understand the relation between the nerves and the pelvic fascia. Dissection should be performed along the loose areolar tissue between the rectal proper fascia and the parietal pelvic fascia.

12.6   Technical Tips for Autonomic Nerve Preservation

In the past open TME era, it was difficult to see the autonomic nerves by eye; therefore, lateral and anterior traction on the rectum was used to produce tenting of the pelvic plexus away from the posterolateral pelvic wall. For subsequent blunt dissection with excessive traction, the dense attachment is usually used to be clamped and ligated. Nowadays, as minimally invasive surgery has evolved, a magnified view has allowed us to see those structures.

One cannot emphasize enough the importance of the technique used for lateral mobilization of the rectum to preserve the autonomic nerves. Usually, the rectal proper fascia surrounding the mesorectum is adhered to the pelvic plexus. The pelvic plexus can be injured directly, or avulsion injury can ensue from excessive traction of the rectum in the narrow pelvic cavity. After the rectosacral fascia is divided, dissection can be continued to the coccyx level. With Denonvilliers' fascia divided, the anterior mesorectum then can be separated from the seminal vesicles. The anterolateral part of the mesorectal fascia is almost directly adhered to the neurovascular bundles and sits down on the pelvic floor; therefore, the mesorectal fascia should be separated carefully to avoid damage to the nerves. Unless posterolateral dissection is continued, the pelvic plexus might not be visualized. At this area, arising sacral nerves can also be seen after the parietal peritoneum is dissected off in a cadaveric dissection [7]. If the tumor is located close to the lateral part of the mesorectum, traction of the rectum and dissection from the pelvic plexus might cause breaching of the covering rectal proper fascia at the narrow true pelvic cavity. If the tumor seems to invade the pelvic wall, en bloc resection should be done including the pelvic plexus. Yamakoshi et al. reported interesting data showing the average distance between the muscularis propria and the pelvic plexus for both autopsied and surgical specimens to be 8.3 mm and 14.7 mm, respectively [18]. The pelvic plexus is located 10 mm from the outer margin of the rectal muscularis propria on average [18]. This observation led us to decide to resect the pelvic plexus concomitantly for curative resection if the middle and lower rectal cancers invade the rectal wall.

Cadaveric dissection with a hemisectioned pelvis shows that the rectal proper fascia is directly adhered to the mesh-like pelvic plexus; this adhered portion used to be regarded as a ligament, the so-called lateral ligament. This ligamentous structure between the mesorectum and the inferior hypogastric nerve and pelvic plexus varies in thickness. This lateral adhesion may contain a middle rectal artery, which is found in approximately 20% of cases, but its incidence varies according to studies [17, 19].

Regarding injury of the pelvic plexus, the surrounding areas should be handled carefully during mobilization of the rectum from the pelvic cavity. With successive dissection of this area, the rectum and mesorectum are finally delivered from the true pelvic cavity, exposing the quadrangular mesh-like structures (pelvic plexus) attached to the rectal proper fascia. It is a matted rhomboid structure that is 4 cm by 2.5 cm in size, lying almost in the sagittal plane lateral to the rectum. Sato reported that the pelvic splanchnic nerves arising more posteromedially from the third and fourth sacral nerves could be considered a component of the lateral ligament [17].

The neurovascular bundles, described by Walsh and Schlegel, run in front of the rectogenital fascia within the parametrium or in the space occupied by the seminal vesicles and the prostate gland [20, 21]. Hollabaugh et al. reported that most of the efferent nerves of the pelvic plexus ran along the prostate surface of Denonvilliers' fascia [22]. Based on Walsh's report on nerve-sparing radical prostatectomy, the seminal vesicles can be used as an intraoperative landmark to identify the pelvic plexus, which is imbedded in the thick fascia and perforated by branches of the inferior vesical artery and vein. The running neurovascular bundles are located at the extreme lateral part of the seminal vesicles, which is a continuation of the pelvic plexus at the lateral pelvic wall [20, 21].

The importance of avoiding damage to the pelvic plexus and the neurovascular bundles to the genitalia during pelvic dissection should be emphasized. For successful separation of the lateral part of the rectum from the pelvic plexus, it is important to incise the rectosacral fascia to continue to dissect down to the coccyx and to separate the mesorectal fascia from the pelvic plexus with meticulous dissection. Proper traction of the rectum is important for preventing avulsion injury of the pelvic plexus. During dissection of this area, the middle rectal artery is sometimes encountered, and it should be ligated with surgical clips and divided or electrocauterized. Mass ligation and too much traction may cause injury to the running third sacral nerve, which is crucial for erectile function. Cutting the rectosacral fascia and opening the retrorectal space laterally usually reveal the nervi erigentes, in which the S3 competent is the largest. Although sharp dissection around this area is necessary, it is difficult to perform in a deep and narrow male pelvis. However, under magnified vision and using gentle traction with a robotic arm instrument, preservation of these structures is more achievable compared to open surgery for rectal cancer.

In summary, regarding autonomic nerve preservation techniques, the superior hypogastric nerve or preaortic sympathetic plexus around the root of the inferior mesenteric artery and the area of the left common iliac artery should be identified, and care should be taken not to damage these structures. Excessive traction on the rectum secondary to posterior mobilization may result in neuropraxia or avulsion of the second, third, and fourth sacral roots. These injuries could result in temporary or permanent bladder and erectile dysfunction.

A high incidence of sexual and bladder dysfunction has been reported after abdominoperineal resection (APR) in comparison to after low anterior resection (LAR). During APR, injury to the cavernous nerves during perineal dissection may result in erectile dysfunction. Division of the rectourethralis muscle and blunt dissection or excessive electrocauterization of the neurovascular bundles at the anterolateral part of the rectum may also contribute to sexual dysfunction. At the perineum, important structural landmarks include the superficial and deep perineal muscles in the anterior perineal body and the posterior anococcygeal ligament [10, 11, 23].

12.7   How to Perform Successful Mobilization of the Rectum from the Pelvic Floor

For a bloodless, sharp pelvic dissection, it is important to understand the embryological fascia plane. The mesorectum and rectum are covered with the rectal proper fascia (visceral pelvic fascia). The parietal pelvic fascia usually covers the bony structures. Between these fascial structures, termed the presacral fascia, the autonomic nervous system is usually present. During posterior pelvic dissection, a dense pelvic fascia, called Waldeyer's fascia, is noted at the S4 level. Unless this fascia is sharply divided, dissection cannot enter the deep pelvic cavity, and presacral venous bleeding can occur with avulsed presacral fascia. During anterior dissection, Denonvilliers' fascia is present at the level of the seminal vesicles and continues to the prostate capsule [7, 12, 14].

The mesorectum is surrounded by the mesorectal fascia in a cylindrical manner, which sits just above the pelvic floor. It is necessary to fully understand the anatomical structures here to perform a complete circumferential sharp pelvic dissection. The mesorectum is tapered down 2 cm above the anorectal ring [7].

Regarding pelvic autonomic nerve preservation, there are some landmark structures that should be identified and preserved, which are the preaortic sympathetic plexus near the root of the inferior mesenteric artery, inferior hypogastric nerves, pelvic plexus, and the neurovascular bundles to the genitalia. From the pelvic plexus, the neurovascular bundles to the genitalia run in the directions of 10 and 2 o'clock from the seminal vesicles. Dissection below the Denonvilliers' fascia is safer to preserve the neurovascular bundles, ensuing preservation of urogenital function [14].

I would like to emphasize that the most important step for completeness of TME for middle and lower rectal cancer will be deep pelvic floor circumferential dissection. This procedure will be the crucial step for better oncologic and functional outcomes. From the level of seminal vesicle or vagina, the Denonvilliers' fascia should be separated from the mesorectal fascia, and mesorectum should be separated from the neurovascular bundle and pelvic plexus. For that, posterior dissection should be continued to the anococcygeal raphe or less, at least reaching Waldeyer's fascia; and then mesorectum should be continued to be separated from the vagina or seminal vesicles circumferentially. After then, you surely meet the gate of the pelvic floor and easily separate rectal wall (in this area, no mesorectum) from the puborectalis muscle and other pelvic floor muscles. So-called deep pelvic dissection from the true pelvis is a very essential technique and concept for colorectal surgeons.

12.8 Technical Tips for Safe Anastomosis

As we pursue curative resection for better oncologic outcomes, it is also important to perform safe colorectal anastomosis. No tension, a good blood supply, and good stapled techniques are essential, and we must know the technical tips for avoiding anastomotic leakage and stenosis. For low ligation, vascular variations of the branches of the inferior mesenteric artery, bifurcation level, and the number of sigmoid arterial branches must be known. The meandering mesenteric artery near the origin of the inferior mesenteric vein at the inferior border of the pancreas is occasionally observed. During ligation of inferior mesenteric vein, it is important to avoid the damage to this arterial arcade, which is a crucial blood supply to the splenic flexure and descending colon.

Conclusion

Sharp pelvic dissection under direct vision with good anatomical knowledge is essential in the field of rectal cancer surgery. The introduction of TME has improved oncologic outcomes in patients with rectal cancer. Functional outcomes should focus on the patients' satisfaction and quality of life. A good understanding of the anatomy of the rectum and of pelvic autonomic nerves and meticulous dissection techniques enable us to achieve both good oncologic and functional

outcomes. With the increase in minimally invasive surgical techniques in current clinical practices, we need more structured education training programs for those skills.

A step-by-step approach with good anatomical knowledge is essential for successful TME. The following are the proposed procedures [24]:

1. *Posterior pelvic dissection*: Posterior dissection is performed along the rectal proper fascia, enveloping the rectum and mesorectum, leaving behind the hypogastric nerves along the pelvic wall; the bilateral ureter and common iliac vessels can be exposed and identified. Dissection is continued down to the rectosacral fascia.
2. *Deep posterior pelvic dissection*: For patients with a very narrow or bulky mesorectum, the sequence of dissection can be changed from the deep posterior dissection into anterior dissection. During this procedure, use of a little broad nylon tape for hanging the rectum to make countertraction upward by an assistant is preferred. Successful TME along the anatomical plane is based on adequate traction and countertraction. After the rectosacral fascia is divided, the attachment between the pelvic plexus and the mesorectal fascia can be dissected off the pelvic wall. Posteriorly, the presacral venous plexus exists.
3. *Anterior pelvic dissection*: After the anterior surface of the peritoneum is divided, the seminal vesicles in males and the posterior vaginal wall in females are identified. The Denonvilliers' fascia is visible at the level of the seminal vesicles, and dissection should be performed behind this fascia. At the 10 and 2 o'clock direction (both tips of the seminal vesicles), neurovascular bundles form the pelvic plexus that runs along the seminal vesicles before going to the genitalia. Finally, after the lower part of the rectum is mobilized from the pelvic floor, pelvic plexus, neurovascular bundles, and pelvic floor muscles are exposed.

4. *Posterolateral or anterolateral pelvic dissection*: This step should be performed carefully before complete rectal mobilization from the pelvic floor. The cylindrical mesorectum with the intact mesorectal fascia should be obtained from the posterolateral dissection, and there should be no breach of the covering mesorectal fascia on the anterolateral side.

5. *Pelvic floor exposure*: The mesorectum is placed on different shapes of the pelvic floor, and some of the pelvic floor muscles, including the puborectalis muscle and anococcygeal raphe, can be identified after full mobilization of the rectum.

References

1. Oh CM, Won YJ, Jung KW, Kong HJ, Cho H, Lee JK, et al. Cancer statistics in Korea: incidence, mortality, survival, and prevalence in 2013. Cancer Res Treat. 2016;48(2):436–50.

2. Shin A, Kim KZ, Jung KW, Park S, Won YJ, Kim J, et al. Increasing trend of colorectal cancer incidence in Korea, 1999–2009. Cancer Res Treat. 2012;44(4):219–26.

3. Heald RJ, Husband EM, Ryall RD. The mesorectum in rectal cancer surgery–the clue to pelvic recurrence? Br J Surg. 1982;69(10):613–6.

4. Kim JY, Kim NK, Lee KY, Hur H, Min BS, Kim JH. A comparative study of voiding and sexual function after total mesorectal excision with autonomic nerve preservation for rectal cancer: laparoscopic versus robotic surgery. Ann Surg Oncol. 2012;19(8):2485–93.

5. Heald RJ, Ryall RD. Recurrence and survival after total mesorectal excision for rectal cancer. Lancet. 1986;1(8496):1479–82.

6. Hohenberger W, Weber K, Matzel K, Papadopoulos T, Merkel S. Standardized surgery for colonic cancer: complete mesocolic excision and central ligation–technical notes and outcome. Color Dis. 2009;11(4):354–64.

7. Kim NK. Anatomic basis of sharp pelvic dissection for curative resection of rectal cancer. Yonsei Med J. 2005;46(6):737–49.

8. Bissett IP, Hill GL. Extrafascial excision of the rectum for cancer: a technique for the avoidance of the complications of rectal mobilisation. Semin Surg Oncol. 2000;18(3):207–15.

9. Church JM, Raudkivi PJ, Hill GL. The surgical anatomy of the rectum–a review with particular relevance

to the hazards of rectal mobilisation. Int J Color Dis. 1987;2(3):158–66.

10. Kim NK. Sharp pelvic dissection for abdominoperineal resection for distal rectal cancer based on anatomical and MRI knowledge. J Korean Soc Coloproctol. 2005;21(4):258–67.

11. Kim NK. Anatomic basis of sharp pelvic dissection for total mesorectal excision with pelvic autonomic nerve preservation for rectal cancer. J Korean Soc Coloproctol. 2004;20(6):424–34.

12. Crapp AR, Cuthbertson AM. William Waldeyer and the rectosacral fascia. Surg Gynecol Obstet. 1974;138(2):252–6.

13. Kourambas J, Angus DG, Hosking P, Chou ST. A histological study of Denonvilliers' fascia and its relationship to the neurovascular bundle. Br J Urol. 1998;82(3):408–10.

14. Heald RJ, Moran BJ, Brown G, Daniels IR. Optimal total mesorectal excision for rectal cancer is by dissection in front of Denonvilliers' fascia. Br J Surg. 2004;91(1):121–3.

15. Liang J, Chang K, Wang S, Havenga K. Anatomical basis of autonomic nerve-preserving total mesorecta exicision for recta cancer. Br J Surg. 1997;84(4):586–7.

16. Havenga K, DeRuiter MC, Enker WE, Welvaart K. Anatomical basis of autonomic nerve-preserving total mesorectal excision for rectal cancer. Br J Surg. 1996;83(3):384–8.

17. Sato K, Sato T. The vascular and neuronal composition of the lateral ligament of the rectum and the rectosacral fascia. Surg Radiol Anat. 1991;13(1):17–22.

18. Yamakoshi H, Ike I, Oki S, Hara M, Shimada H. An assessment of the anatomical relationship between the pelvic plexus and the rectal wall to determine the indications for its preservation in surgery for rectal cancer. Surg Today. 1997;27(11):1005–9.

19. Jones OM, Smeulders N, Wiseman O, Miller R. Lateral ligaments of the rectum: an anatomical study. Br J Surg. 1999;86(4):487–9.

20. Walsh PC, Donker PJ. Impotence following radical prostatectomy: insight into etiology and prevention. J Urol. 1982;128(3):492–7.

21. Walsh PC, Schlegel PN. Radical pelvic surgery with preservation of sexual function. Ann Surg. 1988;208(4):391–400.

22. Hollabaugh RS Jr, Steiner MS, Sellers KD, Samm BJ, Dmochowski RR. Neuroanatomy of the pelvis: implications for colonic and rectal resection. Dis Colon Rectum. 2000;43(10):1390–7.

23. Hur H, Bae SU, Kim NK, Min BS, Baik SH, Lee KY, et al. Comparative study of voiding and male sexual function following open and laparoscopic total mesorectal excision in patients with rectal cancer. J Surg Oncol. 2013;108(8):572–8.

24. Kim NK, Kim YW, Cho MS. Total mesorectal excision for rectal cancer with emphasis on pelvic autonomic nerve preservation: expert technical tips for robotic surgery. Surg Oncol. 2015;24(3):172–80.

Pelvic Autonomic Nerve Preservation and Lateral Pelvic Lymph Node Dissection: Techniques and Oncologic Benefits

Hiroyasu Kagawa and Yusuke Kinugasa

Abstract

The goals of surgery for rectal cancer are to achieve curative resection and maintain quality of life while minimizing the risk of local recurrence and prolonging patient survival. The standard treatment for locally advanced rectal cancer in Japan is TME with lateral lymph node dissection (LLD). Lateral lymph node metastasis was present in 15.6–20.4% of patients with lower rectal cancer and that the risk of pelvic recurrence would decrease by 50% and the 5-year survival rate would improve by 8% when LLD was performed for T3 or T4 lower rectal cancer. The JCOG0212 trial, which is multicenter randomized controlled trial comparing mesorectal excision (ME) with or without LLD, reported that local recurrence was lower in the mesorectal excision (ME) with LLD group (7.4%) compared with the ME-only group (12.6%). The urinary complications and sexual dysfunction rates did not differ between the two groups.

We will describe the surgical procedures needed to perform nerve-sparing LLD in detail. Provided nerve-sparing LLD is performed accurately, local control of rectal cancer is excellent and does not cause urogenital dysfunction. We conclude the procedure appears to be safe and effective.

Keywords

Lateral lymph node dissection · Rectal cancer Autonomic nerve preservation

13.1 Introduction

The goals of surgery for rectal cancer are to achieve curative resection and maintain quality of life while minimizing the risk of local recurrence and prolonging patient survival. Whenever possible, function should also be preserved. These have improved with the development of better surgical techniques and the use of adjuvant therapy. Total mesorectal excision (TME) has been reported to reduce the local recurrence rate [1] and is used with radiotherapy (RT) as the standard treatment for advanced rectal cancer in Western countries. A Dutch trial reported that the 10-year cumulative incidence for local recurrence was lower in a group receiving surgery plus RT than in a group receiving surgery alone but that overall survival did not differ between the groups [2]. Furthermore, RT can be complicated

H. Kagawa (✉)
Division of Colon and Rectal Surgery, Shizuoka
Cancer Center Hospital, Nagaizumi-cho, Sunto-gun,
Shizuoka, Japan
e-mail: h.kagawa@scchr.jp

Y. Kinugasa
Department of Gastrointestinal Surgery,
Tokyo Medical Dental University, Tokyo, Japan
e-mail: kinugasa.srg1@tmd.ac.jp

© Springer Nature Singapore Pte Ltd. 2018
N. K. Kim et al. (eds.), *Surgical Treatment of Colorectal Cancer*,
https://doi.org/10.1007/978-981-10-5143-2_13

by bowel, sexual, or anal dysfunction [3, 4]. Although chemoradiotherapy (CRT) can lower the local recurrence rate, the available evidence shows that it does not improve survival [5, 6]. In contrast to the Western approach of preoperative CRT, the standard treatment for locally advanced rectal cancer in Japan is TME with lateral lymph node dissection (LLD). Moriya et al. described nerve-sparing rectal resection with LLD in the 1980s [7, 8], stating that such an approach could improve the local control, survival, urinary complications, and sexual dysfunction rates [9, 10].

In this chapter, we describe the anatomical characteristics and surgical techniques of LLD and outline the oncological benefits.

13.2 Indications for LLD

In Japan, LLD is the standard treatment for locally advanced lower rectal cancer. According to Japanese Society for Cancer of the Colon and Rectum Guidelines 2016, LLD is indicated when the lower border of a tumor is located distal to the peritoneal reflection and when the tumor has invaded beyond the muscularis propria [11]. This is based on research showing that lateral lymph node (LLN) metastasis has an incidence of 20.1% in lower rectal cancer and that, preoperatively, 7.4% of patients without metastasis on computed tomography or magnetic resonance imaging are subsequently found to have LLN metastasis [12].

13.3 Anatomic Landmarks for LLD

LLNs located between the autonomic nerves and blood vessels are divided into three parts: the common iliac lymph node, the internal iliac lymph node, and the obturator lymph node. They can be dissected en bloc with reference to four planes that surround the LLNs: plane A is the inner side and comprises the hypogastric nerve and pelvic plexus, plane B is the medial side with the visceral branches of the internal iliac artery, plane C is the lateral side with the visceral branches of the internal iliac artery, and plane D is the pelvic wall (Figs.13.1 and 13.2). Thus, the

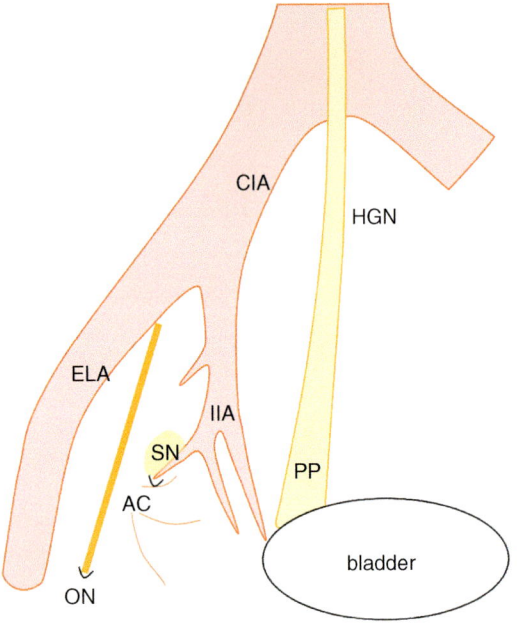

Fig. 13.1 Schematic representation of lateral lymph nodes. *HGN* hypogastric nerve, *PP* pelvic plexus, *CIA* common iliac artery, *IIA* internal iliac artery, *EIA* external iliac artery, *ON* obturator nerve, *SN* sacral nerve, *AC* Alcock's canal

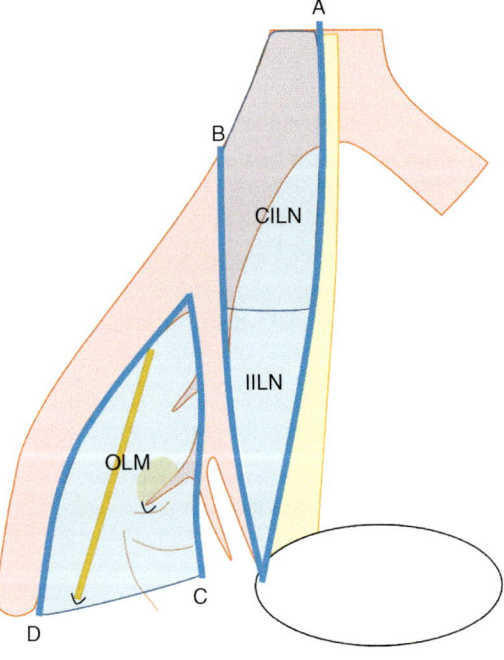

Fig. 13.2 Schematic representation of lateral lymph nodes. A, B, C, D shows four planes surrounding the lymph nodes. *CILN* common iliac node, *IILN* internal iliac lymph node, *OLN* obturator lymph node

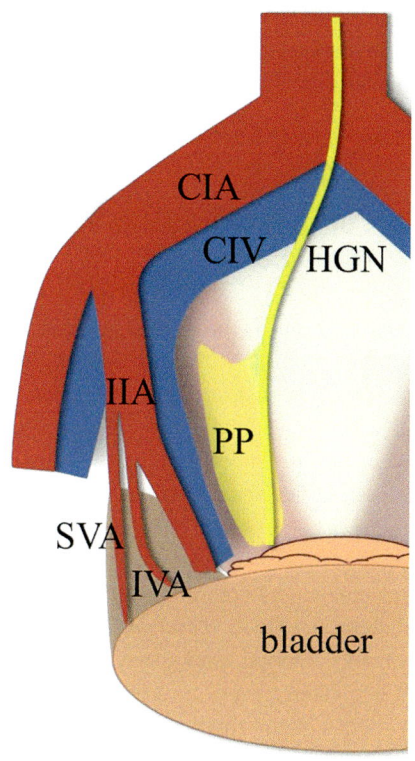

Fig. 13.3 Anatomical landmark of common iliac lymph node dissection and internal iliac lymph node dissection. *HGN* hypogastric nerve, *PP* pelvic plexus, *CIA* common iliac artery, *CIV* common iliac vein, *IIA* internal iliac artery, *SVA* superior vesical artery, *IVA* inferior vesical artery

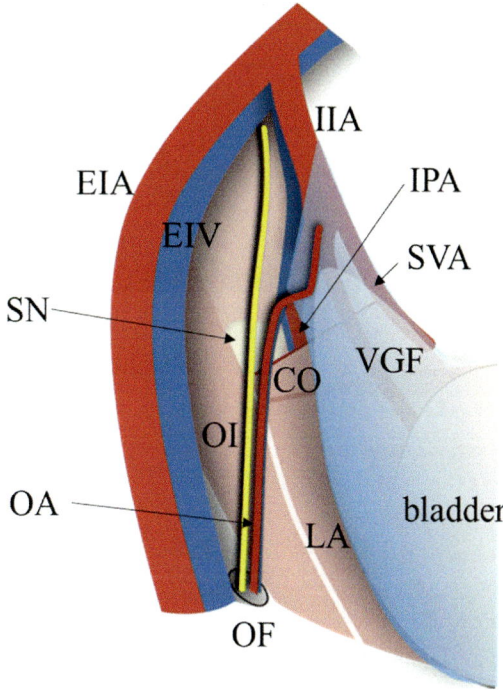

Fig. 13.4 Anatomical landmark of obturator lymph node dissection. *EIA* external iliac artery, *EIV* external iliac vein, *IIA* internal iliac artery, *SVA* superior vesical artery, *IPA* internal pudendal artery, *OA* obturator artery, *VGF* vesicohypogastric fascia, *CO* coccygeal muscle, *OI* internal obturator muscle, *LA* levator ani muscle, *OF* obturator foramen, *SN* sacral nerve

common and internal iliac lymph nodes are located between planes A and B, whereas the obturator lymph nodes are located between planes C and D (Figs. 13.3 and 13.4).

13.4 Surgical Techniques

In our hospital, we perform LLD by laparotomy, laparoscopy, and robotic surgery, with the approach chosen based on patient preference. We have previously reported that robotic surgery improves surgical accuracy, even in the narrow pelvic cavity, making it especially useful for LLD [13]. However,

regardless of the approach chosen, the surgical procedure is the same.

13.4.1 Ureter and Autonomic Nerve Mobilization

The peritoneum is dissected at the level of the common iliac artery, and the entire circumference of the ureter is exposed. Next, the ureter is mobilized and then separated from the retroperitoneum before taping the ureter. An assistant holds the taped ureter and pulls it medially (Fig. 13.5). The ureter is mobilized sufficiently to the point of intersection with the seminal duct in males and round ligament of the uterus in females. When the

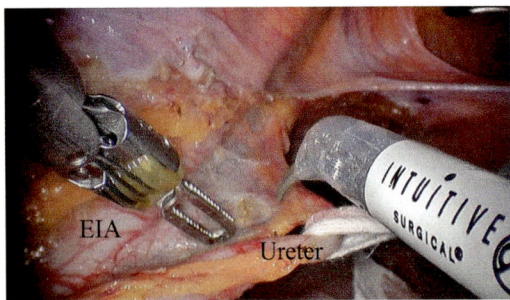

Fig. 13.5 Ureter mobilization. The ureter is identified and mobilized and separated from the retroperitoneum. *EIA* external iliac artery

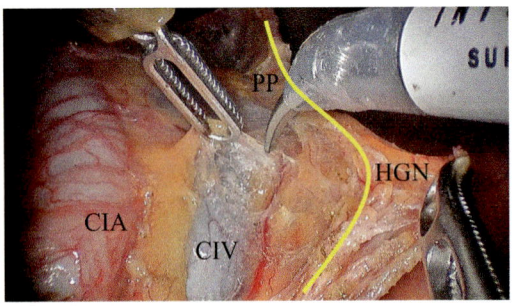

Fig. 13.6 The hypogastric nerve is identified at the level of the aortic bifurcation, and its orientation becomes clear when it is lifted. *HGN* hypogastric nerve, *CIA* common iliac artery, *CIV* common iliac vein, *PP* pelvic plexus

peritoneum is dissected along the seminal duct (round ligament of the uterus) to the external iliac vein, a good surgical field can be obtained for obturator lymph node dissection. The ureter is then mobilized along an avascular space that can be located lateral to the ureter. When the ureter is mobilized in the pelvis, the lateral side of the pelvic plexus and the ureter within the pelvis can be dissected in one layer. The lateral surface of the pelvic plexus is separated so that the autonomic nerves, including the hypogastric nerve, the pelvic splanchnic nerves, and the pelvic plexus, form one layer. The hypogastric nerve is identified at the level of the aortic bifurcation, and its orientation becomes clear when it is lifted (Fig. 13.6). When the nerve is mobilized distally, it extends to the lateral aspect of the already divided pelvic plexus; however, because this is near nerves, an electric scalpel should be avoided, opting for careful blunt dissection instead. The pelvic plexus is separated

until the space between the pelvic splanchnic nerve (S4) and the inferior vesical vessels disappear, or until the TME dissection plane is passed through.

13.4.2 Common Iliac Lymph Node Dissection

The assistant pulls the ureter away laterally, identifying the proximal (the aortic bifurcation), medial (the hypogastric nerve), and lateral (the ventral aspect and medial side of the common iliac artery and vein) borders of the common iliac lymph nodes. The thick lymphatic vessels lie at the proximal border, and dissection is performed after sealing is performed with bipolar forceps or a vessel sealer. The common iliac nodes are dissected along the blood vessel wall to the bifurcation of the internal and external iliac artery (Fig. 13.7). Thin vessels branch directly into the lymph nodes from the common iliac vein, so moderate traction and prior coagulation is needed.

13.4.3 Internal Iliac Lymph Node Dissection

Once again, the assistant pulls the pelvic plexus medially to expand the surgical field for dissection. The medial border of the internal iliac lymph nodes is identified by the lateral pelvic

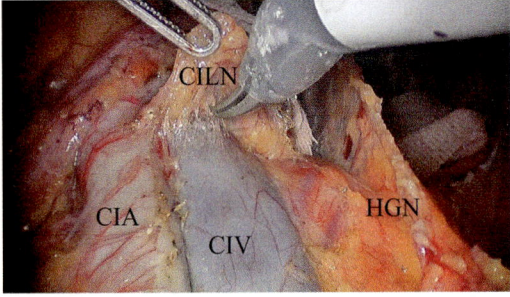

Fig. 13.7 The common iliac nodes are dissected along the blood vessel wall. *HGN* hypogastric nerve, *CILN* common iliac lymph node, *CIA* common iliac artery, *CIV* common iliac vein, *PP* pelvic plexus

plexus, and the lateral border, as the medial side of the internal iliac artery and related visceral branches. To connect the distal dissection of the common iliac lymph node, the nodes are first grasped, and the fatty tissue between the internal iliac artery and the autonomic nerves (the pelvic splanchnic nerves and the pelvic plexus) is dissected while exposing the ventral and medial aspects of the internal iliac artery and vein (Figs. 13.8 and 13.9). The middle rectal artery passes through the dissection plane, and the dissection plane is expanded when it is sectioned. The area before the bifurcation of the superior vesical artery is dissected as the proximal nodes, and the area beyond is dissected as the distal nodes, according to the Japanese Classification of Colorectal Carcinoma [14]. When there is no metastasis to the internal iliac lymph nodes, the nerves and inferior vesical

vessels are preserved to prevent postoperative erectile dysfunction.

13.4.4 Obturator Lymph Node Dissection

The superior vesical artery identified during dissection of the internal iliac lymph nodes is the landmark for identifying the medial border of the obturator lymph nodes (Fig. 13.10). The superior vesical artery is pulled medially, and when distal dissection proceeds, a dissection plane is observed between the surface formed lateral to the internal iliac artery and related visceral branch (the so-called vesicohypogastric fascia) and the obturator lymph nodes (Fig. 13.11). On the proximal side, it is difficult to identify the vesicohypogastric fascia because the obturator artery branches off from the internal iliac artery and passes through the obturator lymph nodes. Therefore, this dissection plane should be found on the bladder side whenever possible. When the visceral branches of the internal iliac artery and vein are dissected as one surface along this plane, the fascia of the levator ani muscle is reached inferiorly. This plane forms the medial border of the obturator lymph nodes, and when mobilized, the vesicohypogastric fascia with the superior vesical artery is pushed aside medially by the assistant and fixed to the wall of the medial border.

Dissection of the lateral border of the obturator lymph nodes is commenced medial to the external iliac vein. The surgical field will have been improved when the peritoneum was dissected to

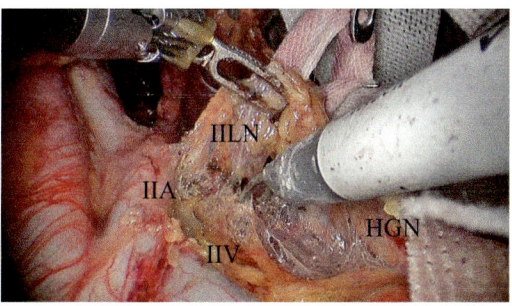

Fig. 13.8 The internal iliac nodes are dissected along the blood vessel wall. *HGN* hypogastric nerve, *IILN* internal iliac lymph node, *IIA* internal iliac artery, *IIV* internal iliac vein

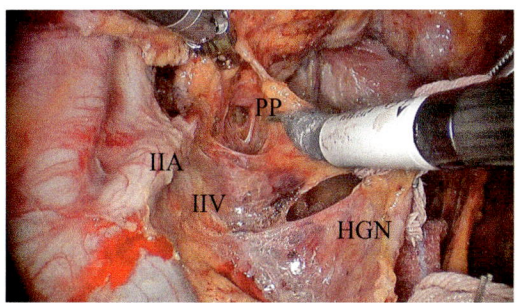

Fig. 13.9 The internal iliac nodes are dissected along the blood vessel wall. *HGN* hypogastric nerve, *IILN* internal iliac lymph node, *IIA* internal iliac artery, *IIV* internal iliac vein, *PP* pelvic plexus

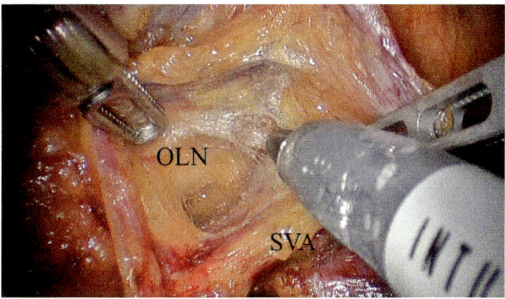

Fig. 13.10 The medial border of the obturator lymph nodes. *SVA* superior vesical artery, *OLN* obturator lymph node

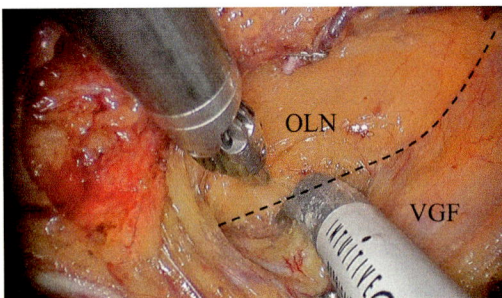

Fig. 13.11 A dissection plane (dot line) is observed between the vesicohypogastric fascia and the obturator lymph nodes. *VGF* vesicohypogastric fascia, *OLN* obturator lymph node

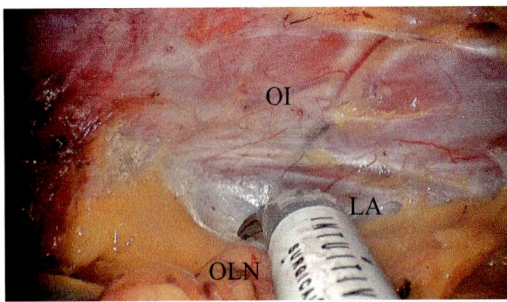

Fig. 13.12 Dissection between the pelvic wall and lateral side of the obturator lymph nodes. *OLN* obturator lymph node, *OI* internal obturator muscle, *LA* levator ani muscle

the point of intersection with the seminal duct or round ligament in males or females, respectively. When identifying the lateral border of the obturator lymph nodes, the assistant pulls the peritoneum of the anterior surface of the external iliac artery laterally and applies tension to facilitate medial and dorsal dissection of the external iliac vein. The external iliac vein is then exposed, and as dissection proceeds laterally and dorsally to the external iliac vein, the iliopsoas muscle is identified and dissected between the pelvic wall and lateral side of the obturator lymph nodes. Eventually, the fascias of the internal obturator and levator ani muscles are reached (Fig. 13.12). Several thin vessels flowing into the pelvic wall can be identified in this dissection plane, and dissection should only be performed after coagulating the vessels.

After the medial and lateral borders of the obturator lymph nodes have been dissected, the assistant can expose the obturator cavity. The

obturator vessels and nerve pass through the fatty tissue together with the obturator lymph nodes, and the obturator nerve can be identified by the obturator foramen at the lower border of the pubic crest as a landmark. Lymphatic vessels from the femur flow into the distal side of the obturator lymph nodes, requiring that dissection be performed using a vessel sealer. The obturator vessels dorsal to the obturator nerve are dissected at the inflow site of the obturator foramen using a vessel sealer.

The proximal side of the obturator lymph nodes is at the site of bifurcation of the internal and external iliac artery. To expand the surgical field with the bifurcation site, the assistant pulls either the internal iliac artery medially or the external iliac artery laterally. The obturator nerve is preserved as it passes through the obturator lymph nodes, and the obturator vessels are clipped and dissected. Lymphatic vessels that flow into the proximal side of the obturator lymph nodes must be dissected using a vessel sealer.

Further dissection proceeds along the internal iliac artery to the base of the obturator cavity. Alcock's canal is then identified, through which the sacral nerve, coccygeus muscle, and internal pudendal vessels pass. As this dissection plane extends caudally, it reaches the TME dissection plane from the levator ani muscle, and the obturator lymph nodes can be completely dissected (Fig. 13.13). To prevent postoperative lymphocysts, the obturator cavity and TME dissection

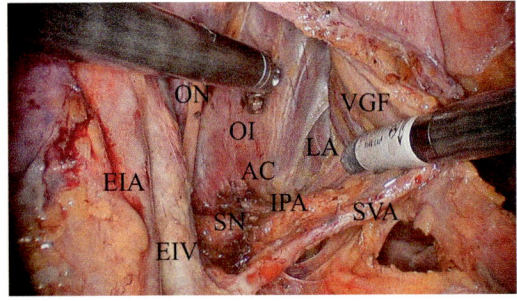

Fig. 13.13 The obturator lymph nodes can be completely dissected. *EIA* external iliac artery, *EIV* external iliac vein, *SVA* superior vesical artery, *IPA* internal pudendal artery, *VGF* vesicohypogastric fascia, *OI* internal obturator muscle, *LA* levator ani muscle, *ON* obturator nerve, *SN* sacral nerve, *AC* Alcock's canal

plane should communicate along the levator ani muscle, preventing lymph accumulation.

13.5 Oncologic Benefit

In Japan, LLD is the standard treatment for cT3 or cT4 stage lower rectal cancer [11]. A retrospective multicenter analysis in Japan reported that LLN metastasis was present in 15.6–20.4% of patients with lower rectal cancer and that the risk of pelvic recurrence would decrease by 50% and the 5-year survival rate would improve by 8% when LLNs dissection was performed for T3 or T4 lower rectal cancer [15]. Furthermore, Akiyoshi et al. reported that LLN could be considered for regional lymph nodes in patients with low rectal cancer. This was because the prognosis of patients with metastasis to the internal iliac lymph nodes was similar to that of patients with N2a (i.e., metastasis to the mesorectal lymph nodes), and because the prognosis of patients with external iliac lymph node metastasis was similar to that for N2b, and better than that of patients with stage IV disease who underwent curative resection [16].

The colorectal cancer study group of the Japan Clinical Oncology Group (JCOG) has also conducted an important multicenter randomized controlled trial comparing mesorectal excision (ME) with or without LLD for clinical stage II or III lower rectal cancer without clinically suspected LLN metastasis (JCOG0212). In a report, Fujita et al. stated that local recurrence was lower in the ME with LLD group (7.4%) compared with the ME-only group (12.6%) ($p = 0.024$). Concerning local recurrence in the lateral pelvis, there were also significantly fewer recurrences in the ME with LLD group (1.1%) compared with the ME-only group (6.5%) [17]. In other research, Kim et al. reported that LLNs were a major cause of local recurrence of rectal cancer when performing curative resection after CRT. They reported a local recurrence rate of 7.9%, with 82.7% of these having recurrence in the lateral pelvic [18]. Based on these results, LLD may be considered effective for the local control of rectal cancer.

13.6 Surgical Data, Complication Details, and Functional Outcomes

Fujita et al. have also reported short-term surgical and outcome data from the JCOG0212 trial. In their report, total surgical time was significantly longer in the ME with LLD group (median 360 min) compared with the ME-only group (254 min; $p < 0.0001$). Also, bleeding was significantly greater in the ME with LLD group (576 mL) compared with the ME-only group (337 mL; $p < 0.0001$). However, the postoperative complication rate (grades 3–4) did not differ between the two groups; equally, at 5% in the ME with LLD group and 3% in the ME-only group, urinary retention rates were not significantly different [12]. In addition, as measured using the International Index of Erectile Function, sexual dysfunction did not differ between the two groups [19].

Conclusion

We have described the surgical procedures needed to perform nerve-sparing LLD. Provided lateral dissection is performed accurately; local control of rectal cancer is excellent and does not cause urogenital dysfunction. We conclude that although LLD increases the time needed for surgery, the procedure appears to be safe and effective.

References

1. Heald RJ, Husband EM, Ryall RD. The mesorectum in rectal cancer surgery—the clue to pelvic recurrence? Br J Surg. 1982;69(10):613–6.
2. van Gijn W, Marijnen CA, Nagtegaal ID, Kranenbarg EM, Putter H, Wiggers T, et al. Preoperative radiotherapy combined with total mesorectal excision for resectable rectal cancer: 12-year follow-up of the multicentre, randomised controlled TME trial. Lancet Oncol. 2011;12(6):575–82. https://doi.org/10.1016/s1470-2045(11)70097-3.
3. Marijnen CA, van de Velde CJ, Putter H, van den Brink M, Maas CP, Martijn H, et al. Impact of short-term preoperative radiotherapy on health-related quality of life and sexual functioning in primary rectal cancer: report of a multicenter randomized trial. J Clin Oncol. 2005;23(9):1847–58. https://doi.org/10.1200/jco.2005.05.256.

4. Peeters KC, van de Velde CJ, Leer JW, Martijn H, Junggeburt JM, Kranenbarg EK, et al. Late side effects of short-course preoperative radiotherapy combined with total mesorectal excision for rectal cancer: increased bowel dysfunction in irradiated patients—a Dutch colorectal cancer group study. J Clin Oncol. 2005;23(25):6199–206. https://doi.org/10.1200/jco.2005.14.779.

5. Sauer R, Liersch T, Merkel S, Fietkau R, Hohenberger W, Hess C, et al. Preoperative versus postoperative chemoradiotherapy for locally advanced rectal cancer: results of the German CAO/ARO/AIO-94 randomized phase III trial after a median follow-up of 11 years. J Clin Oncol. 2012;30(16):1926–33. https://doi.org/10.1200/jco.2011.40.1836.

6. Folkesson J, Birgisson H, Pahlman L, Cedermark B, Glimelius B, Gunnarsson U. Swedish rectal cancer trial: long lasting benefits from radiotherapy on survival and local recurrence rate. J Clin Oncol. 2005;23(24):5644–50. https://doi.org/10.1200/jco.2005.08.144.

7. Moriya Y, Hojo K, Sawada T, Koyama Y. Significance of lateral node dissection for advanced rectal carcinoma at or below the peritoneal reflection. Dis Colon Rectum. 1989;32(4):307–15.

8. Moriya Y, Sugihara K, Akasu T, Fujita S. Nerve-sparing surgery with lateral node dissection for advanced lower rectal cancer. Eur J Cancer. 1995;31A(7–8):1229–32.

9. Sugihara K, Moriya Y, Akasu T, Fujita S. Pelvic autonomic nerve preservation for patients with rectal carcinoma. Oncologic and functional outcome. Cancer. 1996;78(9):1871–80.

10. Moriya Y. Function preservation in rectal cancer surgery. Int J Clin Oncol. 2006;11(5):339–43. https://doi.org/10.1007/s10147-006-0608-z.

11. Watanabe T, Muro K, Ajioka Y, Hashiguchi Y, Ito Y, Saito Y, et al. Japanese Society for Cancer of the colon and Rectum (JSCCR) guidelines 2016 for the treatment of colorectal cancer. Int J Clin Oncol. 2017. https://doi.org/10.1007/s10147-017-1101-6.

12. Fujita S, Akasu T, Mizusawa J, Saito N, Kinugasa Y, Kanemitsu Y, et al. Postoperative morbidity and mortality after mesorectal excision with and without lateral lymph node dissection for clinical stage II or stage III lower rectal cancer (JCOG0212): results from a multicentre, randomised controlled, non-inferiority trial. Lancet Oncol. 2012;13(6):616–21. https://doi.org/10.1016/s1470-2045(12)70158-4.

13. Kagawa H, Kinugasa Y, Shiomi A, Yamaguchi T, Tsukamoto S, Tomioka H, et al. Robotic-assisted lateral lymph node dissection for lower rectal cancer: short-term outcomes in 50 consecutive patients. Surg Endosc. 2015;29(4):995–1000. https://doi.org/10.1007/s00464-014-3760-y.

14. Yasutomi M, Baba S, Hojo K, Kato Y, Kodaira S, Koyama Y. Japanese classification of colorectal carcinoma. 2nd English ed. Tokyo: Kanehara; 2009.

15. Sugihara K, Kobayashi H, Kato T, Mori T, Mochizuki H, Kameoka S, et al. Indication and benefit of pelvic sidewall dissection for rectal cancer. Dis Colon Rectum. 2006;49(11):1663–72. https://doi.org/10.1007/s10350-006-0714-z.

16. Akiyoshi T, Watanabe T, Miyata S, Kotake K, Muto T, Sugihara K. Results of a Japanese nationwide multi-institutional study on lateral pelvic lymph node metastasis in low rectal cancer: is it regional or distant disease? Ann Surg. 2012;255(6):1129–34. https://doi.org/10.1097/SLA.0b013e3182565d9d.

17. Fujita S, Mizusawa J, Kanemitsu Y, Ito M, Kinugasa Y, Komori K, et al. Mesorectal excision with or without lateral lymph node dissection for clinical stage II/III lower rectal cancer (JCOG0212): a multicenter, randomized controlled, noninferiority trial. Ann Surg. 2017;266(2):201–7. https://doi.org/10.1097/sla.0000000000002212.

18. Kim TH, Jeong SY, Choi DH, Kim DY, Jung KH, Moon SH, et al. Lateral lymph node metastasis is a major cause of locoregional recurrence in rectal cancer treated with preoperative chemoradiotherapy and curative resection. Ann Surg Oncol. 2008;15(3):729–37. https://doi.org/10.1245/s10434-007-9696-x.

19. Saito S, Fujita S, Mizusawa J, Kanemitsu Y, Saito N, Kinugasa Y, et al. Male sexual dysfunction after rectal cancer surgery: results of a randomized trial comparing mesorectal excision with and without lateral lymph node dissection for patients with lower rectal cancer: Japan clinical oncology group study JCOG0212. Eur J Surg Oncol. 2016;42(12):1851–8. https://doi.org/10.1016/j.ejso.2016.07.010.

Laparoscopic TME and Sphincter-Saving Procedures

14

William Tzu-Liang Chen and Amar Chand Doddama Reddy

Abstract

This chapter on laparoscopic total mesorectal excision (TME) and sphincter-saving procedures translates hi-tech detailed information for the laparoscopic surgeons enabling them to accomplish advanced laparoscopic colorectal surgery. The indications, operating room set-up, positioning, instruments, techniques, and tips to avoid troubleshooting are disclosed and detailed illustrated material is deciphered step-by-step. It also brings out the different types of coloanal anastomosis and various types of colonic reconstruction that are possible, together with the pros and cons of each procedure.

Keywords

Rectal cancer · Total mesorectal excision · Laparoscopy · Intersphincteric resection

14.1 Introduction

Surgery is an art, and as an artist, a surgeon needs to amalgamate principles of science and technology to make the best progress in surgical care.

For the last two decades, there has been rapid advancement in the surgical techniques needed to treat rectal cancer, from open to laparoscopy and to robotics, but the concepts of surgery remain the same as for any open surgery. The outcome of any cancer surgery depends on complete oncological clearance, and with rectal cancer this depends on the quality of total mesorectal excision (TME). The competence of the surgeon depends on a good-quality specimen that delivers the best oncological outcomes. In the field of developing technology, to demonstrate a good quality of life and functional outcomes, sphincter-saving procedures have recently been demonstrated to be an alternative to many radical abdominoperineal resections (APR) performed in low rectal cancers for achieving satisfactory outcomes.

14.2 History of Laparoscopic TME and Sphincter-Saving Procedures

In the twentieth century, surgeons have struggled to design surgical procedures that gain minimal access to the gastrointestinal tract, and it took a decade to translate these to colorectal procedures. The first laparoscopic colorectal surgery was accomplished by Moises Jacobs in Miami, Florida, in June 1990 [1]. Since then, there has been growing enthusiasm for laparoscopic rectal

W. T.-L. Chen (✉) · A. C. D. Reddy
Division of Colorectal Surgery, Department
of Surgery, Minimally Invasive Surgery Center,
China Medical University Hospital,
Taichung City, Taiwan
e-mail: wtchen@mail.cmuh.org.tw

© Springer Nature Singapore Pte Ltd. 2018
N. K. Kim et al. (eds.), *Surgical Treatment of Colorectal Cancer*,
https://doi.org/10.1007/978-981-10-5143-2_14

surgeries, which, over time, have shown better short-term and equivalent long-term oncological outcomes [2–10]. After the initial success of minimally invasive surgery (MIS) in colon surgeries, owing to the procedure complexity, laparoscopic rectal surgery proceeded at a slower pace as a steep learning curve was required, with deep dissections in the pelvis, difficult stapling in the deep pelvis, and multiple quadrant access, which made rectal surgery complex. Local resection of rectal cancer was first described by Lisfranc in 1826 [11], but as the understanding of the pathogenesis of rectal tumours progressed in the early 1900s, Sir Ernest Miles [12] noted a 95% recurrence rate after perianal resection and emphasised the need for upward, lateral, and downward lymphatic clearance. Thus, in 1908, he reported the first APR. TME was introduced by Heald in 1982 [13, 14] and involved sharp dissection in the narrow pelvis that resulted in a significant decrease in the positivity of the circumferential resection margin (CRM). The primary goal of rectal surgery is to accomplish complete TME, and the secondary goal is to bring about a good quality of life; for these purposes, sphincter-saving surgery came into existence. Table 14.1 displays landmark advancements in rectal cancer surgery [11–37].

14.3 Current Status of Laparoscopy in Rectal Cancer

Rectal surgery is difficult to approach, even with the traditional open approach, as the tumour morphology and patient and surgeon factors determine the technical outcome of the surgery. The laparoscopic technique has played a promising role in rectal surgery, as it provides precise pelvic dissection, better identification of the pelvic structure in a narrow pelvis, and improved magnification and visual angles. Sphincter-preserving surgery has been a recent trend made feasible with adequate pelvic dissection and adequate distal margins using endostapling. Laparoscopic surgery has a technical

Table 14.1 Landmarks in rectal cancer surgery

Rectal surgery

1. First local surgical resection of rectal cancer (perineal approach)—Jacques Lisfranc, 1826
2. Radical rectal resections (perineal approach)—Kraske, Czerny, 1884
3. APRs with lymph node dissections—Ito, Torikata, 1904
4. First transabdominal rectal resection—Carl Gussenbauer, 1879
5. Combined APR—Vincent Czerny
6. TME—Heald, 1982
7. APR + TME—William Ernest Miles, 1908
8. Anterior resection—Claude Dixon, 1948
9. CRM margins—P. Quinke, 1976
10. 5 cm margin—Golinger, Dukes, Buessey
11. J-pouch—Sir Alan Parks, 1978
12. Coloplasty—Zgraggen, 1999
13. Laparoscopic colectomy—Moises Jacobs, 1990
14. Laparoscopic APR—J. Sackier, 1992

Staplers

1. Staples—Hummer Hultl, 1908
2. Reloadable cartridges—Friedrich, 1934
3. L-staplers—Von Seemen
4. E-E circular staplers—Mark Ravitch, 1977
5. Double stapling technique—Knight and Griffin, 1980

Sphincter-saving surgery

1. Pull-through technique—Maunsell, 1892, Cutait, Turnbull, 1960–1970
2. Mucosectomy and coloanal anastomosis—Parks and Peerey, 1980
3. Nerve-sparing TME—Enker, Hojo, and Moriya
4. Intersphincteric resection—Gerald Marks (transabdominal transanal), Schiessel, 1994
5. Laparoscopic ultra-low anterior resection (LAR) with internal sphincter resection (ISR)—M. Watanabe, 2000

advantage in the male pelvis, in the morbid obese, in patients who had undergone previous chemoradiotherapy, and those with bulky distal tumours [5]. Systematic reviews and multiple randomised controlled trials (RCTs; Table 14.2) comparing laparoscopy versus open surgery in rectal cancers have shown the feasibility, safety, better short-term advantages, and similar overall survival and disease-free survival for up to 10 years' follow-up in laparoscopic surgery in rectal cancers [2–10].

Table 14.2 Randomised controlled trials (*RCTs*) comparing open and laparoscopic rectal cancer

RCT	Patients (open/lap)	Follow-up (years)	Overall survival (open/lap)	DFS (open/lap)	Local recurrence (open/lap)	CRM-positive (open/lap)	DRM-positive (open/lap)	Lymph node (open/lap)
CLASICC [2–4]	128/253	10	65.8% vs 82.7% (ns)	67.1% vs 70.8% (ns)	9.9% vs 9.9% (ns)	14% vs 16% (ns)	NA	13.5 vs 12 (ns)
COLOR 2 [5]	345/699	3	83.6% vs 86.7% (ns)	70.8% vs 74.8% (ns)	5% vs 5% (ns)	10% vs 10% (ns)	NA	14 vs 13 (ns)
COREAN [7]	170/170	3	90.4% vs 91.7% (ns)	72.5% vs 79.5% (ns)	4.9% vs 2.3% (ns)	4 vs 3% (ns)	NA	18 vs 17 (ns)
ACOSOG Z6051 [8]	222/240	NA	NA	NA	NA	7.7% vs 12.1% (ns)	1.8% vs 1.7% (ns)	16.5 vs 17.9 (ns)
ALaCaRT [9]	237/238	NA	NA	NA	NA	3% vs 7% (ns)	1% vs 1% (ns)	NA

Abbreviations: *Lap* laparoscopy, *Open* open surgery, *DFS* disease-free survival, *OS* overall survival, *CRM* circumferential resection margins, *DRM* distal resection margins, *CLASICC* conventional versus laparoscopic-assisted surgery in colorectal cancer, *COLOR* colon cancer laparoscopic or open resection, *COREAN* comparison of open versus laparoscopic surgery for mid and low rectal cancer after neoadjuvant chemoradiotherapy, *ALaCaRT* Australasian Laparoscopic Cancer of the Rectum Trial

14.4 Concepts of TME

Total mesorectal excision is defined as "complete removal of lymph node bearing mesorectum along with its intact enveloping fascia" [13, 14]. Complete TME includes:

- High ligation of the inferior mesenteric artery (IMA)
- Mobilisation of the splenic flexure
- Rectosigmoid mobilisation
- Sharp dissection of the avascular plane in the pelvis
- Division of lymphatic and middle haemorrhoidal vessels anterolaterally
- 2-cm distal margin

14.5 Laparoscopic TME

14.5.1 Indications

Indications for laparoscopic rectal surgery are similar to those for open surgery; indications depend on patient habitus, tumour location, depth of penetration, histology, surgeon experience and availability of advancement staplers:

- Anterior resection with partial TME upper rectal tumours
- LAR
- with total TME mid/low rectal tumours
- Ultra-LAR with total TME low rectal tumours
- Intersphincteric resection with coloanal anastomosis (CAA) low rectal cancers with or without internal sphincter involvement

Contraindications for laparoscopic rectal surgery are as follows:

- Poor general condition contraindicating general anaesthesia
- Low rectal cancers with external sphincter complex involvement
- Poor anal tone/function
- Rectal cancer with pelvic side wall/pelvic floor infiltration

14.5.2 Preoperative Evaluation

Preoperative evaluation is important in the stratification of patients into local, locally advanced, and systemic disease as the treatment is tailor-made depending on the tumour stage, patient status, and surgeon expertise available. Evaluation begins with history and digital rectal examination with biopsy to confirm the diagnosis; preoperative digital examination should assess the tumour location (whether anterior, lateral or posterior), tumour size, and distance from the anal verge. Complete colonoscopy should be carried out to assess for synchronous tumours. Local staging is performed by pelvic MRI with a pelvic or endorectal coil or endoscopic ultrasound to assess the depth of penetration of the rectal wall and to assess the regional lymph nodes; any tumours that are T3 lesions and positive lymph nodes should be subjected to neoadjuvant chemoradiotherapy. CT scan of the abdomen and chest should be performed to rule out metastatic disease, preoperative carcinoembryonic antigen should be carried out for postoperative monitoring, preoperative sphincter evaluation should be made by digital examination, and anal manometry should be conducted to assess sphincter tone and function, as poor sphincter tone warrants APR. In any locally advanced tumours, the patient should be warned of the concomitant resection of other pelvic organs such as the prostate, the seminal vesicle, ovary, and bladder. The possibility of postoperative bladder and sexual dysfunction should be discussed with the patient preoperatively. Stoma therapist consultation should be conducted and preoperatively site-marked in all cases of LAR and ISR. In the case of locally advanced tumours with ureteric involvement, preoperative stenting is helpful in identifying ureteric injuries. Preoperative pulmonary and cardiac and renal evaluation should be performed.

14.5.3 Patient Preparation

The patient is placed on a silicone gel sheet at the back and is given shoulder padding for anti-skidding; a bean bag is placed to prevent sliding in a steep position required for laparoscopic surgery (Fig. 14.1). A sandbag is placed behind the pelvis for elevation, to ease insertion of the stapling device and the performance of perineal combined surgeries. Irrigation of the rectum is carried out preoperatively to clear any residual stool, which

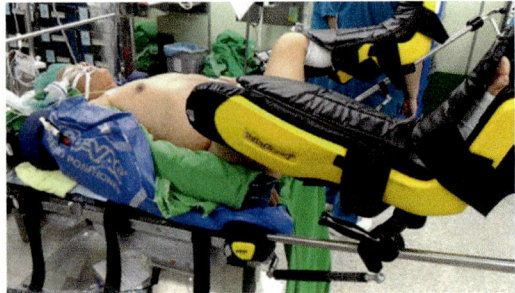

Fig. 14.1 Patient in a modified lithotomy position with shoulder padding, bean bag, and Yellofins stirrups

may hinder during stapling. All patients require general anaesthesia for pelvic surgery. Foley catheterisation to decompress the bladder and intraoperative fluid status monitoring are implemented. Ryle's tube is inserted after induction for gastric decompression and removed immediately post-surgery. DVT prophylaxis with elastic stockings and subcutaneous heparin is performed before induction of anaesthesia. Preoperative antibiotics should be given before intubation and re-dosed appropriately. Mechanical bowel preparation is done the night before surgery.

14.5.4 Operating Room Configuration

A laparoscopic colorectal procedure needs complex equipment and it is advisable to organise the operating room before facilitating the steps of the procedure, which increases the efficacy and shortens the procedure time. Depending on the available area of the operating room and the size of the equipment, the team should decide on the single set-up of the operating room for quick arrangement and adaptation to common procedures for standardisation of the procedure (Fig. 14.2). Each piece of laparoscopic surgical equipment should be functionally tested before the procedure and calibrated according to the schedule of the procedure. Backup instruments and an open set should be kept in case of problems arising during the procedure. It is advisable for the surgeon to train the team in the steps of the procedure and in the instruments and special equipment necessary before the surgical procedure.

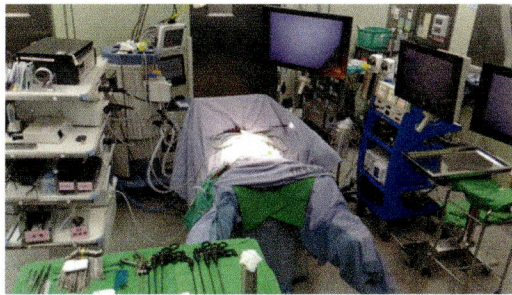

Fig. 14.2 Operating room set up for laparoscopic total mesenteric excision (TME)

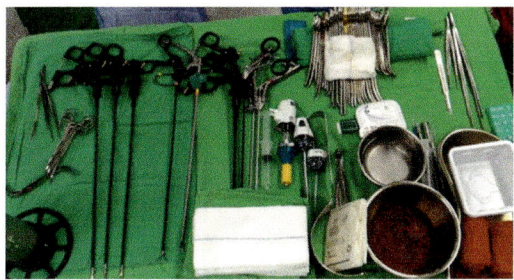

Fig. 14.3 Instrument set for laparoscopic TME

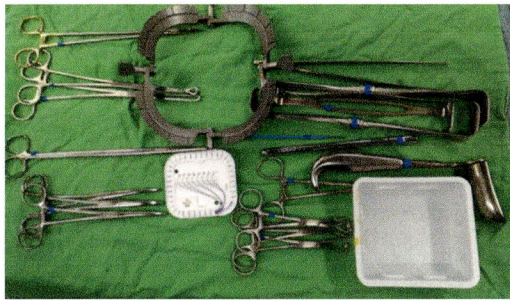

Fig. 14.4 Instruments set up for perianal surgery

14.5.5 Instruments

Advancements in technology have played a pivotal role in laparoscopic colorectal surgery, with high-definition monitors with superior clarity, small diameter and atraumatic ports, advanced stapling instruments, and intraoperative vascular and lymph node mapping, which ultimately translates into improved surgeon comfort and patient outcome. The set-up of the instruments is shown in Figs. 14.3 and 14.4.

Laparoscopic instruments include:

- Veress needle
- Surgical obturator and sleeve—3–5 mm, 2–12 mm
- Endoscopic grasper small and large—4
- Endoscopic Allis clamps—1
- Endoscopic scissors—1
- Endoscopic right-angled dissector/Maryland dissector—1
- Endoscopic clip applicator—1
- Endoscopic retractors
- Energy device—monopolar/bipolar
- Energy device—LigaSure (Covidien, CO, USA), ENSEAL (Ethicon Endo-Surgery, OH, USA), Harmonic scalpel (Ethicon Endo-Surgery, OH, USA)
- Endoscopic needle holder—2
- Endoscopic anvil holder—1
- Atraumatic bowel grasper small, large—4
- Endoscopic port closure needle
- Laparoscopic scope warmer
- Endoscopic staplers and cutters
- Gastrointestinal anastomosis (GIA) and trans-anastomotic stapling device
- Circular staplers—circular end-to-end anastomosis/intraluminal stapler (ILS)

Special instruments used include:

- Colonoscopy
- 3D monitors
- 4K monitors
- Antifogging solution
- Visiport—optical trocar
- Wound protector—S, M, L, XL, XXL size
- Articulating endoscopic linear staplers 45 mm, 60 mm—mechanical/powered
- Nylon tape
- Fluorescence imaging system (SPY/Firefly)
- Infrared fluorescence sentinel lymph node mapping

Perianal procedure instruments needed include:

- Lone star retractor
- End-to-end anastomosis (EEA)/procedure for prolapse and haemorrhoids haemorrhoidal circular staplers

- Transanal endoscopic operation/GelPort path for transanal minimally invasive surgery and transanal endoscopic microsurgery

14.5.6 Surgical Technique

14.5.6.1 Position

The patient is placed in a modified lithotomy position using Allen stirrups with a 15° steep Trendelenburg position air planed slightly to the right side (hip flex 10°, abducted so that the thighs do not interfere with the working hand instruments, and the hip externally rotated 45°, with knees flexed 45°). Both hands are tucked inside and secured. The position of the operating surgeon depends on the step of the surgical procedure; the surgeon stands on the patient's right side, whereas the assistant stands on the opposite side for sigmoid and rectal mobilisation; later, for splenic flexure and T-colon mobilisation, the surgeon stands in the French position. Two monitors are placed in the line of vision, one parallel to the surgeon and the other in the sight of the first assistant. A scrub nurse with a Mayo table is placed at the right foot of the patient, the table should be feet away as the position tilting causes the Mayo stand to interfere with the position. Suction and electrocautery are placed in a bag fixed to the right lateral thigh, as this facilitates easy handling of the instruments and prevents instruments falling away.

14.5.6.2 Port Placement

For anterior resection, four-port placement is used and for LAR, the five-port technique is used. Using open Hasson's technique, a 10-mm incision is made in the umbilicus, the linea alba is grasped with forceps, and the wound is deepened with a knife up to the peritoneum and incised. By using the Hassons-S retractor the abdominal cavity is lifted, a 10-mm trocar is placed, and a pneumoperitoneum of up to 15 mmHg is created; using an Endoflex Olympus 3D camera, careful inspection of the peritoneal cavity is made, including the liver, pelvis, ovary and omentum, small bowel, and mesentery to inspect for tumour dissemination. A 10-mm balloon port (Kii bal-

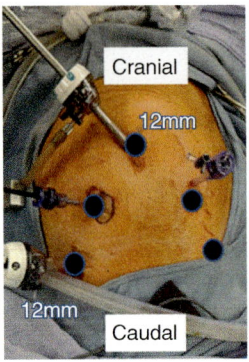

Fig. 14.5 Picture represents the placement of the ports for laparoscopic TME

loon blunt tip system, Applied Medical) is our preference in the umbilicus, as it decreases port slippage and reduces air leakage. A second 12-mm port is placed 2–3 cm medial and superior to the anterior superior iliac spine; another 5-mm port is placed in the right lower quadrant a handbreadth above the 12-mm port. In the case of low rectal dissection, the 12-mm port is placed medially, as it helps in the deep dissection and stapling made at ease in the lower pelvis. An additional 5-mm port in the left lower quadrant is placed above and medial to the anterior superior iliac spine for LARs; an additional 50mm port is placed in the left upper quadrant a handbreadth above the left 5-mm port for deep retraction of the bladder and splenic flexure mobilisation (Fig. 14.5).

14.5.6.3 High Ligation of the Inferior Mesenteric Vein

The patient is positioned in a reverse Trendelenburg position with a right tilt and the surgeon on the right side, retracting the small bowel to the right and making the anatomical landmarks of the ligament of Treitz, inferior mesenteric vein (IMV), IMA, and transverse colon and mesentery clear. The surgery proceeds with the omentum flipped above the T-colon and T-colon retracted cranially by the assistant; identification of the duodenojejunal flexure is done and the ligament of Treitz is completely mobilized. The dissection starts with the surgeon's left hand lifting the mesentery of the descending colon close to the IMV and the mesentery tenting; the surgeon's right hand makes an incision along the lower edge of the IMV, as in Fig. 14.6. With the pneumoperitoneum and the traction applied, the foamy avascular embryological planes along the visceral fascia and Gerota's fascia are clearly appreciated, and using monopolar cautery scissors, the dissection planes are maintained on the upper margin of Toldt's fascia and the parietal fascia is lowered inferiorly. Maintaining a bloodless field is most important to achieve the correct surgical planes; dissection is continued from medial to lateral up to the white line of Toldt laterally. Cranially, the dissection continues until the inferior border of the pancreatic body is identified, up to the tail of the pancreas laterally, and caudally until the IMA is identified. The IMV is skeletonised clear of fibro-fatty tissue all the way along up to the base of the inferior border of the pancreas and is ligated with endoclips, Hem-o-lok or energy-based devices, and is divided.

Tips and Tricks
1. Dissection of the mesentery is performed using monopolar cautery and scissors. With adequate traction, the line of dissection opens, and dissection is progressed further.
2. Identification of the inferior border of the pancreas is critical for entering the lesser sac, as too deep a dissection posteriorly risks entry into the plane posterior to the pancreas. Thus, dissection on the upper border of the advancing edge of the loose areolar tissue helps to maintain the correct plane.

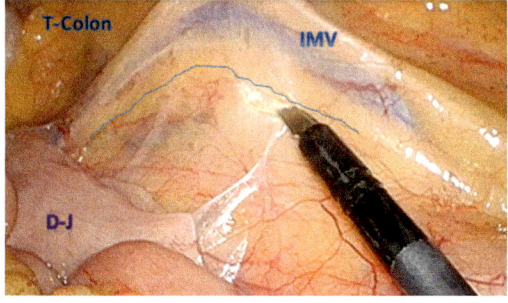

Fig. 14.6 Plane of dissection starts under the IMV. *D* duodenum, *IMV* inferior mesenteric vein, *T* colon-transverse colon)

14.5.6.4   High Ligation of IMA

The patient is positioned in the Trendelenburg position, and the small bowel is retracted in the abdominal cavity, clearing the pelvis, and upward traction of the sigmoid colon is effected by the assistant for inspection of the inferior mesenteric pedicle. Anatomical landmarks such as the sacral promontory, iliac bifurcation, and pulsation at the IMA, which are well appreciated in thin patients, should be clearly noted to identify the plane of dissection. With a left-hand grasper, the sigmoid mesentery is grasped with traction, and the plane of dissection is started from the sacral promontory below and traced cranially to the origin of the IMA. The pneumoperitoneum helps in opening an avascular plane of dissection between the presacral fascia and the mesorectum posteriorly and helps to visualise the hypogastric nerves clearly in the posterior plane; behind the IMA, preserved intact, the hypogastric plexus of nerves is identified as white cord structures at the origin of the IMA. The origin of the IMA is dissected 2 cm above the origin of the aorta to preserve the hypogastric plexus of nerves and is ligated using Hem-o-lok clips. Alternatively, the origin of the IMA can be ligated using an energy-based devices such as Harmonic, LigaSure or Thunderbeat. Alternatively, an Endo GIA vascular stapler can be used, depending on availability and on the preference of the surgeon.

Medial dissection is continued by gentle upward traction by the surgeon's left-hand grasper, and dissection with surgeon's right-hand monopolar scissors is continued along the embryological avascular planes of Toldt's fascia, which is a distinct plane between the mesocolon and underlying retroperitoneum formed by fusion of the visceral peritoneum and parietal peritoneum of the retroperitoneum, as shown in Fig. 14.7. Because the ureter is deep to the parietal peritoneum and medial to the gonadal vessels, it is not visualised if dissection is maintained in the correct planes. In thin patients, the embryological planes are too thin and fused to be separated, and it is easy to lose the dissection planes dissecting deeply posterior. This injures the iliac vessels and ureter, which should be approached meticulously. Identification of the ureter is not necessary if the planes are maintained for dissection, but in the case of reoperative cases, the identification is facilitated by either cranial or caudal dissection from a medial or lateral approach. The site of arterial ligation high or low in rectal surgery is controversial and there is no conclusive evidence, but high ligation, as shown in Fig. 14.8, helps with en-bloc dissection and gives additional length for a low rectal anastomosis. A low ligation of the IMA, as shown in Fig. 14.9, is performed caudal to the origin of the left colic artery, with advantages of increased blood supply to the anastomosis and preservation of the autonomic nerves at the origin of the IMA.

14.5.6.5 Mobilisation of the Descending Colon

Lateral dissection begins with medial traction of the left colon with a left-hand bowel grasper and proceeds along the white line of Toldt in the left

paracolic gutter. Dissection continues to release residual attachments with Gerota's fascia and is incorporated into the medial dissection. The descending colon is completely mobilised, as shown in Fig. 14.10.

14.5.6.6 Splenic Flexure Takedown

Complete mobilisation of the splenic flexure takedown achieves a long length of proximal colon, which is tension-free for anastomosis. This starts with the surgeon positioning himself/herself between the legs of the patient, with the assistant on the right side for retraction of the omentum and T-colon traction laterally. Dissection starts with the surgeon carrying out downward and medial traction of the descending colon and cranial retroperitoneal dissection of the avascular plane from Gerota's fascia to the splenic hilum, and until Gerota's fascia is visualised clearly, as shown in Fig. 14.11. Attachments

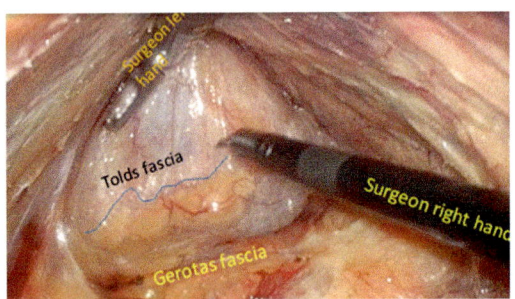

Fig. 14.7 Mobilisation of mesocolon. *Blue line* represents the line of dissection along the advancing margins of Toldt's fascia

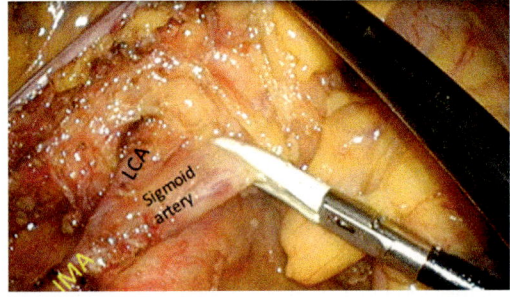

Fig. 14.9 Low ligation of the IMA

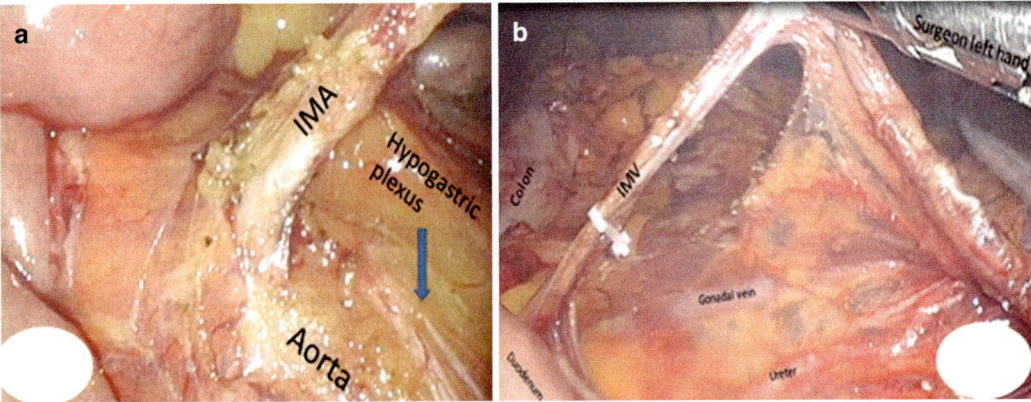

Fig. 14.8 (**a**) Inferior mesenteric artery (IMA) dissection and hypogastric plexus. (**b**) High ligation of the IMA and ureter; the gonadal vein is visualised in the retroperitoneal space

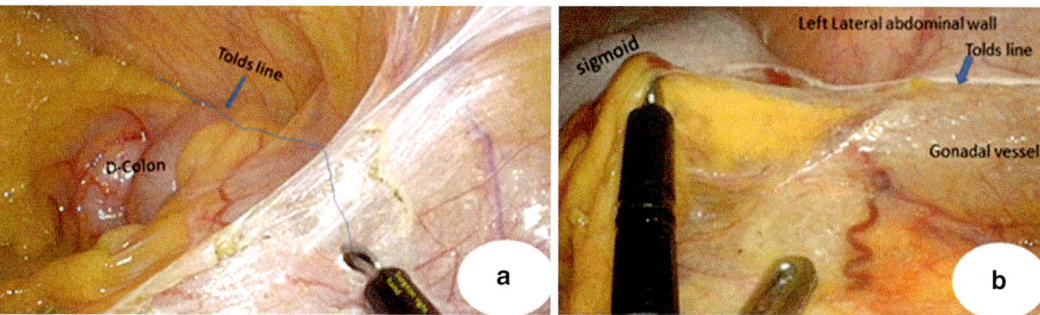

Fig. 14.10 (**a**, **b**) Descending colon mobilised along the white line of Toldt's fascia. *Blue line* in (**a**) demonstrates the line of Toldt's fascia

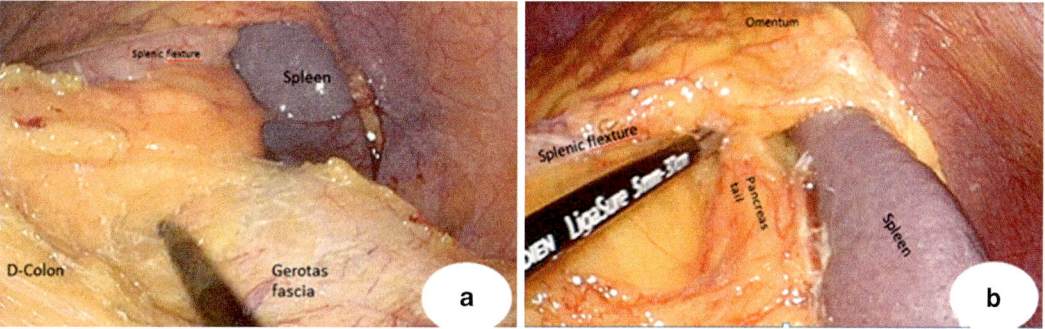

Fig. 14.11 (**a**) Posterior mobilised D-colon from Gerota's fascia. (**b**) Splenic flexure mobilisation with the pancreatic tail visualised at the splenic hilum

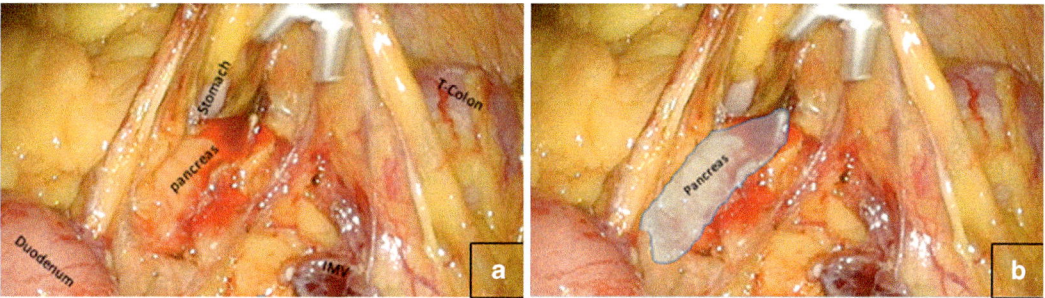

Fig. 14.12 (**a**, **b**) Retroperitoneal approach to a lesser sac with a medial to lateral detachment from the pancreas

of the descending colon are freed up to the spleen by separating the phrenicocolic ligament, lieno-colic ligament, and gastrocolic ligament.

The second step is entry into the lesser sac; one of two approaches can be used: either the medial to lateral or the lateral to medial approach. Separation of the omentum from the T-colon is performed by dissection from medial to lateral, starting from the mid T-colon up to the splenic

flexure. The next step is cranial retraction of the T-colon and identification of the inferior border of the pancreas and the T-colon mesentery, and in the middle colic vessels, the dissection is started to the left of the middle colic vessels and the attachments of the transverse mesocolon to inferior border of the pancreas are detached up to the pancreatic tail, as shown in Fig. 14.12. The dissection continues with detachment of the gastrocolic ligament, with

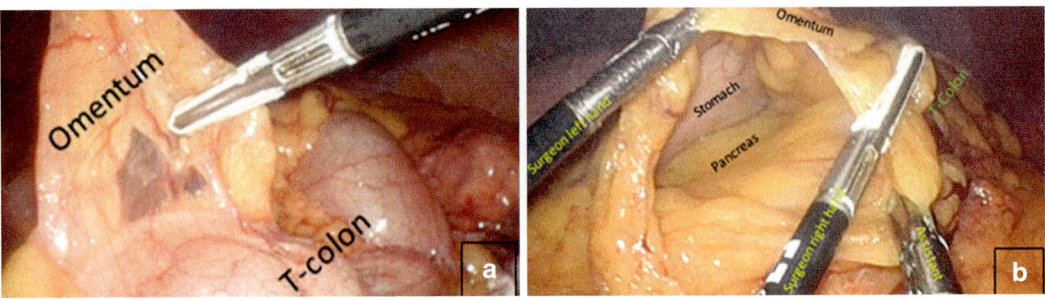

Fig. 14.13 (**a**) Supracolic approach to the lesser sac. (**c**) Medial to lateral dissection of the omentum from the T-colon

Fig. 14.14 Various approach to pancreas and lesser sac. (**a**) Supracolic approach, (**b**) supracolic approach, (**c**) transmesocolic approach, (**d**) retroperitoneal approach

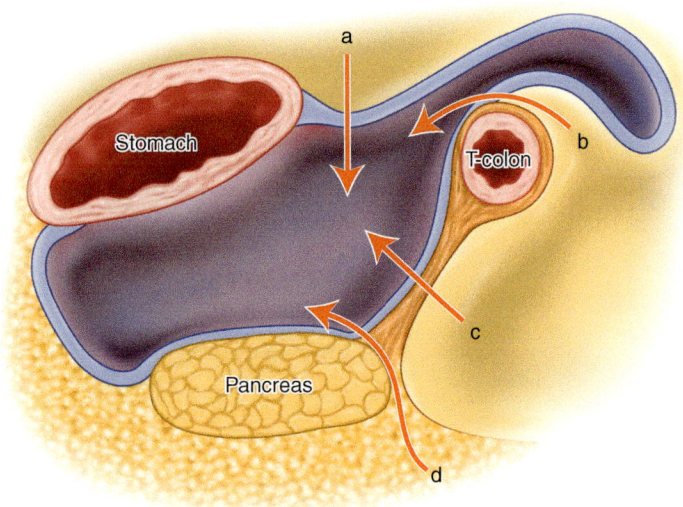

the surgeon's left-hand grasper retracting vertically, and using the right-hand monopolar scissors, the avascular plane is identified, separating close from the T-colon. The final step is caudal traction of the T-colon, and the remaining attachments of the colon to the pancreas are divided.

Tips and Tricks

1. In fatty patients both the medial to lateral and lateral to medial approaches need to be carried out concurrently to achieve a complete flexure takedown.
2. Avoid too much traction of the splenic flexure, as it may cause splenic capsule tear and may occasionally necessitate splenectomy.
3. Various techniques for accessing the lesser sac are explained in Figs. 14.13 and 14.14.

14.5.6.7   Mobilisation of the Rectum

The surgeon repositions to the right side, with an atraumatic bowel grasper in the left hand and monopolar cautery into the right quadrant ports. The patient is airplaned into a reverse Trendelenburg position and the small bowel is positioned to the abdominal cavity for clear visualisation of the pelvis. Dissection is started with traction of the sigmoid colon mesentery vertically and cranially using the assistant's left hand and with assistant's right-hand grasper retracting the redundant sigmoid colon laterally, clearing the field of dissection, with the surgeon's left-hand grasper gently lifting the sigmoid mesocolon vertically at the level of the sacral promontory posterior mesorectal dissection along the avascular "holy plane" of Heald between the visceral

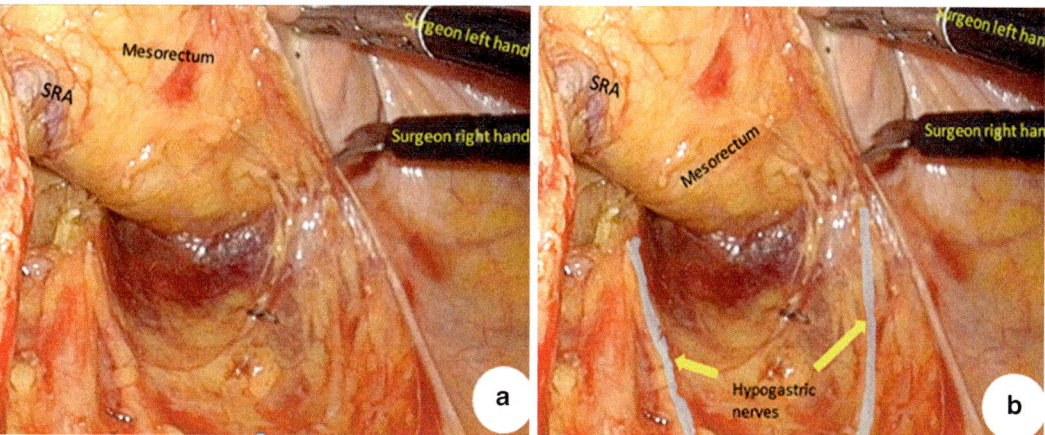

Fig. 14.15 (**a**) Posterior mobilisation of the mesorectum from the retrosacral fascia. (**b**) Preserved hypogastric nerves highlighted in *blue* on the presacral fascia

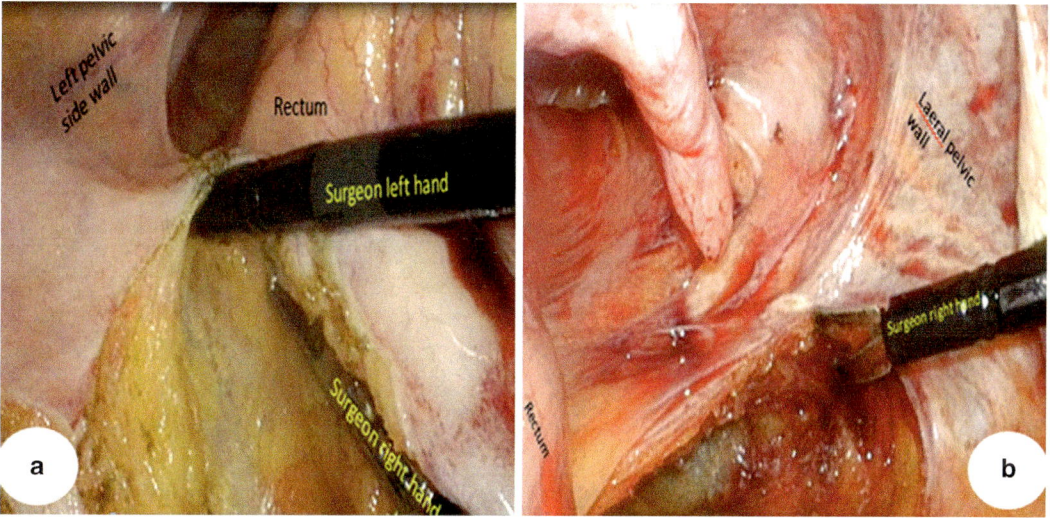

Fig. 14.16 Lateral mobilisation of rectum in pelvis. (**a**) Dissection of the left lateral ligament, (**b**) dissection of the right lateral ligament

and the parietal pelvic fascia, visualising and preserving the hypogastric nerves posteriorly and avoiding dissecting deep into the mesorectal fat superiorly. Planes of dissection are always maintained clear between the endopelvic fascia and retrosacral fascia posteriorly into the presacral plane and from medial to lateral dissection posteriorly; thus, the pelvic nerves are preserved, and the ureter is clearly identified in the lateral pelvic side wall, as shown in Fig. 14.15. Waldeyer's fascia should be cut sharp to enter into the deep pelvic mesorectum.

The next step is lateral dissection, which is started by the assistant retracting the rectum opposite and the surgeon's second hand performing traction on the lateral wall, as in Fig. 14.16, with the jaws of the grasper slightly open, which helps to open the dissection planes along the areolar tissue, with the surgeon's left hand maintaining the traction dissection extending along the lateral ligament, which contains the middle rectal artery. the pelvic autonomic nerves are important in the preservation of these structures; injury to the autonomic nerves is most

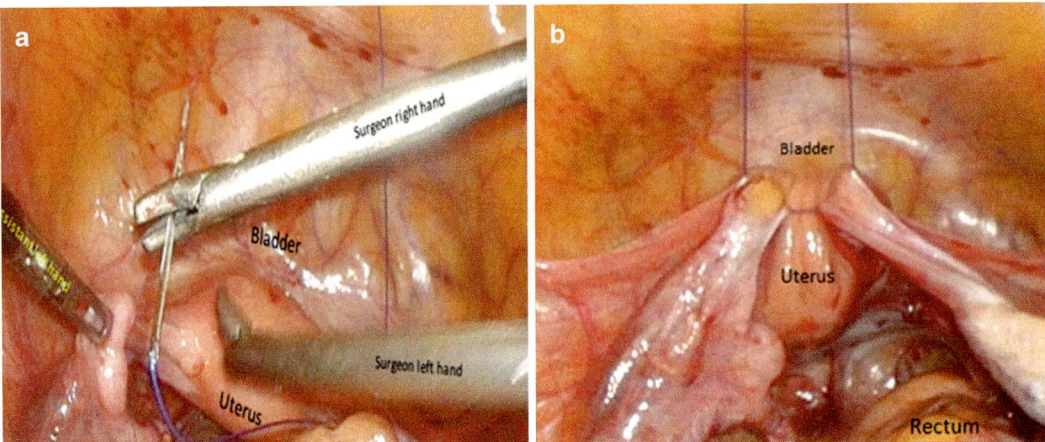

Fig. 14.17 Uterine fundus traction stitch for anterior dissection of the rectum

Fig. 14.18 Anterior dissection of the rectum with dissection of Denovilliers' fascia

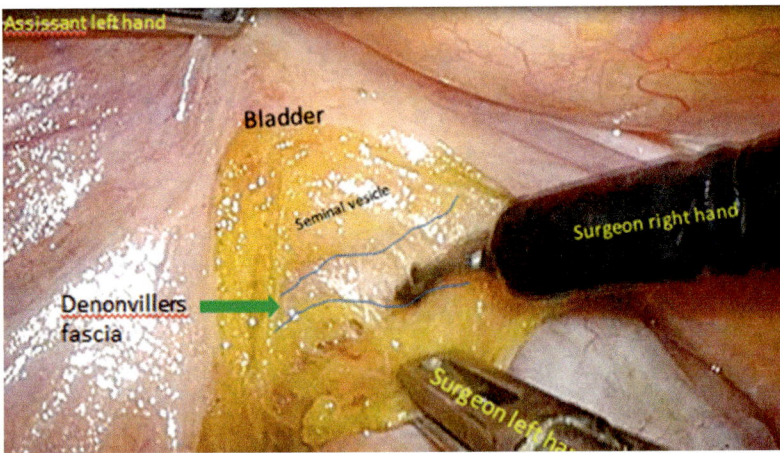

common if the dissection is close to the parietal pelvic fascia. Anterior dissection in women is started in the pouch of Douglas or recto-uterine pouch, with retraction of the uterus and a suture to the abdominal wall fixed on a swab, as shown in Fig. 14.17; in low rectal cancers on the anterior side per vaginal examination and the vagina retracted superiorly helps in identification of the rectovaginal fold. Anterior dissection in males is started by identifying the bladder fold in the pouch of Douglas, incising 1 cm anterior the apex of the pouch, extending the dissection distally, maintaining the plane above Denonvilliers' fascia, as in Fig. 14.18, and identifying the seminal vesicle and the prostrate. Dissection continues up to the lower end of the mesorectum ,which is identified by the muscular pelvic floor muscles.

Denonvilliers' fascia is a double-layered fascia, and distinguishing the layer is not easy during surgery; however, if there are anteriorly placed rectal tumours, care is taken to maintain planes close to the prostate with resection of Denonvilliers' fascia along with the rectum.

Tips and Tricks

1. In difficult anatomy opening the lateral peritoneal fold at the level of the sacral promontory helps to identify the holy plane of Heald.
2. Dissection in the deep rectum needs traction, and this can be achieved with nylon tape tied circumferentially to the upper rectum and cranial traction applied medially or laterally depending on the plane of dissection.

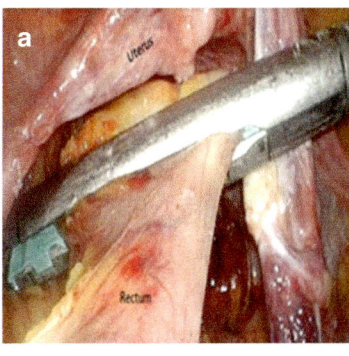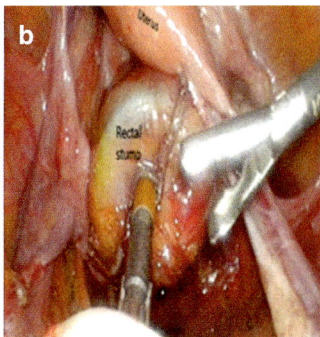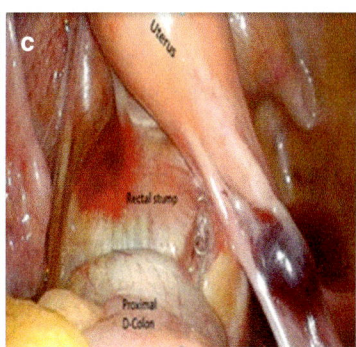

Fig. 14.19 Transection and anastomosis of the rectum with the double stapling technique. (**a**) Intracorporeal articulating staplers for rectal stapling. (**b**) Transanal circular stapler through the rectal stump with locking of the anvil to the cartridge. (**c**) Approximated and complete end-to-end anastomosis

3. Avoid blunt dissection, as only sharp dissection helps to maintain the correct plane.
4. During traction of the lower rectum, a cotton swab in the surgeon's left-hand grasper helps in retraction of the rectum and preventing the breach of TME planes. Violating the TME planes/tumour rupture results in poor oncological outcomes.

14.5.6.8 Rectal Occlusion and Washout

After the colorectal mobilisation, the distal rectum transection is marked with adequate margins from the tumour edge, and an articulating linear stapler is inserted and the rectum occluded. Betadine with saline wash is given to clear the residual stool in the rectum, preventing tumour seeding in the rectal stump.

14.5.6.9 Rectal Transection

The distal rectal transection line is marked with cautery, and 1–2 cm of surrounding mesentery is cleared from the posterior and the lateral surfaces. The stapler is inserted through the right lower quadrant using a 12-mm trocar; the surgeon and the assistant need to be coordinated to make the stapler align with the rectum, as the articulating staplers can maintain a maximum angulation of 65°, as shown in Fig. 14.19. The anvil of the stapler is advanced slowly according to the constant visual line of the camera posteriorly, as there is a chance that the posterior cartridge fork might pierce the rectal wall. After the stapler is locked, re-examination is carried out of the staple edges posteriorly and anteriorly and up to the tip to prevent entanglement of the pelvic side wall structures or the posterior vaginal wall. Most transections need an average of 2–3 staples to complete the transection. Ideally, the number of staples should be minimised to prevent dog ears and a zigzag staple line, as these increase the chances of leakage due to ischaemia [38].

Tips and Tricks

1. In the case of low rectal anastomosis, examination and retraction of the posterior vaginal wall are carried out to prevent involvement in the staple line.
2. In a narrow pelvis and in the male pelvis, it is advisable to use a 45-mm endo-reticulating stapler, as this facilitates the easy articulation of the staples.
3. In bulky rectal tumours, narrow pelvises, and low rectal tumours, a suprapubic 12-mm trocar can be used as an alternative for vertical transection of the rectum.

14.5.6.10 Specimen Extraction

With the era of MIS, further strategies have evolved to minimise the extent of the incision, pain, wound infection, and incisional hernia. There is still no ideal route for extraction of a specimen; new surgical techniques continue to evolve to explore the possible methods of for extracting specimen, which ultimately depend on

the location and size of the tumour, the bulk of
the mesentery, the type of anastomosis performed, the surgeon's preference, and the length
of proximal colon mobilised. All the extraction
sites are protected with wound protectors (Alexis
protector, Applied Medical) to prevent tumour
spillage and also help in the retraction of the
wound. For rectal cancers following LOR, transanal specimen extraction or transabdominal
extraction can be performed, and anastomosis is
completed by either the single-stapling or the
double-stapling technique as in Fig. 14.20. For
low rectal cancers with ISR, specimens are
extracted using transanal and coloanal anastomosis, either handsewn or stapled. The three routes
of specimen extraction are trans-umbilicus,
suprapubic, and transanal.

14.5.6.11 Colorectal Anastomosis

Colorectal Reconstruction

Colorectal surgeons devise new techniques to
preserve adequate length of the rectal stump to
achieve a good quality of life; staples have been
developed to overcome the conventional inade-
quacies of traditional rectal anastomosis. Staples
transformed rectal surgery after the introduction
of the double stapling technique in 1980, with the
convenience of expeditious anastomosis,
decreased contamination, accommodating the
disparity of size, and accessing narrow pelvic
anastomosis. In traditional open colorectal surgery, most anastomoses consisted of end-to-end
coloanal anastomosis; however, symptoms of
anterior resection syndrome prompted surgeons

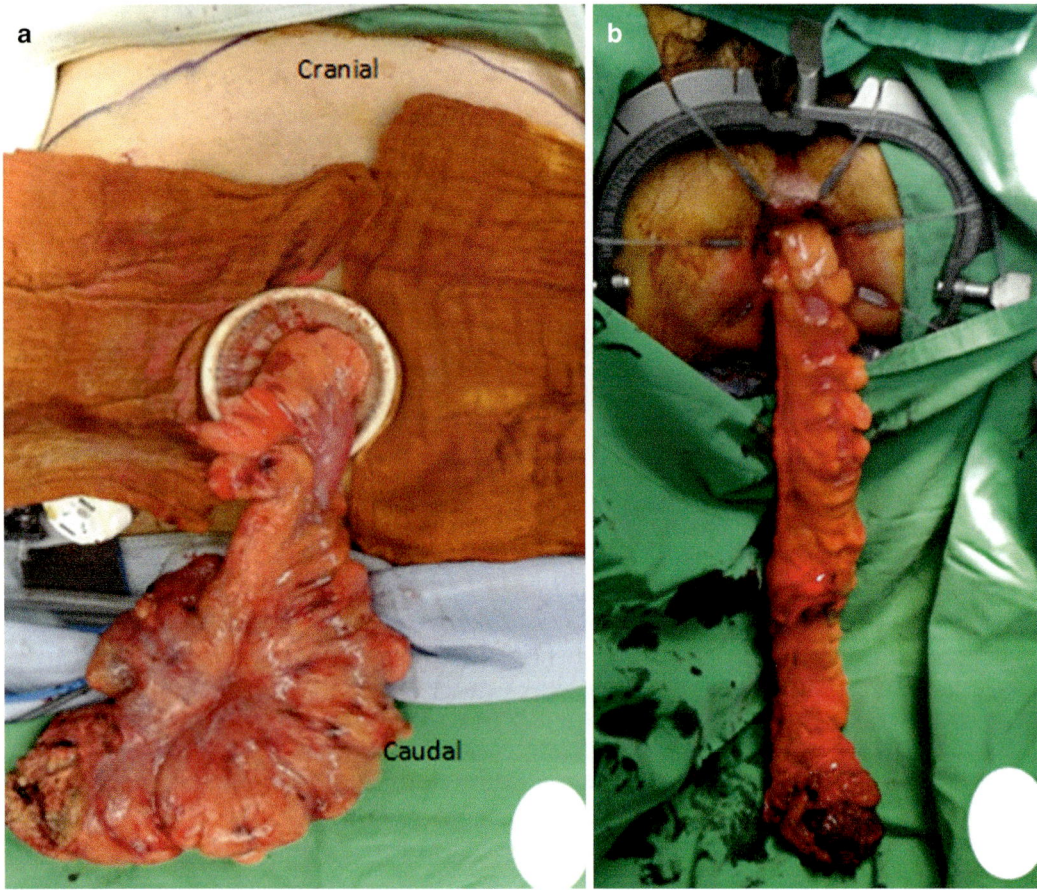

Fig. 14.20 Types of specimen extraction. (**a**) Transumbilical, (**b**) transanal

to search for reservoir techniques and alternative anastomotic methods of preserving the organ and improving functional outcomes. There are four common types of coloanal reconstruction, as shown in Fig. 14.20, which can be either hand-sewn or stapled, although the principles of reconstruction remain the same (Fig. 14.21):

1. End-to-end
2. End-to-side (Baker's technique)
3. J-pouch
4. Transverse coloplasty

The most common type of reconstruction for rectal cancers is end-to-end anastomosis using the double-stapling technique. After the rectal transection distally, the proximal bowel is brought out through the abdominal wound, and Betadine-soaked pads are placed around the wound retractor to prevent wound contamination; the proximal bowel is clamped with non-crushing clamps, and with a sharp knife the bowel is transected. Betadine-soaked gauze is used to clean out the residual stools in the proximal colon. Purse-string sutures are applied, either handsewn or automated (Autosuture, 65-mm purse string device; Covidien, Mansfield, MA, USA). Care should be taken while applying purse string sutures to ensure equidistant bites to produce a good purse string effect, snuggly fitting the anvil and avoiding uneven crumpling. The proximal bowel is dropped back into the abdominal cavity and a hand glove port is used on the wound protector. Then, the curved circular stapler (33-ILS Ethicon Endo-Surgery, USA) is passed through the rectal stump, the shaft is advanced to the stapled end, and the conjoined trocar is advanced through the middle of the blind end of the lumen through the stapler line and positioned in the pelvis. With the anvil holder, the proximal bowel end with anvil is fixed and connected to the trocar with a click. Before closing and firing the stapler, the axis of the proximal colon is checked to prevent any tension, twisting or adjacent organ entrapment such as the mesentery, and epiploicae entrapment in the anastomotic line. Tension-free anastomosis by adequate mobilisation and filling of the pelvis with the colon improves haemostasis and reduces the dead space, which should be practised to prevent leakage.

A J-pouch is created by fashioning a 5- to 6-cm-long pouch predetermined to reach the rectal cuff, and an enterotomy is made in the apex of the pouch 5–6 cm proximal to the stapled end. Linear staplers are applied, and the pouch is created. The anvil of the circular staplers is introduced into the enterotomy and purse string 3–0 Prolene sutures are applied and circular anastomosis carried out to the anal stump using a curved circular stapler (33-ILS Ethicon Endo-Surgery,

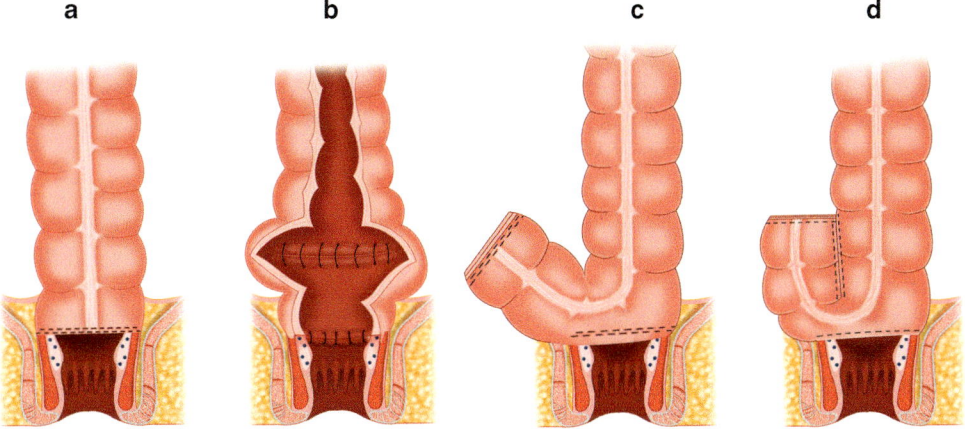

Fig. 14.21 Types of colorectal reconstruction. (**a**) End-to-end, (**b**) transverse coloplasty, (**c**) side-to-end, (**d**) J-pouch

USA). A transverse coloplasty (TP) is performed to create a smaller reservoir than the J-pouch with an 8- to 10-cm vertical colostomy between the two taenias in the antimesenteric border 4–6 cm proximal to the cut end. The colostomy is closed by transverse-like Heineke–Mikulicz pyloroplasty and the EEA completed. End-to-side colorectal anastomosis is carried out, with the anvil of the circular stapler being introduced into the proximal colon 6–8 cm from the end of the divided bowel. From the rectal stump the curved circular stapler (33-ILS Ethicon endo surgery, USA) is introduced and the anastomosis completed. The advantages of end-to-side anastomosis are that it can be beneficial in the case of a narrow pelvis, a thick mesentery, and if there are difficulties in reaching the proximal limb and disparity in the ends.

In conclusion, for reconstructive techniques after rectal resection, systematic reviews and meta-analysis have shown that the colonic J-pouch (CJP) has shown better functional outcomes for 1–2 years compared with straight coloanal anastomosis (SCA) [39–41]. Side-to-end anastomosis, TC, and CJP have better functional outcomes for at least 1 year than the SCA [40, 41].

Types of Colorectal Anastomosis

With regard to colorectal anastomosis in the Achilles heel , every colorectal surgeon strives to maintain an adequate distal margin for oncological outcomes and diminish anastomotic complications. As there are technical difficulties involved in colorectal anastomosis because of a narrow pelvis, a deep field, and a narrow range of mobility, the stapled anastomosis has been commonly used for the colorectal area. There is no difference in outcomes when comparing hand-sewn versus stapled anastomosis in rectal cancers, but stapled anastomoses preserve more of the rectum [41, 42]. The advent of stapling technology in the 1980s has paved way for a decrease in the rates of APR and an increase in sphincter-saving techniques for low rectal cancer with an acceptable safe margin of 1–2 cm of colorectal anastomosis. There are no RCTs to prove which is the best stapling technique, and they depend on

surgeon preference, patient factors, and tumour-related factors. Each technique has unique advantages and disadvantages, and every colorectal surgeon should have an armamentarium for performing colorectal anastomosis to treat low rectal cancer. Staplers provide the advantages of a better blood supply, reduced tissue manipulation, less oedema, uniformity, ease, and rapidity in sutures. Three types of stapled colorectal anastomosis are (Fig. 14.22):

1. Single-stapling technique
2. Double-stapling technique
3. Triple-stapling technique

Single-Stapling Technique

After complete mobilisation of the colon, an adequate margin of the proximal colon is transected using an advanced endostapler (ECHELON FLEX™ GST System) and a distal rectal margin of 5 cm is dissected. The lumen of the rectum is occluded with an intracorporeally free tie suture (silk 1–0) proximal to the proposed line of rectal division, to prevent contamination and tumour spillage into the peritoneal cavity before division. After copious rectal stump irrigation, the rectum is neatly divided with scissors. An extra-small Alexis wound protector (Alexis wound retractor; Applied Medical, Rancho Santa Margarita, CA, USA) is inserted into the peritoneum, and the specimen extracted transanally.

Extracorporeal transanal or trans-umbilical anvil head fixation in the proximal bowel end is decided after intraoperative assessment of the available length of proximal colon and mesentery. If the proximal conduit is of adequate length, then the conduit is extracted transanally, the anvil inserted, and purse string sutures applied. A distal circular stapling device anvil was fixed extracorporeally with a purse string. If the colon length available is short, then the proximal colon was brought through trans-umbilical wound and anvil inserted with purse-string suture around stump edge and then pushed back into the peritoneum. Distal rectal stump was closed with purse-string suture intracorporeally, and single-stapling anastomosis was done using curved intraluminal

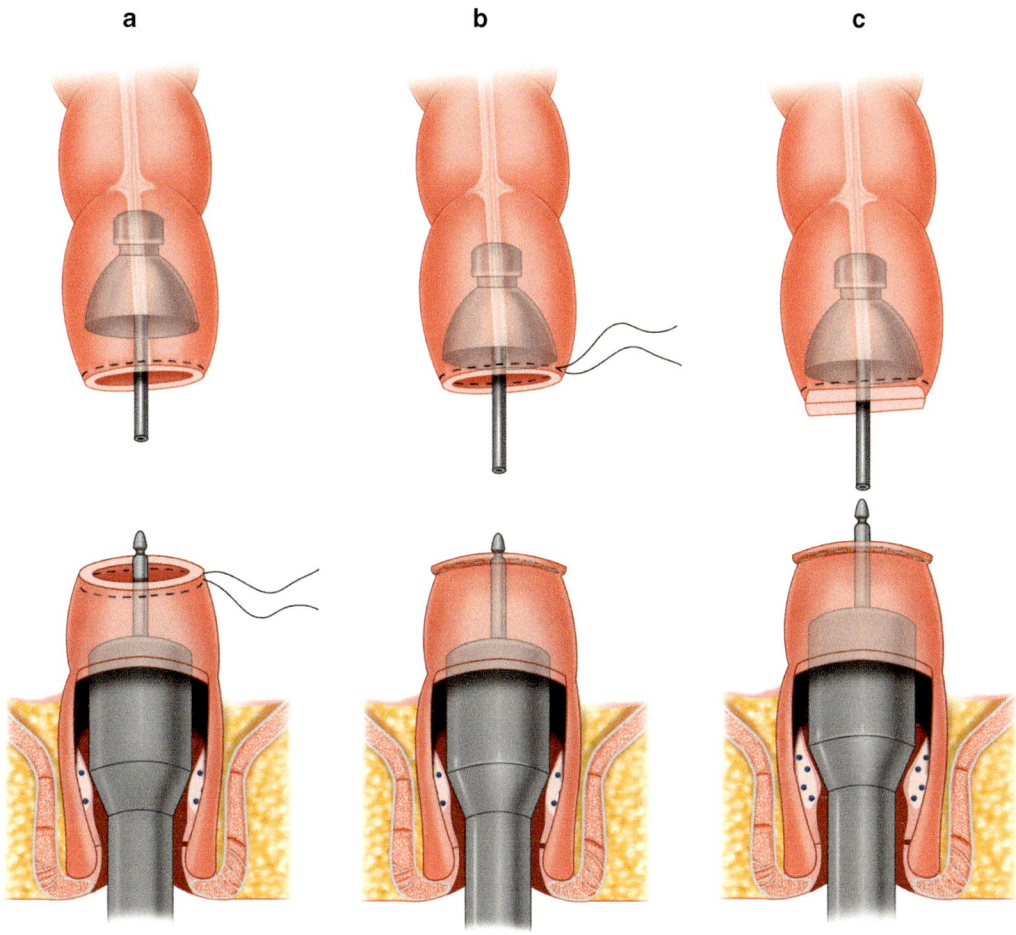

Fig. 14.22 Types of colorectal anastomosis. (**a**) Single-stapling technique, (**b**) double-stapling technique, (**c**) triple-stapling technique

stapler (29 mm, Ethicon Endo-Surgery, USA circular stapler) as in Fig. 14.23. Before the anastomosis is completed, the axis of the proximal bowel should be checked for any twist in the axis and undue tension on the anastomosis. The advantages of the single-stapling technique (SST) are that it gives longer distal transection margins; because it also involves transanal natural orifice specimen extraction, it reduces the extent of the abdominal incision, thereby decreasing pain, decreasing the hospital stay, reducing wound complications, resulting in better cosmesis, and thereby reducing costs [43–46]. The disadvantages are that SST needs technical expertise for intracorporeal suturing, is not suitable for

patients with a higher BMI, and that larger T4 tumours cannot be extracted transanally [43].

Double-Stapling Technique

After colorectal mobilisation, the rectum is transected at least 1–2 cm distal to the tumour using an articulating linear stapler; the mobilised tumour-bearing colonic segment is pulled out via a 3- to 5-cm umbilical incision. The colon was divided at least 10 cm proximal to the tumour, and the anvil head was placed extracorporeally. The bowel was repositioned back into the abdomen, followed by a transanal circular anastomosis, as shown in Fig. 14.24. Directional staple technology (DST) has advantages when there is a

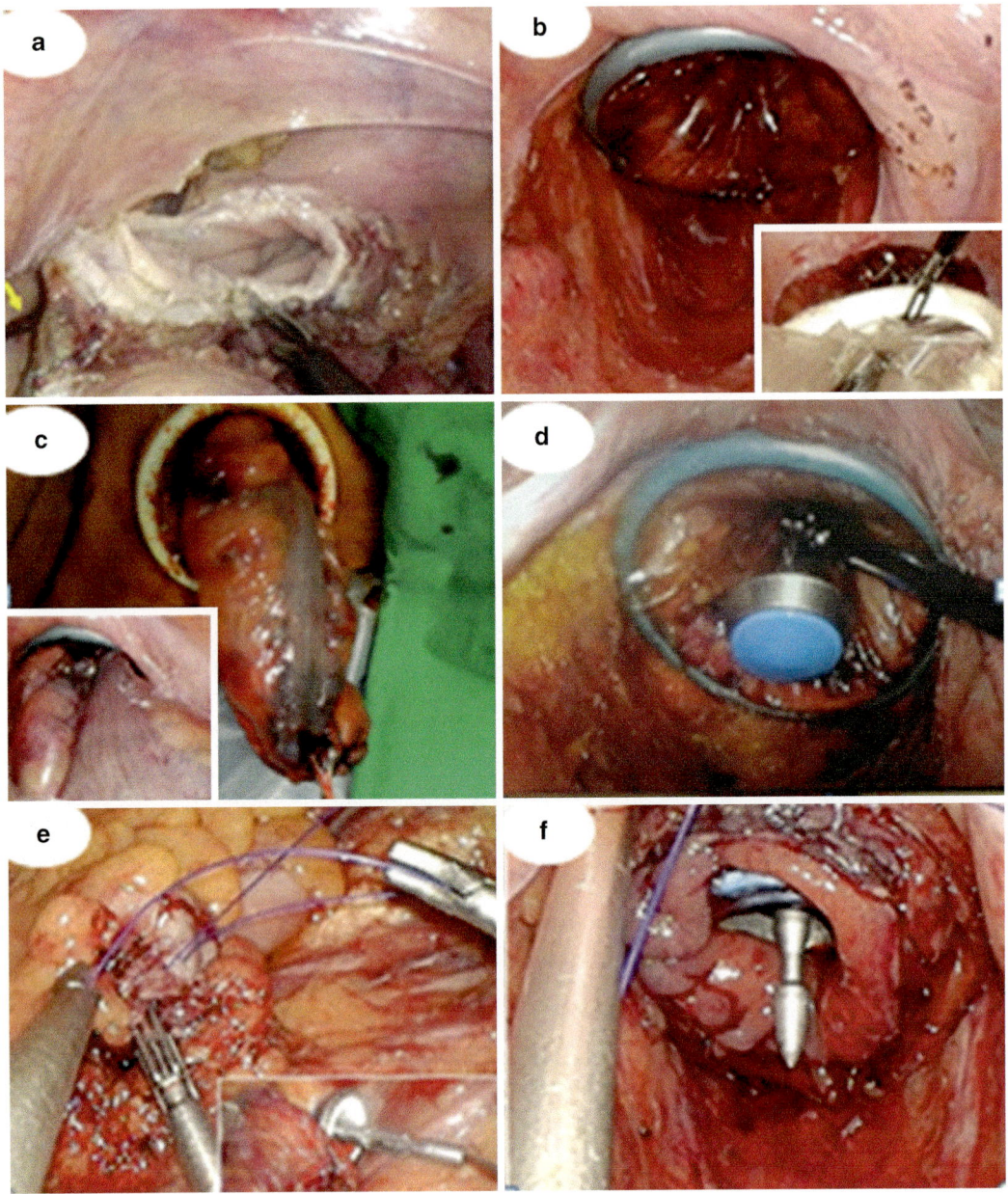

Fig. 14.23 Single-stapling technique with natural orifice specimen extraction. (**a**) Distal stump of the rectum cut with scissors. (**b**) Transanal wound protector device inserted. (**c**) Transanal specimen extraction. (**d**) Transanal anvil insertion. (**e**) Intracorporeal anvil purse string application to the proximal colon. (**f**) Rectal purse string application

discrepancy between the rectal stump and proximal bowel, providing a short operating time and ease of anastomosis, eliminating purse string suturing, and minimising faecal and tumour contamination [47–49]. The disadvantages of DST are that it needs multiple stapler firing, crossing of stapler lines, dog ears, and an additional 12-mm port for stapling [50].

Triple-Stapling Technique

After rectosigmoid mobilisation and transection of the distal rectum using an articulating endosta-

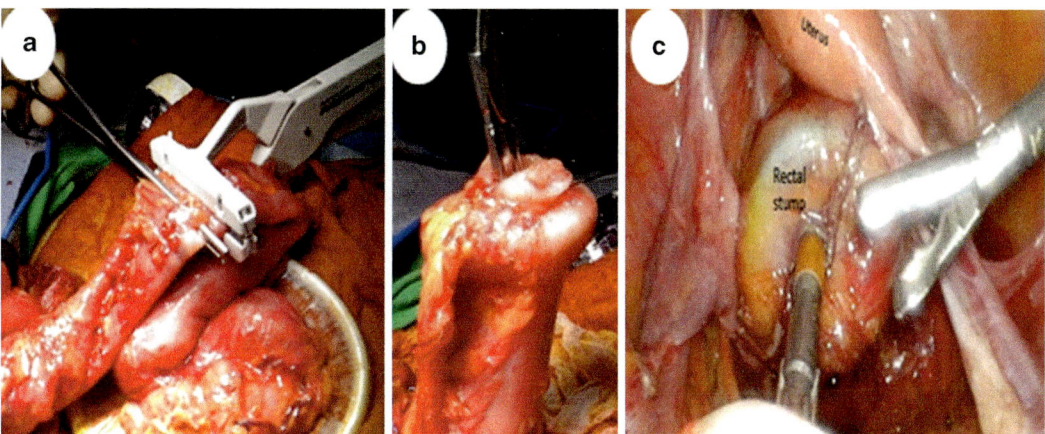

Fig. 14.24 Double-stapling technique. (**a**) Proximal rectal transection and purse string application using an Autosuture device. (**b**) Purse string application on the anvil. (**c**) Locking of the anvil head with a cartridge for a double-stapling anastomosis

pler (60 mm), the colon is delivered extracorporeally and the proximal end is cut with a cold knife. The shaft of the anvil is delivered through the antimesenteric border 5 cm above the proximal colonic end, and the end of the bowel is closed using a linear stapler. A circular anastomosis is performed [51, 52].

14.5.6.12 Assessment of Anastomosis

The anastomosis is assessed for integrity with an intraoperative check colonoscopy after filling the pelvis with saline, the patient being placed in a reverse Trendelenburg position, and looking for an air leak. Anastomotic bleeding should also be noted and if present additional reinforcing sutures are placed over the anastomosis to stem the bleeding. The pelvic wash is completed and a Jackson–Pratt drain is inserted into the pelvis through the lower quadrant port site.

14.5.6.13 Diversion Ileostomy

In the case of low rectal anastomosis, a diversion loop ileostomy is performed by marking the bowel 50–60 cm proximal from the ileocecal junction. The loop is brought through the previously marked stoma site and the stoma is fashioned. Care is taken regarding the orientation to prevent twisting in the exteriorised loop. All port sites >5 mm are closed using 2–0 Vicryl to the fascial and subcuticular levels.

14.5.6.14 Post-Operative Management

The nasogastric tube is removed post-procedure; no antibiotics are administered postoperatively. The urinary catheter is removed after the patient has been mobilised. Early ambulation is encouraged, oral liquids started 8 h after surgery, and the patient progresses to a normal diet as required. The outputs of the ileostomy are monitored and ileostomy diarrhoea treated.

14.5.6.15 Role of Indocyanine Green in Colorectal Anastomosis

Anastomotic leakage in colorectal surgery is a major concern in terms of mortality, morbidity, and long-term outcomes. Most anastomotic leakage occurs because of inadequate perfusion at anastomosis, and there is no reliable tool to confirm the micro-perfusion at the time of anastomosis. Fluorescence angiography is a new tool introduced into laparoscopic MIS to assess perfusion as shown in Fig. 14.25 (the well-vascularised segment is seen in green. The multi-institutional PILLAR II trial of 139 patients on the use of fluorescence angiography showed that the success rate of angiography is 99%, and by performing a fluorescence angiography study, the planned proximal margin of transection changed in 7.9% of patients, with resulting leakage rates of 0% [53]. This is a new

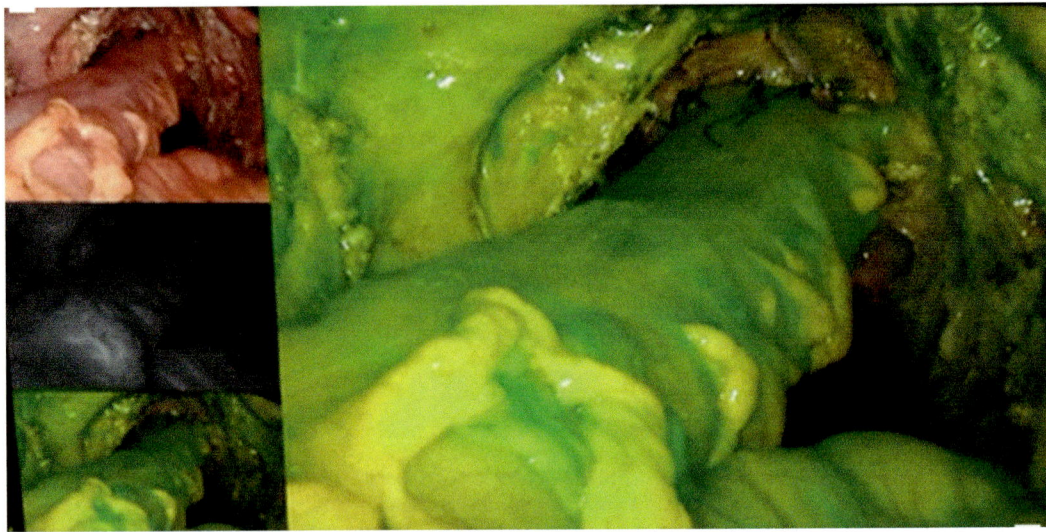

Fig. 14.25 ICG test showing well-vascularised segment of colon, as indicated by the *green colour*

technique, but studies have shown its safety and feasibility. The technique is useful mainly when a high-risk anastomosis is carried out, and in extended resections and re-resections of colorectal cancer where there is a risk of a precarious blood supply [54].

14.6 Intersphincteric Resection

Surgical treatment provides the only chance of a cure for rectal cancer. It is focussed on the preservation of the sphincter complex in low rectal cancers, and the ultimate goal is to achieve a good quality of life. This has been achieved with the best pathophysiological knowledge, surgical techniques, advances in instrumentation technology, and additional chemoradiotherapy, thanks to which there are decreasing rates of APR and increasing rates of sphincter-preserving surgeries for low rectal cancer. Decision-making in cases of low rectal cancer depends on the tumour distance from the anal verge, which gradually decreased from a 5-cm rule to 2 cm, and currently 1 cm is the acceptable distal margin for a good oncological outcome [55].

14.6.1 Patient Selection

Indications:

- Tumour 5 cm from the anal verge
- Tumour 2 cm from the dentate line
- Local spread restricted to the internal anal sphincter
- Adequate sphincter function and continence
- Well-differentiated tumours

Contraindications:

- Faecal incontinence
- T4 lesions
- Tumours invading the puborectalis and external anal sphincter
- Poorly differentiated tumours in low rectum.

14.6.2 Surgical Technique

The procedure is carried out using a combined abdominal and perineal approach, starting with the abdominal approach, with complete dissection of the rectum, followed by total mesorectal resection down to the pelvic floor, and then the anal dissection starts from below. With the patient in the Lloyd–Davies position, a Lone Star self-retaining retractor (Lone Star Medical Products, Houston, TX, USA) is applied, giving complete exposure to the anal canal. The rectal mucosa is infiltrated with 1 mg of diluted epinephrine with 10 ml of saline solution for haemostatic dissection. The anal mucosa is marked by cautery distal to the tumour, and with an adequate margin at least 1 cm from the tumour distal end, a purse string suture is applied to prevent tumour seeding, as in Fig. 14.26a, b. Three of ISR (Fig. 14.27) can be performed with regard to the distal margin of the tumour, with reference to the dentate line and the intersphincteric groove:

- Partial ISR—resection at the dentate line
- Subtotal ISR—resection between the dentate line and the intersphincteric groove
- Total ISR—resection of the internal sphincter at the intersphincteric groove

After mucosal marking, the incision is deepened to identify the intersphincteric plane and the intersphincteric plane is partially or totally preserved, based on the tumour status, the dissection planes the extent proximally to merge with the abdominal team. After dissection of the colon and the rectum from the attachments, the specimen is delivered transanally and the proximal margin is marked by using the ICG fluorescence

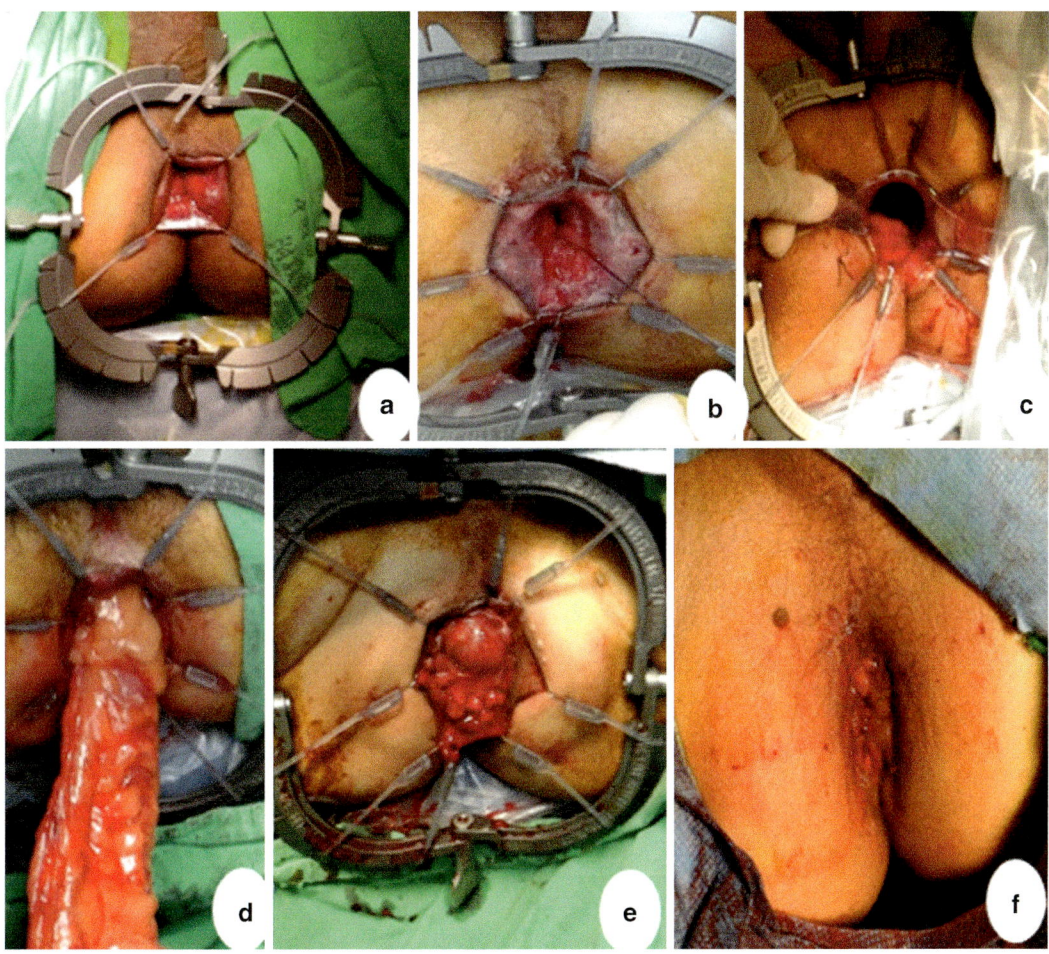

Fig. 14.26 (**a**, **b**) Steps of coloanal anastomosis. (**a**) Position of coloanal anastomosis (CAA) using a lone star retractor. (**b**) Intersphincteric dissection at the level of the dentate line. (**c**) Complete mobilisation of the distal stump. (**d**) Transanal specimen extraction, end-to-end CAA. (**e**) Appearance of the anal verge post-CAA

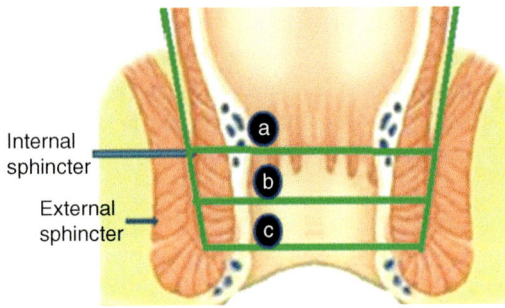

Fig. 14.27 Types of intersphincteric resection. *Green line* represents types of intersphincteric resection

Internal sphincter

External sphincter

angiography test to determine the well-vascularised segment for anastomosis. After the specimen has been removed, copious irrigation of the pelvic cavity is carried out and coloanal anastomosis with or without colonic pouch is performed, either with a stapler or by a single-layer handsewn anastomosis. Protective diversion loop ileostomy is compulsory for the coloanal anastomosis.

Conclusion

Surgery in rectal cancer has faced severe challenges and MIS for rectal cancer has made a phenomenal breakthrough in the momentum of progress in rectal surgery, with more evidence displaying better short-term outcomes and equalling long-term outcomes compared with open surgery. The technological advancement of staplers, minimally invasive instrumentation, and surgeon experience have resulted in more rectum-preserving surgeries and enhancement of patients' quality of life.

References

1. Jacobs M, Verdeja JC, Goldstein HS. Minimally invasive colon resection (laparoscopic colectomy). Surg Laparosc Endosc. 1991;1:144–50.
2. Guillou PJ, Quirke P, Thorpe H, et al. Short-term endpoints of conventional versus laparoscopic-assisted surgery in patients with colorectal cancer (MRC CLASICC trial): multicentre, randomised controlled trial. Lancet. 2005;365:1718–26.
3. Jayne DG, Guillou PJ, Thorpe H, et al. Randomized trial of laparoscopic-assisted resection of colorectal carcinoma: 3-year results of the UK MRC CLASICC trial group. J Clin Oncol. 2007;25:3061–8.
4. Green BL, Marshall HC, Collinson F, et al. Long-term follow-up of the Medical Research Council CLASICC trial of conventional versus laparoscopically assisted resection in colorectal cancer. Br J Surg. 2013;100:75–82.
5. Van der Pas MH, Haglind E, Cuesta MA, et al. Laparoscopic versus open surgery for rectal cancer (COLOR II): short-term outcomes of a randomised, phase 3 trial. Lancet Oncol. 2013;14:210–8.
6. Bonjer HJ, Deijen CL, Abis GA, et al. A randomized trial of laparoscopic versus open surgery for rectal cancer. N Engl J Med. 2015;372:1324–32.
7. Jeong S-Y, et al. Open versus laparoscopic surgery for mid-rectal or low-rectal cancer after neoadjuvant chemoradiotherapy (COREAN trial): survival outcomes of an open-label, non-inferiority, randomised controlled trial. Lancet Oncol. 2014;15:767–74.
8. Fleshman J, Branda M, Sargent DJ, et al. Effect of laparoscopic-assisted resection vs open resection of stage II or III rectal cancer on pathologic outcomes: the ACOSOG Z6051 randomized clinical trial. JAMA. 2015;314:1346–55.
9. Stevenson AR, Solomon MJ, Lumley JW, et al. Effect of laparoscopic-assisted resection vs open resection on pathological outcomes in rectal cancer: the ALaCaRT randomized clinical trial. JAMA. 2015;314:1356–63.
10. Hur H, Bae SU, Kim NK, et al. Comparative study of voiding and male sexual function following open and laparoscopic total mesorectal excision in patients with rectal cancer. J Surg Oncol. 2013;108(8):572.
11. Lisfranc J. Mémoire sur l'éxcision de la partie inférieure du rectum devenue carcinomateuse. Mém Ac R Chir. 1833;3:291–302.
12. Miles WE. A method of performing abdomino-perineal excision for carcinoma of the rectum and of the terminal portion of the pelvic colon. Lancet. 1908;2:1812–3.
13. Heald RJ, Husband EM, Ryall RD. The mesorectum in rectal cancer surgery: the clue to pelvic recurrence? Br J Surg. 1982;67:757–61.
14. Heald RJ. The 'holy plane' of rectal surgery. J R Soc Med. 1988;81:503–33.
15. Kraske P. Zur Exstirpation Hochsitzender Mast Darm Krebse. Verh Deutsch Ges Chir. 1885;14:464–74.
16. Ito H, Kunika H. Zur Kombinierten Exstirpation der hochsitzenden resp.ho hinaufreichenden Mastdarmkarzinome bei Mannern. Deutsche Zeitschrift fur Chirurg. 1904;73:229–48.
17. Torikata R. Beitrag zur kombinierten Exstirpation der hochsitzenden respective ho hinaufriechenden Mastdarmcarcinome bei Mannern. Deutsche Zeitschrift fur Chirurg. 1908;98:162–78.
18. Corman ML. Contributions of eighteenth and nineteenth century French medicine to colon and rectal surgery. Dis Colon Rectum. 2000;43(6 Suppl):S1–S29.

19. Galler AS, Petrelli NJ, Shakamuri SP. Rectal cancer surgery: a brief history. Surg Oncol. 2011;20(4):223–30.

20. Dixon CF. Anterior resection for malignant lesions of the upper part of the rectum and lower part of the sigmoid. Ann Surg. 1948;128:425–42.

21. Quirke P, Durdey P, Dixon MF, Williams NS. Local recurrence of rectal adenocarcinoma due to inadequate surgical resection. Histopathological study of lateral tumour spread and surgical excision. Lancet. 1986;2:996–9.

22. Dukes CE. The spread of cancer of the rectum. Br J Surg. 1930;17:643–8.

23. Parks AG, Nicholls RJ. Proctocolectomy without ileostomy for ulcerative colitis. BMJ. 1978;2:85–8.

24. Z'graggen K, Maurer CA, Buchler MW. Transverse coloplasty pouch. A novel neorectal reservoir. Dig Surg. 1999;16:363–6.

25. Sackier J. Laparoscopic abdominoperineal resection of the rectum. Br J Surg. 1992;79:1207–8.

26. Robicsek F, Konstantinov I. Hümer Hültl: the father of the surgical stapler. J Med Biogr. 2001;9(1):16–9.

27. Friedrich H. Ein eur Magen-Darm-Nahapparat. Zentralbl Chir. 1934;61:304–9.

28. von Seeman H. Zur Operation des Mastdarmkrebses. Eine Nahtquetsche fur due hohe sakrale Amputation. Zentralbl Chir. 1934;61:848.

29. Ravitch MM, Rivarola A. Entero-anastomosis with an automatic instrument. Surgery. 1966;59:270–7.

30. Knight CD, Griffen FD. An improved technique for low anterior resection of the rectum using the EEA stapler. Surgery. 1980;88:710–4.

31. Turnbull RB Jr, Cuthbertson A. Abdominorectal pull-through resection for cancer and for Hirschsprung's disease. Delayed posterior colorectal anastomosis. Cleve Clin Q. 1961;28:109–15.

32. Cutait DE, Figlionlini FJ. A new method of colorectal anastomosis in abdominoperineal resection. Dis Colon Rectum. 1961;4:335–42.

33. Parks AG. Transanal technique in low rectal anastomosis. Proc R Soc Med. 1972;65:975–6.

34. Parks AG, Percy JP. Resection and sutured coloanal anastomosis for rectal carcinoma. Br J Surg. 1982;69:301–4.

35. Moriya Y, Hojo K, Sawada T, Koyama Y. Significance of lateral node dissection for advanced rectal carcinoma at or below the peritoneal reflection. Dis Colon Rectum. 1989;32:307–15.

36. Schiessel R, Karner-Hanusch J, Herbst F, Teleky B, Wunderlich M. Intersphincteric resection for low rectal tumours. Br J Surg. 1994;81:1376–8.

37. Watanabe M, Teramoto T, Hasegawa H, Kitajima M. Laparoscopic ultralow anterior resection combined with peranum intersphincteric rectal dissection for lower rectal cancer. Dis Colon Rectum. 2000;43(Suppl 10):S94–7.

38. Kim JS, Cho SY, Min BS, Kim NK. Risk factors for anastomotic leakage after laparoscopic intracorporeal colorectal anastomosis with a double stapling technique. J Am Coll Surg. 2009;209(6):694–701. https://doi.org/10.1016/j.jamcollsurg.2009.09.021.

39. Brown CJ, Fenech D, McLeod RS. Reconstructive techniques after rectal resection for rectal cancer. Cochrane Database Syst Rev. 2008;2:CD006040. https://doi.org/10.1002/14651858.CD006040.

40. Hüttner FJ, Tenckhoff S, Jensen K, Uhlmann L, Kulu Y, Büchler MW, Diener MK, Ulrich A. Meta-analysis of reconstruction techniques after low anterior resection for rectal cancer. Br J Surg. 2015;102(7):735–45. https://doi.org/10.1002/bjs.9782.

41. Slieker JC, Daams F, Mulder IM, Jeekel J, Lange JF. Systematic review of the technique of colorectal anastomosis. JAMA Surg. 2013;148(2):190–201. https://doi.org/10.1001/2013.

42. McGinn FP, Gartell PC, Clifford PC, Brunton FJ. Staples or sutures for low colorectal anastomoses: a prospective randomized trial. Br J Surg. 1985;72:603–5.

43. Saurabh B, Chang SC, Ke TW, Huang YC, Kato T, Wang HM, Chen WT, Fingerhut A. Natural orifice specimen extraction with single stapling colorectal anastomosis for laparoscopic anterior resection: feasibility, outcomes, and technical considerations. Dis Colon Rectum. 2017;60:43–50. https://doi.org/10.1097/DCR.0000000000000739.

44. Huang YC, Chang SC, Chiang HC, Ke TW, Wang HM, Chen WT. Natural orifice specimen extraction with single-stapling anastomosis for distal colon resection: feasibility and outcomes. Formos J Surg. 2017;50:16–20.

45. Hisada M, Katsumata K, Ishizaki T, Enomoto M, Matsudo T, Kasuya K, et al. Complete laparoscopic resection of the rectum using natural orifice specimen extraction. World J Gastroenterol. 2014;20:16707–13.

46. Kim HJ, Choi GS, Park JS, Park SY. Comparison of intracorporeal single-stapled and double-stapled anastomosis in laparoscopic low anterior resection for rectal cancer: a case-control study. Int J Colorectal Dis. 2013;28(1):149–56. https://doi.org/10.1007/s00384-012-1582-8.

47. Moritz E, Achleitner D, Holbing N, Miller K, Speil T, Weber F. Single versus double stapling technique in colorectal surgery. Dis Colon Rectum. 1991;34:495–7.

48. Moore JWE, Chapuis PH, Bokey EL. Morbidity and mortality after single- and double-stapled colorectal anastomoses in patients with carcinoma of the rectum. Aust N Z J Surg. 1996;66:820–3. https://doi.org/10.1111/j.1445-2197.1996.tb00757.

49. Chiarugi M, Buccianti P, Sidoti F, Franceschi M, Goletti O, Cavina E. Single and double stapled anastomoses in rectal cancer surgery; a retrospective study on the safety of the technique and its indication. Acta Chir Belg. 1996;96(1):31–6.

50. Ito M, Sugito M, Kobayashi A, et al. Relationship between multiple numbers of stapler firings during rectal division and anastomotic leakage after laparoscopic rectal resection. Int J Colorectal Dis. 2008;23:703–7.

51. O'Rourke N, Moran BJ, Heald RJ. A laparoscopic tri-
    ple stapling technique that facilitates anterior resection
    for rectal cancer. J Laparoendosc Surg. 1994;4:261–3.
52. Julian TB, Kolachalam RB, Wolmark N. The triple-
    stapled colonic anastomosis. Dis Colon Rectum.
    1989;32:989–95.
53. Jafari MD, Wexner SD, Martz JE, et al. Perfusion
    assessment in laparoscopic left-sided/anterior resec-
    tion (PILLAR II): a multi-institutional study. J Am
    Coll Surg. 2015;220:82–92.

54. Chand A, Chen WT, Li MK. Current status of mini-
    mally invasive surgery in colorectum. Ann Laparosc
    Endosc Surg. 2016;11:23. https://doi.org/10.21037/
    ales.2016.
55. Rullier E, Laurent C, Bretagnol F, Rullier A, Vendrely
    V, Zerbib F. Sphincter-saving resection for all rectal
    carcinomas: the end of the 2-cm distal rule. Ann Surg.
    2005;241:465–9.

Robotic Total Mesorectal Excision and Sphincter-Saving Operation

15

Jin Cheon Kim

Abstract

The concept of total mesorectal excision (TME), which is the standard technique in rectal cancer operations, was established by Heald and Ryall in 1978. Overall local recurrence rates vary widely from 3% to 33% in conventional surgery, whereas TME has consistently achieved LR rates below or equal to 10%. Otherwise, neoadjuvant chemoradiotherapy and technical advances with stapling devices facilitate sphincter-saving operation (SSO) in lower rectal cancer (LRC) patients with competent oncological and functional outcomes. The SSO consists of anterior resection and low anterior resection (LAR) including ultra-LAR with intersphincteric resection (ISR), according to the level of dissection and anastomosis. With the advent of laparoscopic rectal cancer surgery, robot-assisted SSO appears to be a promising technique with its minimal invasiveness and clear visualization into the deep pelvic cavity. Robot-assisted TME and SSO have become recognized as being safe and feasible in comparison with open and laparoscopic approaches. The robot approach possesses many advantages over the latter two approaches, including its magnified view, dexterity supported by wristed instruments and stable traction, and ergonomic excellence. Robot-assisted TME could therefore enable deeper dissection and lower anastomosis in the pelvic region than is possible with a laparoscopy or open approach, with slightly better functional recovery. Several comparative studies reported robot-assisted ISR showing an equivalent oncological outcome with a little improved immediate postoperative outcome compared with open ISR. However, further studies including randomized controlled trials are needed to complement and establish the evidence for the oncological superiority of robot-assisted SSO compensating its financial burden.

Electronic Supplementary Material The online version of this chapter https://doi.org/10.1007/978-981-10-5143-2_15 contains supplementary material, which is available to authorized users.

J. C. Kim
Department of Surgery, University of Ulsan College of Medicine and Asan Medical Center,
Seoul, South Korea
e-mail: jckim@amc.seoul.kr

Keywords

Robot · Rectal cancer · Total mesorectal excision (TME) · Sphincter-saving operation (SSO) · Intersphincteric resection (ISR) Operative method · Complications · Outcomes

© Springer Nature Singapore Pte Ltd. 2018
N. K. Kim et al. (eds.), *Surgical Treatment of Colorectal Cancer*,
https://doi.org/10.1007/978-981-10-5143-2_15

15.1   Introduction

Korea has unexpectedly recorded the greatest incidence of colorectal cancer (CRC) in the world, followed by the European Union in second place. In recent years, a trend toward an increasing proportion of cases occurring in the right colon has been found, as recorded for other countries, while the absolute number of rectal cancer patients does not appear to have reduced. In this regard, we should consider several items of practical relevance. Firstly, the universal use of colonoscopy enables more colonic polyps and cancers to be detected in the right colon. Secondly, considering rectal length as being only 1/10 of the entire colon length, the proportion of rectal cancer (>1/3 of colorectal cancers) still overwhelms that of colon cancer. Thirdly, colon and rectal cancers present the same genomic constitution, except for 16% hypermutated cancer, as reported by the Cancer Genome Atlas in 2012 [1]. With consideration of all these facts, the substantial occurrence of rectal cancer cannot be underestimated, even in the era of the right shift of CRC.

We cannot help but reminisce over the role of surgery, which has been consistently positioned as the best treatment for rectal cancer. Since the historical accomplishment of abdominoperineal resection (APR) by Dr. Miles in the year 1904, sphincter-saving operations (SSOs) have merely tried to preserve anal function 60 years thereafter. However, recent approaches for rectal cancer surgery have diversified into open, laparoscopy-assisted, and robot-assisted ones. Although the latter two approaches take advantage of minimal invasiveness, the appropriate approach in terms of practical efficacy and long-term outcome remains to be determined.

The concept of total mesorectal excision (TME), which is the standard technique in rectal cancer operations, was established by Heald and Ryall in 1978 [2]. TME principally includes a sharp dissection at the mesorectal fascial envelope, according to the notion that the lateral mesorectal spread of small tumor foci (which

tends to be excluded in the classical anterior resection) can cause local recurrence (LR). As the procedure is inevitably accompanied by some technical challenges due to the restrictive operative field in the pelvis, a crucial parameter for the quality control of this procedure is identification of the complete mesorectal envelope [3]. Overall LR recurrence rates vary widely from 3% to 33% in conventional surgery, whereas TME has consistently achieved LR rates below or equal to 10% [4, 5].

SSOs are considered as a procedure of choice in patients with rectal cancer. A comparative study using a treatment trade-off method found that most patients preferred low anterior resection (LAR) rather than APR, even if LAR was accompanied by fecal incontinence [6]. Neoadjuvant treatments, the precise acquisition of surgical anatomy, technological advances, and stapling devices have concurrently facilitated a significant reduction in the rate of APR. SSOs are mostly confined to radical LAR operations and ultra-LAR, including intersphincteric resection (ISR). The use of ISR has recently been increasing with the knowledge that the levator muscle and external anal sphincter (EAS) are separated from the internal anal sphincter (IAS) and rectal proper muscle by the conjoined longitudinal muscle [7]. Despite possible dysfunctions in bowel due to injuries of anal sphincter muscles and pelvic nerves, a meta-analysis on ISR revealed that most patients were satisfied with acceptable bowel movement [8]. One Japanese study achieved a 93% rate of SSO (including ISR) in 1033 consecutive rectal cancer patients [9]. However, APR still remains an indispensable surgical tool for the treatment of lower rectal cancer (LRC) when tumors are situated very low down in the rectum, particularly in the case of large tumors, sphincter invasion, poor sphincter function, and patients with a deep or narrow pelvis.

Laparoscopy-assisted (LA) approaches are increasingly replacing open resection in SSOs for rectal cancer, as in other colon operations, although major clinical guidelines have not yet endorsed

LA resection outside of a clinical trial (the American Society of Colon and Rectal Surgeons, National Comprehensive Cancer Network: www. nccn.org). One meta-analysis showed no significant differences in oncological outcomes between LA and open rectal cancer surgery [10]. Although the LA approach enables a magnified view within the pelvic cavity, the technical validity, including optimal retraction in the pelvis, inadequate TME occurring from the leverage effect, frequent conversion, and ergonomic discomfort, remains particularly challenging. With the advent of robotic surgery platforms, robot-assisted (RA) SSO appears to be a promising technique, with its high dexterity and clear visualization enabling efficient retraction and fine dissection in the deep pelvic cavity, while, at the same time, minimizing invasiveness. Several comparative studies of case series have reported on RA ISR, and these have shown equivalent oncological outcomes with a little improvement in immediate postoperative outcome when compared with open ISR [11–13]. However, no haptic feedback, longer operative time, and higher cost than open and LA SSOs are the limitations.

15.2 Operative Methods

15.2.1 General Principles of TME and SSO

TME has been established as the standard procedure during rectal cancer surgery, obviating blunt dissection of the rectum along the retrorectal fascia. The lateral and posterior borders of the TME should include the fascia propria of the rectum along the prehypogastric nerve fascia, leaving the mesorectal envelope intact (Fig. 15.1). Anteriorly, there is an avascular plane between the seminal vesicles and Denonvilliers' fascia, which means the fascia needs to be retained on the specimen, along with the lateral and posterior mesorectal envelope [14]. If TME includes an adequate block dissection of the rectal lymphatics, efficient local control may be achieved, even in cases with lymph node metastasis [15]. Apart from distant metastasis, several inevitable conditions escape the TME field, for example, extramural invasion of the circumferential margin (tumor budding, extramural venous invasion, and extranodal

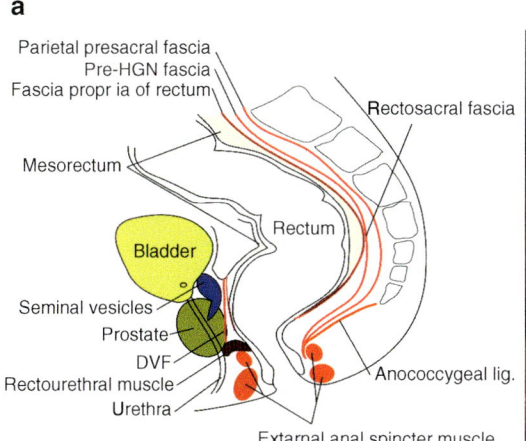

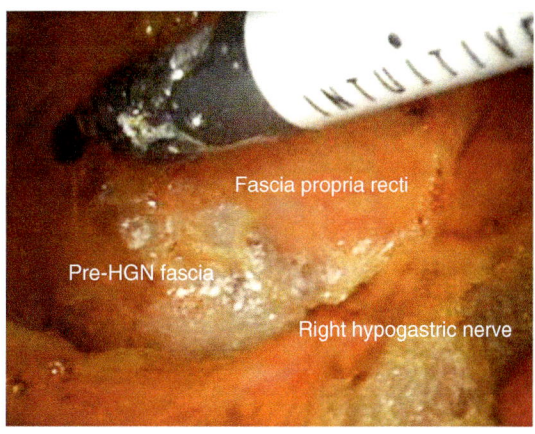

Fig. 15.1 (**a**) Layered structure of the pelvic fascia. (**b**) (Courtesy of Dr. Yusuke Kinugasa). Total mesorectal excision along the prehypogastric nerve fascia, preserving pelvic autonomic nerves. *HGN* hypogastric nerve, *DVF* Denonvilliers' fascia

extension), remnant mesorectal involvement during distal transaction, lateral spread of pelvic lymph nodes beyond the mesorectum, and possible seeding into the pelvis during dissection.

The caudal mesorectum ends at the apical level of the levator ani. This part of the rectum was previously called "the rectal no man's land," as it could not be reached from the abdomen, and remained as a relatively inviolate area during surgical exploration [16]. This concept should be abandoned, particularly in the era of minimally invasive approaches using LA and RA, which enable fine exposure and dissection into the pelvic cavity. TME practically consists of the two types of resection in accordance with the resection level, namely, a resection at or below the mesorectal end as complete TME and a resection above that level leaving a part of the mesorectum as tumor-specific mesorectal excision (TSME). As careful evaluation of the mesorectal envelope has important implications for reducing LR, the resected specimen must be thoroughly evaluated, both grossly and microscopically. Quirke et al. suggested different grades for the quality and completeness of the mesorectal envelope in TME, i.e., gross architecture, defects (≤5 mm), coning, and shape of circumferential resection margin (CRM) [3]; these are also recommended in the American Joint Committee on Cancer (AJCC) Cancer Staging (8th ed., 2017).

The rectum is approximately 12–16 cm in length, and half of this is covered by the peritoneum. The SSO consists of anterior resection or LAR, according to whether the level of the anastomosis is, respectively, above or below the peritoneal reflection. LAR can be further divided into LAR and ultra-LAR including ISR, according to whether the level of dissection and anastomosis is, respectively, above or below the mesorectal end. The extent of ISR has been conveniently classified into partial, subtotal, and total, according to the position of the IAS excision, i.e., above the dentate line, between the dentate line and the intersphincteric groove, or total excision of the IAS (Fig. 15.2).

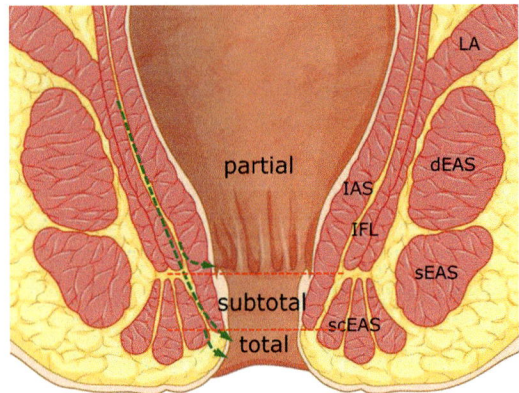

Fig. 15.2 Various types of intersphincteric resection classified into partial, subtotal, and total, according to the position of the IAS excision, i.e., above the dentate line, between the dentate line and the intersphincteric groove, and total excision of the IAS, respectively. The green dotted line indicates the excision line, and the red dotted line indicates the dentate line (upper) and intersphincteric groove (lower). *IAS* internal anal sphincter, *IFL* intersphincteric fibromuscular layer, *sc/s/d EAS* subcutaneous, superficial, deep external anal sphincter, *LA* levator ani

15.2.2 Cart Installation and Port Placement for RA SSO

Features of the robot platform, including magnified 3-D imaging, a surgeon-controlled stable camera system, EndoWrist instruments, and a fixed third-arm retraction, are particularly beneficial when performing SSO. The hybrid approach, composed of LA and RA approaches for the abdominal and pelvic procedures, respectively, was the first approach to be accomplished in a considerable number of centers. Recently, RA SSO has mostly adopted a totally robotic colorectal mobilization, using the four-arm da Vinci S, Si, and Xi surgical systems (Intuitive Surgical, Sunnyvale, CA, USA). The latest Xi system gives a widened range of motion with its rotational (±171°) overhead Boom and Flex systems. Efficient port placement appears to be a crucial determinant for successful SSO and varies in accordance with the robot system, surgeons' convenience, and type of operation.

For example, the author uses six ports including two assistant's ports, with the cart placed either obliquely at the anterosuperior iliac spine in the Si system or vertically at the left flank in the Xi system (Fig. 15.3). The initial endoscope port is placed adjacent to the umbilicus to visualize the entire colon, maintaining 10–15 cm from the lesion for both the Si and Xi systems. In the Si system, arm 1 is equipped with dissecting instruments during the entire procedure, while arms 2 and 3 are furnished with retraction and grasping instruments, moving from the right upper port to the left upper port, and from the left upper to left lower port, during abdominopelvic and pelvic procedures, respectively (Fig. 15.3a). However, the movement of arms during SSO is generally unnecessary for the entire procedure in the Xi system (Fig. 15.3b). Along the horizontal umbilical line, the first port (arm 1) for the retraction instrument is placed 2 cm lateral to the left midclavicular line, and the second port (for the arm 2) is placed 6–8 cm from the first port. The fourth port (for arm 4) is placed at the oblique line crossing the right midclavicular line. Arms 2 and 4 can be moved to ipsilateral lower ports in the case of a deep pelvic cavity or intersphincteric dissection. The two ports unoccupied by robotic arms can alternatively substitute for the assistant's ports, for suction, auxiliary supplies, and stapling.

15.2.3 Operative Procedures

The author's RA SSO uses a totally robotic colorectal mobilization, which consists of abdominopelvic and pelvic approaches using a da Vinci Si or Xi surgical system (Intuitive Surgical; Fig. 15.4). The procedure starts with an abdominopelvic procedure, in which the mesocolic fascia is incised from the root of the inferior mesenteric artery (IMA) into the right peritoneal reflection along the medial margin of the right common iliac and internal iliac arteries. The IMA is divided and ligated as high- or low-type, followed by the inferior mesenteric vein ligation and excision, mostly preserving the left colic artery. A medial to lateral dissection for sufficient colonic mobilization is

continued near the level of IMA up to the distal border of the pancreas, leaving the left gonadal vessels and left ureter along the retrofacial plane. The TME is continued into the pelvic cavity along the prehypogastric nerve fascia, preserving the hypogastric trunk, the hypogastric nerves, and the right pelvic plexus. The left peritoneal excision is then followed from the white fusion line up to the splenocolic ligament and greater omentum, further separating the left colon (sometimes including the transverse colon) from the retroperitoneum. The left colonic dissection continues into the pelvic cavity, resecting the left lateral peritoneal border along the medial margin of the left common iliac and internal iliac arteries, leaving the left pelvic plexus intact. The pelvic procedure follows the abdominopelvic procedure to accomplish the complete TME. Using a stable robot retraction at the right side of the urinary bladder, a sharp dissection is carried out to separate the rectum from the seminal vesicles, and the prostate (vagina in females) from the Denonvilliers' fascia, followed by separation of the levator muscles. After the right side dissection, a similar maneuver is repeated on the left side of the pelvis, followed by completion of pelvic dissection at the anococcygeal ligament. Otherwise, in TSME, the pelvic dissection is progressed up to 3–5 cm caudal to the scheduled anastomotic line, followed by distal mesorectal excision at the anastomotic site.

In the case of possible metastatic lymph nodes by imaging studies, the lateral pelvic lymph node dissection can be accompanied after completion of the pelvic dissection. The distal resection can be conveniently carried out using a robot stapler; otherwise, an articulating endoscopic linear stapler may be used. A proximal resection is continued along the mesocolon. The Si and Xi systems are equipped with an indocyanine green fluorescence imaging (IFI) system to identify real-time vascular perfusion (Fig. 15.5a). As this procedure does not require much extra time or a high cost, it may be helpful to prevent anastomotic leakage (AL) in cases of questionable perfusion. The bowel continuity is mostly established by the double-stapling technique, without any type of

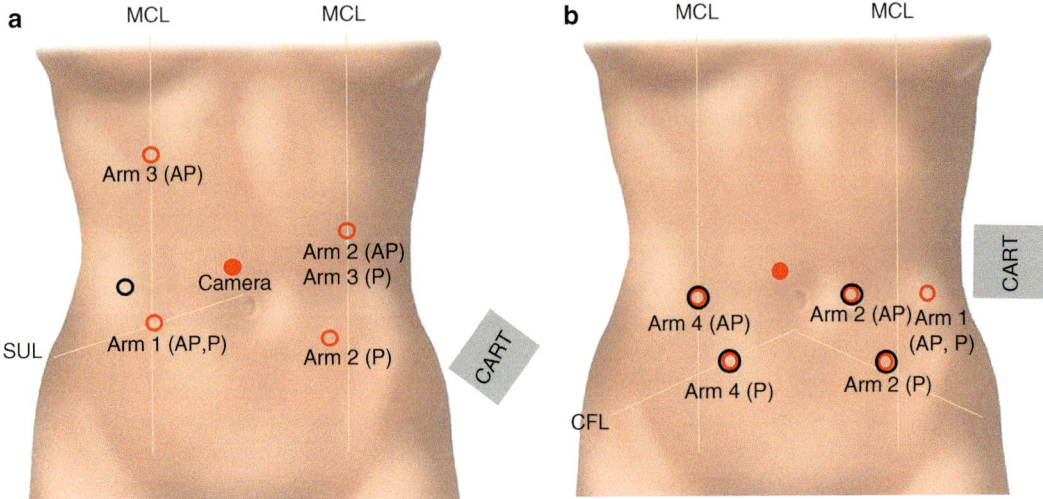

Fig. 15.3 Cart installation and port placement for RA SSO. (**a**) Si system. (**b**) Xi system. Red and black circles indicate robot port and assistant's port, respectively. *SUL* spinoumbilical line, *CFL* costo-femoral line, *MCL* midclavicular line, *AP* abdominopelvic procedure, *P* pelvic procedure

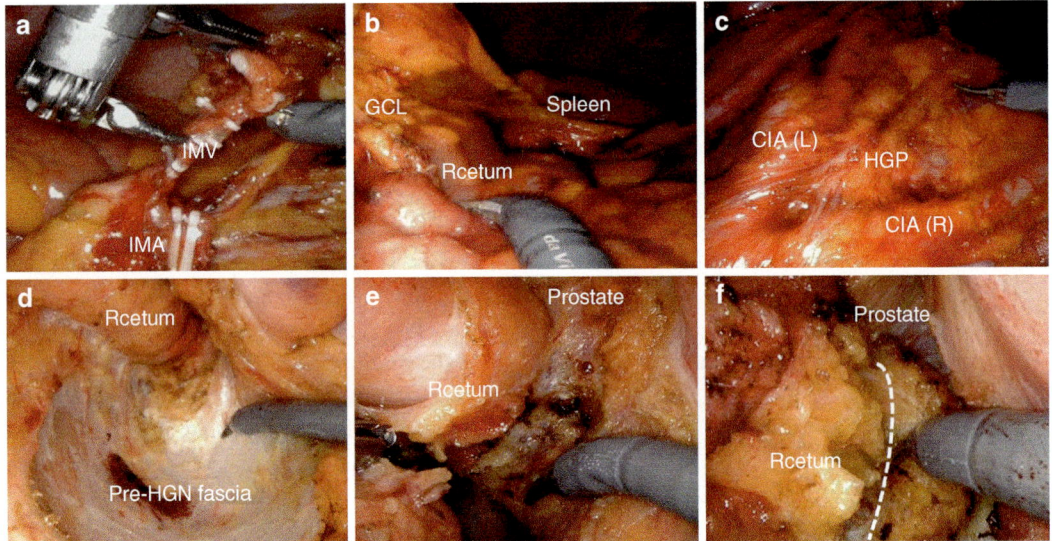

Fig. 15.4 Robot-assisted sphincter-saving operation. (**a**) Ligation and excision of inferior mesenteric artery and vein. (**b**) Left colon mobilization with splenic flexure takedown. (**c**, **d**) Pelvic dissection observing the principles of total mesorectal excision and pelvic autonomic nerve preservation. (**e**) Mobilization of the distal rectum on the right side. (**f**) Distal mesorectal excision in a case of tumor-specific mesorectal excision at the scheduled anastomotic site. *IMA* inferior mesenteric artery, *IMV* inferior mesenteric vein, *GCL* gastrocolic ligament, *HGP* hypogastric plexus, *CIA(R) and CIA(L)* common iliac artery, right and left, *HGN* hypogastric nerve

coloplasty. Robotic linear stapling has recently enabled efficient accessibility and safe grasping during double-stapling (Fig. 15.5b). The cross or weak points of the double-stapling anastomosis can be safely strengthened by reinforcing sutures to prevent AL. A diverting ileostomy is added at the surgeon's discretion. After clinical and radiological confirmation of freedom from leakage or stricture, the bowel continuity is resumed 1 month after completion of postoperative adjuvant treatment, or 3 months postoperatively in cases without adjuvant treatment.

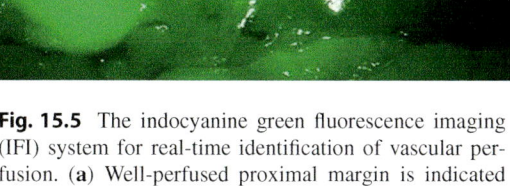
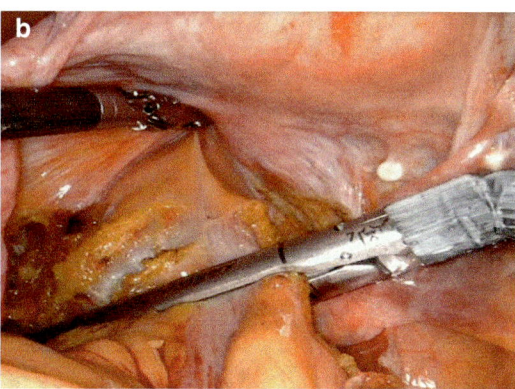

Fig. 15.5 The indocyanine green fluorescence imaging (IFI) system for real-time identification of vascular perfusion. (**a**) Well-perfused proximal margin is indicated (white dotted line, scheduled line of proximal resection).

(**b**) The recent introduction of robotic linear stapling enables efficient accessibility and safe grasping during double-stapling

In ISR, a sharp dissection is particularly required at the end point of the TME where the mesorectal fascia merges with the distal rectum, the so-called Morson's waist, and this is further advanced into the intersphincteric space. The intersphincteric plane, which is composed of longitudinal fibromuscular tissues, can be comfortably entered via an RA fine dissection between the pubococcygeus/puborectalis and IAS. Through the transabdominal approach, the RA procedure conveniently enables intersphincteric dissection up to the level of the subcutaneous EAS, except for cases with severe anatomical restriction. The EAS needs to be fundamentally preserved, although partial excision of the deep EAS muscles can be combined in the case of tumor invasion. Finally, coloanal anastomosis is accomplished by either the double-stapled or hand-sewn method. Transanal intersphincteric dissection is included in some cases of subtotal and total ISR. The current procedure for RA ISR is shown in the supplementary material (Supplementary Video 15.1).

15.3 Operation-Associated Outcomes

Operative outcomes allowing comparison of TME by the three approaches are shown in Table 15.1 [11–13]. In the three studies described, few operative mortalities (i.e., within 1 month of surgery) occurred in the LA and RA groups after

TME, except for one case using the open approach. The three studies exhibited a very low rate of conversion to the open approach and were probably reporting from large-volume centers with abundant experience. Unfortunately, the relatively well-designed ROLARR trial (https://clinicaltrials.gov/ct2/show/NCT01736072) did not suggest any remarkable differences between RA and LA rectal cancer surgery in its early report, except for possible benefits in the particular subgroups of male gender, high body mass index, and LAR; it did, however, note the heterogeneity in the technical skills of the participating surgeons (minimal requirement of ten LA and ten RA cases). One meta-analysis that included seven publications presented a significantly lower conversion rate for RA TME than for LA TME, with an absolute risk reduction of 7% ($p < 0.001$) [17]. Another study using 2868 propensity-matched patients from the USA National Cancer Database reported a significantly lower conversion rate for RA LAR than for LA LAR, with rates of 9.5% vs. 16.4%, respectively ($p < 0.001$) [18]. Total operative time is consistently longer in RA than in LA TME. This is primarily due to the elapsed time for docking and port placement, mostly included in the measurement, which may be reduced with accumulated experience. Additionally, the general use of robotic stapling may conveniently reduce the extra time required for RA SSO during anastomosis. The RA could address an impact on learning curve for rectal cancer operation, requiring lesser

Table 15.1 Operative and postoperative outcomes among open vs. laparoscopy-assisted vs. robot-assisted approaches for sphincter-saving operations

Parameters	Park et al. [11]				Kang et al. [12]				Kim et al. [13]			
	Open	LA	RA	p-value	Open	LA	RA	p-value	Open	LA	RA	p-value
No. of patients, M/F	27/31	70/53	28/24	0.367	110/55	97/68	104/61	0.333	700/395	302/184	333/200	0.74
Site, U/M/L, %	58/42[a]	56/44[a]	40/60[a]	0.077	59/41[b]	67/33[b]	66/35[b]	0.295	10/51/39	26/56/18	9/43/49	**<0.001**
Preop CRT, %	10.2	8.1	23.1	**0.017**	32.7	21.8	23.6	0.054	50.5	12.6	32.3	**<0.001**
pStage, 0–I/II/III	31/36/33	28/42/30	29/29/42	0.46	42/25/33	38/29/33	36/31/33	0.148	39/30/31	48/21/31	44/24/32	**<0.001**
Op time, min	239 ± 59	158 ± 49	233 ± 52	**<0.001**	253 ± 88	278 ± 82	310 ± 115	**<0.001**	126 ± 43	127 ± 39	189 ± 52	**<0.001**
Diversion, %	4.5	4.1	1.9	0.72	31.8	27.2	25	0.403	40.3	13.7	39.8	**<0.001**
Conversion, %	n. a.	0	0	1	n. a.	1.8	0.6	0.623	n. a.	5.1	0.2	**<0.001**
LN harvest	18 ± 10	15 ± 10	19 ± 10	0.06	17 ± 10	15 ± 9	15 ± 9	0.075	21 ± 9	20 ± 8	23 ± 10	**<0.001**
DRM, mm	23 ± 15	32 ± 21	28 ± 19	**0.002**	22 ± 17	20 ± 17	19 ± 14	0.1/8	24 ± 16	24 ± 18	27 ± 16	**0.019**
CRM+, %	5.7	5.8	4.5	0.89	10.3	6.7	4.2	0.097[c]	1.2	1.2	0.9	0.878
Leakage, %	9.1	5.6	9.6		3.4	10.8	7.3	**0.042**	3.1	4.3	2.1	0.117[d]
Flatus passage, d	4.4 ± 3	3 ± 1.1	3.2 ± 1.8	**<0.001**	3 ± 1.4	2.4 ± 1.2	2.2 ± 1.1	**<0.001**	2.5 ± 1	1.9 ± 0.9	1.8 ± 0.9	**<0.001**
Urinary debility, %	2.2	1.6	0		8.5	4.2	4.2	**0.034**[e]	7	6	5.4	0.429
Postop mortality	1.1	0	0	0.373	0	0	0	1	0	0	0	1

LA laparoscopy-assisted, *RA* robot-assisted, *M/F* male/female, *U/M/L* upper/middle/lower, *preop* preoperative, *op* operation, *pStage* pathologic stage in accordance with AJCC 7th ed. *DRM* distal resection margin, *CRM* circumferential resection margin, *postop* postoperative, *n. a.* not applicable or available

Bold font, $p < 0.05$

[a]Intraperitoneal/extraperitoneal

[b]>6 cm/≤6 cm

[c]Open vs. RA, $p = 0.034$

[d]Open vs. RA, $p = 0.002$

[e]Open vs. RA, $p = 0.015$

number of cases in a study using the cumulative sum method using seven studies [19]. The physical burden on surgeons may be reduced in the RA approach, because of reductions to the three common ergonomic errors in the posture of surgeons, namely, a forward head position, improper shoulder elevation, and pelvic girdle asymmetry [20].

Operative outcomes comparing TME by the three approaches are shown in Table 15.1 [11–13]. The number of lymph nodes harvested only presented a significant difference in one study (Table 15.1). Lymph node yield is significantly less in patients with preoperative chemoradiotherapy (CRT) than in those who have not undergone it [21]. Otherwise, a TME including pelvic lymph node dissection or the extent of bowel resection in the respective approach might be implicated in the lymph node retrieval. Most RA SSO investigations achieved at least 1 cm of distal resection margin. In a study including 107 LRC patients, Mezhir et al. found viable tumors via intramural spread in three patients (2.7%) whose tumor nest was limited to less than 1 cm from the gross tumor edge [22]. Moreover, one meta-analysis reported that clinical evidence does not support the 1-cm rule in patients with LRC undergoing pre- or postoperative radiotherapy [23]. A CRM of at least 1 mm is generally accepted [24]. The CRM+ rate has been recorded as 2.3–9.6% in RA SSO, and only a few patients presented with marginal benefits compared with open SSO. Although CRM+ is probably implicated in tumor characteristics, including pT4 and lymphovascular or perineural invasion, it is not necessarily a reflection of the operative quality: perfect TME must be observed as a minimum requirement to prevent CRM+.

Two meta-analyses did not find any remarkable differences in general complication rates between open and LA and RA CRC operations [17, 25]. However, a previous study by the author found that early general complications (≤ 1 month postsurgery) occurred more frequently in open TME than in LA and RA TME (19.3% vs. 13.0% vs. 12.2%; $p < 0.001$), with the rate of ileus and wound infection being particularly marked in the open group [13]. Some SSOs are inevitably accompanied by AL, with an average rate of 9.5% of patients (range, 2.5–45.6%) showing AL, although no significant differences have been demonstrated between the three approaches [12, 14, 26]. AL is known to increase the LR rate and, according to a recent meta-analysis, a concurrently poor disease-free survival (DFS) [26]. The diverse risk factors for AL have been suggested to include male gender, old age, preoperative CRT, the absence of protective stoma, and a lower tumor location or anastomosis level, although the quality of the evidence for these was mostly moderate to low [27, 28]. As concurrent diversion has been accepted to reduce AL (at least significant AL), temporary ileal diversion is recommended in cases with preoperative CRT, a complicated operation including coloanal anastomosis, or inadequate perfusion. With the exception of some technical failures, poor local tissue oxygenation due to inadequate vascular perfusion has been implicated in all of the causes of AL [29]. To examine the perfusion status at the anastomotic site, Jafari et al. used laser fluorescence angiography (LFA); they made changes to the initial surgical plans in 11% of cases, with no occurrences of AL [30]. LFA using IFI appears to be helpful to reduce AL during RA SSO. One study using RA IFI reported a change in the proximal transection site in 16 of 40 patients with SSO, resulting in an AL rate of 5% [31]. The author experienced the AL rate to be 89% lower in the IFI+ group than in the IFI− group, at 0.6% vs. 5.2% ($p < 0.001$) [28].

15.4 Postoperative Functional Outcomes

Bowel movement generally recovers earlier in minimally invasive TME than in the open approach, although its practical value may not be assessable [11–13]. In a multivariate analysis, the author found that RA was one of the significant parameters determining SSO (odds ratio, 2.458; $p < 0.001$; Table 15.2) [13]. Most bowel function will have settled down 6–12 months after SSO, but some patients suffer from a disorder of defecation termed anterior resection syndrome [32]. Long-term functional impairment of the bowel

Table 15.2 Parameters associated with achievement of a sphincter-saving operation [13]

Parameters[a]	SSO achievement	*p*-value[b]	OR	95% CI	*p*-value[c]
Tumor location, U + M vs. L	1337/1440 vs. 620/773 (99.8 vs. 80.2)	**<0.001**	74.594	21.852–254.64	**<0.001**
Preoperative CRT, no vs. yes	1316/1328 vs. 642/786 (99.1 vs. 81.7)	**<0.001**	0.139	0.067–0.292	**<0.001**
Procedure, Open + LA vs. RA	1451/1581 vs. 507/553 (91.8 vs. 95.1)	**0.01**	2.458	1.497–4.036	**<0.001**
pT, 1–3 vs. 4	1897/2042 vs. 61/72 (92.9 vs. 84.7)	**0.018**	0.108	0.032–0.366	**<0.001**
Tumor growth, E/I	1315/1353 vs. 623/737 (97.2 vs. 84.5)	**<0.001**	1.017	0.622–1.662	0.946
LVI, no vs. yes	1501/1633 vs. 420/442 (91.9 vs. 95)	**0.030**	0.544	0.3–0.988	**0.046**
Transfusion >400 ml, no vs. yes	1890/2028 vs. 68/86 (93.2 vs. 79.1)	**<0.001**	0.46	0.216–0.978	**0.044**

SSO sphincter-saving operation, *OR* odds ratio, *CI* confidence interval, *U/M/L* upper/middle/lower, *CRT* chemoradiotherapy, *LA* laparoscopy-assisted, *RA* robot-assisted, *pT* pathologic T category, *E/I* expanding/infiltrative, *LVI* lymphovascular invasion
Bold font, $p < 0.05$
[a]Values in parentheses are percentages
[b]All parameters were compared using Fisher's exact test with two-sided verification
[c]Potential variables were verified by multivariate analysis using binary logistic regression

occurs mostly from pelvic sepsis, AL, or anastomotic stricture. Additionally, risk factors for a permanent stoma include LR, pelvic sepsis including AL and anastomotic stricture, male gender, and perioperative CRT, with their incidence ranging from 3% to 9.5% [33, 34]. It is hoped that RA SSO will reduce permanent stoma by decreasing these risk factors.

Genitourinary dysfunction appears to occur more frequently in open TME than in RA TME [13, 35, 36]. Although one meta-analysis did not find any detrimental effects of CRT on genitourinary dysfunction [37], it may be associated with preoperative CRT. Kim et al. reported an earlier recovery (3 months postsurgery) of erectile function in patients treated with RA TME than in those treated with LA TME [36]. Otherwise, Luca et al. reported that in their 74 patients who underwent RA TME, both urinary and sexual competence increased progressively until 1 year postsurgery [38]. Taken together, RA TME enables a reduction in the damage to the pelvic autonomic nerves, particularly to susceptible cavernosal fibers at the level of the prostate, with the benefits probably resulting from the fine dissection with magnified view, efficient traction, and wristed instruments.

15.5 Recurrences and Survival Outcomes

Heald, a founder of the concept "holy plane and TME," reported that in 405 rectal cancer patients who underwent open curative resections over the period 1978–1997, the 5-year LR and DFS rates were 3% and 4%, and the 10-year rates were 80% and 78%, respectively [39]. LA TME has been tried since the 1990s, with several randomized trials having demonstrated good outcomes [40, 41]. For example, the CLASICC trial showed 5-year LR, overall survival (OS), and DFS rates of open TMEs vs. LA TMEs as 7.6% vs. 9.4%, 56.7% vs. 62.8%, and 52.1% vs. 53.2%, respectively, without demonstrating any statistically significant differences between the two groups. It also mentioned a previously reported difference in CRM+ rates (open vs. LA, 12% vs. 6%), which did not translate into the 5-year LR rate [40]. The COREAN trial reported that LA TME for locally advanced rectal cancer after preoperative CRT provided non-inferior survival outcomes to open TME, suggesting LA TME to be justified when performed by well-qualified colorectal surgeons [41]. To the contrary, the two randomized trials ACOSOG Z6051 and ALaCaRT report that LA TME failed to meet the criterion for non-inferiority for pathologic outcomes when compared with TME, but these studies need a longer follow-up for recurrence and survival outcomes [42, 43].

A few investigations have compared the recurrence and survival outcomes of LA and RA TME (Table 15.3). According to a recent case series study using propensity score matching, the 5-year OS, cancer-specific survival (CSS), and DFS rates for RA TME vs. LA TME were 90.5% vs. 78.0%, 90.5% vs. 79.5%, and 72.6% vs. 68.0%, respectively, with the differences between the two procedures not being statistically significant [44], although RA TME was a significant prognostic factor for OS and CSS (hazard ratio = 0.033, $p = 0.004$; hazard ratio = 0.367, $p = 0.0161$, respectively) in a multivariate analysis. Another

study involving 288 rectal cancer patients with TME also found no differences in OS, DFS, and LR rates between RA TME and LA TME [45]. A previous study by the author also found no significant differences in the group comparisons of open TME vs. LA TME vs. RA TME for 3-year LR rates, 7% vs. 3.4% vs. 2.5%; 3-year OS rates, 91.9% vs. 94.4% vs. 94.6%; or 3-year DFS rates, 82.2% vs. 83.1% vs. 82.2% [13].

15.6 Intersphincteric Resection

ISR categorized as ultralow LAR (uLAR) is considered the most extreme type of SSO. It involves partial or complete resection of the IAS to achieve an acceptable distal margin for tumors located at

Table 15.3 Recurrence and survival outcomes among open vs. laparoscopy-assisted vs. robot approaches in total mesorectal excision and intersphincteric resection

Operations	Investigator (y)	Study type	Groups	5-year (3-year) LR, %	5-year (3-year) SR, %	5-year (3-year) OS, %	5-year (3-year) DFS, %
		Mean FU ± SD, m	No. of patients	p-value	p-value	p-value	p-value
TME[a]	Kim et al. (2017) [44]	Case series (PSM)[b]	LA vs. RA	n. a.	n. a.	78 vs. 90.5	68 vs. 72.6
		40.3 (18–58)	192 vs. 196			0.323	0.641
TME[a]	Park et al. (2015) [45]	Case series[b]	LA vs. RA	1.2 vs. 3.3	16.7 vs. 12	93.5 vs. 92.8	78.7 vs. 81.9
		54 ± 17	84 vs. 33	0.649	0.42	0.829	0.547
TME[a]	Kim et al. (2016) [13]	Case series[b]	Open vs. LA vs. RA	(2.7 vs. 3.4 vs. 2.5)	(16.7 vs. 13.6 vs. 17.8)	(91.9 vs. 94.4 vs. 94.6)	(82.1 vs. 83.1 vs. 82.2)
		42 ± 10	101	0.85	0.5	0.352	0.944
ISR	Park et al. (2015) [47]	Case series (PSM)	LA vs. RA	(5.7 vs. 6.7)	n. a.	(94.8 vs. 93.8)	(90.5 vs. 89.6)
		52 vs. 56	106 vs. 106	8.2 vs. 8.7		88.4 vs. 88.5	82.8 vs. 80.6
				0.935		0.899	0.298
ISR	Yoo et al. (2015) [48]	Case series	LA vs. RA	n. a.	n. a.	88.5 vs. 95.2	75 vs. 76.7
		34 vs. 37	26 vs. 44			0.174	0.946

LR local recurrence, *SR* systemic recurrence, *OS* overall survival, *DFS* disease-free survival, *FU* follow-up, *SD* standard deviation, *TME* total mesorectal excision, *ISR* intersphincteric resection, *PSM* propensity score matching, *LA* laparoscopy-assisted, *RA* robot-assisted, *n. a.* not available
Bold font, $p < 0.05$
[a]Including abdominoperineal operation cases of 20.8% (Kim et al. 2017), 3.9% vs. 7.4% (Park et al. 2015), and 11% vs. 2.1% vs. 4.9% (Kim et al. 2016)
[b]Median values (interquartile range)

the intersphincteric groove. Although the depth of invasion for ISR is preferably confined to ≤T2, some T3 and T4a lesions could also be amenable to ISR, depending on the tumor location and size, and in combination with partial excision of the EAS or preoperative CRT. Generally, the operative procedure consists of two approaches, i.e., transabdominal and trans-anal procedures. The transabdominal procedure ends with dissection at the mesorectal fascia down to the pelvic floor and is followed by the trans-anal procedure, which includes ISR and a hand-sewn anastomosis. The pioneer study recorded an LR rate of 5.3% in 113 LRC patients, including 31% with Dukes stage C [46]. One meta-analysis examining 14 ISR studies involving 1289 patients presented the operative mortality rate as 0.8% and the cumulative morbidity rate as 25.8% [8]. This meta-analysis demonstrated satisfactory oncological and functional outcomes, comparable with those of LAR, presenting the LR rate as 6.7%, the 5-year OS rate as 86.3% (62–97%), the 5-year DFS rate as 78.6% (70–87%), and the mean bowel movement as 2.7 times/day.

With the advent of minimally invasive rectal cancer surgery, LA and RA ISRs appear to be promising techniques with clear visualization into the deep pelvic cavity. Laparoscopic dissection of the anal canal via a transabdominal approach has been technically challenging for even experienced surgeons, particularly in the setting of a narrow male pelvis, visceral obesity, and previous irradiation. Additionally, the dissection into the intersphincteric space below the end of the mesorectal plane cannot be safely performed via a transabdominal route in open or LA methods, even with the use of magnified vision. Therefore, the completion of an open or LA ISR is inevitably accompanied by a trans-anal approach. These dual approaches may result in an uneven contour of the resected specimen and may be prone to destroying the CRM and EAS. Contrary to the open or LA ISRs, the author has experienced a totally transabdominal ISR with double-stapled anastomosis to be feasible in more than 90% of RA ISR groups, even if the mean level of the anastomosis was 1.9 cm from the anal verge in cases of RA ISR [35]. In the study, the mean fecal incontinence score (FIS) was within the satisfactory anorectal function range (≤10) at 12 months postoperation in both the open and RA ISR groups but was significantly higher in the open group up to 12 months postsurgery. Additionally, sexual dysfunction in male patients under 65 years occurred 2.7 times more frequently in the open group than in the RA group (34.1 vs. 12.5%; p = 0.023). However, two recent comparative studies demonstrated no significant differences between the two groups in terms of perioperative and oncological outcomes (Tables 15.3 and 15.4) [47, 48].

Conclusion

Through a little more than 10 years of experience, RA TME and SSO have become recognized as being safe and feasible in comparison with open and LA approaches. The robot approach possesses many advantages over the latter two approaches, including its magnified view, dexterity supported by wristed instruments and stable traction, and ergonomic excellence. In LRC, the RA approach appears to be an important parameter for achieving an SSO, thereby maximizing sphincter preservation. Current progress in robot systems allows the provision of embedded real-time perfusion imaging and stapling systems. Although the mechanical merits of robot systems have not presently been translated into satisfactory progress in respect to oncological outcome in rectal cancer surgery, RA TME could enable deeper dissection and lower anastomosis in the pelvic region than is possible with an LA or open approach, with slightly better functional recovery. Well-designed randomized trials are still required to confirm or refute the efficiency and oncological superiority of RA TME and SSO.

Table 15.4 Operative and postoperative outcomes in open or laparoscopy-assisted vs. robot-assisted approaches for intersphincteric resection

Parameters	Kim et al. [13]			Park et al. [47]			Yoo et al. [48]		
	Open	RA	p-value	LA	RA	p-value	LA	RA	p-value
No. of patients, M/F	78/36	64/44	0.165	71/35	75/31	0.148	17/9	35/9	0.533
Tumor distance, cm	4 ± 0.9	3.8 ± 1.2	0.262	3.3 ± 1.1	3.2 ± 1	0.444	3.7 ± 0.9	3.2 ± 0.8	**0.031**
Preop CRT, %	83.3	45.4	**<0.001**	56.2	64.2	0.261	26.9	54.5	**0.025**
pStage, 0–I/II/III	59/18/24	45/21/33	0.144	70/30[a]	69/31[a]	0.882	30/31/31/8[b]	43/25/21/11[b]	0.673
Op time, min	124 ± 29	191 ± 39	**<0.001**	233 ± 79	272 ± 84	**0.001**	287 ± 51	316 ± 65	**0.038**
Diversion, %	48.2	46.3	0.789	68.9	71.1	0.652	n. a.	n. a.	
Conversion, %	n. a.	0		1.9	0.9	0.511	n. a.	n. a.	
LN harvest	16 ± 7	18 ± 7	0.062	15 ± 10	13 ± 7	0.126	21 ± 15	13 ± 9	**0.043**
DRM, mm (DRM+, %)	(0)	(0)	(1)	1.2 ± 0.7	1.2 ± 0.8	0.739	1.7 ± 3	1.3 ± 1	0.291
CRM+, %	0	0.9	0.486	9	8	0.976	19.2	9.1	0.277
Leakage, %	8.8[c]	9.3[c]	1	5.7	3.8	0.517	0	11.4	0.15
Flatus passage, d	2.7 ± 1.1	1.8 ± 0.9	**<0.001**	5.2 ± 4[d]	4.6 ± 2.9[d]	0.251	2.5 ± 1.5[d]	2.6 ± 1.6[d]	0.312
Urinary debility, %	5.3	9.3	0.49	9.4	40.7	0.06	3.8	9.1	**0.044**
FIS at 12 m postop, %	10.3	7.7	**0.004**	17[e]	19[e]	n. s.	14	14	0.835
Postop mortality	0	0	1	0	0	0	0	0	1

LA laparoscopy-assisted, *RA* robot-assisted, *M/F* male/female, *preop* preoperative, *op* operation, *pStage* pathologic stage in accordance with AJCC 7th ed. *DRM* distal resection margin, *CRM* circumferential resection margin. *FIS* fecal incontinence score (measured using Wexner's scoring method). *n. a.* not applicable or available. *n. s.* not significant

Bold font, $p < 0.05$

[a] pStage I–II/III

[b] pStage 0–I/II/III/IV

[c] Including delayed leakage

[d] Time to toleration of diet, days

[e] Bowel movement/day during 24 months postsurgery

References

1. Cancer Genome Atlas Network. Comprehensive molecular characterization of human colon and rectal cancer. Nature. 2012;487:330–7.
2. Heald RJ, Husband EM, Ryall RD. The mesorectum in rectal cancer surgery–the clue to pelvic recurrence? Br J Surg. 1982;69:613–6.
3. Campa-Thompson M, Weir R, Calcetera N, Quirke P, Carmack S. Pathologic processing of the total mesorectal excision. Clin Colon Rectal Surg. 2015;28:43–52.
4. Abulafi AM, Williams NS. Local recurrence of colorectal cancer: the problem, mechanisms, management and adjuvant therapy. Br J Surg. 1994;81:7–19.
5. Martling AL, Holm T, Rutqvist LE, et al. Effect of a surgical training programme on outcome of rectal cancer in the county of Stockholm: Stockholm colorectal cancer study group. Basingstoke bowel cancer research project. Lancet. 2000;356:93–6.
6. Bossema E, Stiggelbout A, Baas-Thijssen M, et al. Patients' preferences for low rectal cancer surgery. Eur J Surg Oncol. 2008;34:42–8.
7. Fritsch H, Brenner E, Lienemann A, Ludwikowski B. Anal sphincter complex: reinterpreted morphology and its clinical relevance. Dis Colon Rectum. 2002;45:188–94.
8. Martin ST, Heneghan HM, Winter DC. Systematic review of outcomes after intersphincteric resection for low rectal cancer. Br J Surg. 2012;99:603–12.
9. Saito N, Ito M, Kobayashi A, Nishizawa Y, et al. Long-term outcomes after intersphincteric resection for low-lying rectal cancer. Ann Surg Oncol. 2014;21:3608–15.
10. Ohtani H, Tamamori Y, Azuma T, et al. A meta-analysis of the short- and long-term results of randomized controlled trials that compared laparoscopy-assisted and conventional open surgery for rectal cancer. J Gastrointest Surg. 2011;15:1375–85.
11. Park JS, Choi GS, Lim KH, Jang YS, Jun SH. S052: a comparison of robot-assisted, laparoscopic, and open surgery in the treatment of rectal cancer. Surg Endosc. 2011;25:240–8.
12. Kang J, Yoon KJ, Min BS, Hur H, et al. The impact of robotic surgery for mid and low rectal cancer: a case-matched analysis of a 3-arm comparison— open, laparoscopic, and robotic surgery. Ann Surg. 2013;257:95–101.
13. Kim JC, Yu CS, Lim SB, Park IJ, Kim CW, Yoon YS. Comparative analysis focusing on surgical and early oncological outcomes of open, laparoscopy-assisted, and robot-assisted approaches in rectal cancer patients. Int J Color Dis. 2016;31:1179–87.
14. Nagtegaal ID, van de Velde CJ, van der Worp E, Kapiteijn E, Quirke P, van Krieken JH, Cooperative Clinical Investigators of the Dutch Colorectal Cancer Group. Macroscopic evaluation of rectal cancer resection specimen: clinical significance of the pathologist in quality control. J Clin Oncol. 2002;20:1729–34.
15. Colquhoun P, Wexner SD, Cohen A. Adjuvant therapy is valuable in the treatment of rectal cancer despite total mesorectal excision. J Surg Oncol. 2003;83:133–9.
16. Williams NS. The rectal 'no man's land' and sphincter preservation during rectal excision. Br J Surg. 2010;97:1749–51.
17. Memon S, Heriot AG, Murphy DG, Bressel M, Lynch AC. Robotic versus laparoscopic proctectomy for rectal cancer: a meta-analysis. Ann Surg Oncol. 2012;19:2095–101.
18. Speicher PJ, Englum BR, Ganapathi AM, Nussbaum DP, Mantyh CR, Migaly J. Robotic low anterior resection for rectal cancer: a national perspective on short-term oncologic outcomes. Ann Surg. 2015;262:1040–5.
19. Jiménez-Rodríguez RM, Rubio-Dorado-Manzanares M, Díaz-Pavón JM, et al. Learning curve in robotic rectal cancer surgery: current state of affairs. Int J Color Dis. 2016;31:1807–15.
20. Rosenblatt PL, McKinney J, Adams SR. Ergonomics in the operating room: protecting the surgeon. J Minim Invasive Gynecol. 2013;20:744.
21. Lykke J, Roikjaer O, Jess P, Danish Colorectal Cancer Group. Tumour stage and preoperative chemoradiotherapy influence the lymph node yield in stages I-III rectal cancer: results from a prospective nationwide cohort study. Color Dis. 2014;16:O144–9.
22. Mezhir JJ, Shia J, Riedel E, Temple LK, et al. Whole-mount pathologic analysis of rectal cancer following neoadjuvant therapy: implications of margin status on long-term oncologic outcome. Ann Surg. 2012;256:274–9.
23. Pahlman L, Bujko K, Rutkowski A, Michalski W. Altering the therapeutic paradigm towards a distal bowel margin of <1 cm in patients with low-lying rectal cancer: a systematic review and commentary. Color Dis. 2013;15:e166–74.
24. Lin HH, Lin JK, Lin CC, et al. Circumferential margin plays an independent impact on the outcome of rectal cancer patients receiving curative total mesorectal excision. Am J Surg. 2013;206:771–7.
25. Biffi R, Luca F, Bianchi PP, et al. Dealing with robot-assisted surgery for rectal cancer: Current status and perspectives. World J Gastroenterol. 2016;22:546–56.
26. Mirnezami A, Mirnezami R, Chandrakumaran K, Sasapu K, Sagar P, Finan P. Increased local recurrence and reduced survival from colorectal cancer following anastomotic leak: systematic review and meta-analysis. Ann Surg. 2011;253:890–9.
27. Pommergaard HC, Gessler B, Burcharth J, Angenete E, Haglind E, Rosenberg J. Preoperative risk factors for anastomotic leakage after resection for colorectal cancer: a systematic review and meta-analysis. Color Dis. 2014;16:662–71.

28. Kim JC, Lee JH, Park SH. Interpretative guidelines and possible indications for indocyanine green fluorescence imaging in robot-assisted sphincter-saving operations. Dis Colon Rectum. 2017;60:376–84.

29. Vignali A, Gianotti L, Braga M, Radaelli G, Malvezzi L, Di Carlo V. Altered microperfusion at the rectal stump is predictive for rectal anastomotic leak. Dis Colon Rectum. 2000;43:76–82.

30. Jafari MD, Wexner SD, Martz JE, et al. Perfusion assessment in laparoscopic left-sided/anterior resection (PILLAR II): a multi-institutional study. J Am Coll Surg. 2015;220:82–92.

31. Hellan M, Spinoglio G, Pigazzi A, Lagares-Garcia JA. The influence of fluorescence imaging on the location of bowel transection during robotic left-sided colorectal surgery. Surg Endosc. 2014;28:1695–702.

32. Brown SR, Seow Choen F. Preservation of rectal function after low anterior resection with formation of a neorectum. Semin Surg Oncol. 2000;19:376–85.

33. Seo SI, Yu CS, Kim GS, et al. Characteristics and risk factors associated with permanent stomas after sphincter-saving resection for rectal cancer. World J Surg. 2013;37:2490–6.

34. Kim MJ, Kim YS, Park SC, et al. Risk factors for permanent stoma after rectal cancer surgery with temporary ileostomy. Surgery. 2016;159:721–7.

35. Kim JC, Lim SB, Yoon YS, Park IJ, Kim CW, Kim CN. Completely abdominal intersphincteric resection for lower rectal cancer: feasibility and comparison of robot-assisted and open surgery. Surg Endosc. 2014;28:2734–44.

36. Kim JY, Kim NK, Lee KY, Hur H, Min BS, Kim JH. A comparative study of voiding and sexual function after total mesorectal excision with autonomic nerve preservation for rectal cancer: laparoscopic versus robotic surgery. Ann Surg Oncol. 2012;19:2485–93.

37. Loos M, Quentmeier P, Schuster T, et al. Effect of preoperative radio(chemo)therapy on long-term functional outcome in rectal cancer patients: a systematic review and meta-analysis. Ann Surg Oncol. 2013;20:1816–28.

38. Luca F, Valvo M, Ghezzi TL, et al. Impact of robotic surgery on sexual and urinary functions after fully robotic nerve-sparing total mesorectal excision for rectal cancer. Ann Surg. 2013;257:672–8.

39. Heald RJ, Moran BJ, Ryall RD, Sexton R, MacFarlane JK. Rectal cancer: the Basingstoke experience of total mesorectal excision, 1978-1997. Arch Surg. 1998;133:894–9.

40. Jayne DG, Thorpe HC, Copeland J, Quirke P, Brown JM, Guillou PJ. Five-year follow-up of the medical research council CLASICC trial of laparoscopically assisted versus open surgery for colorectal cancer. Br J Surg. 2010;97:1638–45.

41. Kang SB, Park JW, Jeong SY, et al. Open versus laparoscopic surgery for mid or low rectal cancer after neoadjuvant chemoradiotherapy (COREAN trial): short-term outcomes of an open-label randomised controlled trial. Lancet Oncol. 2010;11:637–45.

42. Fleshman J, Branda M, Sargent DJ, et al. Effect of laparoscopic-assisted resection vs open resection of stage II or III rectal cancer on pathologic outcomes: the ACOSOG Z6051 randomized clinical trial. JAMA. 2015;314:1346–55.

43. Stevenson AR, Solomon MJ, Lumley JW, et al. Effect of laparoscopic-assisted resection vs open resection on pathological outcomes in rectal cancer: the ALaCaRT randomized clinical trial. JAMA. 2015;314:1356–63.

44. Kim J, Paek SJ, Kang DW, et al. Robotic resection is a good prognostic factor in rectal cancer compared with laparoscopic resection: long-term survival analysis using propensity score matching. Dis Colon Rectum. 2017;60:266–73.

45. Park EJ, Cho MS, Baek SJ, et al. Long-term oncologic outcomes of robotic low anterior resection for rectal cancer: a comparative study with laparoscopic surgery. Ann Surg. 2015;261:129–37.

46. Schiessel R, Novi G, Holzer B, et al. Technique and long-term results of intersphincteric resection for low rectal cancer. Dis Colon Rectum. 2005;48:1858–65.

47. Park JS, Kim NK, Kim SH, et al. Multicentre study of robotic intersphincteric resection for low rectal cancer. Br J Surg. 2015;102:1567–73.

48. Yoo BE, Cho JS, Shin JW, et al. Robotic versus laparoscopic intersphincteric resection for low rectal cancer: comparison of the operative, oncological, and functional outcomes. Ann Surg Oncol. 2015;22:1219–25.

Extralevator APR (ELAPE)

16

Jin-Tung Liang

Abstract

Extralevator APR has become a popular procedure for patients with distal rectal cancer requiring an APR procedure. In contrast to conventional APR, extralevator APR is characterized by that the dissection of levators is performed close to their attachment on the lateral pelvic sidewall, thus making the resected anorectal specimen cylindrical rather than with a waist in shape. Technically, extralevator APR would seem to be probably more effective in reducing the positivity of circumferential resection margin and intraoperative rectal perforation but is associated with the disadvantage of more extensive tissue removal from around the anorectum, which leaves a large cavity to close. To date, systematic reviews and meta-analyses comparing extralevator APR with conventional APR were inconclusive. In this chapter, we present the knack and pitfall in performing the extralevator APR. In our view, although the evidences for the oncologic superiority of extralevator APR are still weak, it does benefit for some carefully selected patients with locally invasive diseases.

Keyword

Extralevator APR

16.1 Introduction

With the improvement of surgical technique and the refinement of surgical instruments, sphincter preservation operation (SPO) instead of abdominoperineal resection (APR) has become the mainstay surgical modality for the treatment of distal rectal cancer. Currently, the percentage of APR for distal rectal cancer represented only less than 10% in "center of excellence" worldwide. It has been reported that the oncological outcome is poorer in patients with distal rectal cancer undergoing a traditional APR procedure, in comparison with those treated by a standard total mesorectal excision (TME) followed by a SPO procedure. It is generally considered that the poorer oncological efficacy of the traditional APR results from the inadequate circumferential resection margin (CRM) around anal sphincter muscles, the spillage of cancer cells due to overexposure around the junctional area between internal and external anal sphincter, or the perforation of the rectum during surgical manipulation [1–3].

Remarkably, Holm and colleagues [4–6] proposed a more extensive procedure, the extralevator abdominoperineal resection (ELAPE), with a view to improving local tumor control and reducing

J.-T. Liang
Department of Surgery, National Taiwan University
Hospital, Taipei City, Taiwan
e-mail: jintung@ntu.edu.tw

local recurrence [6–8]. ELAPE results in cylindrical specimen without a "waist," common after traditional APR, to minimize the risk of inadvertent tumor involvement of the circumferential resection margin (CRM) and to reduce the risk of intraoperative tumor perforation.

In our institution, we have abandoned the traditional open surgery for an APR; instead, the vast majority of patients with distal rectal cancer requiring an APR procedure were performed by the laparoscopic or robotic approach [1–3]. Because ELAPE was more complex in the process of cancer resection and perineal reconstruction, it is specifically performed only for locally advanced distal rectal cancer with or without a preoperative concurrent chemoradiation therapy (CCRT). Herein, we present the standardized surgical procedures of ELAPE in our institution.

16.2   Surgical Techniques

Basically, the laparoscopic and robotic approaches for an APR are the same in the surgical procedures but with a little difference in port configurations [1–3]. In laparoscopic APR, the camera port was set at the right periumbilicus; two working ports were set at the right upper and lower abdominal in consideration of the surgeons' personal ergonomics; and two assistant ports were set at the left side with the designing of the upcoming colostoma in the port site over the left lower abdomen to save the wound size. For a robotic APR, five abdominal ports were set:

A 12-mm camera port is placed 3 cm to the right and 3 cm above the umbilicus.

A 12-mm port is placed to the right lower quadrant (midclavicular line) through which is telescoped an 8-mm robotic port designated as R1 for the right robotic working arm (the 8-mm port can be removed to place an endostapler).

An 8-mm port is placed to the left upper quadrant just to the right of the midclavicular line midway between the umbilicus and left subcostal region designated as R3 for the left robotic working arm.

A 12-mm assistant port is placed to the right lateral mid-abdomen for retracting and suctioning by an assistant.

An 8-mm port is set to the left lower quadrant which is placed at the same height and positioned as the right lower quadrant port for counter-traction as R2 robotic arm.

The robotic cart was placed in left hip position. During the entire APR procedure, each robotic working arm and assistant instrument was inserted through its respective uniform abdomen port cited above, and the position of the robotic cart was remained unchanged.

The dissection sequence of abdominal phase of APR in robotic approach was similar to that of APR performed by traditional laparoscopic surgery [1–3] (Fig. 16.1), comprising the following:

1. Medial-to-lateral mesenteric dissection along the preaortic plane
2. Optional ligation and transection of inferior mesenteric vein
3. N3 lymph node dissection over the root of inferior mesenteric artery
4. Low ligation of vascular pedicle with preservation of the left colic artery and autonomic nerve plexus
5. Mobilization of the sigmoid colon and sometimes the mobilization up to the descending colon
6. Dissection of the presacral fascia downward to the anococcygeal rhaphae with preservation of paired hypogastric nerves and pelvic autonomic nerve plexus
7. Incision of the peritoneal reflection laterally and then anteriorly
8. Separation of the rectum and the vagina/prostate circumferentially to the level of levators with the appreciation of Denonvilliers' fascia

To ensure the en bloc resection of cancer in cylindrical style, i.e., the ELAPE (Fig. 16.2), the

Fig. 16.1 (**a**)
Traditional
abdominoperineal
resection (APR). APR is
indicated for tumor
located around dentated
line (D). (**b**) Surgical
specimen of traditional
APR, in which a "waist"
can be seen. Traditional
APR seems to be still
appropriate for this
patient, whose tumor did
not penetrate the muscle
layer

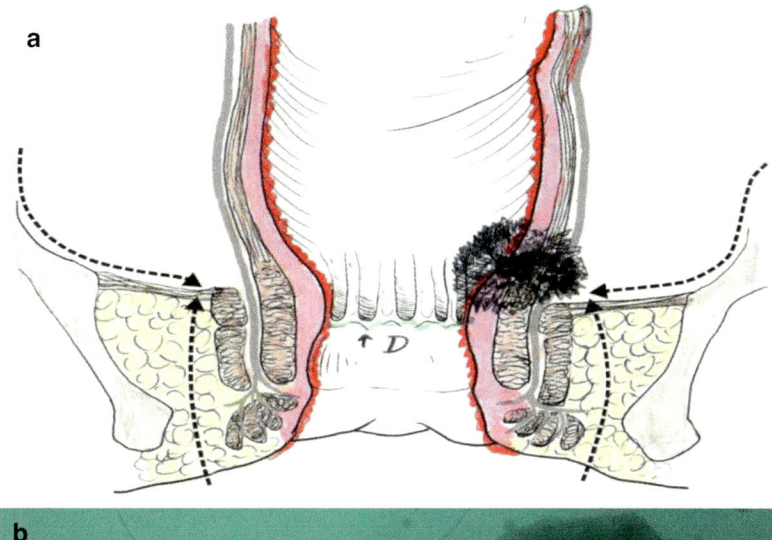

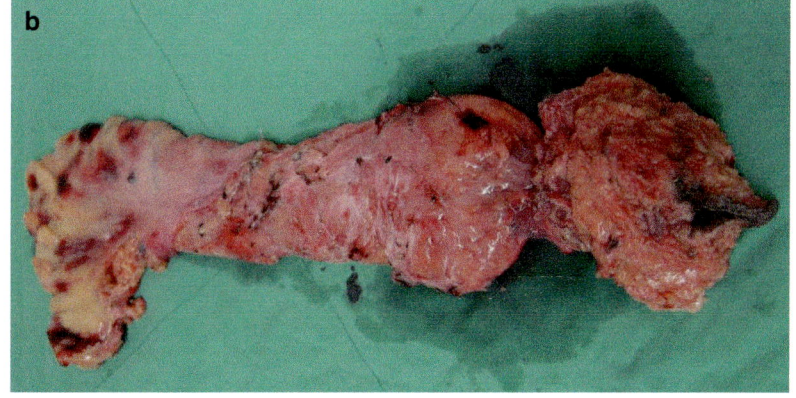

lateral dissection is from the transection of lateral ligament vertically downward until the levator muscle is visualized, and, posteriorly, the dissection is halted when the coccygeal tip is exposed (Fig. 16.3). We emphasize that the junctional area between the internal and external sphincter should not be intentionally exposed.

After the completion of the robotic total mesorectal excision (TME), the robotic cart is removed, and a colostoma was shaped over the left low abdominal quadrant. Then, we undertook the perineal dissection, and finally the rectal cancer was extirpated in cylindrical style.

In the perineal phase of dissection, we first make an elliptical incision around the anal verge in consideration of upcoming perineal wound closure without tension. Thereafter, undermining the subcutaneous fatty tissue was developed within the triangular area circumscribed by the coccygeal tip and bilateral ischial tuberosity. Subsequently, we attempted to make an en bloc resection of the fatty tissues over the ischiorectal fossa until the levator ani muscle was exposed. Finally, the pelvic floor over the coccygeal tip is opened, and the rectosigmoid colon was everted outside the pelvic cavity. After resection of the levator ani muscle attached to the anorectum with adequate margin, the perineal phase for the ELAPE is completed (Fig. 16.3).

Fig. 16.2 (**a**) Extralevator APR (ELAPE). (**b**) ELAPE is the cylindrical anorectal excision. ELAPE is mandatory for this distal rectal cancer with perineal fistula formation, which is opened in the right figure

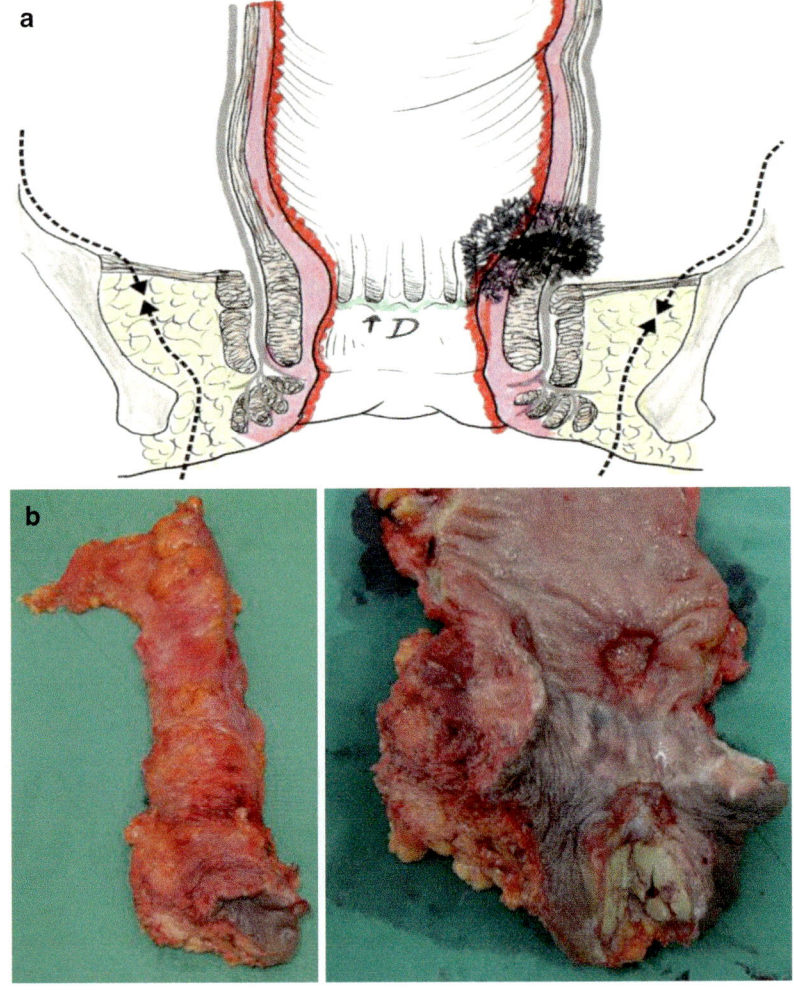

Fig. 16.3 (**a**) For a ELAPE, the lateral perirectal fatty tissues are incise vertically and halted when the levator ani muscle is exposed (arrow, L). (**b**) Posteriorly, the dissection is halted when the coccygeal bone (C) is exposed lest it should overexpose the internal and external anal sphincters, and the fatty tissues over the bilateral ischiorectal (I) fossa are removed. (**c**) A shrunken ulcer crater (blue arrow) of rectal cancer was at 0.5 cm above dentate line. (**d**) Laparoscopic view of the perineum after the completion of perineal phase of APR. The CRM was created outside the levators (blue arrow) to give wider clearance. The prostate (*p*) and indwelled pelvic rubber drain tube were also seen. (**e**) When anococcygeal ligament (*ano*) was reached, the dissection was stopped in time to obviate overexposure of the internal anal sphincter. The planned resection margin was shown as a white dotted line at the tip of coccygeal bone (*c*). (**f**) The wide dissection over levators (blue arrow) to ensure an adequate perineal resection margin. Anteriorly, the vaginal (*v*) and retroverted uterus (*ut*) were seen. (**g**) The posterior mesorectal fascia was kept intact, and the levator ani muscle was severed just at its insertion to the coccygeal bone (*c*) to ensure an adequate cylindrical resection margin. (**h**) An ulcerative tumor was within 0.5 cm above dentate line

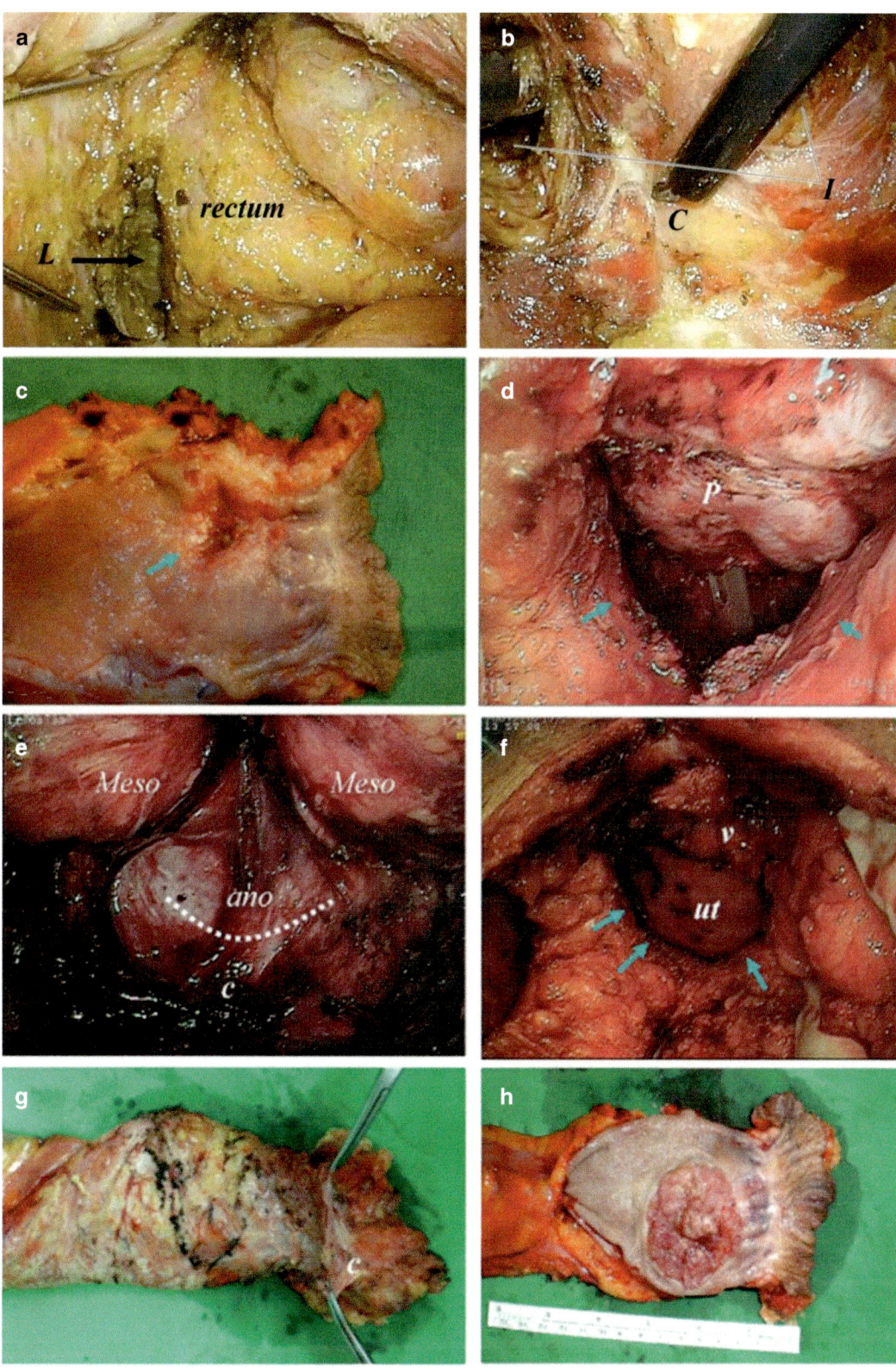

16.3　Comments on the ELAPE

Previous reports on ELAPE have been varying; West et al. [4, 5] described lower perforation rates and fewer cases with involved CRM using ELAPE in a comparison with historical controls with high rates of both perforations and involved margins. Stelzner et al. [9] suggested from a systematic review of 14 nonrandomized studies in the time frame of 1997–2011 on "extended APE" and 50 studies on traditional APE from 1991 to 2011 that "extended APE" had a reduced risk of intraoperative perforation. It was not possible to analyze the effects on local recurrence and survival rates in their review. Other reports of case series with historical controls have been unable to confirm these findings [10, 11]. More recently, Ortiz and colleagues [12] present propensity score-matched data on 914 patients from 2008 to 2013 with no advantage for ELAPE on intraoperative perforations, involved CRM, local recurrence, or mortality. Their study is a prospectively registered, large, multicenter study. The fact that not all Spanish centers took part may represent a possible selection bias. In addition, a recently presented study from Denmark [13] on all Danish patients operated with standard APE or ELAPE from 2009 to August 2012 shows no benefit for ELAPE regarding short-term oncological outcomes (involved CRM). One randomized controlled trial by Han et al. [14] reported reduced recurrence rates after ELAPE, suggesting that there is an oncological advantage with ELAPE in comparison with traditional APE in patients with T3 and T4 tumors. However, their study was small (n ¼ 67) and lacked details of external and internal validity. Because of these methodological weaknesses, their findings may be regarded as interesting but not conclusive. Zhou et al. [15] have published a meta-analysis recently and did not indicate a statistically significant superiority of ELAPE over conventional APE in terms of CRM positivity and intraoperative bowel perforation. Remarkably, Prytz et al. [16] made a registry-based, observational national cohort study in Sweden and showed that ELAPE results in a significantly increased 3-year local recurrence rate as compared with standard APE. Intraoperative perforation seems to be an important risk factor for local recurrence. In addition to significantly increased 3-year local recurrence rates, the significantly increased incidence of wound complications leads to the conclusion that ELAPE should only be considered in selected patients at risk of intraoperative perforation.

It has been generally accepted that ELAPE leaves a huge perineal defect which cannot be closed. However, although the patients undergoing ELAPE frequently complained of a bulging out over the perineum, especially when weight-bearing or doing Valsalva maneuver, incarcerated bowel herniation or painful sensation infrequently occurred, because the bowel was not redundant enough to descend to the perineum. However, some surgeons still cooperated with plastic surgeons to use rotational myocutaneous flaps or autologous aponeurosis graft from fascia tensor lata to reconstruct the pelvic floor.

16.4　In Conclusions

The oncological efficacy of ELAPE remains inconclusive. However, to achieve adequate CRM and R0 resection for the treatment of locally advanced distal rectal cancer, the ELAPE still plays some roles in the context of personalized precision surgery.

References

1. Liang JT, Lee PH. Multimedia article. Laparoscopic abdominoperineal resection for lower rectal cancers: how do we do it? Surg Endosc. 2006;20:695–6.
2. Liang JT, Lai HS. Robotic abdominoperineal resection for lower rectal cancers…how we do it? J Laparoendosc. 2013;20:213–20.
3. Liang JT, Cheng JC, Huang KC, Lai HS, Sun CT. Comparison of tumor recurrence between laparoscopic total mesorectal excision with sphincter preservation and laparoscopic abdominoperineal resection for low rectal cancer. Surg Endosc. 2013;27:3452–64.
4. West NP, Finan PJ, Anderin C, et al. Evidence of the oncologic superiority of cylindrical abdominoperineal excision for low rectal cancer. J Clin Oncol. 2008;26:3517–22.
5. West NP, Anderin C, Smith KJ, et al. Multicentre experience with extralevator abdominoperineal excision for low rectal cancer. Br J Surg. 2010;97:588–99.

6. Holm T, Ljung A, Haggmark T, et al. Extended abdominoperineal resection with gluteus maximus flap reconstruction of the pelvic floor for rectal cancer. Br J Surg. 2007;94:232–8.

7. Moore TJ, Moran BJ. Precision surgery, precision terminology: the origins and meaning of ELAPE. Color Dis. 2012;14:1173–4.

8. Shihab OC, Heald RJ, Holm T, et al. A pictorial description of extralevator abdominoperineal excision for low rectal cancer. Color Dis. 2012;14:e655–60.

9. Stelzner S, Koehler C, Stelzer J, et al. Extended abdominoperineal excision vs. standard abdominoperineal excision in rectal cancer—a systematic overview. Int J Color Dis. 2011;26:1227–40.

10. Krishna A, Rickard MJ, Keshava A, et al. A comparison of published rates of resection margin involvement and intra-operative perforation between standard and 'cylindrical' abdominoperineal excision for low rectal cancer. Color Dis. 2013;15:57–65.

11. Asplund D, Haglind E, Angenete E. Outcome of extralevator abdominoperineal excision compared with standard surgery. Results from a single centre. Color Dis. 2012;14:1191–6.

12. Ortiz H, Ciga MA, Armendariz P, et al. Multicentre propensity score-matched analysis of conventional versus extended abdominoperineal excision for low rectal cancer. Br J Surg. 2014;101: 874–82.

13. Klein M, Fischer A, Rosenberg J, et al. ExtraLevatory AbdominoPerineal excision (ELAPE) does not result in reduced rate of tumor perforation or rate of positive circumferential resection margin: a nationwide database study. Ann Surg. 2015;261:933–8.

14. Han JG, Wang ZJ, Wei GH, et al. Randomized clinical trial of conventional versus cylindrical abdominoperineal resection for locally advanced lower rectal cancer. Am J Surg. 2012;204:274–82.

15. Zhou X, Sun T, Xie H, et al. Extralevator abdominoperineal excision for low rectal cancer: a systematic review and meta-analysis of the short-term outcome. Color Dis. 2015;17:474–81.

16. Prytz M, Angenete E, Bock D, Haglind E. Extralevator abdominoperineal excision for low rectal cancer—extensive surgery to be used with discretion based on 3-year local recurrence results. Ann Surg. 2016;263:516–21.

Intersphincteric Resection and Coloanal Anastomosis

17

Min Soo Cho and Nam Kyu Kim

Abstract

Radical resection for low rectal cancer is the mainstay among the treatment modalities. Intersphincteric resection (ISR) is considered a relatively new but effective surgical treatment for low-lying rectal tumor. With the advance of treatment modality, patients who have undergone abdominoperineal resection in the past can be treated with ISR. Furthermore, preoperative chemoradiation induces tumor downstaging and facilitates anal sphincter-preserving surgery. To achieve good oncologic outcomes, appropriate patient selection based on magnetic resonance imaging (MRI) is also important because MRI provides accurate information on the extent of tumor invasion and the anal canal structures. On top of all, meticulous surgical technique based on anatomical dissection is essential. Future investigations should be directed in improving functional outcomes after ISR.

Keywords

Rectal neoplasm · Intersphincteric resection Coloanal anastomosis · Operative technique Operative outcome

M. S. Cho • N. K. Kim (✉)
Department of Surgery, Yonsei University College of Medicine, Seoul, South Korea
e-mail: namkyuk@yuhs.ac

Abbreviations

3-D	Three-dimensional
APR	Abdominoperineal resection
CAA	Coloanal anastomosis
CRM	Circumferential resection margin
CRT	Chemoradiation therapy
ISR	Intersphincteric resection
MRI	Magnetic resonance imaging
TME	Total mesorectal excision
TRUS	Transrectal ultrasonography
uLAR	Ultralow anterior resection

17.1 Introduction

The primary goal for the surgical treatment of rectal cancer is to achieve an oncologic cure while preserving function. Total mesorectal excision (TME) is the standard surgical procedure for rectal cancer. The concept of TME is the elimination of potential sources of local recurrence by completely excising the mesorectum through sharp pelvic dissection [1]. TME has evolved to include the tailored removal of the mesorectum with adequate mucosal margins that are determined according to the distance of the tumor from the anal verge [2]. However, surgical treatment for low rectal cancer remains challenging, particularly with regard to the preservation of the anal sphincter. Anatomically, the mesorectum disappears at a distance of 1–2 cm above the anorectal sling, and only the rectal wall remains to the anal hiatus. Thus, there are greater risks of direct tumor invasion of the adjacent structures and of a positive circumferential resection margin (CRM) in low rectal lesions.

In 1977, Lyttle and Parks [3] used the term "intersphincteric excision" in the context of surgical treatment for inflammatory bowel disease, and the authors described the dissection of the anal canal and rectum via the intersphincteric plane. In 1981, Shafix [4] also described a technique for anorectal mobilization through the intersphincteric plane for the treatment of benign and malignant rectal diseases. In 1982, Parks and Percy [5] described an ultralow anterior resection (uLAR) with a coloanal anastomosis (CAA) for low rectal cancers. This technique involves dissecting away the mucosa from just above the dentate line, followed by a hand-sewn anastomosis within the anal canal. With improvements in technique, double-stapled CAA can also be performed within a wide pelvis using a circular stapler.

In 1994, Schiessel et al. [6] described ISR for low rectal cancers. The underlying concept is a proctectomy based on the TME technique and the extension of the dissection through the intersphincteric plane. This technique involves a perianal approach through the intersphincteric plane, the partial or complete removal of the internal anal sphincter, and the restoration of intestinal continuity by a hand-sewn anastomosis.

Traditionally, a distal resection margin of at least 5 cm has been recommended for anal sphincter-preserving surgery [7]. However, numerous reports have established that rectal tumors rarely spread more than 1–2 cm distally and that oncologic outcomes are not compromised with a 2-cm distal margin in rectal cancer patients who are undergoing surgery alone [8–11]. Moreover, findings from recent studies support the oncologic safety of a shorter distal margin of only 1 cm when it is combined with multimodality treatment [12].

Recent advances in surgical techniques and multimodal treatments would have led to the possibility of sphincter preservation in patients who

have undergone abdominoperineal resection (APR) in the past. In this regard, intersphincteric resection (ISR) has been described by Schiessel et al. [6] as the definitive surgical technique for anal sphincter preservation, and now, ISR in combination with preoperative chemoradiation therapy (CRT) is increasingly being performed in patients with low rectal cancers. In this chapter, we will discuss ISR and coloanal reconstruction in terms of its surgical indications, the operative techniques, and its oncologic and functional outcomes.

Several surgical options can be considered for low rectal cancer. The uLAR and CAA without ISR include a total proctectomy to the level of the anorectal ring just above the level of the puborectalis muscle and the restoration of bowel continuity using either a double-stapled or a hand-sewn anastomosis [13]. ISR can be considered for low rectal cancers that are close to the dentate line unless the tumor involves the external sphincter. The ISR procedure includes the partial or complete removal of the internal sphincter by dissecting within the intersphincteric plane [14–17]. After resection, coloanal reconstruction is performed using an end-to-end CAA, a J-pouch, coloplasty, or an end-to-side CAA, using either a hand-sewn or a stapled anastomosis. Because of technical advances and greater surgical experience, a combined resection of the external sphincter or levator ani muscle can be performed in highly selected patients in whom the tumor has invaded the external sphincter or the levator ani muscle [18–22].

17.2 Normal Anatomy of the Anal Canal and Indication of ISR

The anal canal is the last part of the digestive tract, and the anatomical anal canal refers to a zone between the dentate line and the anal verge, and it is approximately 2–3 cm long. The surgical anal canal refers to the zone between the anorectal ring and the anal verge. It is about 4–5 cm long and is shorter in women. The anorectal ring refers the site where the rectum goes into the pelvic floor. The levator ani muscle forms the pelvic floor and it is attached to the pelvic sidewall. The levator ani muscle is composed of the pubococcygeus, puborectalis, and iliococcygeus muscles. During rectal dissections, the U-shaped puborectalis muscle and the surrounding levator ani muscles are easily seen in the form of a membranous sheet and they sometimes adhere to the proper rectal fascia [23]. The anorectal ring is angled by the puborectalis muscle and is pulled anteriorly by the contraction of the puborectalis muscle [24]. The levator ani muscle is innervated by branches of the pudendal, inferior rectal, perineal, and sacral nerves [25, 26]. The anal canal is surrounded by the internal sphincter and the longitudinal rectal muscle layer, and the external sphincter [27] and the coccyx are located posteriorly, the ischiorectal fossa is located laterally, and the urethra is located anteriorly in men and the lower part of the vagina is located anteriorly in women.

The internal sphincter is connected from the inner circular smooth muscle of the rectum supplied by autonomic nerve. The length of the internal sphincter muscle is about 2 cm and 3 cm on the anterior and posterior sides, respectively [28]. The mean thickness is 4.5–5.9 mm [29], and the internal sphincter muscle ends with a thickened edge that is 1–1.5 cm from the anal verge and constitutes the intersphincteric or Hilton's groove. The intersphincteric groove is an important surgical landmark for proctology procedures that is well palpated during digital rectal examination. The outer longitudinal muscle of the rectum gets thinner in the distal rectum and meets the fibers from the puborectalis muscle and forms a thin band. This band runs between the internal and external sphincters, and it spreads radially and penetrates the subcutaneous portion of the external sphincter and, finally, ends as a supporting structure for the hemorrhoidal plexus. The external sphincter muscle is a striated muscle that forms a cylinder around the internal sphincter. While it acts in concert with the puborectalis muscle, its innervation is different. The anal canal receives both sympathetic and parasympathetic innervation that controls the action of the internal anal sphincter. The external sphincter is innervated by the perineal branch of the sacral

nerve and the inferior rectal branch of the internal pudendal nerve [30].

During operations for low rectal cancer, the anterior dissection is the most difficult part, and sometimes, surgeons may miss the proper dissection plane. Uchimoto et al. [31] emphasized the importance of the rectourethralis muscle based on a histologic study. They demonstrated that Denonvilliers' fascia is absent at the level of the rectourethralis muscle and that the rectal wall is directly attached to the rectourethralis muscle. The anorectal veins and cavernous nerve are present around the rectourethralis muscle; thus, deeper dissection to the anterior surface of Denonvilliers' fascia may cause unwanted bleeding or nerve injury. Neurovascular bundles cross the seminal vesicles in the 10 o'clock and 2 o'clock directions; therefore, unless the tumor is located anteriorly, the correct dissection plane is between the posterior side of Denonvilliers' fascia and the proper rectal fascia [32–35]. Kinugasa et al. [36] highlighted that surgeons may overlook the correct surgical plane that lies between the ventral and dorsal layers of the anococcygeal ligament during perianal dissections (Fig. 17.1).

17.2.1 Definitions of ISR Procedure

The ISR procedure should be differentiated from uLAR and CAA based on whether the internal sphincter is removed. The ISR procedure is classified according to the amount of the internal sphincter that is removed. Schiessel et al. [6] described two types of ISR that involved either the complete or partial excision of the internal sphincter. Rullier et al. [14] proposed three types of ISR, namely, the total, subtotal, and partial ISR (Fig. 17.2). In Japan, three subtypes of ISR are defined. A total ISR occurs at the level of the intersphincteric groove, a subtotal ISR occurs between the dentate line and the intersphincteric groove, and a partial ISR occurs at the level of the dentate line [37]. These classifications are supported by the histological observations of Akagi et al. [38] who measured the lengths of the resected internal sphincters in specimens from CAA, ISR, and APR procedures. The mean

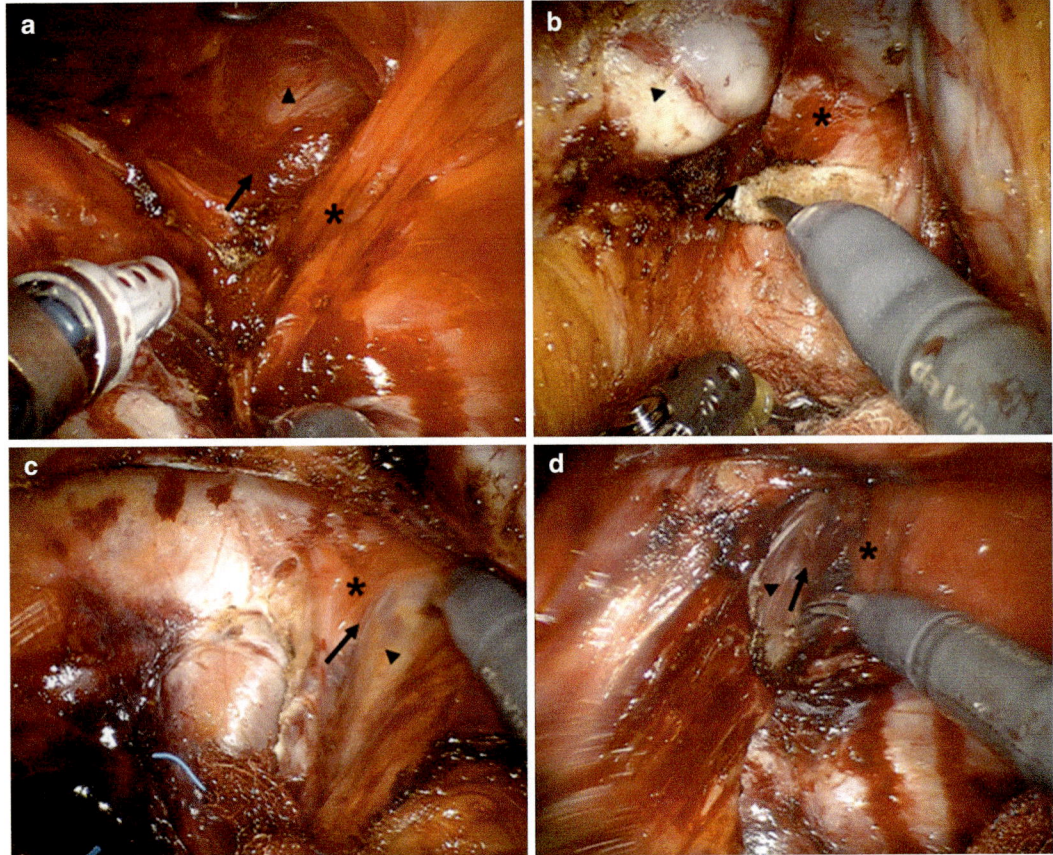

Fig. 17.1 Essential surgical anatomy for intersphincteric resection. Operative pelvic anatomy by robotic three-dimensional vision. (**a**) Posterior dissection through the intersphincteric plane (arrow) between the rectum (arrowhead) and the puborectalis muscle (asterisk). (**b**) Anterior surgical plane (arrow) behind the Denonvilliers' fascia (asterisk). Seminal vesicle (arrowhead). (**c, d**) Left and right lateral dissection around the anal hiatus. Intersphincteric plane (arrow) is identified between the rectum (arrowhead) and the medial side of the puborectalis muscle (asterisk)

lengths of the internal sphincters were 1.3 mm in the CAA, 11.5 mm in the partial ISR, 17.1 mm in the subtotal ISR, 21.3 mm in the total ISR, and 28.4 mm in the APR specimens. In recent years, ISR in combination with resection of the deep or superficial external anal sphincter is described in selected cases [18–20, 22].

17.2.2 Indications

The ISR procedure is primarily indicated for patients with low rectal tumors within the surgical anal canal and where the tumor involves the internal sphincter [16, 38–55]. If the tumor is located at the level of the puborectalis muscle and involves the external anal sphincter or levator ani muscle, APR remains the gold standard for surgical treatment. However, in some specific cases, more extensive resection techniques, including levator muscle excision and external sphincter excision, have been explored to preserve the anal sphincter [18–20, 22].

Good surgical outcomes can be anticipated when the tumor is staged at T1–T3, mobile, confined to less than 50% of the rectal circumference, and a well-to-moderately differentiated adenocarcinoma and when the patient has a good performance status, with an Eastern Cooperative Oncology Group score of 0–2, and good anal function.

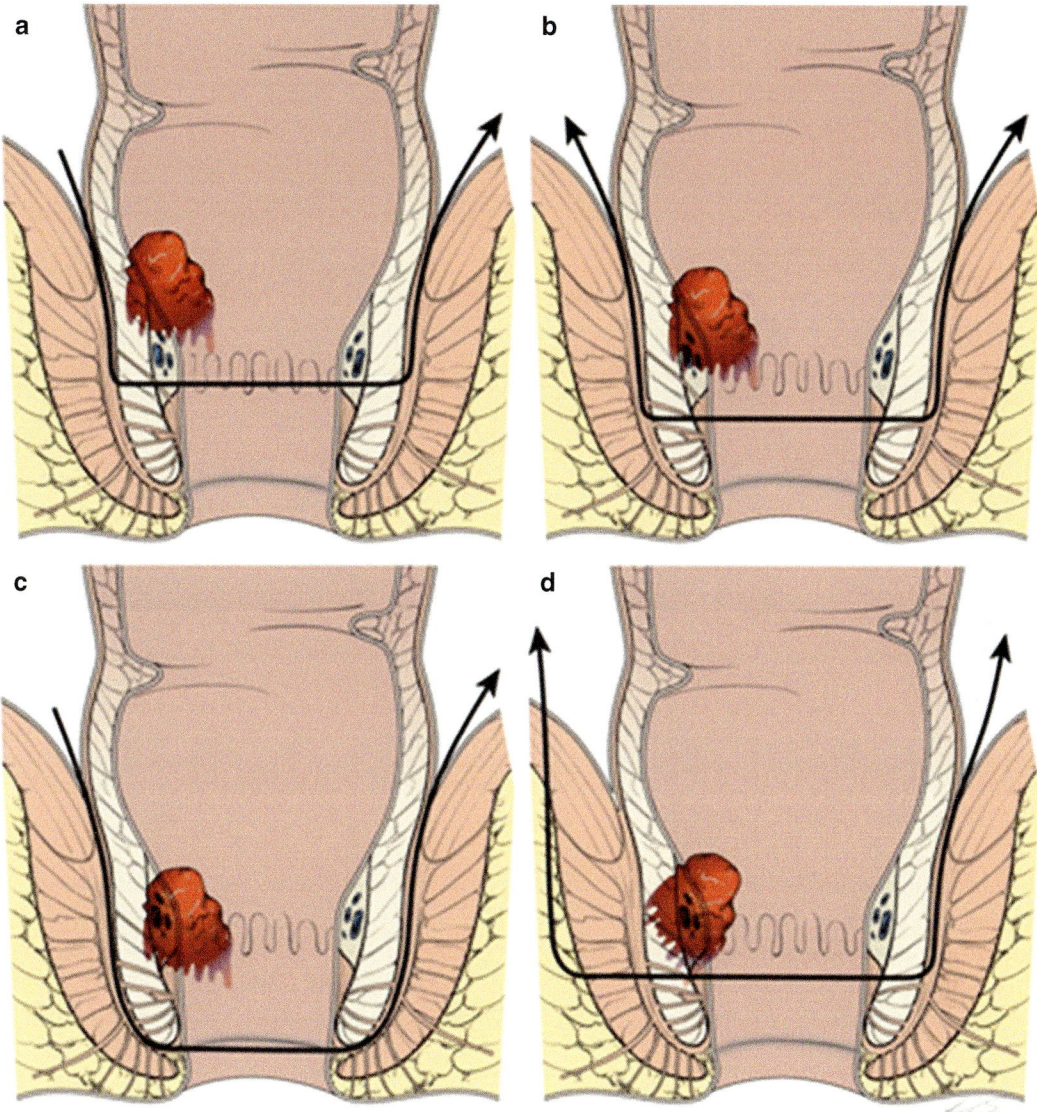

Fig. 17.2 Types of intersphincteric resection (ISR). (**a**) Partial ISR. (**b**) Subtotal ISR. (**c**) Total ISR. (**d**) ISR in combination with resection of deep or superficial external anal sphincter in selected cases [18–20, 22]

Standard management of locally advanced rectal cancer now comprises preoperative CRT followed by radical resection [56, 57]. Preoperative CRT reduces tumor bulk and increases the probability of sphincter-preserving surgery. Indeed, sphincter-preserving surgery can be achieved in a large proportion of patients who undergo CRT [58]. Preoperative CRT is associated with a pathologic complete response rate of 4–31%, which is a good oncologic outcome in terms of both recurrence and survival [59] (Fig. 17.3).

17.2.3 Baseline Image Study

The preoperative staging workup includes digital rectal examinations, transrectal ultrasonography (TRUS), colonoscopy, abdominopelvic computed tomography scanning, pelvic magnetic

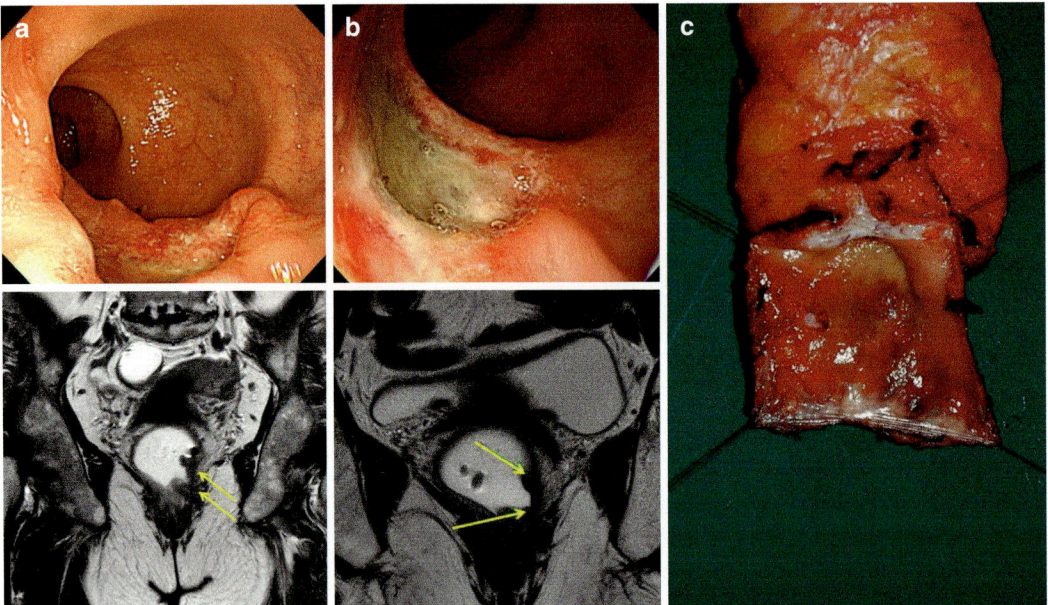

Fig. 17.3 Preoperative chemoradiation therapy (CRT) and intersphincteric resection (ISR) in a 64-year-old female patient with low rectal cancer. (**a**) Before preoperative CRT, the rectal tumor was located 3 cm from the anal verge and pretreatment magnetic resonance imaging (MRI) shows suspected tumor invasion to the internal anal sphincter muscle on T2-weighted coronal image. (**b**) After preoperative CRT, the depth of main tumor invasion was downstaged based on post-treatment colonoscopy and MRI. T2-weighted coronal image shows posttreatment fibrosis with decreased signal intensity. (**c**) Surgical specimen after ISR. Suspicious invasion on preoperative MRI was replaced with fibrosis. Final pathology report confirmed 4-mm tumor-free circumferential margin

resonance imaging (MRI), and positron emission tomography scanning. Preoperative CRT is considered for patients with bulky and/or tethered tumors that TRUS and pelvic MRI determine to be at clinical stages T3–T4 or if clinically positive lymph node metastases are detected.

17.2.3.1 Transrectal Ultrasonography (TRUS)

TRUS is useful when determining T1 or T2 disease because the higher-frequency sonoprobe has a higher resolution [60]. Katsura et al. [61] reported that the positive predictive values were 96.2% and 85.7% for T1 and T2 disease, respectively. Three-dimensional (3-D) ultrasound has become popular in recent years [62]. The 360° rotating ultrasound transducers have higher frequencies (6–16 MHz), and the system has an automated image reconstruction function. Multiplanar images can be obtained with 3-D TRUS, and it provides more comprehensive information with respect to the depth of tumor invasion and the relationships among the adjacent structures [63].

17.2.3.2 Pelvic MRI

Pelvic MRI is widely used for preoperative regional staging of rectal cancer to determine the depth of rectal wall invasion, the presence of nodal metastases, and CRM involvement. The coronal and axial MRI planes reveal whether the anal sphincter or the levator muscle is involved in low rectal cancer that is very close to the anorectal ring around the level of the levator ani muscle [64, 65]. It is important to assess the depth of tumor invasion in low rectal cancer using MRI. T1 is defined as a tumor that is confined to the mucosa and submucosa, T2 is defined as a tumor that is confined to the muscularis propria, and T3 is defined as a tumor that has penetrated the rectal wall and involves the mesorectal fat. T4 is defined as a tumor that involves the visceral peritoneum (T4a) or the adjacent tissues (T4b), including those of the prostate, vagina, sacrum, and pelvic sidewall. Caution should be exercised when interpreting the depth of tumor invasion located at or below the levator muscles. Tumor invasion of the external anal sphincter is interpreted as stage T3, and tumor invasion of the levator muscles is interpreted as stage T4 [66–68]. To standardize MRI reporting, the MERCURY group suggested that low rectal cancer is defined when the lowest margin of the tumor is located at or below the upper border of the puborectalis muscle [68, 69].

17.3 Coloanal Reconstruction Techniques

To date, several methods for coloanal reconstruction after proctectomy have been described (Table 17.1). In terms of the shape of the proximal colon, the current options for coloanal reconstruction include straight CAA (end-to-end), J-pouch reconstruction, coloplasty, and side-to-end anastomoses, and either hand-sewn or stapled anastomoses are performed. When performing a stapled anastomosis, 10–15 mm of distal remnant anoderm is incorporated into the circular stapler. In addition, the external anal sphincter may become entrapped within the stapler and the pelvic cavity should be wide enough for the creation of a stapled anastomosis. Accordingly, the hand-sewn anastomosis is the gold standard following subtotal or total ISR. A hand-sewn anastomosis has the advantages of being easy, simple, and familiar to surgeons. In addition, it can be performed conveniently in a narrow and deep pelvis.

Since its first description by Parks and Percy [5], the straight (end-to-end) anastomosis has been the most commonly used method for CAA. In their study, 69 of the 70 patients were either fully continent ($n = 39$) or they had only minor bowel dysfunction ($n = 30$), and only one patient was incontinent. The main symptoms of bowel dysfunction were frequency and irregular bowel movements. Anterior resection syndrome refers to a broad spectrum of bowel habit changes that range from irregular bowel movements to fecal incontinence or defecation difficulty following low anterior resection. The incidence of anterior resection syndrome has been reported to be about 30% among patients who have undergone low anterior resection, and the quality of life is likely to be impaired in affected individuals [70, 71]. A reduction in the reservoir capacity is thought to be one reason for anterior resection syndrome; therefore, a colonic pouch is devised to increase the neorectal reservoir capacity [72, 73].

A colonic pouch is a surgically constructed neorectal reservoir. A J-shaped pouch is commonly used because it is simple and easy to construct. Lazorthes et al. [72] observed that a colonic J-pouch increased the maximum tolerated volume and reduced the frequency of bowel movements. In their study, 60% of the patients

Table 17.1 Methods of coloanal reconstruction

	Colon configuration	Anastomosis	Fecal diversion (%)	Type of stoma
Schiessel et al. [6]	End-to-end	Hand-sewn	100	Colostomy
Braun et al. [55]	End-to-end	Hand-sewn, stapled	NS	Colostomy, ileostomy
Rullier et al. [14]	End-to-end, J-pouch	Hand-sewn, stapled	100	Colostomy, ileostomy
Teramoto et al. [109]	End-to-end	Hand-sewn	100	Colostomy
Watanabe et al. [110]	End-to-end	Hand-sewn	100	Ileostomy
Akasu et al. [111]	End-to-end, J-pouch, coloplasty	Hand-sewn	87	NS
Kim et al. [107]	End-to-end, J-pouch	Hand-sewn	100	Ileostomy

NS not specified

with pouches and 33% of the patients without pouches produced one or two stools per day during the first year. After 1 year, 86% of the patients with pouches and 33% of the patients without pouches had one or two bowel movements per day. Parc et al. [73] evaluated the functional results from 31 patients who had J-pouches, and they found that there was no incontinence and that the mean number of bowel movements was 1.1 per day; however, 25% of the patients eventually required enemas to defecate.

Some controversies remain regarding the use of J-pouches in relation to the optimal length of the pouch, the use of the sigmoid colon, and long-term functional outcomes. The length of the J-pouch has varied from 5 cm [74], 6 cm [72], 7 cm [75], 8 cm [73], 9 cm [76], 10 cm [74], to 12 cm [72]. However, lengthy pouches develop defecation dysfunction, including the inability to evacuate bulky stools, tenesmus, or the need for regular enemas [72, 73, 75–80]; hence, the length has been reduced to 5–6 cm. Indeed, Ho et al. [81] demonstrated that small J-pouches that are 5-cm-long retain liquid stools well, and 6–8-cm-long pouches are now recommended.

The use of the sigmoid colon for the creation of J-pouches is another issue. Traditionally, both the sigmoid and descending colon have been used; however, disadvantages associated with the use of the sigmoid colon have been suggested, and these include diverticular disease, bulky mesentery, and motility problems. Seow-Choen [82] suggested that the sigmoid colon contributes to evacuatory dysfunction because defecation difficulties were observed in 25% of patients who had pouches created using the sigmoid colon [83], but these difficulties were not seen in patients who had pouches created using the descending colon [79, 84].

It is unclear whether the beneficial effects of J-pouches on bowel function are maintained in the long term [85, 86]. Defecatory function improves with time, even after straight CAA, because of an increase in the neorectal reservoir volume, the improvement in sphincter function, the recovery of the rectoanal inhibitory reflex, and improvements in neorectal sensations [87, 88]. Ho et al. [89] observed that stool frequency and the incidence of incontinence were lower at

6 months in patients with pouches, but that the benefit was not sustained 2 years after surgery. Meanwhile, Harris et al. [90] demonstrated that 5–9 years after surgery, patients with J-pouches had better long-term outcomes with respect to their Kirwan continence scores, their evacuation difficulties, and urgency associated with defecation compared with patients with straight CAA.

The colonic J-pouch is created as described next. The two loops of the descending colon are anastomosed in a "J" configuration using a linear stapler. The appropriate pouch length is 5–8 cm, and the linear stapler may be inserted through the uppermost or lowermost parts of the J-pouch. The enteroenterostomy site is carefully inspected for any bleeding along the staple line, and hemostatic sutures are applied at the site of any bleeding. Then, hand-sewn or stapled anastomoses are performed.

Coloplasty refers to a colonic reservoir that is created by a longitudinal incision with a transverse closure using a method that is analogous to that of the Heineke-Mikulicz pyloroplasty. Z'graggen et al. [91, 92] originally described this technique in a pig model, and Fazio et al. [93, 94] applied it to low colorectal or coloanal anastomoses. A reservoir for the coloplasty is made by a longitudinal incision, which is 8–10 cm long, along the teniae coli on the antimesenteric side. The colonic incision is stopped 4–6 cm proximal to the distal end of the colon, the colostomy is closed transversely using absorbable sutures, and then a stapled or hand-sewn anastomosis is performed with a prepared reservoir. Remzi et al. [95] demonstrated that the coloplasty group had fewer night bowel movements, fewer bowel movements per day, less clustering, and less antidiarrheal agent use than the straight anastomosis group. Coloplasty is now considered a good alternative technique when a colonic J-pouch is technically difficult.

The side-to-end anastomosis was described for colorectal anastomoses in 1950, and its theoretical advantages include technical ease, a blood supply, and a larger anastomosis lumen [96]. Huber et al. [97] compared colonic pouches with side-to-end anastomoses after low anterior resections. The defecation frequencies were 2.2 and 5.4 per day at 3 months and 2.3 and 3.1 per day at 6 months in the pouch and side-to-end anastomosis groups, respec-

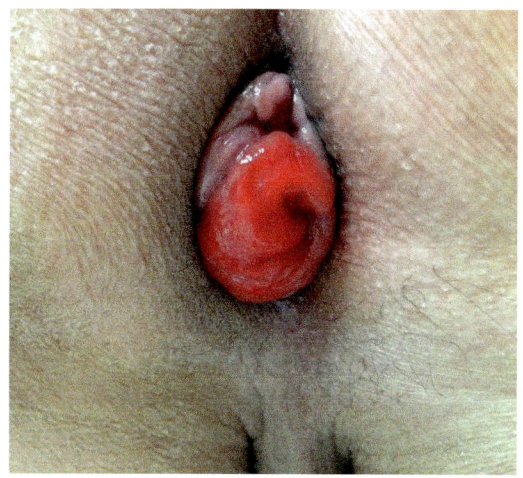

Fig. 17.4 Postoperative mucosal prolapse after intersphincteric resection

tively. The investigators pointed out that the side-to-end anastomoses showed satisfactory long-term function and that the major benefit associated with the colonic pouches was seen during the immediate postoperative period. Machado et al. [98] observed that the colonic J-pouch and side-to-end anastomosis had comparable functional outcomes 2 years after low anterior resections.

When considering coloanal reconstruction, a straight (end-to-end) CAA is an easy, simple, and convenient reconstruction method, which is preferred after ISR. While J-pouch construction is performed to improve defecation function, it is not always possible, particularly in patients who have a narrow pelvis or bulky mesentery. Accordingly, surgeons should be cautious about the selection of the optimal coloanal reconstruction technique. While the J-pouch may be the first choice as opposed to the end-to-end CAA, coloplasty or side-to-end CAA can be also considered as second options.

Some additional techniques deserve to be mentioned. The use of irradiated sigmoid colons may cause anastomotic strictures or leakages [99]. Kim et al. [100] suggested that hand-sewn sutures between the levator muscles and the distal anorectal stumps may improve postoperative defecatory function. Yamada et al. [41] reported that 4 out of 20 patients who underwent total ISR experienced postoperative mucosal prolapses of the neorectum, and mucosal excisions were later

performed in all 4 patients. In my opinion, a redundant proximal colon may be a source of a prolapse, and the appropriate length of the proximal colon is just beyond the symphysis pubis (Fig. 17.4). Furthermore, anchoring sutures between the proximal colon and the levator muscles may prevent prolapses.

17.4 Combined Excision of the External Sphincter or Levator Ani Muscles

More extensive resections in addition to ISR have been described in the literature (Fig. 17.5). In 2002, Fucini et al. [22] described the excision of the levator muscles and the preservation of the part of internal sphincter and the external sphincter and its innervation for low T4 rectal cancers. Shirouzu et al. [18] described the excision of the puborectalis muscle, deep and superficial external sphincter, and the internal sphincter muscles while preserving the subcutaneous external sphincter muscle. Cong et al. [20] described the partial longitudinal resection of the anorectal and sphincter muscles. This technique involves the unilateral removal of the sphincter complex as occurs in APR. Alasari et al. [19] described a hemi-levator excision through the intersphincteric plane by removing the levator ani and the deep external sphincter muscles. All of these new techniques need to be scrutinized with respect to oncologic safety and functional outcomes. A diverting stoma is created by either a loop transverse colostomy or an ileostomy after ISR with CAA for rectal cancer. Although a diverting stoma does not prevent anastomotic leakages, the use of a diverting loop stoma does reduce symptomatic anastomotic leakages [2, 101]; thus, fecal diversion is cautiously considered after ISR.

17.5 Details of Essential Operative Technique

The operative procedures comprise three essential steps, namely, the first abdominal procedure, the second perianal procedure, and the third second abdominal procedure.

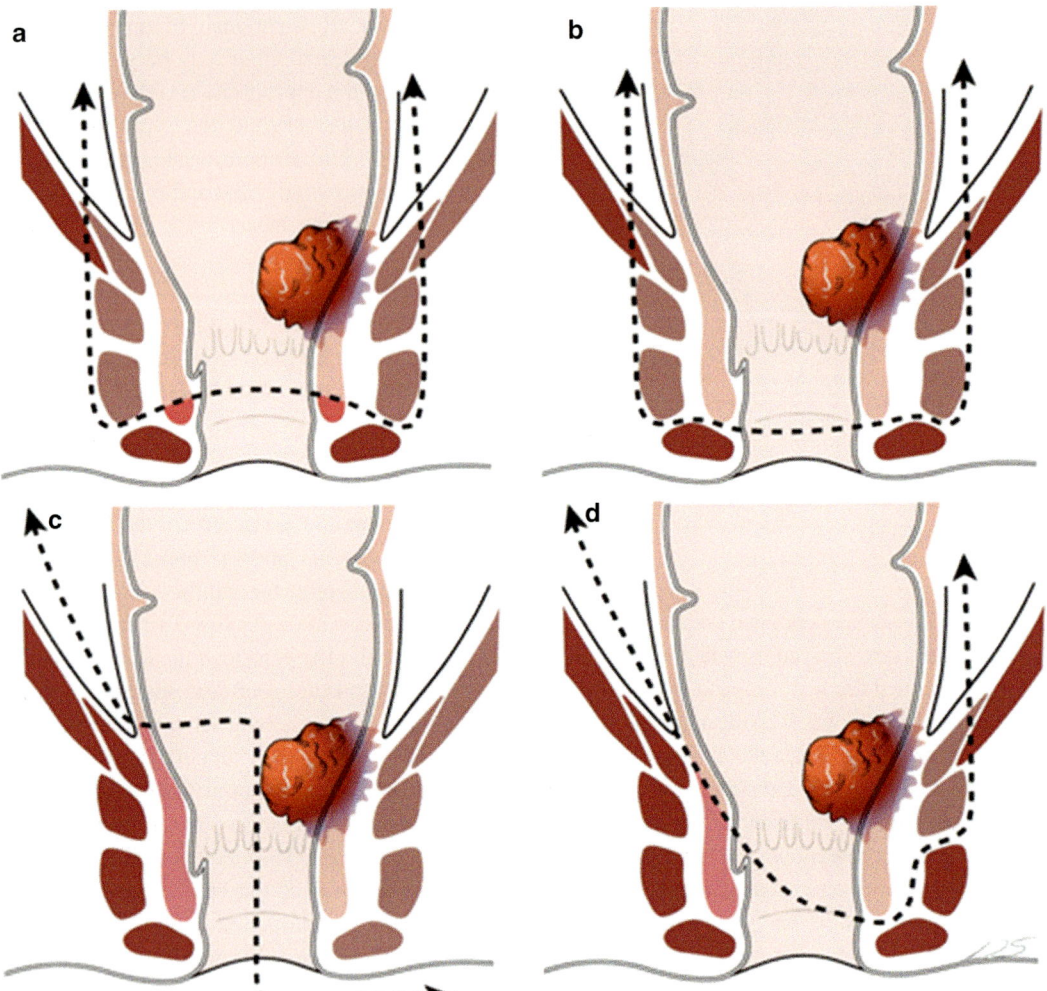

Fig. 17.5 External anal sphincter resection and levator muscle excision. (**a**) Excision of the levator, internal, and external anal sphincter muscles while preserving distal parts of the internal and external sphincters and its innervation for low T4 rectal cancers described by Fucini et al. [22]. (**b**) Excision of the puborectalis muscle, deep and superficial external sphincter as well as internal sphincter muscles while preserving subcutaneous external sphincter muscle described by Shirouzu et al. [18]. (**c**) Partial longitudinal resection of the anorectum and sphincter muscles described by Cong et al. [20]. This technique involves removal of all sphincter complex unilaterally such as abdominoperineal resection. (**d**) Hemi-levator excision through the intersphincteric plane by removal of the levator ani and deep external sphincter muscles described by Alasari et al. [19]

17.5.1 Abdominal Procedure

1. Patient position and skin incision

    The patient is placed in the lithotomy-Trendelenburg position with the legs supported by Lloyd-Davies stirrups. The laparotomy for the ISR procedure begins with a midline abdominal skin incision. After abdominal exposure, the small bowel is protected by a bowel bag, and a mechanical self-retaining retractor is placed in position.

2. Ligation of the inferior mesenteric artery

    An incision is made at the level of the sacral promontory. A peritoneal incision extends along the right side of the rectal mesentery and the avascular plane is exposed. The pedicle of the inferior mesenteric vessel is visualized, and the colonic mesentery is separated from the underlying fascia propria of the rectum and the inferior hypogastric nerves. The superior hypogastric plexus is carefully preserved around the aortic bifurcation, the inferior mesenteric artery is ligated at the root of its origin from the abdominal aorta, and the lymph nodes along the inferior mesenteric artery are cleared from just above the superior hypogastric nerves overlying the aorta. The inferior mesenteric vein is divided immediately beneath the pancreas. Older patients or patients with questionable blood supplies may be candidates for low ties of the inferior mesenteric artery.

3. Descending and sigmoid colon mobilization via the medial to lateral or lateral to medial approaches

   During mobilization of the descending colon and the sigmoid colon, the locations of the ureter and the gonadal vessels are assessed and preserved.

4. Splenic flexure mobilization

   The splenic flexure of the colon is routinely mobilized to gain a sufficient length for coloanal anastomosis. After ligation of the inferior mesenteric vein just below the inferior border of the pancreas, an avascular retroperitoneal space between the mesentery and Gerota's fascia, including the perirenal fat, is developed. The loose attachment of the transverse mesocolon is separated from the lower border of the pancreas, and the lesser sac is entered. The left paracolic gutter is dissected, and the previously dissected retroperitoneal plane of Toldt's fascia is identified. The greater omentum overlying the transverse colon is divided to enter the lesser sac, and the previous surgical plane is met at this point. Finally, any loose connective tissue is freed to complete the colonic mobilization, and the medial part of colonic mesentery is divided carefully, avoiding any injury to the marginal artery.

5. Total mesorectal excision

   The pelvic dissection is continued along the parietal pelvic fascia, leaving the hypogastric nerve intact over the aorta. The proper rectal fascia enveloping the mesorectum should remain intact during the pelvic dissection. The autonomic pelvic plexus is also preserved. The rectum is sharply dissected to the anal hiatus of the pelvic diaphragm. The posterior rectal dissection is performed in the retrorectal avascular space along the visceral pelvic fascia plane. The rectosacral fascia or Waldeyer's fascia is encountered at the S4 level between the presacral fascia and the proper rectal fascia. Division of the rectosacral fascia enables the surgeon to reach down to the level of the coccyx. The anterior rectal dissection involves the identification of Denonvilliers' fascia in males.

   Techniques to preserve the autonomic nerves are performed to preserve postoperative sexual and voiding functions. It is important to perform a U-shaped incision during the excision of Denonvilliers' fascia in the anterior part of the rectum to avoid injury of the genitourinary neurovascular bundles. In females, the rectum and the vaginal wall should be dissected carefully. The lateral part of the rectum is mobilized after the anterior and posterior dissections while avoiding excessive traction of the rectum. The pelvic plexus and the arising sacral nerves are assessed and preserved [24]. The three common sites of nerve injury are the superior hypogastric plexus, the inferior hypogastric plexus, and the pelvic plexus.

6. Dissection to the anal canal through the intersphincteric plane

   The puborectalis muscle sling is exposed laterally, and the anococcygeal ligament is divided at the posterior side of the anal canal. The intersphincteric space is identified between the puborectalis muscle and the rectal wall. The dissection continues through the puborectalis muscle and in the deep part of the external anal sphincter at the intra-anal canal.

17.5.2 Transanal Procedures

1. Assessment of the lower margin of the tumor and the distal resection margin.

   A Lone Star retractor (Lone Star Medical Products, Inc., Houston, TX, USA) is applied to the anus, and a profuse rectal washout is performed using a solution of betadine and saline. Then, 0.25% bupivacaine mixed with epinephrine is injected below the dentate line. The lower tumor margin is assessed, and a distal resection margin that is at least 1–2 cm long is obtained whenever possible.

2. Determine which type of ISR (partial, subtotal, or total) is appropriate and circumferential incision around the distal margin. A digital rectal examination is performed to identify the intersphincteric groove, and the circumferential incision is made (Fig. 17.6). The incised distal rectum is closed with absorbable sutures to prevent contamination of the intraluminal contents.

3. Full mobilization of the rectum to the level of the levator ani muscle.

   The posterior dissection begins at the level of the dentate line for partial ISR cases, between the dentate line and the intersphincteric groove for subtotal ISR cases, or at the intersphincteric groove for total ISR cases. The lateral and anterior dissections continue through the intersphincteric plane. Before further circumferential resection, the distal rec-

tum is closed with sutures to prevent fecal contamination. Further posterior and lateral dissections continue, and the anterior attachment of the prostate or the vagina is eventually dissected. The rectal wall and the internal sphincter are sharply dissected just above the puborectalis sling along the surgical plane developed via the abdominal approach. The muscular rectal wall is freed using cautery at the level of the anorectal ring, and full mobilization is confirmed using the index finger.

4. Specimen is delivered via transanal pull-through or the abdominal route.

   The specimen can be delivered either through the anus or through the abdominal wound. For patients with bulky mesorectums or narrow pelvises, it is difficult to deliver the specimen via the anus. The specimen is then transected with an adequate proximal margin.

5. Coloanal reconstruction.

   The reconstruction type (J-pouch, end-to-end, side-to-end, or coloplasty) and method (hand-sewn or stapled) are selected. Splenic

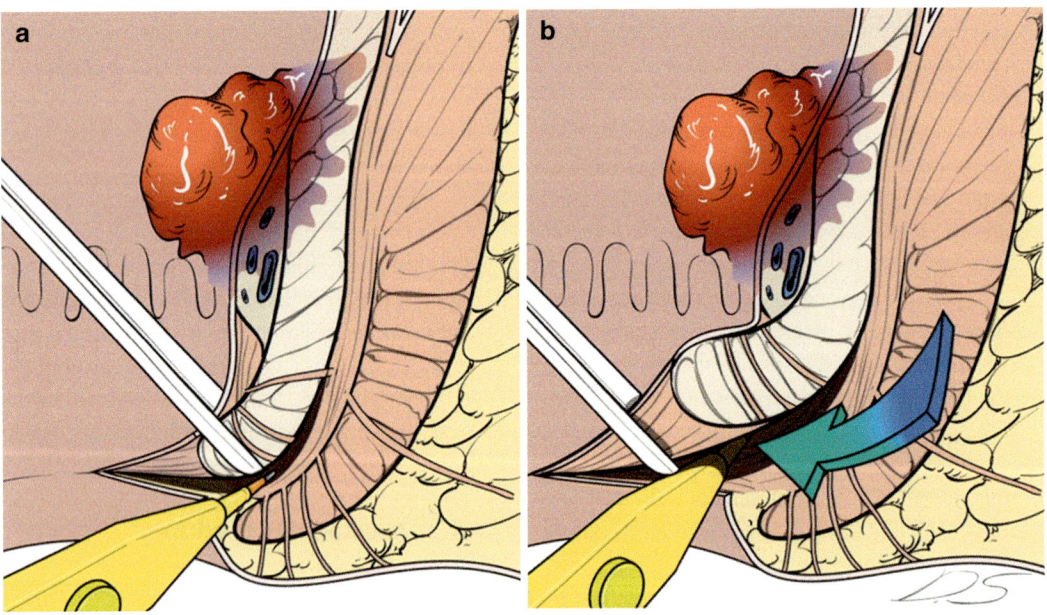

Fig. 17.6 Perianal procedure for intersphincteric resection (ISR). (**a**) Lower margin of the tumor is assessed, and proper type of ISR (partial, subtotal, or total) is selected. Digital rectal examination is performed to identify inter-sphincteric groove, and 0.25% bupivacaine mixed with epinephrine is injected below the dentate line. (**b**) Circumferential incision is made along the intersphincteric groove

flexure mobilization is beneficial to ensure the acquisition of a sufficient colonic length. Anastomotic tension should be avoided. The mesocolon should not be twisted when the pouch is delivered into the pelvic cavity. The prepared proximal colon is pulled down through the anus. Unnecessary colonic appendages, namely, the appendices epiploicae, are trimmed for the anastomosis. For hand-sewn anastomoses, a CAA is performed using absorbable 3-0 sutures placed in an interrupted fashion. Anastomosis is positioned at the level of intersphincteric groove, not at the dentate line. Each suture should incorporate either external or internal sphincter muscles to provide anastomotic strength (Fig. 17.7). The proximal colon is then anastomosed to the anal mucosa or the external sphincter. For the double-stapling technique, a manual purse-string suture is made around the anoderm to facilitate the use of the circular stapler. The stapling technique is quick and technically convenient compared with hand-sewn anastomoses. However, as mentioned previously, stapled anastomoses are difficult to perform in subtotal or total ISR cases.

17.5.3 Abdominal Procedure

1. Placement of pelvic and colonic drains before closure of the abdominal wall.

2. A temporary protective stoma is made in the right lower quadrant area using the terminal ileum. A diverting ileostomy is closed 2 months later or when the planned adjuvant chemotherapy is completed.

17.5.4 Minimally Invasive Surgery

17.5.4.1   Laparoscopic Approach

The operative principles underlying the laparoscopic approach are the same as ISR through laparotomy. The patient is placed in the lithotomy-Trendelenburg position, and five trocars are positioned after a carbon dioxide pneumoperitoneum has been established at 12-mm Hg. One camera port with an 11-mm trocar is placed in the umbilicus using the open technique, one 12-mm port is placed in the left lower quadrant area, one 12-mm port is placed in the right lower quadrant area, and two 5-mm ports are placed in the left and right upper quadrant areas. High or low ligation of the inferior mesenteric artery, splenic flexure mobilization, total mesorectal excision, and intersphincteric dissection are then performed sequentially. After the perianal procedures, the specimen is brought out through the anus or through a minilaparotomy wound. Coloanal reconstruction is undertaken in the same manner as that used for ISR through laparotomy.

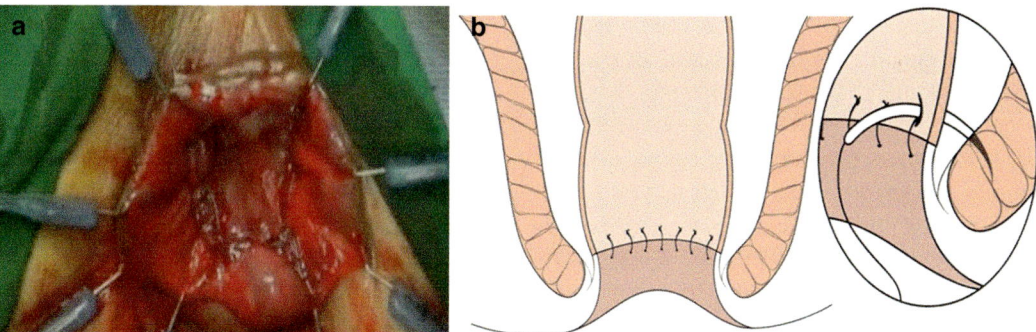

Fig. 17.7 Hand-sewn coloanal anastomosis. (**a**) Lone Star retractor (Lone Star Medical Products, Inc., Houston, TX, USA) is applied to the anus. End-to-end coloanal reconstruction with hand-sewn anastomosis is performed by absorbable 3-0 sutures in an interrupted fashion. (**b**) Anastomosis is positioned at the level of intersphincteric groove, not at the dentate line. Each suture should incorporate either external or internal sphincter muscles to provide anastomotic strength

17.5.4.2 Robotic Approach

There is growing interest in the da Vinci Surgical System (Intuitive Surgical, Sunnyvale, CA, USA), and robotic systems have been adopted in a variety of surgical fields, including urology, gynecology, and gastrointestinal surgery. The robotic surgical system provides a 3-D view of the surgical site, tremor-filtering, and more ergonomic instrumentation compared with conventional laparoscopic surgical systems [102]. Pelvic surgery can benefit from the advantages of robotic systems, and indeed, robotic prostate surgery has quickly become a standard minimally invasive approach.

We evaluated outcomes after robotic ($n = 47$) and laparoscopic ($n = 37$) uLAR with CAA [103]. The demographic and operative data did not differ significantly between the two patient groups, but the rate of conversion to open surgery was lower in the robotic surgery group (2.1%) compared with the laparoscopic surgery group (16.2%, $p = 0.02$). In addition, the mean duration of the hospital stay was shorter in the robotic surgery group (9 days) than in the laparoscopic surgery group (11 days). No postoperative mortality occurred.

For robotically assisted ISR with CAA, the perianal approach is performed first before docking the robotic system [13]. The perianal dissection is performed at the beginning of the operation. After an injection of bupivacaine, the dissection begins at the intersphincteric groove. A meticulous dissection is performed from the intersphincteric groove to the lower rectum. After suturing the dissected rectum, the gauze is packed into the anal canal to maintain the pneumoperitoneum during the robotic procedure.

The robotic procedure then begins, and the surgical principles include high or low ties of the inferior mesenteric vessels and routine splenic flexure mobilization. Next, a total mesorectal excision is performed. The robotic arms provide solid and stable anterior and lateral traction. Rectal retraction is performed using cotton tape with an endosuture device. The anatomical pelvic dissection is performed using the robotic EndoWrist® Instruments. It is important not to injure the neurovascular bundles. After completing the total mesorectal excision, further dissection continues to the pelvic floor. The pelvic dissection is completed when the previously packed gauze is seen at the puborectalis sling. The muscular wall of the rectum is divided at the level of the puborectalis muscle, which is facilitated by the robotic arms. While performing ISR with CAA, a secure and meticulous dissection through to the pelvic floor is critical for oncological safety, and this can easily be achieved with the aid of the robotic ergonomic instruments and the magnified 3-D view, even in a narrow pelvic cavity. Specimen is delivered through the anus or through an additional mini-laparotomy wound. Caution should be exercised when patients have bulky mesocolons or mesorectums because it is difficult to pull specimens through the anal route. After undocking the robotic arms, the coloanal reconstruction is performed.

Recently, Kim et al. [104] described ISR technique with a complete abdominal approach. They pointed that a robotic approach facilitates visualization of the embryonic intersphincteric plane between the rectum and the surrounding pelvic floor musculatures in the abdominal side.

17.6 Short-Term and Long-Term Outcomes

17.6.1 Morbidity and Mortality

TME for rectal cancer is associated with significant postoperative morbidity and mortality. It has been reported that the wound infection rate is 7%, the anastomotic leak rate is 11%, and the postoperative mortality rate is 2% [105]. The overall morbidity rate associated with ISR is reportedly 4.8–65%, while the anastomotic leak rate is 5.1–25.8%, the anastomotic stricture rate is 3–15.8%, and the mortality rate is 0–5% [106].

17.6.2 Oncologic Outcomes

Schiessel et al. [6] reported a local recurrence rate of 10% and a disease-free survival rate of 83.2%. Rullier et al. [16] reported a local recurrence rate of 2% and a disease-free survival rate of 70%. Saito et al. [49] analyzed data from several Japanese institutions and reported that the local recurrence rate was 5.8% and that the overall and disease-free survival rates were 91.9% and 83.2%, respectively.

Portier et al. [47] compared outcomes between CAA without ISR (n = 105) and CAA with ISR (n = 173) over a mean follow-up period of 66.8 months. The 5-year local recurrence rate did not differ between the CAA without ISR (6.7%) and the CAA with ISR (10.6%) groups. Furthermore, the 5-year overall survival rate did not differ between the CAA without ISR (80%) and the CAA with ISR (86.1%) groups.

Weiser et al. [42] compared outcomes from three surgical techniques, namely, CAA, ISR, and APR, for low rectal cancer, and they determined that the local recurrence rates were 2% (2/28), 0%

(0/44), and 9% (6/63) in the CAA, ISR, and APR groups, respectively. The 5-year recurrence-free survival rates for the CAA, ISR, and APR groups were 85%, 83%, and 47%, respectively, and the 5-year disease-specific survival rates for the CAA, ISR, and APR groups were 97%, 96%, and 59%, respectively. They concluded that sphincter preservation in combination with preoperative CRT for low rectal cancer did not compromise the oncologic outcomes. In addition, Saito et al. [43] compared the oncologic outcomes between ISR and APR. They found that the local recurrence rates were 10.6% (14/132) and 15.7% (11/70) in the ISR and APR groups, respectively; the 5-year local relapse-free survival rates were 83% and 80% in the ISR and APR groups, respectively; and the 5-year disease-free survival rates were 69% and 63% in the ISR and APR groups, respectively. They also found that the 5-year overall survival rates were 80% and 61.5% in the ISR and APR groups, respectively. Saito et al. [43] suggested that ISR is an oncologically acceptable surgical approach compared with APR for very low rectal cancers (Table 17.2).

Table 17.2 Oncologic outcomes

	Year	N	FU (month)	R0 (%)	LR (%)	CSS or OS (%)	DFS (%)
Braun et al. [55]	1992	63	80	100	11	62	–
Bannon et al. [54]	1995	109	40	NR	11	87	–
Kohler et al. [53]	2000	31	82	100	10	79	–
Rullier et al. [16]	2005	92	40	89	2	81	70
Schiessel et al. [17]	2005	121	94	96.7	5.3	88	NR
Saito et al. [49]	2006	228	41	98.7	5.3	92	83
Hohenberger et al. [50]	2006	65	70	92	23	–	–
Chamlou et al. [48]	2007	90	56	94	7	82	75
Akasu et al. [46]	2008	120	42	96.7	6.7	91	77
Krand et al. [44]	2009	47	68	98	2	85	82
Han et al. [45]	2009	40	43	100	11	62	NR
Weiser et al. [42]	2009	44	47	92	0	96	83
Yamada et al. [41]	2009	107	41	100	2.5	92	87
Baek et al. [103]	2013	84[a]	32	100	6	87–91	81
Akagi et al. [38]	2013	83	60	100	11	87	74
Saito et al. [108]	2014	199	78	100	14	78	67

FU follow-up, *LR* local recurrence, *CSS* cancer-specific survival, *OS* overall survival, *DFS* disease-free survival, *NR* not reported
[a]Including ultralow anterior resection with coloanal anastomosis

17.6.3 Functional Outcomes

Functional outcomes, for example, defecation, are important clinical outcome measures following ISR for low rectal cancer. We reviewed the literature and found that the mean stool frequency varies from 2.2 to 5.1 times per day and that urgency was noted in 2–50% of patients. Perfect continence was achieved in 30–80%, fecal soiling was observed in 11–63%, and incontinence of flatus was observed in 9–88% of patients [6, 38, 41, 44, 45, 48, 51, 53, 55, 107, 108]. Saito et al. [49] evaluated functional outcomes in 110 patients using the Wexner score, and the mean score was 7.8 after a 24-month follow-up period. Using the Kirwan classification, perfect continence was observed in 36 patients, incontinence of flatus was observed in 32 patients, occasional minor soiling was observed in 25 patients, and frequent major soiling was observed in 7 patients. None of the patients needed a colostomy for fecal incontinence. In a recent study by the same group [108], the median Wexner score at 5 years was 8 and 10 in the surgery alone and in the surgery plus preoperative CRT groups, respectively. Risk factors for poor postoperative functional outcomes were being a man and the use of preoperative CRT (Table 17.3).

Conclusions

ISR is a safe and effective surgical technique for low rectal cancer. Now, patients who have undergone APR in the past can be treated with ISR. In addition, preoperative CRT induces tumor downstaging and facilitates anal sphincter-preserving surgery. To achieve good oncologic outcomes, appropriate patient selection based on MRI is important, because MRI provides accurate information about the extent of tumor invasion and the anal canal structures. On top of all, a meticulous surgical technique based on anatomical dissections is essential. Recent developments in robotic technology provide an enhanced surgical view and ergonomic instrumentation; hence, fine dissections with effective traction are possible. Future investigations should be directed to improve functional outcomes after ISR.

Table 17.3 Functional outcomes

	Year	N	Stool frequency/day	Urgency (%)	Perfect continence (%)	Soiling (%)	Incontinence of flatus (%)
Braun et al. [55]	1992	63	2.2	22	75	15	17
Kohler et al. [53]	2000	31	3.3	–	30	63	11
Schiessel et al. [17]	2005	121	2.2	–	86	14	–
Chin et al. [51]	2006	10	a	50	30	20	20
Chamlou et al. [48]	2007	90	2.3	19	41	59	25
Krand et al. [44]	2009	47	2.3	2	80	11	9
Han et al. [45]	2009	40	2.2	31	43	29	29
Yamada et al. [41]	2009	107	3.7	–	42	28	–
Kim et al. [107]	2009	21	b	0	50	25	25
Akagi et al. [38]	2013	83	5.1	33	60	16–22	88
Saito et al. [108]	2014	104	4	32	–	26–30	55

a50% had less than three times per day
b75% had less than two times per day

Acknowledgments The authors are deeply grateful to Dong-Su Jang, MFA, (Medical Illustrator, Medical Research Support Section, Yonsei University College of Medicine, Seoul, Korea) for his outstanding medical illustrations.

References

1. Heald RJ, Husband EM, Ryall RDH. The mesorectum in rectal cancer surgery—the clue to pelvic recurrence? Br J Surg. 1982;69(10):613–6.
2. Kim NK, Kim YW, Min BS, Lee KY, Sohn SK, Cho CH. Operative safety and oncologic outcomes of anal sphincter-preserving surgery with mesorectal excision for rectal cancer: 931 consecutive patients treated at a single institution. Ann Surg Oncol. 2009;16(4):900–9.
3. Lyttle JA, Parks AG. Intersphincteric excision of the rectum. Br J Surg. 1977;64(6):413–6.
4. Shafik A. A new concept of the anatomy of the anal sphincter mechanism and the physiology of defecation. XII. Anorectal mobilization: a new surgical access to rectal lesions. Preliminary report. Am J Surg. 1981;142(5):629–35.
5. Parks AG, Percy JP. Resection and sutured coloanal anastomosis for rectal carcinoma. Br J Surg. 1982;69(6):301–4.
6. Schiessel R, Karner-Hanusch J, Herbst F, Teleky B, Wunderlich M. Intersphincteric resection for low rectal tumours. Br J Surg. 1994;81(9):1376–8.
7. Goligher JC, Dukes CE, Bussey HJ. Local recurrences after sphincter saving excisions for carcinoma of the rectum and rectosigmoid. Br J Surg. 1951;39(155):199–211.
8. Karanjia ND, Schache DJ, North WR, Heald RJ. 'Close shave' in anterior resection. Br J Surg. 1990;77(5):510–2.
9. Shirouzu K, Isomoto H, Kakegawa T. Distal spread of rectal cancer and optimal distal margin of resection for sphincter-preserving surgery. Cancer. 1995;76(3):388–92.
10. Andreola S, Leo E, Belli F, Lavarino C, Bufalino R, Tomasic G, et al. Distal intramural spread in adenocarcinoma of the lower third of the rectum treated with total rectal resection and coloanal anastomosis. Dis Colon Rectum. 1997;40(1):25–9.
11. Kim YW, Kim NK, Min BS, Huh H, Kim JS, Kim JY, et al. Factors associated with anastomotic recurrence after total mesorectal excision in rectal cancer patients. J Surg Oncol. 2009;99(1):58–64.
12. Bujko K, Rutkowski A, Chang GJ, Michalski W, Chmielik E, Kusnierz J. Is the 1-cm rule of distal bowel resection margin in rectal cancer based on clinical evidence? A systematic review. Ann Surg Oncol. 2012;19(3):801–8.
13. Kang J, Hur H, Min BS, Lee KY, Kim NK. Robotic coloanal anastomosis with or without intersphincteric resection for low rectal cancer: starting with the perianal approach followed by robotic procedure. Ann Surg Oncol. 2012;19(1):154–5.
14. Rullier E, Zerbib F, Laurent C, Bonnel C, Caudry M, Saric J, et al. Intersphincteric resection with excision of internal anal sphincter for conservative treatment of very low rectal cancer. Dis Colon Rectum. 1999;42(9):1168–75.
15. Saito N, Ono M, Sugito M, Ito M, Morihiro M, Kosugi C, et al. Early results of intersphincteric resection for patients with very low rectal cancer: an active approach to avoid a permanent colostomy. Dis Colon Rectum. 2004;47(4):459–66.
16. Rullier E, Laurent C, Bretagnol F, Rullier A, Vendrely V, Zerbib F. Sphincter-saving resection for all rectal carcinomas: the end of the 2-cm distal rule. Ann Surg. 2005;241(3):465–9.
17. Schiessel R, Novi G, Holzer B, Rosen HR, Renner K, Holbling N, et al. Technique and long-term results of intersphincteric resection for low rectal cancer. Dis Colon Rectum. 2005;48(10):1858–65. discussion 65-7
18. Shirouzu K, Ogata Y, Araki Y, Kishimoto Y, Sato Y. A new ultimate anus-preserving operation for extremely low rectal cancer and for anal canal cancer. Tech Coloproctol. 2003;7(3):203–6.
19. AlAsari SF, Lim D, Kim NK. Hemi-levator excision to provide greater sphincter preservation in low rectal cancer. Int J Color Dis. 2013;28(12):1727–8.
20. Cong JC, Chen CS, Zhang H, Qiao L, Liu EQ. Partial longitudinal resection of the anorectum and sphincter for very low rectal adenocarcinoma: a surgical approach to avoid permanent colostomy. Color Dis. 2012;14(6):697–704.
21. Shelygin YA, Vorobiev GI, Pikunov DY, Markova EV, Djhanaev YA, Fomenko OY. Intersphincteric resection with partial removal of external anal sphincter for low rectal cancer. Acta Chir Lugoslav. 2008;55(3):45–53.
22. Fucini C, Elbetti C, Petrolo A, Casella D. Excision of the levator muscles with external sphincter preservation in the treatment of selected low T4 rectal cancers. Dis Colon Rectum. 2002;45(12):1697–705.
23. Diop M, Parratte B, Tatu L, Vuillier F, Brunelle S, Monnier G. "Mesorectum": the surgical value of an anatomical approach. Surg Radiol Anat. 2003;25(3–4):290–304.
24. Kim NK. Anatomic basis of sharp pelvic dissection for curative resection of rectal cancer. Yonsei Med J. 2005;46(6):737–49.
25. Grigorescu BA, Lazarou G, Olson TR, Downie SA, Powers K, Greston WM, et al. Innervation of the levator ani muscles: description of the nerve branches to the pubococcygeus, iliococcygeus, and puborectalis muscles. Int Urogynecol J Pelvic Floor Dysfunct. 2008;19(1):107–16.
26. Lazarou G, Grigorescu BA, Olson TR, Downie SA, Powers K, Mikhail MS. Anatomic variations of the pelvic floor nerves adjacent to the sacrospinous

ligament: a female cadaver study. Int Urogynecol J Pelvic Floor Dysfunct. 2008;19(5):649–54.

27. Fritsch H, Brenner E, Lienemann A, Ludwikowski B. Anal sphincter complex: reinterpreted morphology and its clinical relevance. Dis Colon Rectum. 2002;45(2):188–94.

28. Fenner DE, Kriegshauser JS, Lee HH, Beart RW, Weaver A, Cornella JL. Anatomic and physiologic measurements of the internal and external anal sphincters in normal females. Obstet Gynecol. 1998;91(3):369–74.

29. Huebner M, Margulies RU, Fenner DE, Ashton-Miller JA, Bitar KN, DeLancey JO. Age effects on internal anal sphincter thickness and diameter in nulliparous females. Dis Colon Rectum. 2007;50(9):1405–11.

30. Barleben A, Mills S. Anorectal anatomy and physiology. Surg Clin North Am. 2010;90(1):1–15.

31. Uchimoto K, Murakami G, Kinugasa Y, Arakawa T, Matsubara A, Nakajima Y. Rectourethralis muscle and pitfalls of anterior perineal dissection in abdominoperineal resection and intersphincteric resection for rectal cancer. Anat Sci Int. 2007;82(1):8–15.

32. Kim JY, Kim NK, Lee KY, Hur H, Min BS, Kim JH. A comparative study of voiding and sexual function after total mesorectal excision with autonomic nerve preservation for rectal cancer: laparoscopic versus robotic surgery. Ann Surg Oncol. 2012;19(8):2485–93.

33. Kinugasa Y, Murakami G, Suzuki D, Sugihara K. Histological identification of fascial structures posterolateral to the rectum. Br J Surg. 2007;94(5):620–6.

34. Kinugasa Y, Murakami G. The contents of lateral ligaments: is organized connective tissue present? Dis Colon Rectum. 2006;49(8):1243–4. author reply 4-5

35. Kinugasa Y, Murakami G, Uchimoto K, Takenaka A, Yajima T, Sugihara K. Operating behind Denonvilliers' fascia for reliable preservation of urogenital autonomic nerves in total mesorectal excision: a histologic study using cadaveric specimens, including a surgical experiment using fresh cadaveric models. Dis Colon Rectum. 2006;49(7):1024–32.

36. Kinugasa Y, Arakawa T, Abe S, Ohtsuka A, Suzuki D, Murakami G, et al. Anatomical reevaluation of the anococcygeal ligament and its surgical relevance. Dis Colon Rectum. 2011;54(2):232–7.

37. Yamada K, Ogata S, Saiki Y, Fukunaga M, Tsuji Y, Takano M. Functional results of intersphincteric resection for low rectal cancer. Br J Surg. 2007;94(10):1272–7.

38. Akagi Y, Kinugasa T, Shirouzu K. Intersphincteric resection for very low rectal cancer: a systematic review. Surg Today. 2013;43(8):838–47.

39. Martin ST, Heneghan HM, Winter DC. Systematic review of outcomes after intersphincteric resection for low rectal cancer. Br J Surg. 2012;99(5):603–12.

40. Kuo LJ, Hung CS, Wu CH, Wang W, Tam KW, Liang HH, et al. Oncological and functional outcomes of intersphincteric resection for low rectal cancer. J Surg Res. 2011;170(1):e93–8.

41. Yamada K, Ogata S, Saiki Y, Fukunaga M, Tsuji Y, Takano M. Long-term results of intersphincteric resection for low rectal cancer. Dis Colon Rectum. 2009;52(6):1065–71.

42. Weiser MR, Quah HM, Shia J, Guillem JG, Paty PB, Temple LK, et al. Sphincter preservation in low rectal cancer is facilitated by preoperative chemoradiation and intersphincteric dissection. Ann Surg. 2009;249(2):236–42.

43. Saito N, Sugito M, Ito M, Kobayashi A, Nishizawa Y, Yoneyama Y, et al. Oncologic outcome of intersphincteric resection for very low rectal cancer. World J Surg. 2009;33(8):1750–6.

44. Krand O, Yalti T, Tellioglu G, Kara M, Berber I, Titiz MI. Use of smooth muscle plasty after intersphincteric rectal resection to replace a partially resected internal anal sphincter: long-term follow-up. Dis Colon Rectum. 2009;52(11):1895–901.

45. Han JG, Wei GH, Gao ZG, Zheng Y, Wang ZJ. Intersphincteric resection with direct coloanal anastomosis for ultralow rectal cancer: the experience of People's republic of China. Dis Colon Rectum. 2009;52(5):950–7.

46. Akasu T, Takawa M, Yamamoto S, Ishiguro S, Yamaguchi T, Fujita S, et al. Intersphincteric resection for very low rectal adenocarcinoma: univariate and multivariate analyses of risk factors for recurrence. Ann Surg Oncol. 2008;15(10):2668–76.

47. Portier G, Ghouti L, Kirzin S, Guimbaud R, Rives M, Lazorthes F. Oncological outcome of ultra-low coloanal anastomosis with and without intersphincteric resection for low rectal adenocarcinoma. Br J Surg. 2007;94(3):341–5.

48. Chamlou R, Parc Y, Simon T, Bennis M, Dehni N, Parc R, et al. Long-term results of intersphincteric resection for low rectal cancer. Ann Surg. 2007;246(6):916–21. discussion 21-2

49. Saito N, Moriya Y, Shirouzu K, Maeda K, Mochizuki H, Koda K, et al. Intersphincteric resection in patients with very low rectal cancer: a review of the Japanese experience. Dis Colon Rectum. 2006;49(10 Suppl):S13–22.

50. Hohenberger W, Merkel S, Matzel K, Bittorf B, Papadopoulos T, Gohl J. The influence of abdominoperanal (intersphincteric) resection of lower third rectal carcinoma on the rates of sphincter preservation and locoregional recurrence. Color Dis. 2006;8(1):23–33.

51. Chin CC, Yeh CY, Huang WS, Wang JY. Clinical outcome of intersphincteric resection for ultra-low rectal cancer. World J Gastroenterol. 2006;12(4):640–3.

52. Vorobiev GI, Odaryuk TS, Tsarkov PV, Talalakin AI, Rybakov EG. Resection of the rectum and total excision of the internal anal sphincter with smooth mus-

cle plasty and colonic pouch for treatment of ultralow rectal carcinoma. Br J Surg. 2004;91(11):1506–12.

53. Kohler A, Athanasiadis S, Ommer A, Psarakis E. Long-term results of low anterior resection with intersphincteric anastomosis in carcinoma of the lower one-third of the rectum: analysis of 31 patients. Dis Colon Rectum. 2000;43(6):843–50.

54. Bannon JP, Marks GJ, Mohiuddin M, Rakinic J, Jian NZ, Nagle D. Radical and local excisional methods of sphincter-sparing surgery after high-dose radiation for cancer of the distal 3 cm of the rectum. Ann Surg Oncol. 1995;2(3):221–7.

55. Braun J, Treutner KH, Winkeltau G, Heidenreich U, Lerch MM, Schumpelick V. Results of intersphincteric resection of the rectum with direct colo-anal anastomosis for rectal carcinoma. Am J Surg. 1992;163(4):407–12.

56. Benson AB III, Bekaii-Saab T, Chan E, Chen YJ, Choti MA, Cooper HS, et al. Rectal cancer. J Natl Compr Cancer Netw. 2012;10(12):1528–64.

57. Silberfein EJ, Kattepogu KM, Hu CY, Skibber JM, Rodriguez-Bigas MA, Feig B, et al. Long-term survival and recurrence outcomes following surgery for distal rectal cancer. Ann Surg Oncol. 2010;17(11):2863–9.

58. Sauer R, Becker H, Hohenberger W, Rodel C, Wittekind C, Fietkau R, et al. Preoperative versus postoperative chemoradiotherapy for rectal cancer. N Engl J Med. 2004;351(17):1731–40.

59. Garcia-Aguilar J, de Anda Hernandez E, Sirivongs P, Lee SH, Madoff RD, Rothenberger DA. A pathologic complete response to preoperative chemoradiation is associated with lower local recurrence and improved survival in rectal cancer patients treated by mesorectal excision. Dis Colon Rectum. 2003;46(3):298–304.

60. Kim NK, Kim MJ, Yun SH, Sohn SK, Min JS. Comparative study of transrectal ultrasonography, pelvic computerized tomography, and magnetic resonance imaging in preoperative staging of rectal cancer. Dis Colon Rectum. 1999;42(6):770–5.

61. Katsura Y, Yamada K, Ishizawa T, Yoshinaka H, Shimazu H. Endorectal ultrasonography for the assessment of wall invasion and lymph node metastasis in rectal cancer. Dis Colon Rectum. 1992;35(4):362–8.

62. Hunerbein M, Pegios W, Rau B, Vogl TJ, Felix R, Schlag PM. Prospective comparison of endorectal ultrasound, three-dimensional endorectal ultrasound, and endorectal MRI in the preoperative evaluation of rectal tumors. Preliminary results. Surg Endosc. 2000;14(11):1005–9.

63. Ryu JG, Kim YW, Kim NK, Huh H, Min BS, Lee KY, et al. Early experience of three dimensional transrectal ultrasonography: comparison of diagnostic accuracy between two dimensional transrectal ultrasonography, computed tomography and magnetic resonance imaging in rectal cancer patients with preoperative chemoradiation therapy. Korean J Clin Oncol. 2010;6(2):43–51.

64. Kim YW, Kim NK, Min BS, Kim H, Pyo J, Kim MJ, et al. A prospective comparison study for predicting circumferential resection margin between preoperative MRI and whole mount sections in mid-rectal cancer: significance of different scan planes. Eur J Surg Oncol. 2008;34(6):648–54.

65. Chang GJ, You YN, Park IJ, Kaur H, Hu CY, Rodriguez-Bigas MA, et al. Pretreatment high-resolution rectal MRI and treatment response to neoadjuvant chemoradiation. Dis Colon Rectum. 2012;55(4):371–7.

66. Dewhurst CE, Mortele KJ. Magnetic resonance imaging of rectal cancer. Radiol Clin N Am. 2013;51(1):121–31.

67. Brown G, Kirkham A, Williams GT, Bourne M, Radcliffe AG, Sayman J, et al. High-resolution MRI of the anatomy important in total mesorectal excision of the rectum. AJR Am J Roentgenol. 2004;182(2):431–9.

68. Mercury Study Group. Diagnostic accuracy of preoperative magnetic resonance imaging in predicting curative resection of rectal cancer: prospective observational study. BMJ. 2006;333(7572):779.

69. Shihab OC, Moran BJ, Heald RJ, Quirke P, Brown G. MRI staging of low rectal cancer. Eur Radiol. 2009;19(3):643–50.

70. Otto IC, Ito K, Ye C, Hibi K, Kasai Y, Akiyama S, et al. Causes of rectal incontinence after sphincter-preserving operations for rectal cancer. Dis Colon Rectum. 1996;39(12):1423–7.

71. Williamson ME, Lewis WG, Finan PJ, Miller AS, Holdsworth PJ, Johnston D. Recovery of physiologic and clinical function after low anterior resection of the rectum for carcinoma: myth or reality? Dis Colon Rectum. 1995;38(4):411–8.

72. Lazorthes F, Fages P, Chiotasso P, Lemozy J, Bloom E. Resection of the rectum with construction of a colonic reservoir and colo-anal anastomosis for carcinoma of the rectum. Br J Surg. 1986;73(2):136–8.

73. Parc R, Tiret E, Frileux P, Moszkowski E, Loygue J. Resection and colo-anal anastomosis with colonic reservoir for rectal carcinoma. Br J Surg. 1986;73(2):139–41.

74. Hida J, Yasutomi M, Fujimoto K, Okuno K, Ieda S, Machidera N, et al. Functional outcome after low anterior resection with low anastomosis for rectal cancer using the colonic J-pouch. Prospective randomized study for determination of optimum pouch size. Dis Colon Rectum. 1996;39(9):986–91.

75. Drake DB, Pemberton JH, Beart RW Jr, Dozois RR, Wolff BG. Coloanal anastomosis in the management of benign and malignant rectal disease. Ann Surg. 1987;206(5):600–5.

76. Kusunoki M, Shoji Y, Yanagi H, Hatada T, Fujita S, Sakanoue Y, et al. Function after anoabdominal rectal resection and colonic J pouch--anal anastomosis. Br J Surg. 1991;78(12):1434–8.

77. Dehni N, Parc R, Church JM. Colonic J-pouch-anal anastomosis for rectal cancer. Dis Colon Rectum. 2003;46(5):667–75.

78. Nicholls RJ, Lubowski DZ, Donaldson DR. Comparison of colonic reservoir and straight colo-anal reconstruction after rectal excision. Br J Surg. 1988;75(4):318–20.

79. Ho YH, Tan M, Seow-Choen F. Prospective randomized controlled study of clinical function and anorectal physiology after low anterior resection: comparison of straight and colonic J pouch anastomoses. Br J Surg. 1996;83(7):978–80.

80. Hallbook O, Nystrom PO, Sjodahl R. Physiologic characteristics of straight and colonic J-pouch anastomoses after rectal excision for cancer. Dis Colon Rectum. 1997;40(3):332–8.

81. Ho YH, Yu S, Ang ES, Seow-Choen F, Sundram F. Small colonic J-pouch improves colonic retention of liquids--randomized, controlled trial with scintigraphy. Dis Colon Rectum. 2002;45(1):76–82.

82. Seow-Choen F. Colonic pouches in the treatment of low rectal cancer. Br J Surg. 1996;83(7):881–2.

83. Berger A, Tiret E, Parc R, Frileux P, Hannoun L, Nordlinger B, et al. Excision of the rectum with colonic J pouch-anal anastomosis for adenocarcinoma of the low and mid rectum. World J Surg. 1992;16(3):470–7.

84. Seow-Choen F, Goh HS. Prospective randomized trial comparing J colonic pouch-anal anastomosis and straight coloanal reconstruction. Br J Surg. 1995;82(5):608–10.

85. Joo JS, Latulippe JF, Alabaz O, Weiss EG, Nogueras JJ, Wexner SD. Long-term functional evaluation of straight coloanal anastomosis and colonic J-pouch: is the functional superiority of colonic J-pouch sustained? Dis Colon Rectum. 1998;41(6):740–6.

86. Hida J, Yoshifuji T, Tokoro T, Inoue K, Matsuzaki T, Okuno K, et al. Comparison of long-term functional results of colonic J-pouch and straight anastomosis after low anterior resection for rectal cancer: a five-year follow-up. Dis Colon Rectum. 2004;47(10):1578–85.

87. O'Riordain MG, Molloy RG, Gillen P, Horgan A, Kirwan WO. Rectoanal inhibitory reflex following low stapled anterior resection of the rectum. Dis Colon Rectum. 1992;35(9):874–8.

88. Nakahara S, Itoh H, Mibu R, Ikeda S, Oohata Y, Kitano K, et al. Clinical and manometric evaluation of anorectal function following low anterior resection with low anastomotic line using an EEA stapler for rectal cancer. Dis Colon Rectum. 1988;31(10):762–6.

89. Ho YH, Seow-Choen F, Tan M. Colonic J-pouch function at six months versus straight coloanal anastomosis at two years: randomized controlled trial. World J Surg. 2001;25(7):876–81.

90. Harris GJ, Lavery IC, Fazio VW. Function of a colonic J pouch continues to improve with time. Br J Surg. 2001;88(12):1623–7.

91. Z'Graggen K, Maurer CA, Mettler D, Stoupis C, Wildi S, Buchler MW. A novel colon pouch and its comparison with a straight coloanal and colon J-pouch--anal anastomosis: preliminary results in pigs. Surgery. 1999;125(1):105–12.

92. Maurer CA, Z'Graggen K, Zimmermann W, Hani HJ, Mettler D, Buchler MW. Experimental study of neorectal physiology after formation of a transverse coloplasty pouch. Br J Surg. 1999;86(11):1451–8.

93. Fazio VW, Mantyh CR, Hull TL. Colonic "coloplasty": novel technique to enhance low colorectal or coloanal anastomosis. Dis Colon Rectum. 2000;43(10):1448–50.

94. Mantyh CR, Hull TL, Fazio VW. Coloplasty in low colorectal anastomosis: manometric and functional comparison with straight and colonic J-pouch anastomosis. Dis Colon Rectum. 2001;44(1):37–42.

95. Remzi FH, Fazio VW, Gorgun E, Zutshi M, Church JM, Lavery IC, et al. Quality of life, functional outcome, and complications of coloplasty pouch after low anterior resection. Dis Colon Rectum. 2005;48(4):735–43.

96. Baker JW. Low end to side rectosigmoidal anastomosis; description of technic. Arch Surg. 1950;61(1):143–57.

97. Huber FT, Herter B, Siewert JR. Colonic pouch vs. side-to-end anastomosis in low anterior resection. Dis Colon Rectum. 1999;42(7):896–902.

98. Machado M, Nygren J, Goldman S, Ljungqvist O. Functional and physiologic assessment of the colonic reservoir or side-to-end anastomosis after low anterior resection for rectal cancer: a two-year follow-up. Dis Colon Rectum. 2005;48(1):29–36.

99. Matthiessen P, Hallbook O, Andersson M, Rutegard J, Sjodahl R. Risk factors for anastomotic leakage after anterior resection of the rectum. Color Dis. 2004;6(6):462–9.

100. Kim JC, Kim CW, Yoon YS, Lee HO, Park IJ. Levator-sphincter reinforcement after ultralow anterior resection in patients with low rectal cancer: the surgical method and evaluation of anorectal physiology. Surg Today. 2012;42(6):547–53.

101. Matthiessen P, Hallbook O, Rutegard J, Simert G, Sjodahl R. Defunctioning stoma reduces symptomatic anastomotic leakage after low anterior resection of the rectum for cancer: a randomized multicenter trial. Ann Surg. 2007;246(2):207–14.

102. Park IJ, You YN, Schlette E, Nguyen S, Skibber JM, Rodriguez-Bigas MA, et al. Reverse-hybrid robotic mesorectal excision for rectal cancer. Dis Colon Rectum. 2012;55(2):228–33.

103. Baek SJ, Al-Asari S, Jeong DH, Hur H, Min BS, Baik SH, et al. Robotic versus laparoscopic coloanal anastomosis with or without intersphincteric resection for rectal cancer. Surg Endosc. 2013;27(11):4157–63.

104. Kim JC, Lim SB, Yoon YS, Park IJ, Kim CW, Kim CN. Completely abdominal intersphincteric resection for lower rectal cancer: feasibility and comparison of robot-assisted and open surgery. Surg Endosc. 2014;28(9):2734–44.

105. Paun BC, Cassie S, MacLean AR, Dixon E, Buie WD. Postoperative complications following surgery for rectal cancer. Ann Surg. 2010;251(5):807–18.
106. Tilney HS, Tekkis PP. Extending the horizons of restorative rectal surgery: intersphincteric resection for low rectal cancer. Color Dis. 2008;10(1):3–15. discussion -6
107. Kim JS, Lee CR, Kim NK, Hur H, Min BS, Ahn JB, et al. Intersphincteric resection and coloanal anastomosis for very low lying rectal cancer. J Korean Surg Soc. 2009;76(1):28–35.
108. Saito N, Ito M, Kobayashi A, Nishizawa Y, Kojima M, Nishizawa Y, et al. Long-term outcomes after intersphincteric resection for low-lying rectal cancer. Ann Surg Oncol. 2014;21(11):3608–15.
109. Teramoto T, Watanabe M, Kitajima M. Per anum intersphincteric rectal dissection with direct coloanal anastomosis for lower rectal cancer: the ultimate sphincter-preserving operation. Dis Colon Rectum. 1997;40(10 Suppl):S43–7.
110. Watanabe M, Teramoto T, Hasegawa H, Kitajima M. Laparoscopic ultralow anterior resection combined with per anum intersphincteric rectal dissection for lower rectal cancer. Dis Colon Rectum. 2000;43(10 Suppl):S94–7.
111. Akasu T, Takawa M, Yamamoto S, Yamaguchi T, Fujita S, Moriya Y. Risk factors for anastomotic leakage following intersphincteric resection for very low rectal adenocarcinoma. J Gastrointest Surg. 2010;14(1):104–11.

Transanal Total Mesorectal Excision

18

Masaaki Ito

Abstract

1. Transanal total mesorectal excision (taTME)—a down-to-up surgery in which traditional TME that was performed from the abdominal cavity side is endoscopically performed from the perineum side—was proposed, and its safety and efficacy were shown.

2. taTME could offer a unique anatomical recognition different from traditional TME. Especially when dissecting the anterior wall, recognition of rectourethral muscle and Denonvilliers' fascia is characteristic of this technique.

3. Though there are some issues with taTME that need to be solved, it is expected to be effective in patients with severe obesity or a huge uterine fibroid that makes expansion of the visual field and dissecting with standard laparoscopic surgery difficult.

Keywords

TME · Trans-anal TME · Rectal cancer · ISR

M. Ito
Department of Colorectal Surgery, National Cancer Center Hospital East,
Kashiwa, Chiba Prefecture, Japan
e-mail: maito@east.ncc.go.jp

18.1 Introduction

Treatment of low rectal cancer has made rapid progress in the last 20 years. Anus-preserving surgery with intersphincteric resection (ISR) and minimally invasive laparoscopic surgery are good examples of rapid progress in this field. The essence of these advancements is based on the expansion of the visual field and real-time sharing of surgical information.

Rectal cancer surgeries that were previously visible only to the surgeon became open to every surgeon as if a play in a theater with the arrival of endoscopic surgery so that people can see every move the surgeon makes.

Especially, laparoscopic ISR symbolizes the progress in the last 10 years. Near the beginning of the year 2000, this surgical method was initiated with laparotomy and became recognized in providing a delicate dissection technique in the pelvic floor under an expanded visual field in endoscopic surgery. As a result, the surgical anatomy near the anal canal that was vague before the use of this technique had become clear, leading to the development of a new surgical method.

With the development of transanal total mesorectal resection (taTME) that we have introduced here, history will be repeated. In other words, the present method that utilizes the reduced-port surgery (RPS) technique from the anus using an endoscope has the potential to expand even further as a modern surgical method. Rectal cancer surgery that has been developed with various restrictions was considered "the furthest surgery from the abdomen," but looking at it from another perspective, it is "the closest surgery to the anus."

18.2 Transanal Minimally Invasive Surgery (TAMIS)

TAMIS is an acronym for transanal minimally invasive surgery. Previously, transanal endoscopic microsurgery (TEM) was used as an endoscopic surgery from the anus. This surgery was developed by Buess et al. and is widely acknowledged worldwide. It had a major impact on local resections from the anus, rectum, and sigmoid colon. However, this surgical method had some restrictions: (1) devices are expensive, (2) there are restrictions on optical equipment, and (3) there are restrictions on energy devices used by the surgeon.

Subsequently, as the time changed, endoscopic surgeries became further developed, wherein the number and diameter of ports were reduced gradually. In other words, it led to RPS. A representative single-port surgery is a unique surgical technique that is applied effectively to TAMIS.

TAMIS that was first reported in 2009 was used to resect polyp in a transanal manner instead of TEM. However, this surgical technique was later applied and developed toward a surgical method that fully removes rectal cancer or a down-to-up surgical method of performing TME from the anus.

In 2013, a review of TAMIS in its dawn was presented [1]. It discussed the initial status of TAMIS between 2010 and 2013.

According to this 2013 paper, this surgical method is being implemented in 16 countries and was mostly applied to local resections with 390 cases reported worldwide. On the other hand, down-to-up TME has been performed in 78 cases.

Presently, in regard to transanal endoscopic surgeries, TAMIS is used for intestinal surgeries, while taTME is used to perform down-to-up TME after leaving the intestinal tract.

18.3 taTME

With the application of TAMIS, traditional TME could be performed in a retrograde manner.

According to a report on 20 cases from Spain in 2013 [2], the surgical method was proposed as "down-to-up TME." The clinical background was as follows: 11 males and 9 female patients, with the mean distance from the anus to the lower edge of the tumor being 6.5 cm, 3/10/7 cases of upper/middle/lower rectal lesions, respectively, and preoperative chemoradiotherapy for 14 patients.

The mean duration of surgery was 234 min, with the volume of bleeding being 45 mL. The reconstruction method was manual sewing for 13 patients (65%) and stapling for 7 (35%). This report concluded that this surgical method is safe for a well-educated team.

A similar report was presented from the USA in 2014 [3]. In this paper, the same surgical technique was proposed as TAMIS-TME, and the clinical course of 20 cases was reported. This report especially discussed about subjects for whom this surgical method was advantageous and concluded that it is an effective surgical method for obese patients with body mass index (BMI) >30.

18.4 Surgical Technique of taTME and Anatomical Recognition

18.4.1 Preparation

Let us discuss the specific preparation for this surgical method.

The surgery is started with patient in a lithotomy position and under general anesthetic. In the lithotomy position, the lower limbs are a little elevated. If the limbs are elevated more, the monitor from the anus side becomes difficult to view; thus, the elevation of the lower limbs is slightly different from the typical anal operation (Fig. 18.1a). Upon thoroughly disinfecting the area around the anus, a cover cloth is placed around the anus to prepare for the anal operation.

With the use of the Lone Star retractor, the distances from the anal verge, pectinate line, and anorectal line to the tumor are confirmed.

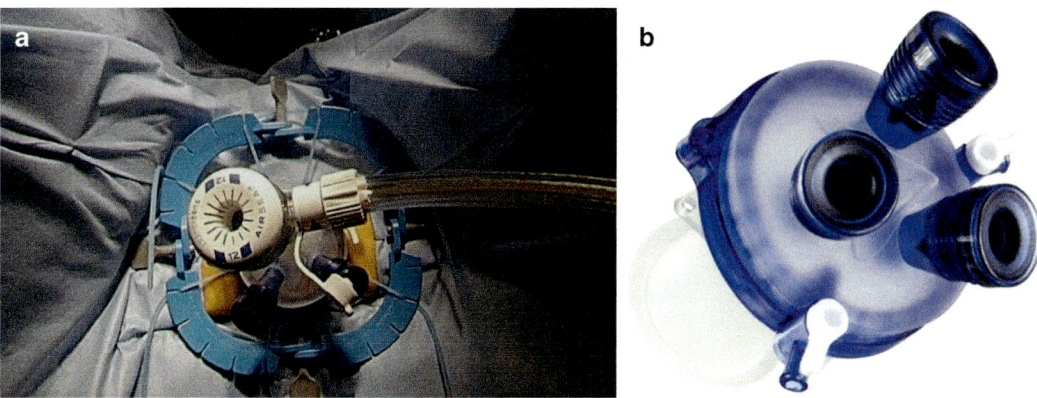

Fig. 18.1 Preparation for anal operation. (**a**) Anal operation. The area around the anus is cleaned, and with the use of a Lone Star retractor, a platform for taTME is applied. (**b**) GelPOINT path. This is a platform for taTME. It allows the use of three ports. The surgical technique is similar to a single-port surgery

Table 18.1 Two types of taTME procedure

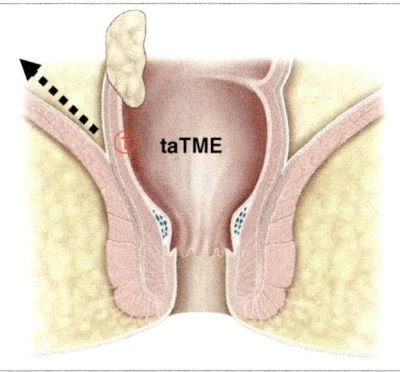
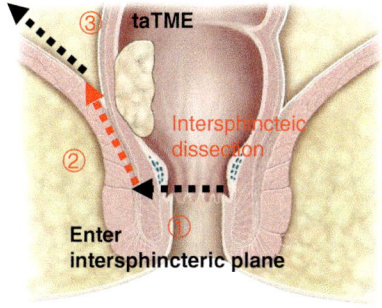

	1. taTME
	– Purse-string suture
	– Initially GelPOINT placement
	– Down-to-up TME under pneumo-rectum or pneumo-pelvis
	– Resectable rectal adenocarcinoma with a tumor edge more than 5 cm from the anal verge (AV)
	2. Transanal intersphincteric dissection followed by taTME
	– Transanal intersphincteric dissection in anal canal
	– Closure of distal stump
	– GelPOINT placement
	– Down-to-up TME under pneumo-pelvis
	– Resectable rectal adenocarcinoma with a tumor edge less than 5 cm from the anal verge (AV)

18.4.2 Applying GelPOINT (Fig. 18.1b)

There are two points of applying GelPOINT depending on the position of the rectal tumor: (1) after intersphincteric dissection from the anal side and closure of the anal-side stump and (2) before starting the taTME technique. The former is the same as the anal operation of ISR and is used when the tumor is near the anus, specifically within 5 cm from the anal verge. If the tumor is positioned in more oral side, first, GelPOINT is applied, and then, endoscopic surgery is performed. In other words, depending on the position of the tumor, the timing of GelPOINT application differs (Table 18.1).

GelPOINT is applied perfectly to the anal canal so that the pneumoperitoneum will not leak. It also allows for the use of three ports.

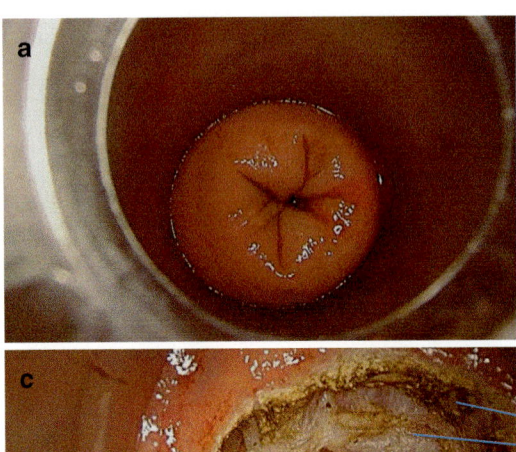
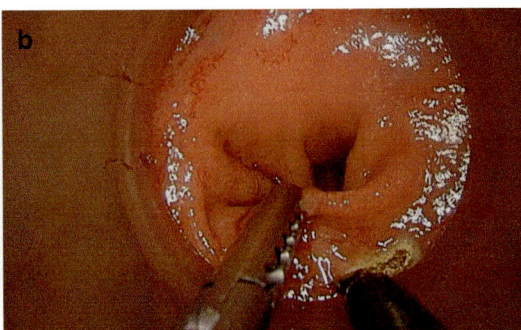

It clearly shows the rectal muscularis propria burned with an electric knife.

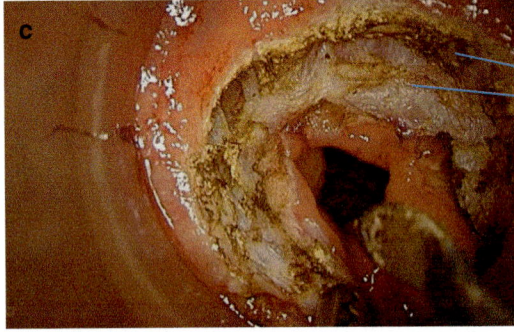

Fig. 18.2 Beginning of the taTME technique. (**a**) GelPOINT use in taTME. A rectal tumor was located about 3 cm from the upper end of the anal canal; thus, without dissecting the anal canal, GelPOINT is applied first, and taTME is planned. (**b**) Dissection of the rectal mucosa. While maintaining a 2-cm distal margin from the tumor, the rectal mucosa is dissected across the whole perimeter. (**c**) Full thickness of the rectal wall is dissected across the whole perimeter. The rectal wall is dissected across the whole perimeter. It clearly shows the rectal muscularis propria burned with an electric knife. After making an incision across the whole perimeter, the anorectal stump is closed. It not only prevents spread of tumor cells but also cleans the anal canal

Thus, it is a surgical method similar to the single-port method, but compared to the single-port method, the surgical field is limited, and since the rectum is fixed with the surrounding tissues, it is easy to build traction. As such, this is a relatively easy surgical operation.

In this paper, we will explain taTME wherein GelPOINT was applied from the start.

18.4.3 Rectal Wall Dissection Across the Whole Perimeter and Closure of the Distal Stump (Fig. 18.2a)

Securing sufficient distal margin from the tumor, the rectal wall is dissected across the whole perimeter with a monopolar cautery. The white layer of the rectal muscularis propria is recognized as the brown-colored burned trace (Fig. 18.2c).

The anal-side stump should be closed as early as possible, and the anal canal is cleaned with saline if possible. Careful attention should be paid to preventing the spread of the tumor.

18.4.4 Dissection of the Anterior Wall of the Rectum

In a rectal cancer surgery, dissection of the anterior wall is very difficult. Especially with the narrow pelvis of male patients, the dissecting procedure is anatomically often restricted. The most advantageous surgical aspect of taTME is indeed the dissection of the anterior wall.

1. Identification of rectourethral muscle

First, an important landmark is the "rectourethral muscle," as an accurate dissecting proce-

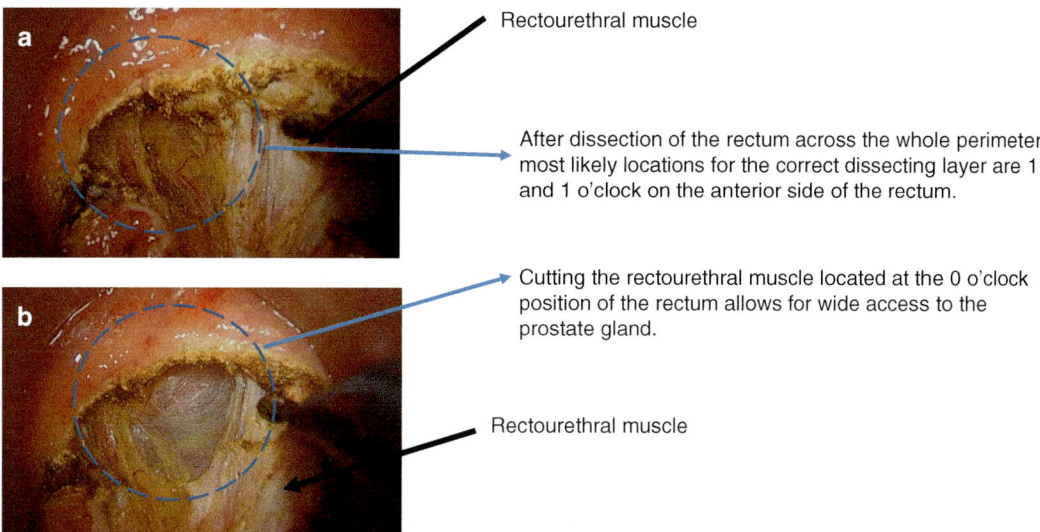

Rectourethral muscle

After dissection of the rectum across the whole perimeter, most likely locations for the correct dissecting layer are 11 and 1 o'clock on the anterior side of the rectum.

Cutting the rectourethral muscle located at the 0 o'clock position of the rectum allows for wide access to the prostate gland.

Rectourethral muscle

Fig. 18.3 Dissecting points of the anterior wall—identification and dissection of the rectourethral muscle. (**a**) Find a space on the left and right anterior wall where it is easy to enter the prostate gland. After dissection of the rectum across the whole perimeter, most likely locations for the correct dissecting layer are 11 and 1 o'clock on the anterior side of the rectum. This space allows an easy access to the prostate gland through blunt dissecting. "Rectourethral muscle," a smooth muscle fiber, is identified on the immediate anterior wall. (**b**) Cutting the rectourethral muscle. Cutting the rectourethral muscle located at the 0 o'clock position of the rectum allows for wide access to the prostate gland

dure is not possible without this recognition. We felt that in the past perineal manipulation in the Miles operation, this "rectourethral muscle" was not recognized. In taTME, identification of this anatomy is performed with high reproducibility.

When the rectum is dissected across the whole perimeter, small amounts of the longitudinal fibers are found at 11 and 1 o'clock positions on the anterior side. If we apply blunt dissecting in these areas, the lower part of the prostate gland covered in membrane is recognized (Fig. 18.3a).

Then, white smooth muscle fibers become clearly visible on the just anterior wall. This is the smooth muscle fiber that connects the rectum and urethra, in other words, the rectourethral muscle. The area called the perineal body may also be closed from here. It is unlikely that intraperitoneal operation can clearly recognize the rectourethral muscle (Fig. 18.3b).

The rectourethral muscle is a structure that needs to be resected so that the prostate gland is clearly recognized on the anterior wall of the rectum.

2. Dissecting of the posterior aspect of the prostate gland and dissection of Denonvilliers' fascia

When the rectourethral muscle is resected, the prostate gland becomes exposed (Fig. 18.4a). When dissecting is along the posterior side of the prostate gland, Denonvilliers' fascia adhered to the prostate gland becomes fixed (Fig. 18.4b). Since this fascia strongly adheres to the prostate gland, incision in this fascia becomes a necessary surgical procedure (Fig. 18.4c). When Denonvilliers' fascia is resected, part of the prostate gland and the whole seminal vesicle can be seen (Fig. 18.4d).

After Denonvilliers' fascia resection, countertraction is applied in the inferior direction, which allows for separation between the seminal vesicle and Denonvilliers' fascia, leading to the peritoneal reflection (Fig. 18.5).

When summarizing dissecting points of the anterior wall of the rectum (Fig. 18.6), there are two large landmarks, the rectourethral muscle and Denonvilliers' fascia, and by resecting these, we reach the peritoneal reflection.

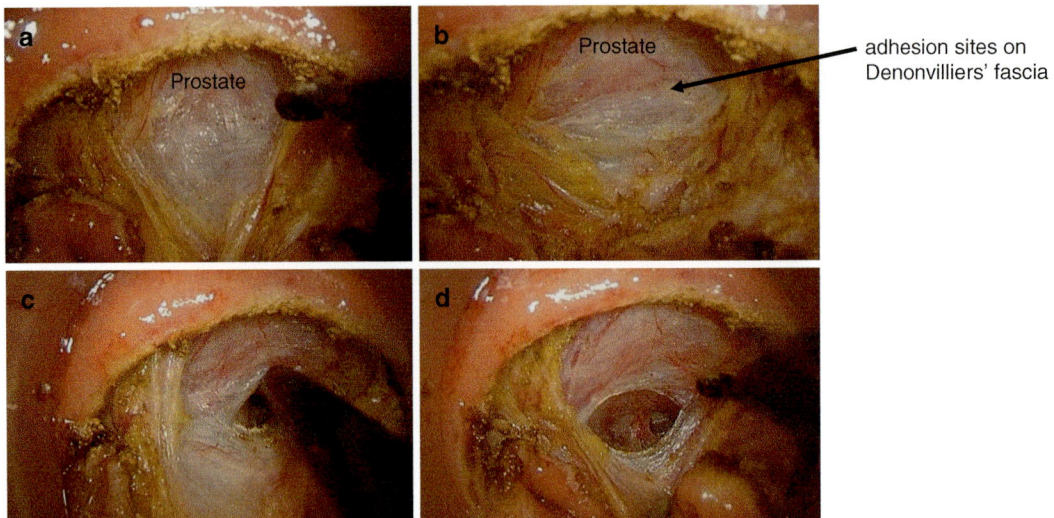

Fig. 18.4 Dissecting points of the anterior wall—identification and dissection of Denonvilliers' fascia. (**a**) Anterior wall dissecting after rectourethral muscle dissection. If the rectourethral muscle is removed, the posterior side of the prostate gland is exposed. (**b**) Identification of prostate gland adhesion sites on Denonvilliers' fascia. If the posterior side of the prostate gland is peeled, the area where Denonvilliers' fascia adheres to the prostate gland becomes clear. (**c**) Beginning the dissection of Denonvilliers' fascia. If Denonvilliers' fascia is not removed, the level of the seminal vesicle cannot be achieved. (**d**) Identification of seminal vesicle after Denonvilliers' fascia dissection. By removing Denonvilliers' fascia, the upper end of the prostate gland and seminal vesicle become visible

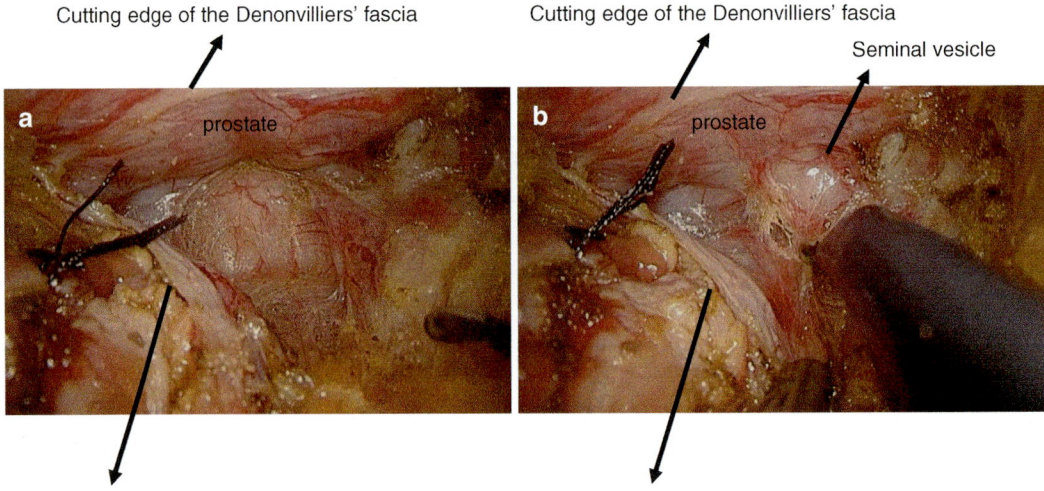

Fig. 18.5 Anatomical recognition after Denonvilliers' fascia dissection on the anterior wall of the rectum. (**a**) Denonvilliers' fascia adhesion position. By removing Denonvilliers' fascia, the position at which it adheres with the prostate gland is recognized. It shows that Denonvilliers' fascia adheres to the upper part of pros- tate gland. (**b**) Dissecting between the seminal vesicle and Denonvilliers' fascia. Once the seminal vesicle is recognized, it is peeled between Denonvilliers' fascia, reaching the peritoneal reflection. This dissecting layer is recognized in a similar manner as the dissecting layer from the abdominal side in laparoscopic surgery

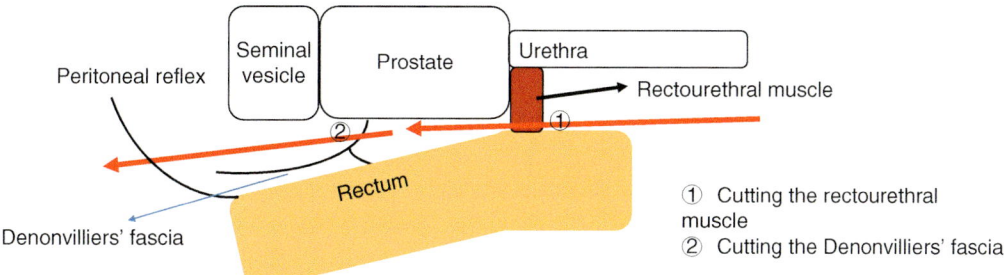

Fig. 18.6 Important anatomical landmarks on the anterior wall in taTME. There are two anatomical landmarks in the anterior wall of the rectum in taTME. One is the rectourethral muscle, and the other is Denonvilliers' fascia. These are structures that need to be dissected. Roughly, when the rectourethral muscle is dissected, the prostate gland and seminal vesicle become visible

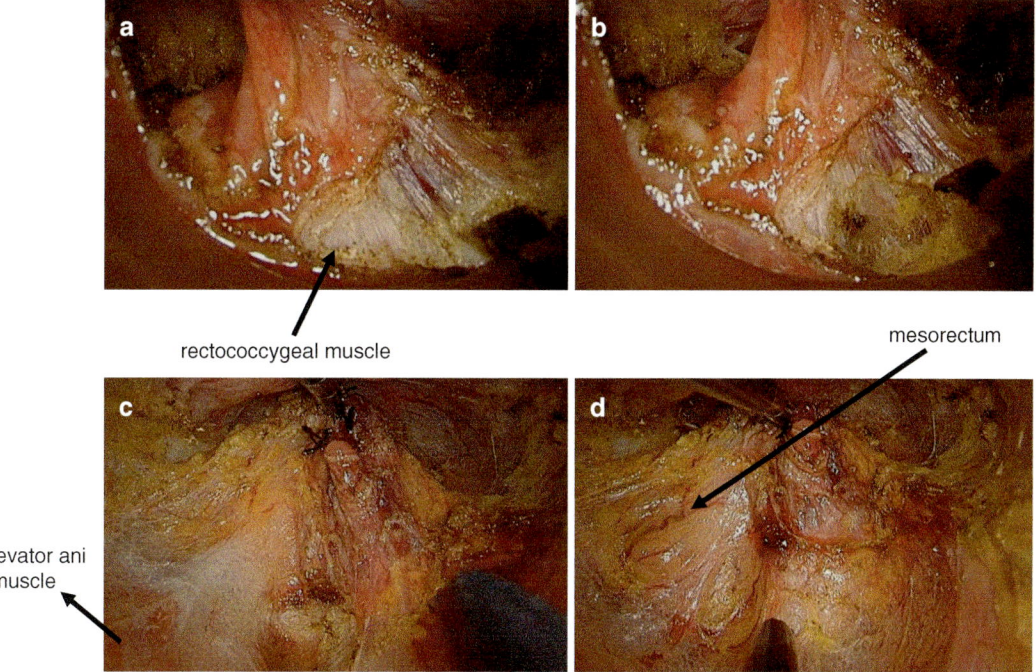

Fig. 18.7 Dissecting the posterior wall of the rectum in taTME. (**a**) Identification of the rectococcygeal muscle. The structure that needs to be identified immediately in the posterior wall of the rectum is the hiatal ligament. (**b**) Dissection of the rectococcygeal muscle. On the posterior wall of the rectum, it is easier to find the dissecting layer at 5 and 7 o'clock of the posterior wall than in the true posterior wall where the hiatal ligament is. The hiatal ligament is a smooth muscle fiber histologically and needs to be dissected. (**c**) Identification of the levator ani muscle and endopelvic fascia. When the rectococcygeal muscle is dissected, the posterior wall of the rectum is widely expanded, but it is easier to identify the levator ani muscle, the external structure, first instead of the mesorectum. (**d**) Identification of the mesorectum. Recognizing the endopelvic fascia that covers the surface layer of the levator ani muscle, each layer is carefully dissected as if dissecting inside over each layer, in order to identify the yellow-colored fascia of the mesorectum

18.4.5 Dissecting Procedure of the Posterior Wall of the Rectum

The landmark for the dissecting procedure of the posterior wall is the rectococcygeal muscle which might be some part of the pelvic hiatal ligament, and it is a white muscle fiber that appears directly behind the resected rectum wall on the posterior side (Fig. 18.7a). It is a smooth muscle fiber histologically and needs to be resected (Fig. 18.7b). The posterior side of the rectum allows for a good

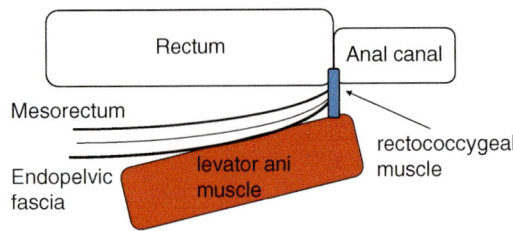

Fig. 18.8 Important anatomical landmark on the posterior wall in taTME. After the rectococcygeal muscle is dissected near the upper edge of the anal canal, even if it enters a deeper layer once, the mesorectum needs to be identified while making the dissecting layer shallow. If the dissection continues in the deep layer, venous injury around the anterior side of sacrum and straying the lateral cavity may occur

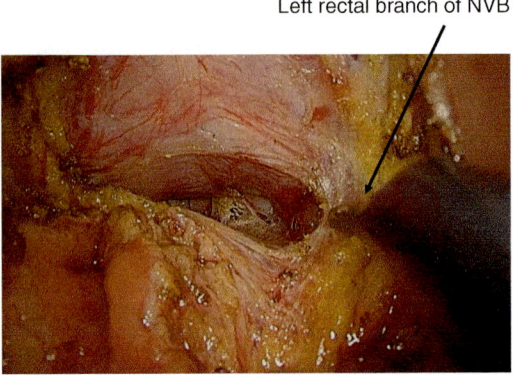

Fig. 18.9 Identifying the NVB. By dissecting the anterior wall to the level of seminal vesicle and applying strong tension to the rectum, the NVB and dissection site that preserves nerves are identified

visual field, and dissecting is relatively easy; however, it is often difficult to select the correct layer to dissect in the early stage of surgery. This is probably because it is an area where fascias such as the endopelvic fascia and fascia propria of the rectum are closely adhered. The dissecting layer is easier to find at 5 and 7 o'clock of the posterior wall instead of directly posterior to it. In some cases, it often gets included in the dissecting layer outside of the endopelvic fascia.

When an incision is made to the rectococcygeal muscle, the posterior wall of the rectum is widely exposed, but instead of immediately identifying the mesorectum, an exterior structure, the levator ani muscle, is identified first (Fig. 18.7c), and the endopelvic fascia covering the anterior side is recognized. It is dissected carefully as if dissecting inside over each layer. It may lead to few errors if the yellow-colored fascia of mesorectum is identified (Fig. 18.7d).

In any case, even if it enters a deeper layer near the upper edge of the anal canal, the mesorectum needs to be identified while making the dissecting layer shallow.

If dissection continues at the deeper layer, venous injury on the anterior side of the sacrum and the nerve injury in the lateral side could happen. Therefore, to achieve good nerve conservation, it needs to return to the correct layer immediately (Fig. 18.8).

In a posterior wall procedure, once the correct dissection plane along the mesorectum is identified, the dissecting procedure becomes relatively

easy. Once dissection reaches the S2–S3 level through good upward traction of the rectum, dissecting is completed.

18.4.6 Dissection on the Anterior and Lateral Sides

1. Identification of the neurovascular bundle (NVB) on the anterior side (Fig. 18.9)

The anterior wall is dissected to the level of the seminal vesicle, and through strong traction of the rectum to inside, the NVB is identified, also recognizing the resection site while preserving the nerves.

2. Identification of the pelvic plexus and dissection of the lateral ligament (Fig. 18.10)

A more common pitfall of taTME is straying the lateral cavity due to dissecting the layer too deep.

To prevent this, the most important aspect is to identify the mesorectum on the posterior wall, and without straying the identified the mesorectum, the lateral side is also dissected. It was notable that traction of the rectum must be performed well during separation of the lateral ligament during the procedure from abdominal side, but it is the same with taTME. With strong traction of the

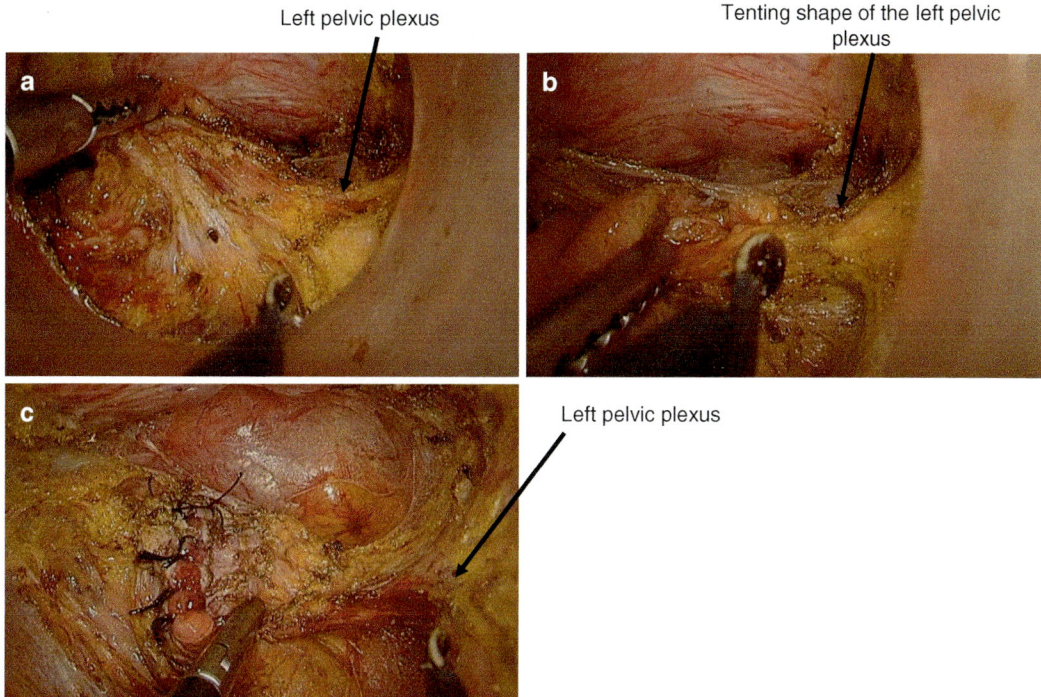

Fig. 18.10 Identification of pelvic plexus and lateral dissection. When dissecting the lateral ligament from abdominal side, thorough traction of the rectum is important. It is exactly the same in taTME. By applying strong traction to the rectum toward the median side, layers of the mesorectum and pelvic plexus are revealed and dissected

rectum, planes of the mesorectum and pelvic plexus are revealed and dissected.

18.4.7 Opening of the Peritoneal Reflection

On the anterior wall of the rectum, if dissection goes beyond the seminal vesicle, a relatively thick peritoneum is recognized (Fig. 18.11a). Through opening, it connects with the abdominal cavity (Fig. 18.11b). The release of pneumoperitoneum pressure that was maintained on the perineal side confirms the connection.

When taTME is performed, a laparoscope is used to create a quick visual confirmation of the peritoneal incision of the peritoneal reflection on the anterior side of the rectum. Based on this, when connections are made from the dissecting layer of the perineum through the whole perimeter, dissecting is completed.

In many cases, since a temporary colostomy is used, specimens can be collected from the stoma sites.

18.5 Present Issues with TME and Those Solved by taTME

In normal rectal cancer surgeries, performing TME in patients with a narrow pelvis is considered difficult. This mainly applies to male patients. Furthermore, in patients with high visceral fat accumulation and high BMI, quality of the surgery is difficult to secure, and curability could be affected.

In such difficult cases, the dissecting operation of the anterior wall is always difficult, potentially causing erroneous identification of layers and unexpected bleeding.

On the other hand, massive uterine fibroids in women become a major obstacle in the normal

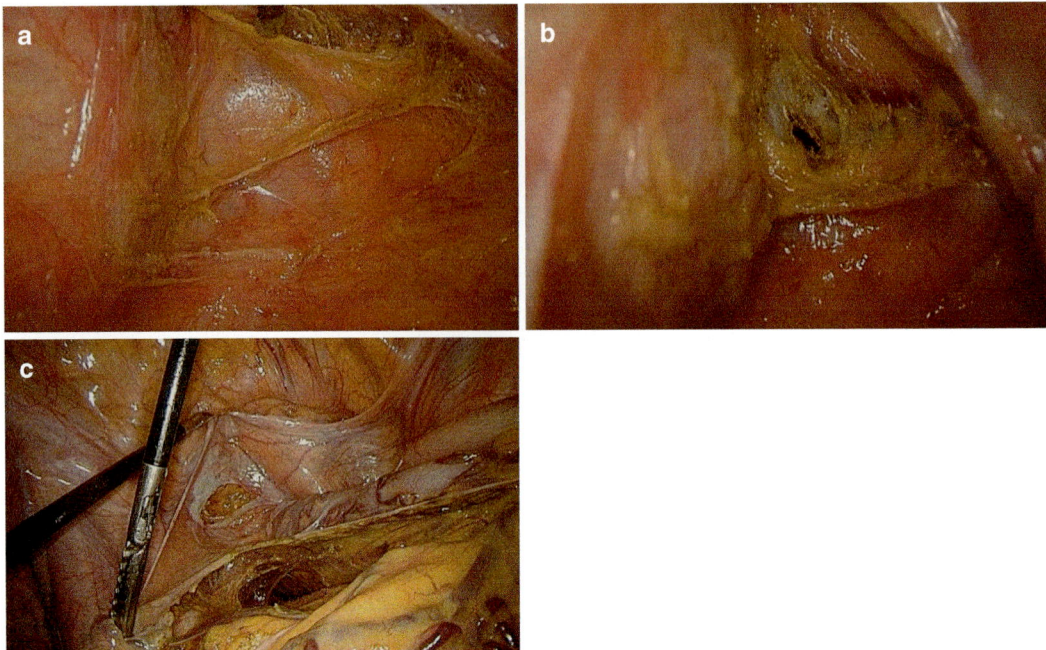

Fig. 18.11 Opening of the peritoneal reflection in the anterior wall. (**a**) Identification of the peritoneal reflection. If dissected beyond the seminal vesicle on the anterior wall of the rectum, the relatively thick peritoneum near the peritoneal reflection is recognized. (**b**) Opening of the peritoneal reflection. Through peritoneotomy of the peritoneal reflection, a connection is made with the abdominal cavity. The release of pneumoperitoneum pressure that was maintained in the perineal side confirms the connection. (**c**) Identification of the dissection site of the peritoneal reflection from the abdominal cavity. When taTME is performed, a laparoscope can visually confirm the peritoneal incision of the peritoneal reflection on the anterior side of the rectum

TME operation, and good visual field expansion cannot be achieved. In patients with a history of pelvic surgery and localized recurrences in the pelvis, identification of the dissecting layer in the normal TME operation is difficult.

As such, with rectal cancer surgery, there are inherent variations in the degree of difficulties in surgery due to diverse pelvic shapes. Furthermore, history of surgery and presence of uterine fibroid that inhibits expansion of good visual field make surgery difficult.

In these cases, taTME is an extremely effective method. taTME will come up with an answer for a simple truth that sites that are even further from the abdominal cavity are very close to the anus.

taTME may lead to the following possibilities:

1. Useful in rectum cancer cases in which expansion of the visual field with a normal laparoscope and dissecting are difficult

2. Useful in the surgical procedure of the anterior wall where anatomical recognition and dissecting are difficult
3. Shorter operation time
4. Recognition of a new surgical anatomy

18.6   Problems with taTME

Though there are many clinical advantages of taTME, there remain problems that need to be solved:

1. Concern of spreading tumor cells by opening the rectum
2. Erroneous confirmation of the dissecting plane, especially in the lateral cavity
3. Difficult identification of the NVB
4. Difficulty in maintenance of pneumoperitoneum pressure after connection with the abdominal cavity

5. Understanding of anatomy specific to taTME
6. Learning is needed before performing taTME

Conclusions

taTME is a technique that is an extension of the perineal operation that was previously performed with the naked eye in ISR and Miles operation. However, as the number of taTME cases increases, this surgery performed endoscopically from the anus begins to feel like a new surgical technique.

With the appearance of laparoscopic surgery, rectal surgeons such as us were shocked with this surgical method that made "invisible" visible; taTME is said to be a surgery that stands on the extension of a similar history. In other words, taTME is a revolutionary surgery that makes "invisible" with laparoscopic surgery "visible."

TAMIS still has various issues that need to be addressed. We hope to solve each of these issues and lead to a breakthrough in the new rectal cancer surgery to effectively treat many patients with rectal cancer.

References

1. Martin-Perez B, Andrade-Ribeiro GD, Hunter L, Atallah S. A systematic review of transanal minimally invasive surgery (TAMIS) from 2010 to 2013. Tech Coloproctol. 2014;18(9):775–88. https://doi.org/10.1007/s10151-014-1148-6.
2. de Lacy AM, Rattner DW, Adelsdorfer C, Tasende MM, Fernández M, Delgado S, Sylla P, Martínez-Palli G. Transanal natural orifice transluminal endoscopic surgery (NOTES) rectal resection: "down-to-up" total mesorectal excision (TME)–short-term outcomes in the first 20 cases. Surg Endosc. 2013;27(9):3165–72. https://doi.org/10.1007/s00464-013-2872-0.
3. Atallah S, Martin-Perez B, Albert M, deBeche-Adams T, Nassif G, Hunter L, Larach S. Transanal minimally invasive surgery for total mesorectal excision (TAMIS-TME): results and experience with the first 20 patients undergoing curative-intent rectal cancer surgery at a single institution. Tech Coloproctol. 2014;18(5):473–80. https://doi.org/10.1007/s10151-013-1095-7.

Functional Outcomes in Rectal Cancer Patients After Surgical Treatment

Sung-Bum Kang and Sung Il Kang

Abstract

Functional outcomes are clinically important in the treatment of rectal cancer patients as they provide clinicians with important information to judge the patient's status. Quality of life is based on the patient's functional status; these two terms are often synonymous in healthcare. The function or quality of life is affected by rectal cancer itself and by its treatment. Clinicians must manage the patient's quality of life and the patient's concerns about disease symptoms and adverse effects. Because statistically significant differences in quality of life subscales may not be clinically important, it is critical to define what differences are clinically relevant. In addition, response shift phenomenon should be considered when interpreting quality of life in longitudinal studies. Although preoperative chemoradiotherapy has shifted the treatment paradigm toward organ preservation, its impact on quality of life is somewhat controversial when compared with no radiotherapy. Minimally invasive surgery may have clinical benefits on quality of life compared with open surgery, but no randomized controlled trials have demonstrated whether laparoscopic, robot-assisted, or transanal total mesorectal excision provides superior effects on quality of life. Sphincter-preserving surgery does not appear to be superior to a permanent stoma. Rectal cancer patients usually suffer from postoperative bowel dysfunction and sexual-urinary dysfunction, but we lack effective tools to preventive these dysfunctions. Therefore, patients should receive information about postoperative dysfunction before undergoing surgery. More work is needed to develop tools to prevent postoperative dysfunction related to rectal cancer treatment and to manage the quality of life of rectal cancer patients.

Keywords

Rectal cancer · Functional outcomes · Quality of life · Bowel dysfunction · Sexual-urinary dysfunction · Chemoradiotherapy · Minimally invasive surgery · Sphincter-preserving surgery · Permanent stoma

19.1 Introduction

Multimodal treatment of rectal cancer has improved its local control and long-term oncologic outcomes over the last three decades. The anal sphincter is preserved in about 84% of patients with rectal cancer [1] owing to the surgeon's craftmanship and to preoperative chemoradiotherapy.

S.-B. Kang (✉) • S. Il Kang
Department of Surgery, Seoul National University
College of Medicine, Seoul National University
Bundang Hospital, Seongnam, South Korea
e-mail: kangsb@snubh.org

© Springer Nature Singapore Pte Ltd. 2018
N. K. Kim et al. (eds.), *Surgical Treatment of Colorectal Cancer*,
https://doi.org/10.1007/978-981-10-5143-2_19

However, up to 90% of patients who undergo sphincter-preserving surgery (SPS) experience changes in bowel habits that range from changes in bowel frequency to fecal incontinence, urgency, or evacuatory dysfunction; this is known as low anterior resection syndrome (LARS) [2, 3]. Although there has been a shift in the treatment paradigm toward organ preservation and cancer control, which have been trialed in selected patients for advanced rectal cancer, quality of life (QoL) remains a controversial issue [2, 3]. Preoperative chemoradiotherapy is also associated with adverse effects and negative effects on the patient's QoL, as well as bowel and sexual-urinary functions [4]. Patient-reported outcomes, such as QoL, are now regarded as key outcomes when assessing interventions for rectal cancer [5].

The previous studies of QoL in rectal cancer patients had many limitations. The results of these studies are difficult to interpret for several reasons [6], including a lack of prospective cohort studies, heterogeneity of tumor location, different instruments used to evaluate QoL, and potential artifacts caused by multiple testing. Furthermore, the previous studies did not report baseline data, especially QoL, age, tumor stage, and preoperative anal function. There are still no definitive strategies for managing functional problems like fecal incontinence and sexual-urinary dysfunction [7], even though they are major problems after rectal cancer surgery [8–10]. Clinicians must manage the patient's QoL and concerns about disease symptoms and adverse effects after rectal cancer treatment [11].

This review focuses on the functional outcomes, bowel dysfunction after SPS, sexual-urinary dysfunction, the effects of chemoradiotherapy and minimally invasive surgery on QoL, and differences between SPS and abdominoperineal resection (APR).

19.2 Measurement and Considerations of Functional Outcomes

Functional outcomes refer to a person's ability to perform tasks. QoL is mostly evaluated in terms of physical, social/role, emotional/psychological,

and cognitive functions [5]. QoL, as discussed in this chapter, is based on functional status, and the two terms are synonymous in healthcare. QoL can be measured during and any time after treatment. QoL is clinically relevant to the treatment of cancer patients as it provides clinicians with important information used to judge patient management [12]. Owing to the inaccuracies of physician-based assessment of QoL, patient-reported outcomes are now accepted in clinical practice [13]. Therefore, validated and reliable tools are needed to ascertain QoL. Measurements are obtained by asking patients to rate their impression of QoL using either a generic or a disease-specific instrument [5]. Generic instruments are designed to evaluate the generalized effects of health problems felt by the patient, whereas disease-specific instruments examine the effects of a specific condition [5]. The type of instrument used depends on the purpose and context of QoL being measured. QoL instruments allow standardized quantification of QoL that can readily support treatment decision-making, evaluation, and follow-up in clinical research and routine practice [5].

The European Organization for Research and Treatment of Cancer (EORTC) QoL Group created a combined system to assess QoL that comprises a generic core questionnaire such as the EORTC QLQ-C30 to evaluate issues common to different cancer sites and treatments [14] and modules specific to different cancers. The EORTC QLQ-CR38 module, for example, was developed to assess QoL questions in patients with colorectal cancer and has been translated and validated for use in several languages. However, the QLQ-CR38 questionnaire may not cover the symptomatic side effects and/or functional advantages of current treatments because of changes in the treatment of colorectal cancer and the questionnaire's limited specificity [15, 16]. Accordingly, work to revise the QLQ-CR38 began several years ago and resulted in the development of a shorter questionnaire, the QLQ-CR29 [17]. Korean versions of the QLQ-C30 and QLQ-CR29 are now available [18, 19].

Because a statistically significant difference does not necessarily indicate clinical importance, it is critical to determine what differences are clinically relevant. In clinical trials, this should be done a priori [5]. Although some investigators have examined this issue by measuring the patient's perceived extent using arbitrary values, some guidelines were recently published to help researchers interpret the results of the QLQ-C30 instrument [20]. In addition, on a review of 152 relevant articles [21], guidelines for the size of effects were provided for the QLQ-C30 subscales and can be used to calculate the sample sizes of clinical trials and facilitate the interpretation of differences in QLQ-C30 scores [21].

Most of the studies found limited differences in the QoL subscales between rectal cancer patients and the general population [5]. In some studies, the QoL subscales were better after surgery than before surgery. For example, in the COREAN trial [22], sexual function had improved at 3 months after open surgery or laparoscopic surgery compared with baseline. This improvement might be associated with a tendency toward a shift in patient responses. This phenomenon is explained by patient's psychological state and methodological aspects [4]. First, the relatively high QoL might be caused by the feeling of rejoice [23]. The diagnosis of a life-threatening disease and successful treatment may positively influence the patient's perception of life, resulting in higher patient-reported QoL values [24]. Another explanation involves the patient's adaptation to the disease and a consequent shift in the patient's reference point. In fact, disease adaptation might cause a change in internal standard values, resulting in underestimation of QoL before treatment and/or in overestimation of previous symptoms [25, 26]. Patients may reconceptualize QoL during the disease course to accommodate their illness.

19.3   Bowel Dysfunction After Sphincter-Preserving Surgery

Rectal cancer patients may experience a spectrum of bowel dysfunction symptoms after rectal cancer surgery that includes fecal incontinence, urgency, frequent bowel movement, bowel fragmentation, and rectal evacuatory dysfunction.

This wide spectrum of symptoms is known as LARS [3] and affects 25–80% of patients [27]. The latest follow-up of patients in the Dutch total mesorectal excision trial revealed that 46% of surviving patients experienced "major LARS," as long as 14 years after treatment [28], depending on tumor location and anastomosis height [28–30]. In a prospective study of 266 patients, Ihn et al. used a validated bowel function scoring system, the Memorial Sloan Kettering Cancer Center questionnaire, and reported that only tumor location was independently associated with impaired bowel function after SPS [30]. They suggest that preoperative counseling should be implemented to inform patients of the risk of bowel dysfunction, especially in patients with lower rectal cancer.

The mechanism of LARS is multifactorial and involves sphincter injury, alterations in anorectal physiology, the onset of pudendal neuropathy, denervation of the autonomic nerve, lumbar plexopathy with anastomotic sepsis, or the use of neoadjuvant chemoradiotherapies [27, 28]. Neurological or structural damage to the internal anal sphincter leads to unconscious leakage of rectal contents, whereas injury to the external anal sphincter usually results in fecal urgency and conscious awareness of impending leakage beyond voluntary control. Rectal evacuatory disorder is associated with loss of rectoanal coordination, manifesting as impaired rectal contraction and paradoxical anal contraction [31, 32]. Anal sensation at the anal transitional zone changes after surgery and is important for maintaining continence, preserving anorectal sampling, and controlling the urge to defecate [33]. The speed at which stool moves through the large bowel reflects contractile activity. Of note, hindgut denervation significantly increases colonic motility in rats [34].

Although there are no specific treatments for LARS, preventive measures should be considered, including nerve-sparing surgery, patient education, the dose/duration of pelvic irradiation [3], and reconstruction after rectal transection. Reconstructive techniques include constructing a side-to-end anastomosis, colonic pouch, and transverse coloplasty. The effects of neorectal volume on function remain unclear, and there are no obvious long-term benefits of any of these techniques [35]. In a meta-analysis of 21 trials comprising data from 1636 patients, colonic J-pouch and side-to-end colo-anal anastomosis or transverse coloplasty were associated with better functional outcomes than straight colo-anal anastomosis, in the first year after surgery [36, 37].

19.4 Sexual-Urinary Dysfunction After Rectal Cancer Surgery

Although sexual problems are common, the impact of rectal cancer treatment on sexual function is poorly understood because the majority of earlier studies were limited by their low response rates. Injury to the autonomic pelvic nerves is one of the most important causes of sexual dysfunction. The incidence of sexual dysfunction after rectal cancer surgery varies widely in prior studies, from 5% to 90%. In female patients, the incidence of sexual dysfunction ranged from 65% to 80%, which is more than expected [38]. Patients feel that sexual function is relevant and needs to be discussed before and after surgery [39–41]. However, more than half of patients perceive that they do not receive satisfactory preoperative information [42, 43], and <10% of patients with postoperative sexual dysfunction were referred to a specialist [44]. Therefore, preoperative consultations should provide patients with information about the risk of sexual dysfunction [45].

Approaches to prevent or treat urinary dysfunction have not been established, even though urinary dysfunction is common and persists for a long time after rectal cancer surgery. Urinary dysfunction is mainly related to autonomic nerve damage during surgery or preoperative radiotherapy. Lee et al. showed that in the study of 352 rectal cancer patients with mild preoperative urinary symptoms, 13.6% experienced acute urinary retention after surgery [46]. This study suggests that it is important to keep a urinary catheter in place for >2 days and consider intraoperative fluid restriction to prevent acute urinary retention after rectal cancer surgery. A randomized clinical trial investigated the efficacy of the selective α1-adrenoceptor antagonist tamsulosin to prevent acute voiding difficulty after rectal cancer surgery [47]. However, administration of tamsulosin at a dose of 0.2 mg/day, as recommended for studies in Asian populations, did not prevent acute voiding difficulty after rectal cancer surgery.

19.5 Impact of Chemoradiotherapy

Multimodal treatment of rectal cancer is based on advances in surgical pathology, refinements in surgical techniques and instrumentation, new imaging modalities, and the widespread use of neoadjuvant therapy [2]. However, preoperative chemoradiotherapy of rectal cancer is associated with adverse effects, which have negative effects on the patient's QoL, bowel function, and sexual-urinary function [4]. Wiltink et al. reported some statistical differences in functioning and symptoms at 14 years after surgery in patients who underwent surgery only and patients who underwent neoadjuvant therapy [48]. In a randomized controlled study of 102 men with stage II–III rectal cancer, erectile and urinary functions were significantly worsened by neoadjuvant chemoradiotherapy compared with chemotherapy alone [49]. A Cochrane review published in 2013 concluded that the effects of preoperative chemoradiotherapy on function outcome and QoL are incompletely understood and should be addressed in future trials [50].

19.6 Impact of Minimally Invasive Surgery

Following the advent of laparoscopic surgery, postoperative QoL has become a controversial issue. In the COREAN trial, which compared open and laparoscopic surgery after chemoradiotherapy in patients with mid- or low rectal cancer [22], the laparoscopic group had better physical functioning scores, less fatigue, and fewer micturition, gastrointestinal, and defecation problems than the open group at 3 months after proctectomy or ileostomy takedown. Although QoL data were not reported in the ACOSOG Z6051 trial and the ALaCaRT trial [51, 52], subgroup analyses of the COLOR II trial [53] revealed that the QoL after rectal cancer surgery was not affected by the surgical approach (i.e., open or laparoscopic surgery). A systematic review [54] showed that neither laparoscopy nor open surgery was superior in terms of preserving sexual and bladder function. In meta-analyses comparing the outcomes of robot-assisted surgery and laparoscopic surgery for rectal cancer, robot-assisted surgery was associated with earlier recovery of urogenital function in men [55]. However, there are no randomized controlled trials showing whether robot-assisted surgery is associated with better urogenital function than laparoscopic surgery [56]. In addition, although the transanal approach for low rectal cancer did not adversely affect bowel or urologic functions compared with conventional laparoscopy, larger well-designed studies are required to investigate these issues further [57].

19.7 Quality of Life with or Without Permanent Stoma

To date, no large-scale prospective studies have compared QoL between APR and SPS for lower rectal cancer, even though a permanent stoma following rectal cancer excision is believed to have detrimental effects on QoL [15, 58]. There is still no evidence supporting routine use of SPS for low rectal cancer, while it is increasingly being used instead of APR for low rectal cancer [59–61]. Previous studies suggested that the rate of SPS for rectal cancer might be a marker for surgical quality [60, 62] and that SPS provided better QoL and sexual or urinary function compared with APR. [15, 58] Nevertheless, many controversies remain, and these studies are limited by selection bias and measurement bias [6].

Some prospective studies have compared QoL between APR and SPS for rectal cancer. The National Surgical Adjuvant Breast and Bowel Project (NSABP) R-04 trial was a randomized controlled trial of neoadjuvant chemoradiotherapy in patients with resectable stage II–III rectal cancer located <12 cm from anal verge that evaluated QoL at 1 year after surgery [63]. Patients who underwent APR reported worse body image at 1 year than patients who underwent SPS, but the latter group reported worse gastrointestinal tract symptoms [63], similar to other studies in rectal cancer [64, 65]. In a prospective study of 100 rectal cancer patients, SPS is a chance for better quality of life than APR, although at 6 months after surgery, the QoL of patients improved regardless of the surgical approach [64]. However, these studies were not specific to low rectal cancer [63–65]. A recent prospective study of patients with low rectal cancer showed that overall QoL was comparable between APR and SPS and that APR was associated with better cognitive and social function, and fewer adverse symptoms compared with SPS [66], as reported in another study [67]. However, those studies involved a small number of patients and did not consider the differences in preoperative QoL between the APR and SPS groups [66, 67]. Unfortunately, a Cochrane review could not provide definitive conclusions on this topic because of the paucity of high-quality studies, and the authors highlighted the need for further prospective studies [68]. Considering these findings, the superiority of SPS may be less clear than commonly believed. The formation of a stoma should not be deemed a failure of surgical treatment, and APR does not reflect suboptimal surgical treatment or quality. A randomized controlled trial comparing the outcomes of APR and SPS may provide strong support for either these approaches in patients with low rectal cancer, but such studies are not feasible because most patients prefer SPS rather than other methods. For this reason, a large-scale prospective cohort study is ongoing, the abdominoperineal resection versus sphincter-preserving surgery for lower rectal cancer (ASPIRE) study, which is comparing QoL and patient outcomes between APR and SPS among Korean patients with low rectal cancer (ClinicalTrials.gov ID: NCT01461525).

Conclusion

The patient's function or QoL is affected by rectal cancer itself and its treatment. Clinicians must manage the patient's QoL and concerns about disease symptoms and adverse effects.

The effect size and a shift in responses should be considered when designing and interpreting studies focusing on QoL. The impact of preoperative chemoradiotherapy, minimally invasive surgery, and permanent stoma on QoL remains controversial. Although rectal cancer patients suffer from bowel dysfunction and sexual-urinary dysfunction after surgery, we do not have tools to prevent or treat such disorders. Therefore, before surgery, patients should be informed about the risk of postoperative bowel and sexual-urinary dysfunction. More studies are required to develop tools to prevent postoperative dysfunction related to rectal cancer treatment and to manage the QoL issues in rectal cancer patients.

Disclosure The author has no potential conflicts of interest to declare. The author received no commercial support for this study.

References

1. Jorgensen ML, Young JM, Dobbins TA, Solomon MJ. Assessment of abdominoperineal resection rate as a surrogate marker of hospital quality in rectal cancer surgery. Br J Surg. 2013;100:1655–63.
2. Smith JJ, Garcia-Aguilar J. Advances and challenges in treatment of locally advanced rectal cancer. J Clin Oncol. 2015;33:1797–808.
3. Bryant CL, Lunniss PJ, Knowles CH, Thaha MA, Chan CL. Anterior resection syndrome. Lancet Oncol. 2012;13:e403–8.
4. Giandomenico F, Gavaruzzi T, Lotto L, et al. Quality of life after surgery for rectal cancer: a systematic review of comparisons with the general population. Exp Rev Gastroenterol Hepatol. 2015;9:1227–42.
5. Juul T, Thaysen H, Chen T. Quality of life in rectal cancer patients. In: Longo WE, Reddy V, Audisio RA, editors. Modern management of cancer of the rectum. London: Springer; 2015. p. 349–66.
6. Ho VP, Lee Y, Stein SL, Temple LK. Sexual function after treatment for rectal cancer: a review. Dis Colon Rectum. 2011;54:113–25.
7. Lundby L, Duelund-Jakobsen J. Management of fecal incontinence after treatment for rectal cancer. Curr Opin Support Palliat Care. 2011;5:60–4.
8. Martin ST, Heneghan HM, Winter DC. Systematic review of outcomes after intersphincteric resection for low rectal cancer. Br J Surg. 2012;99:603–12.
9. Saito N, Sugito M, Ito M, et al. Oncologic outcome of intersphincteric resection for very low rectal cancer. World J Surg. 2009;33:1750–6.
10. Schiessel R, Karner-Hanusch J, Herbst F, Teleky B, Wunderlich M. Intersphincteric resection for low rectal tumours. Br J Surg. 1994;81:1376–8.
11. van Duijvendijk P, Slors JF, Taat CW, et al. Prospective evaluation of anorectal function after total mesorectal excision for rectal carcinoma with or without preoperative radiotherapy. Am J Gastroenterol. 2002;97:2282–9.
12. Gotay CC. Assessing cancer-related quality of life across a spectrum of applications. J Natl Cancer Inst Monogr. 2004;2004:126–33.
13. Bottomley A. The cancer patient and quality of life. Oncologist. 2002;7:120–5.
14. Aaronson NK, Ahmedzai S, Bergman B, et al. The European Organization for Research and Treatment of Cancer QLQ-C30: a quality-of-life instrument for use in international clinical trials in oncology. J Natl Cancer Inst. 1993;85:365–76.
15. Engel J, Kerr J, Schlesinger-Raab A, Eckel R, Sauer H, Hölzel D. Quality of life in rectal cancer patients: a four-year prospective study. Ann Surg. 2003;238:203–13.
16. Neuman HB, Schrag D, Cabral C, et al. Can differences in bowel function after surgery for rectal cancer be identified by the European Organization for Research and Treatment of Cancer quality of life instrument? Ann Surg Oncol. 2007;14:1727–34.
17. Gujral S, Conroy T, Fleissner C, et al. Assessing quality of life in patients with colorectal cancer: an update of the EORTC quality of life questionnaire. Eur J Cancer. 2007;43:1564–73.
18. Yun YH, Park YS, Lee ES, et al. Validation of the Korean version of the EORTC QLQ-C30. Qual Life Res. 2004;13:863–8.
19. Ihn MH, Lee SM, Son IT, et al. Cultural adaptation and validation of the Korean version of the EORTC QLQ-CR29 in patients with colorectal cancer. Support Care Cancer. 2015;23:3493–501.
20. Fayers P, Aaronson N, Bjordal K, et al. The EORTC QLQ-C30 scoring manual. 3rd ed. Brussels: European Organisation for Research and Treatment of Cancer; 2001.
21. Cocks K, King MT, Velikova G, Martyn St-James M, Fayers PM, Brown JM. Evidence-based guidelines for determination of sample size and interpretation of the European Organisation for the Research and Treatment of Cancer Quality of Life Questionnaire Core 30. J Clin Oncol. 2011;29:89–96.
22. Kang SB, Park JW, Jeong SY, et al. Open versus laparoscopic surgery for mid or low rectal cancer after neoadjuvant chemoradiotherapy (COREAN trial): short-term outcomes of an open-label randomised controlled trial. Lancet Oncol. 2010;11:637–45.
23. Nord E. The significance of contextual factors in valuing health states. Health Policy. 1989;13:189–98.
24. Gosselink MP, Busschbach JJ, Dijkhuis CM, Stassen LP, Hop WC, Schouten WR. Quality of life after total mesorectal excision for rectal cancer. Color Dis. 2006;8:15–22.

25. Sprangers MA. Response-shift bias: a challenge to the assessment of patients' quality of life in cancer clinical trials. Cancer Treat Rev. 1996;22(Suppl A):55–62.

26. Schwartz CE, Sprangers MA. Methodological approaches for assessing response shift in longitudinal health-related quality-of-life research. Soc Sci Med. 1999;48:1531–48.

27. Ziv Y, Zbar A, Bar-Shavit Y, Igov I. Low anterior resection syndrome (LARS): cause and effect and reconstructive considerations. Tech Coloproctol. 2013;17:151–62.

28. Chen TY, Wiltink LM, Nout RA, et al. Bowel function 14 years after preoperative short-course radiotherapy and total mesorectal excision for rectal cancer: report of a multicenter randomized trial. Clin Colorectal Cancer. 2015;14:106–14.

29. Denost Q, Laurent C, Capdepont M, Zerbib F, Rullier E. Risk factors for fecal incontinence after intersphincteric resection for rectal cancer. Dis Colon Rectum. 2011;54:963–8.

30. Ihn MH, Kang SB, Kim DW, et al. Risk factors for bowel dysfunction after sphincter-preserving rectal cancer surgery: a prospective study using the Memorial Sloan Kettering Cancer Center bowel function instrument. Dis Colon Rectum. 2014;57:958–66.

31. O'Riordain MG, Molloy RG, Gillen P, Horgan A, Kirwan WO. Rectoanal inhibitory reflex following low stapled anterior resection of the rectum. Dis Colon Rectum. 1992;35:874–8.

32. Rao SS, Welcher KD, Leistikow JS. Obstructive defecation: a failure of rectoanal coordination. Am J Gastroenterol. 1998;93:1042–50.

33. Miller R, Bartolo DC, Cervero F, Mortensen NJ. Anorectal sampling: a comparison of normal and incontinent patients. Br J Surg. 1988;75:44–7.

34. Lee WY, Takahashi T, Pappas T, Mantyh CR, Ludwig KA. Surgical autonomic denervation results in altered colonic motility: an explanation for low anterior resection syndrome? Surgery. 2008;143:778–83.

35. Brown CJ, Fenech DS, McLeod RS. Reconstructive techniques after rectal resection for rectal cancer. Cochrane Database Syst Rev. 2008;16:CD006040. https://doi.org/10.1002/14651858.

36. Hüttner FJ, Tenckhoff S, Jensen K, Uhlmann L, Kulu Y, Büchler MW, Diener MK, Ulrich A. Meta-analysis of reconstruction techniques after low anterior resection for rectal cancer. Br J Surg. 2015;102:735–45.

37. Park JG, Lee MR, Lim SB, et al. Colonic J-pouch anal anastomosis after ultralow anterior resection with upper sphincter excision for low-lying rectal cancer. World J Gastroenterol. 2005;11:2570–3.

38. Celentano V, Cohen R, Warusavitarne J, Faiz O, Chand M. Sexual dysfunction following rectal cancer surgery. Int J Color Dis. 2017. https://doi.org/10.1007/s00384-017-2826-4.

39. da Silva GM, Hull T, Roberts PL, et al. The effect of colorectal surgery in female sexual function, body image, self-esteem and general health: a prospective study. Ann Surg. 2008;248:266–72.

40. Sanoff HK, Morris W, Mitcheltree AL, Wilson S, Lund JL. Lack of support and information regarding long-term negative effects in survivors of rectal cancer. Clin J Oncol Nurs. 2015;19:444–8.

41. Leon-Carlyle M, Schmocker S, Victor JC, et al. Prevalence of physiologic sexual dysfunction is high following treatment for rectal cancer: but is it the only thing that matters? Dis Colon Rectum. 2015;58:736–42.

42. Chorost MI, Weber TK, RJ LEE, Rodriguez-Bigas MA, Petrelli NJ. Sexual dysfunction, informed consent and multimodality therapy for rectal cancer. Am J Surg. 2000;179:271–4.

43. Hendren SK, O'Connor BI, Liu M, et al. Prevalence of male and female sexual dysfunction is high following surgery for rectal cancer. Ann Surg. 2005;242:212–23.

44. Angenete E, Asplund D, Andersson J, Haglind E. Self reported experience of sexual function and quality after abdominoperineal excision in a prospective cohort. Int J Surg. 2014;12:1221–7.

45. Duran E, Tanriseven M, Ersoz N, et al. Urinary and sexual dysfunction rates and risk factors following rectal cancer surgery. Int J Color Dis. 2015;30:1547–55.

46. Lee SY, Kang SB, Kim DW, HK O, Ihn MH. Risk factors and preventive measures for acute urinary retention after rectal cancer surgery. World J Surg. 2015;39:275–82.

47. Jang JH, Kang SB, Lee SM, Park JS, Kim DW, Ahn S. Randomized controlled trial of tamsulosin for prevention of acute voiding difficulty after rectal cancer surgery. World J Surg. 2012;36:2730–7.

48. Wiltink LM, Chen TY, Nout RA, et al. Health-related quality of life 14 years after preoperative short-term radiotherapy and total mesorectal excision for rectal cancer: report of a multicenter randomised trial. Eur J Cancer. 2014;50:2390–8.

49. Huang M, Lin J, Yu X, et al. Erectile and urinary function in men with rectal cancer treated by neoadjuvant chemoradiotherapy and neoadjuvant chemotherapy alone: a randomized trial report. Int J Color Dis. 2016;31:1349–57.

50. De Caluwé L, Van Nieuwenhove Y, Ceelen WP. Preoperative chemoradiation versus radiation alone for stage II and III resectable rectal cancer. Cochrane Database Syst Rev. 2013;28:CD006041. https://doi.org/10.1002/14651858.CD006041.pub3.

51. Fleshman J, Branda M, Sargent DJ, et al. Effect of laparoscopic-assisted resection vs open resection of stage II or III rectal cancer on pathologic outcomes: the ACOSOG Z6051 randomized clinical trial. JAMA. 2015;314:1346–55.

52. Stevenson AR, Solomon MJ, Lumley JW, et al. Effect of laparoscopic-assisted resection vs open resection on pathological outcomes in rectal cancer: the ALaCaRT randomized clinical trial. JAMA. 2015;314:1356–63.

53. Andersson J, Angenete E, Gellerstedt M, et al. Health-related quality of life after laparoscopic and open surgery for rectal cancer in a randomized trial. Br J Surg. 2013;100:941–9.

54. Lim RS, Yang TX, Chua TC. Postoperative bladder and sexual function in patients undergoing surgery for rectal cancer: a systematic review and meta-analysis of laparoscopic versus open resection of rectal cancer. Tech Coloproctol. 2014;18:993–1002.

55. Panteleimonitis S, Ahmed J, Harper M, Parvaiz A. Critical analysis of the literature investigating urogenital function preservation following robotic rectal cancer surgery. World J Gastrointest Surg. 2016;8:744–54.

56. Broholm M, Pommergaard HC, Gögenür I. Possible benefits of robot-assisted rectal cancer surgery regarding urological and sexual dysfunction: a systematic review and meta-analysis. Color Dis. 2015;17:375–81.

57. Pontallier A, Denost Q, Van Geluwe B, Adam JP, Celerier B, Rullier E. Potential sexual function improvement by using transanal mesorectal approach for laparoscopic low rectal cancer excision. Surg Endosc. 2016;30:4924–33.

58. Sideris L, Zenasni F, Vernerey D, et al. Quality of life of patients operated on for low rectal cancer: impact of the type of surgery and patients' characteristics. Dis Colon Rectum. 2005;48:2180–91.

59. Temple LK, Romanus D, Niland J, et al. Factors associated with sphincter-preserving surgery for rectal cancer at national comprehensive cancer network centers. Ann Surg. 2009;250:260–7.

60. Morris E, Quirke P, Thomas JD, Fairley L, Cottier B, Forman D. Unacceptable variation in abdominoperineal excision rates for rectal cancer: time to intervene? Gut. 2008;57:1690–7.

61. Lim SB, Heo SC, Lee MR, et al. Changes in outcome with sphincter preserving surgery for rectal cancer in Korea, 1991-2000. Eur J Surg Oncol. 2005;31:242–9.

62. Tilney HS, Heriot AG, Purkayastha S, et al. A national perspective on the decline of abdominoperineal resection for rectal cancer. Ann Surg. 2008;247:77–84.

63. Russell MM, Ganz PA, Lopa S, et al. Comparative effectiveness of sphincter-sparing surgery versus abdominoperineal resection in rectal cancer: patient-reported outcomes in National Surgical Adjuvant Breast and Bowel Project randomized trial R-04. Ann Surg. 2015;261:144–8.

64. Monastyrska E, Hagner W, Jankowski M, Głowacka I, Zegarska B, Zegarski W. Prospective assessment of the quality of life in patients treated surgically for rectal cancer with lower anterior resection and abdominoperineal resection. Eur J Surg Oncol. 2016;42:1647–53.

65. Näsvall P, Dahlstrand U, Löwenmark T, Rutegård J, Gunnarsson U, Strigård K. Quality of life in patients with a permanent stoma after rectal cancer surgery. Qual Life Res. 2017;26:55–64.

66. How P, Stelzner S, Branagan G, et al. Comparative quality of life in patients following abdominoperineal excision and low anterior resection for low rectal cancer. Dis Colon Rectum. 2012;55:400–6.

67. Kasparek MS, Hassan I, Cima RR, Larson DR, Gullerud RE, Wolff BG. Quality of life after coloanal anastomosis and abdominoperineal resection for distal rectal cancers: sphincter preservation vs quality of life. Color Dis. 2011;13:872–7.

68. Pachler J, Wille-Jorgensen P. Quality of life after rectal resection for cancer, with or without permanent colostomy. Cochrane Database Syst Rev. 2005;18:CD004323.

Part V

Anatomic Consideration for Colon Cancer Surgery

Anatomic Basis Based on Embryologic Plane and Vascular Variation

20

Yojiro Hashiguchi

Abstract

One of the main technical difficulties in the performance of colon cancer surgery derives from the fusion of the mesocolon with the duodenum, the pancreas, and the greater omentum during embryological development. Another difficulty is due to the innate variation of feeding arteries and drainage veins. From the technical aspect, understanding the embryologic plane helps achieve successful complete mesocolic excision (CME), and knowledge of vascular variation contributes to safe and appropriate central vascular ligation (CVL). For CME, a dissection plane between the fusion fascia of Toldt and the subperitoneal fascia is recommended in order to ensure the preservation of the integrity of the entire mesocolon. For CVL in a right-side colon cancer surgery, the superior mesenteric vein and its branches such as the gastrocolic trunk of Henle and the middle colic vein should be carefully treated due to their anatomic complexity and vascular variations.

Keywords

CME · CVL · Fusion fascia · Subperitoneal fascia · Gastrocolic trunk

Y. Hashiguchi
Department of Surgery, Teikyo University,
Tokyo, Japan
e-mail: yhashi@med.teikyo-u.ac.jp

20.1 Background

Total mesorectal excision (TME) for rectal cancer has been established as an optimal procedure to reduce local recurrence [1]. Similarly, it has been advocated that complete mesocolic excision (CME) with central vascular ligation (CVL) be performed as a standard procedure for colon cancer surgery [2, 3]. The concept of CME is the en bloc removal of the tumor along with a sufficient length of the colon, regional lymph nodes, lymph vessels, and fat tissue within the mesocolon. To accomplish a CME, sharp dissection following embryological anatomic planes [4] is required for the mobilization of the colon and mesocolon. The feeding artery of the tumor should be ligated and cut at the root for complete removal of the regional vessels. This concept has been well recognized among Asian surgeons as a D3 dissection [5], which is described in the Japanese Classification of Colorectal Carcinoma [6] and is recommended in the Japanese Society for Cancer of the Colon and Rectum (JSCCR) guidelines 2016 for the treatment of colorectal cancer [7].

A comparison of D3 specimens with CME specimens indicated that both methods provide sufficiently high rates of successful mesocolic plane surgery and long distances from the high vascular tie to the bowel wall [8]. To achieve effective colon cancer surgery, it is essential to understand the anatomy based on embryology. One of the main technical difficulties in the performance of colon cancer surgery derives from the fusion of the mesocolon with the duodenum, the pancreas, and the greater omentum during embryological development. Another difficulty is due to the innate variation of feeding arteries and drainage veins. From the technical aspect, understanding the embryologic plane helps achieve successful CMEs, and knowledge of vascular variation contributes to safe and appropriate CVLs.

20.2 Embryologic Plane

There are many publications concerning fascial composition, and the names used for the fasciae are not consistent among these publications, with variations in accord with the authors' specialties. For example, publications concerning urology usually call the subperitoneal fascia "renal fascia." Herein I have used the names of fasciae according to Mike and Kano [9], who proposed clear definitions and explanations of the fascial composition for laparoscopic colorectal surgery.

20.3 Embryological Development

The primitive gut forms during the fourth week of gestation. Ventral folding of lateral sides forms the midgut, and the cranial and caudal ends form the

foregut and the hindgut. In the subsequent week of gestation, the foregut, the midgut, and the hindgut are suspended from the abdominal wall by the dorsal mesentery [10]. Over the following weeks, the midgut becomes the primary intestinal loop and rotates 270°counterclockwise around the superior mesenteric artery (SMA) and the superior mesenteric vein (SMV), until the third month [9]. Some portions of the gastrointestinal tract develop adjacent to the body wall during development, and the dorsal mesentery becomes incorporated into the body wall, making the organ secondarily retroperitoneal. These secondarily peritoneal organs such as the duodenum, pancreas, ascending colon, and descending colon are especially important in surgical procedures used for colon cancer.

The right fusion fascia of Toldt is formed by the fusion of the ascending colon and its mesentery with the retroperitoneum, while the left fusion fascia of Toldt is formed by the fusion of the descending colon and its mesentery with the retroperitoneum. The embryologic rotation of the bowel and the formation of the fusion fascia are illustrated in Fig. 20.1. The inside of fusion fascia cannot be dissected in surgical procedures.

The central area (pancreaticoduodenal portion) is much more complicated. First, the mesentery of the second portion of the duodenum is attached to the parietal peritoneum and thus

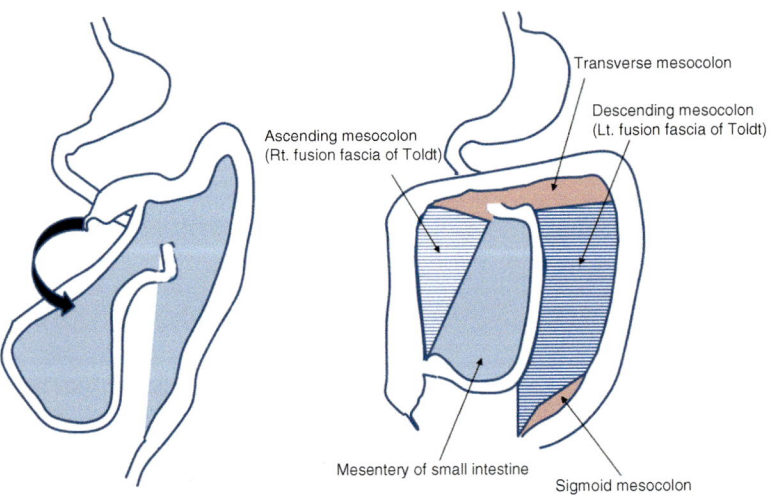

Fig. 20.1 Embryologic rotation and formation of the fascia of Toldt

Transverse mesocolon

Descending mesocolon (Lt. fusion fascia of Toldt)

Ascending mesocolon (Rt. fusion fascia of Toldt)

Mesentery of small intestine

Sigmoid mesocolon

forms the posterior pancreatic fascia of Treitz. The ascending colon and its mesentery then cover the head of the pancreaticoduodenal region and form the right fusion fascia of Toldt and the anterior pancreatic fascia. Thus, the ventral side of the second portion of the duodenum and the pancreas head are covered by the anterior pancreatic fascia, while their dorsal side is covered by the posterior pancreatic fascia [9]. As the right fusion fascia of Toldt separates into these two planes in the pancreaticoduodenal portion, it is not easy to identify the appropriate planes of dissection to perform a CME. The basic concept of surgery for colorectal cancer is to strictly separate the entire mesocolon off the retroperitoneal plane, preserving its integrity. The recognition of the fascia during surgery leads to the correct dissection along the right plane.

20.4 Selection of Dissection Plane

To avoid unnecessary bleeding and tumor exposure, surgical procedures for colon cancer should be performed in accordance with the embryonic fascial anatomy. West et al. [4] proposed a grading system of colon surgery on the basis of the presence and extent of any identifiable mesocolic defects. The grading includes dissection in the mesocolic plane (when an intact mesocolon is present), the intramesocolic plane (when there are significant mesocolic defects that do not expose the muscularis propria), or the muscularis propria plane (when significant and extensive defects that expose areas of muscularis propria are observed). The final grading is based on the poorest area, regardless of its relationship to the area of the tumor [4]. Throughout the embryological development, there are fusions of fascia and complicated layers surrounding the colon. If the dissection plane develops close to the colon and mesocolon, there is a greater chance that significant mesocolic defects will develop and/or that the muscularis propria of the colon will be observed. The appropriate dissection plane should thus be selected.

20.5 The Fascial Composition of the Right Side of the Colon with Respect to the Dissection Plane

The fascial composition of the right side of the colon is described in Fig. 20.2a–c. The caudal side is simple, and the cranial pancreaticoduodenal portion is more complexed due to the embryologic rotation of the bowel.

For CME, a dissection plane between the right fusion fascia of Toldt and the subperitoneal fascia is recommended in order to ensure the preservation of the integrity of the entire mesocolon. In this case, the procedure begins with the incision of the peritoneum at the base of the mesentery of the terminal ileum and then proceeds cranially to the lower portion of the right colon, dissecting between the Toldt's fusion fascia and the subperitoneal fascia. The dissection should proceed medially to the second portion of the duodenum.

When this dissection plane is taken, the plane should be intentionally shifted ventrally by incising the Toldt's fusion fascia or the posterior pancreatic fascia when the dissection reaches the second or third portion of the duodenum, because the right fusion fascia of Toldt divides into two planes and the dorsal side becomes the posterior pancreatic fascia of the Treitz (Fig. 20.1b). If the original dissection plane (between the Toldt's fusion fascia and the subperitoneal fascia) is continued cranially, the dissection can proceed toward the dorsal side of the duodenum and pancreas. The dissection should be continued cranially along the ventral and medial sides of the second portion of the duodenum. The transverse mesocolon is separated from the pancreas and gastroepiploic veins by dividing the greater omentum. By taking this plane, the dissection is performed along the ventral side of the subperitoneal fascia and the surface of the duodenum and pancreas. This is considered the ideal plane for the en bloc resection of colon cancer. The ideal dissection plane for the right side of the colon is demonstrated in the Fig. 20.2a–c. The pancreaticoduodenal

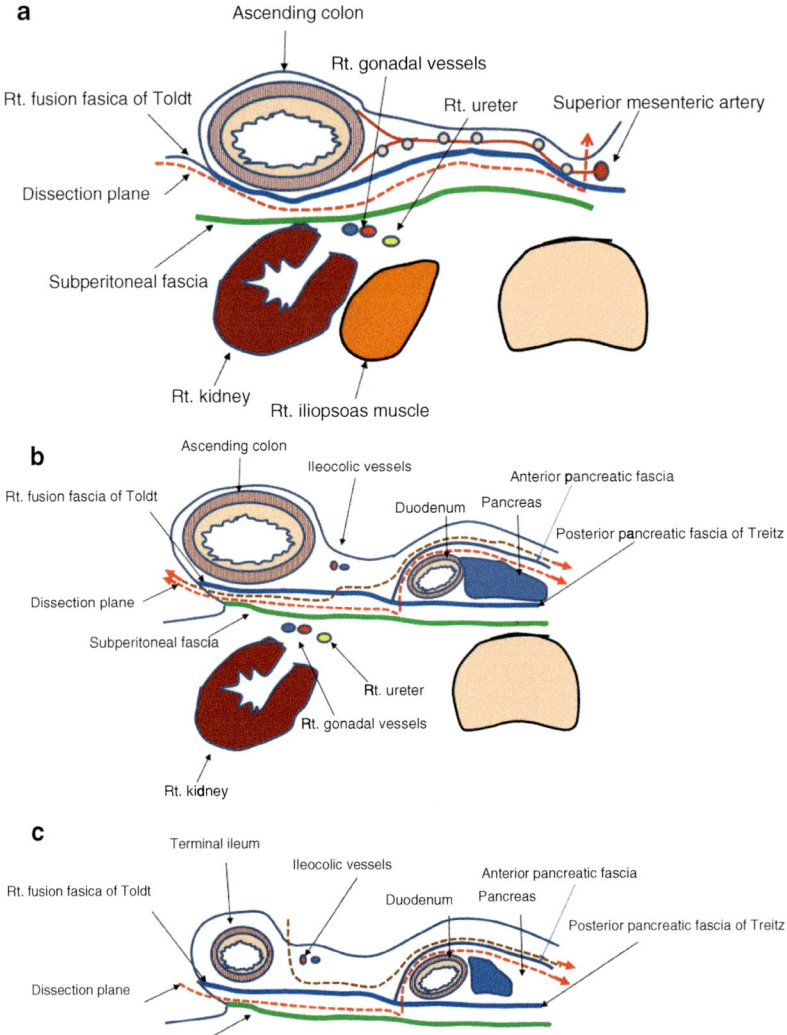

Fig. 20.2 (**a**) Dissection plane for the caudal portion of the right-side colon. Dissection plane should be between the right fusion fascia of Toldt and the subperitoneal fascia (red dotted line). (**b**) The dissection plane for the cranial portion of the right side of the colon. The ideal dissection plane is between the right fusion fascia of Toldt and the subperitoneal fascia and then ventrally shifted between the anterior pancreatic fascia and the duodenum (red dotted line). In the median approach used for a laparoscopic right hemicolectomy, the shallower dissection plane is usually selected (brown dotted line). (**c**) Sagittal view of the dissection plane for the right side of the colon. The ideal dissection plane is started at the base of the terminal ileum between the right fusion fascia of Toldt and the subperitoneal fascia and then ventrally shifted between the anterior pancreatic fascia and the duodenum (red dotted line). In the median approach used for the laparoscopic right hemicolectomy, the dissection is usually started bellow the ileocolic vessels and continues dissecting the ventral plane of the fusion fascia of Toldt cranially, following the shallower dissection plane (brown dotted line)

portion and surgical trunk after a CME and CVL are shown in Fig. 20.3a.

There is a trend for the selection of a shallower dissection plane in the medial approach in laparoscopic surgery. In this case, the dissection is begun by lifting the ileocolic vessels and then continued by dissecting the ventral plane of the Toldt's fusion fascia. The plane of this dissection

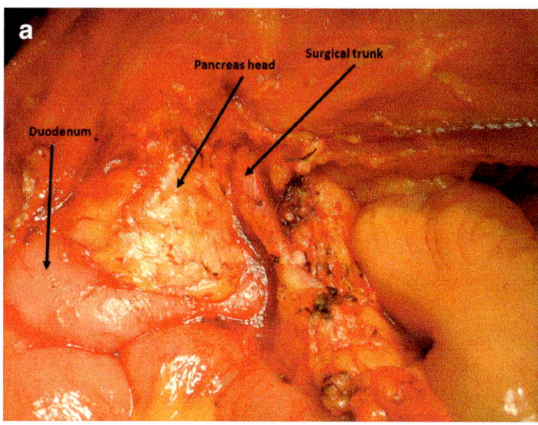
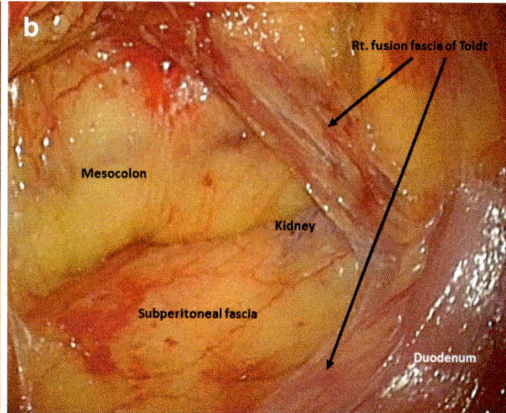

Fig. 20.3 (**a**) The view of the pancreaticoduodenal portion after CME and CVL by open right hemicolectomy. The duodenum and pancreas head are exposed without the fascia. (**b**) The relationship among the subperitoneal fascia, right fusion fascia of Toldt, and mesocolon in the cranial portion of right-side colon observed by laparoscopy

is performed within the mesentery, leaving the fusion fascia with the retroperitoneum. With the use of this plane, the duodenum and pancreas are automatically left on the dorsal side of the dissection layer. However, when the dissection approaches the ascending colon or transverse colon, it becomes difficult to separate the fusion fascia and colon. Thus, the dissection plane is eventually shifted to the plane between the fusion fascia and the subperitoneal fascia. This plane of dissection may not be appropriate for maintaining the integrity of the entire mesocolon. The laparoscopic view of the subperitoneal fascia, the right fusion fascia of Toldt, and the mesocolon are shown in Fig. 20.3b.

20.6 The Fascial Composition of the Left-Side Colon with Respect to the Dissection Plane

Although the descending colon loses its mobility due to the formation of the left fusion fascia of Toldt, the sigmoid colon maintains a degree of mobility that varies among individuals. When a sigmoidectomy is performed, a lateral approach is common for open surgery, and a medial approach is common for laparoscopic surgery.

Either way, the dissection should be performed between the left fusion fascia of Toldt and the subperitoneal fascia to sufficiently mobilize the left side of the colon. The dissection plane between the fusion fascia and the subperitoneal fascia is shown in Fig. 20.4.

As the subperitoneal fascia continues to the fascia propria of the rectum, this "fascia propria" should be identified at the level of promontorium in the medial approach. The incision of the retroperitoneum and the dissection between the fusion fascia and the subperitoneal fascia should be extended cranially and then toward the left, leaving the left ureter and gonadal vessels under the subperitoneal fascia. After the sufficient dissection from the medial side, the lateral approach should be started by incising the white line of Toldt. The integrity is maintained by the resection of the fusion fascia with the mesocolon (Fig. 20.5).

In the case of a patient with cancer at the splenic flexure, left hemicolectomy is selected as the standard surgery. In this case, the dissection between the fusion fascia and subperitoneal fascia is extended cranially to the pancreas. As the subperitoneal fascia continues to the dorsal side of the pancreas, the dissection plane should be shifted ventrally at the lower border of the pancreas. This shift is relatively difficult in fatty patients.

Fig. 20.4 Dissection plane for the caudal portion of the left-side colon. Dissection plane should be between the left fusion fascia of Toldt and the subperitoneal fascia (red dotted line)

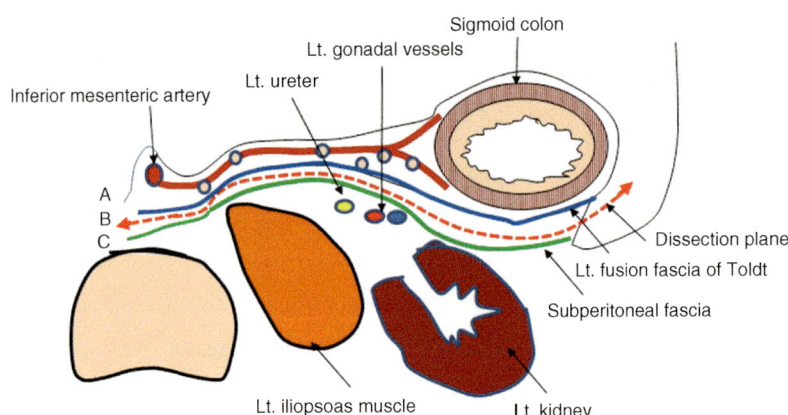

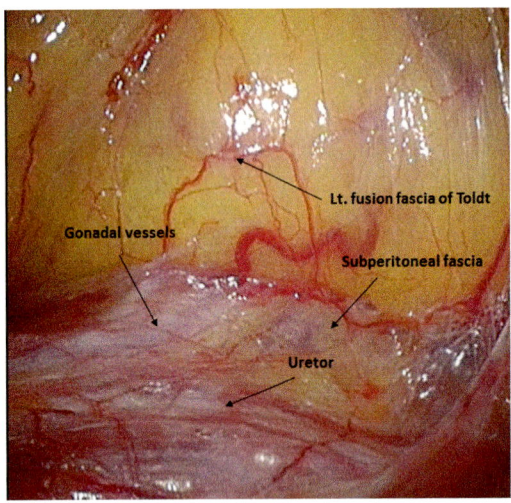

Fig. 20.5 Dissection plane for the caudal portion of the sigmoid colon during a median approach by laparoscopic sigmoidectomy. The dissection was performed between the left fusion fascia of Toldt and the subperitoneal fascia

anastomotic leakage after a CVL of the inferior mesenteric artery (IMA) or middle colic artery (MCA). Knowing the potential vascular variations is essential for the safe and effective ligation of feeding arteries and draining veins. It is also important when considering the optimal margins for bowel resection and the blood supply for anastomotic reconstruction.

20.8 Right-Side Colon

The inferior mesenteric vein (IMV), which is called "surgical trunk" in cases of colon cancer surgery, should be exposed to perform a CVL and to remove the regional lymph nodes at the root of feeding arteries. The typical appearance of the surgical trunk is shown in Fig. 20.6. However, there are many variations in the right-side colon.

20.7 Vascular Variation

There are a large number of vascular variations in the colon as compared to the rectum. As the proximal two-thirds of the transverse colon originate from the midgut and the distal third of the transverse colon to rectum from the hindgut, there is a clear separation of the blood-supplying and blood-draining routes between these two parts of the colon. The connection between the right-side colon and the left-side colon is sometimes loose and becomes the cause of

20.8.1 Arteries

The right-side colon is supplied by the SMA. There are three major branches of SMA: the ileocolic artery (ICA), the right colic artery (RCA), and the MCA. The ICA always directly arises from the SMA and is constantly present. In contrast, the RCA much less frequently arises from the SMA and may arise from the ICA or the MCA. This variation of the RCA should be taken into consideration while dissection is performed along the surgical trunk. The MCA usually arises

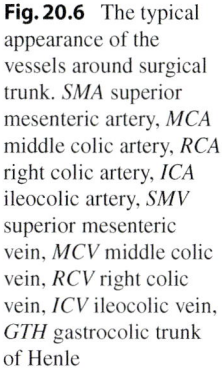
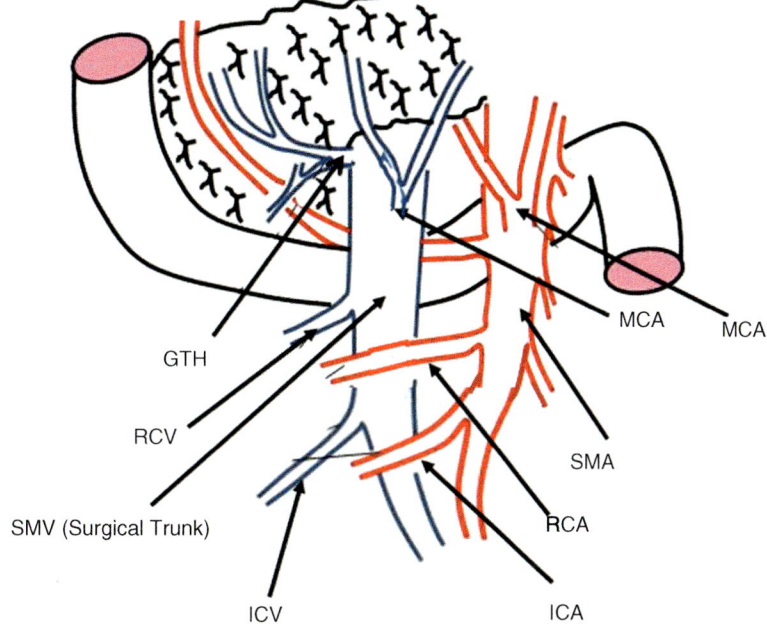

Fig. 20.6 The typical appearance of the vessels around surgical trunk. *SMA* superior mesenteric artery, *MCA* middle colic artery, *RCA* right colic artery, *ICA* ileocolic artery, *SMV* superior mesenteric vein, *MCV* middle colic vein, *RCV* right colic vein, *ICV* ileocolic vein, *GTH* gastrocolic trunk of Henle

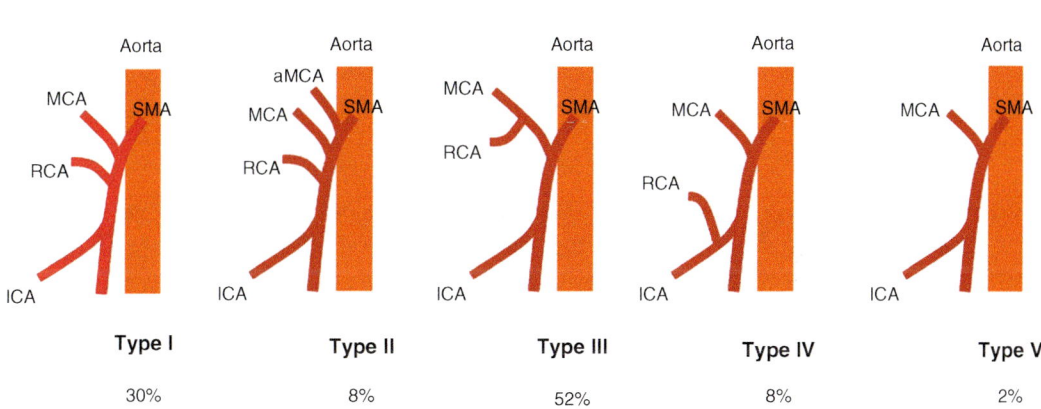

Fig. 20.7 Variation of the right colic and middle colic arteries. Type I, RCA and MCA from SMA (30%). Type II, RCA, MCA, and accessory (a)MCA from SMA (8%). Type III, RCA from MCA (52%). Type IV, RCA from ICA (8%). Type V, no RCA (2%) [11]

directly from the SMA and is divided into two (right and left) branches or three branches (right, left, and accessory). In some cases, the right MCA and the left MCA separately and directly arise from the SMA, resulting in the absence of the MCA. Anatomic variations of the RCA and MCA with the incidences are shown in Fig. 20.7 [11].The incidences are largely in accordance with the recent data from cadavers [12, 13].

20.8.2 Veins

Performing a CVL has the potential to injure a vein. Vein injury during a laparoscopic surgery for right-sided colon cancer may result in massive bleeding and is one of the leading causes of conversion to open surgery. The risk of inadvertent vascular injury is particularly increased when vessels for CVL are exposed. The SMV and its branches such as the gastrocolic trunk of Henle (GTH) and the middle colic vein (MCV) should be carefully treated due to their anatomic complexity and vascular variations.

The unexpected variation of the GTH is one of the factors contributing to the incidence of serious bleeding during colon cancer surgery [14]. Alsabilah et al. [15] reported their intraoperative charting of right colonic arteriovenous anatomy. They suggested five types of GTH based on venous tributaries from the right colon: type I, no venous tributaries (58.1%); type II, RCV only (16.1%); type III, RCV and accessory (a)MCV (8.1%); type IV, RCV and MCV (3.2%); and type V, MCV only (3.2%) (Fig. 20.8) [15].

The relationship of the ICA and the SMV is important for the central vascular ligation of an ICA. Several studies noted that the ICA passes the SMV anteriorly or posteriorly at similar incidences [16]. When the ICA passes the SMV posteriorly, ligation of the ICA at the root from the SMA is much more difficult for laparoscopic surgery, and the ligation is performed at the left side of the SMV. The required level of D3 lymph node dissection for patients whose ICA passes the SMV posteriorly is an unsettled matter.

20.9 Left-Side Colon

For left-sided colon cancer, the central vessels are the IMA and the IMV. However, the IMA is often preserved for descending colon cancer surgery, whereas the left colic artery (LCA) is often preserved for sigmoid colon or rectal cancer surgery. In such cases, the variation of the feeding arteries is more important.

20.9.1 Arteries

The IMA arises from the abdominal aorta. The main branches are the LCA and the superior rectal artery (SRA). Two or more sigmoid branches originate from the LCA or SRA. The pattern of IMA variation is shown in Fig. 20.9 [11]. The distance

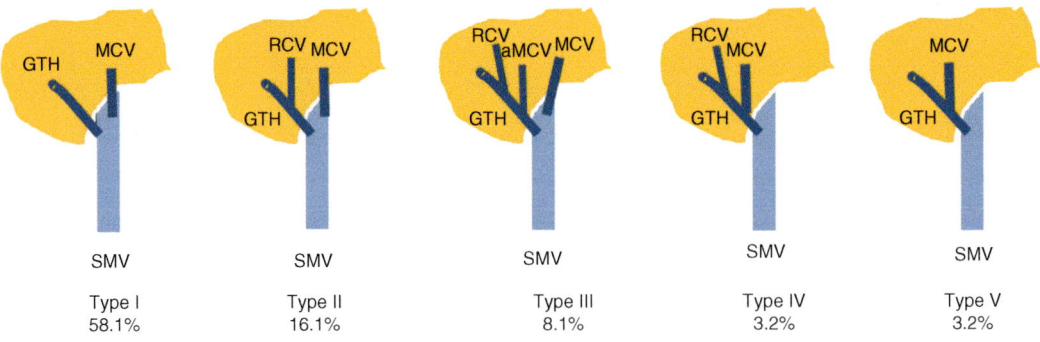

Fig. 20.8 Variation of gastrocolic trunk of Henle (GTH). Type I, no venous tributaries (58.1%). Type II, RCV only (16.1%). Type III, RCV and aMCV (8.1%). Type IV, RCV and MCV (3.2%). Type V, MCV only (3.2%) [15]

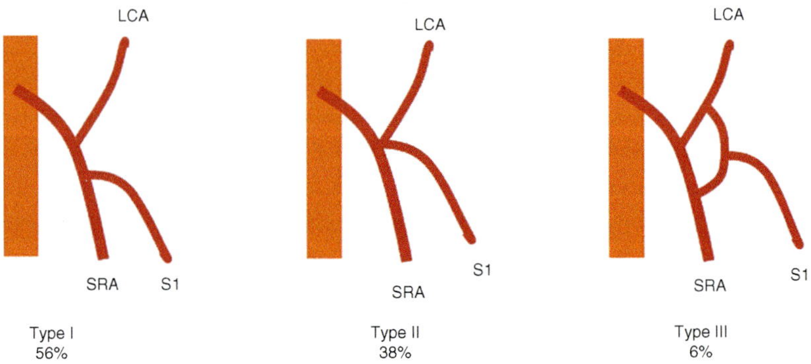

Fig. 20.9 Variation of left colic artery. Type I, isolated divergence from IMA (56%). Type II, common divergence with S1 from IMA (38%). Type III, formation of small arch (6%) [11]

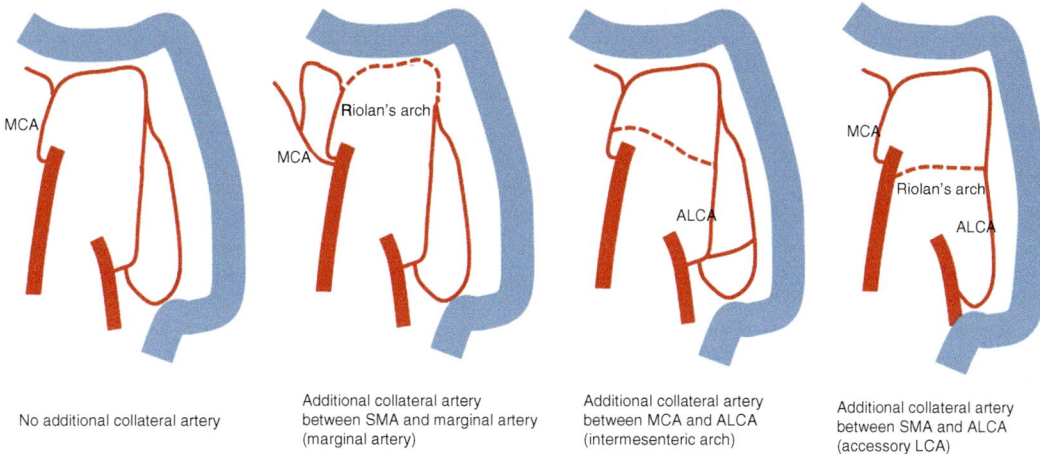

No additional collateral artery

Additional collateral artery between SMA and marginal artery (marginal artery)

Additional collateral artery between MCA and ALCA (intermesenteric arch)

Additional collateral artery between SMA and ALCA (accessory LCA)

Fig. 20.10 Variations of Riolan's arch. Riolan's arch may be identical to the marginal artery connecting the SMA and the IMA. Otherwise, Riolan's arch may repre-sent a rare artery, connecting the MCA to an ascending left colic artery (ALCA) or the SMA to an ALCA

from the origin of the IMA to the branch of the LCA or the first sigmoid branch (S1) also varies considerably among individuals. These variations are particularly important when a CVL is not per-formed and the LCA or S1 is intentionally pre-served for patients with early-stage cancer or for patients with a high risk of complications.

20.9.2 Veins

The left-side colon has also shown variations of drainage vein, but these variations are not usually the cause of serious hemorrhage and are thus clinically less important.

20.10 Riolan's Arch

The connection of the SMA and IMA is impor-tant when the IMA is ligated and cut at the root as the CVL procedure. The term "Riolan's arch" is often used as the name of the artery connect-ing the SMA and the IMA, but Riolan's arch may be identical to the marginal artery connect-ing the SMA and the IMA. Otherwise, Riolan's arch may represent a rare artery connecting the MCA to the ascending LCA. It is suggested that the marginal artery is usually sufficient for left colic circulation after ligation of the IMA. However, the connection of the marginal

artery with the ascending LCA at the level of the left transverse colon might be important in chronic atherosclerotic obstructive disease of the SMA, IMA, and/or celiac trunk [17]. Therefore, it is recommended that ligation of the IMA should be avoided if a hypertrophic ascending LCA is identified. Riolan's arch is described in Fig. 20.10.

References

1. Heald RJ. Total mesorectal excision. The new European gold standard. G Chir. 1998;19(6–7):253–5.
2. Hohenberger W, Weber K, Matzel K, Papadopoulos T, Merkel S. Standardized surgery for colonic can-cer: complete mesocolic excision and central liga-tion – technical notes and outcome. Color Dis. 2009; 11(4):354–64. discussion 64-5.
3. West NP, Hohenberger W, Weber K, Perrakis A, Finan PJ, Quirke P. Complete mesocolic excision with central vascular ligation produces an oncologi-cally superior specimen compared with standard sur-gery for carcinoma of the colon. J Clin Oncol. 2010; 28(2):272–8.
4. West NP, Morris EJ, Rotimi O, Cairns A, Finan PJ, Quirke P. Pathology grading of colon cancer sur-gical resection and its association with survival: a retrospective observational study. Lancet Oncol. 2008;9(9):857–65.
5. Xie D, Yu C, Gao C, Osaiweran H, Hu J, Gong J. An optimal approach for laparoscopic D3 lymphadenec-tomy plus complete mesocolic excision (D3+CME) for right-sided colon cancer. Ann Surg Oncol. 2017;24(5): 1312–3.

6. Japanese Society for Cancer of the Colon and Rectum. Japanese classification of colorectal carcinoma (second English edition). Tokyo: Kanehara; 2009.

7. Watanabe T, Muro K, Ajioka Y, Hashiguchi Y, Ito Y, Saito Y, et al. Japanese Society for Cancer of the Colon and Rectum (JSCCR) guidelines 2016 for the treatment of colorectal cancer. Int J Clin Oncol. 2017. https://doi.org/10.1007/s10147-017-1101-6. [Epub ahead of print].

8. West NP, Kobayashi H, Takahashi K, Perrakis A, Weber K, Hohenberger W, et al. Understanding optimal colonic cancer surgery: comparison of Japanese D3 resection and European complete mesocolic excision with central vascular ligation. J Clin Oncol. 2012;30(15):1763–9.

9. Mike M, Kano N. Laparoscopic surgery for colon cancer: a review of the fascial composition of the abdominal cavity. Surg Today. 2015;45(2):129–39.

10. Sadler TW. Langman's medical embryology. 12th ed. Philadelphia: Lippincott; 2012.

11. Michels NA. The variant blood supply to the small and large intestines. Its import in regional resections. A new anatomic study based on four hundred dissections with a complete review of the literature. J Int Coll Surg. 1963;39:127–70.

12. Acar HI, Comert A, Avsar A, Celik S, Kuzu MA. Dynamic article: surgical anatomical planes for complete mesocolic excision and applied vascular anatomy of the right colon. Dis Colon Rectum. 2014;57(10):1169–75.

13. Kuzu MA, Ismail E, Celik S, Sahin MF, Guner MA, Hohenberger W, et al. Variations in the vascular anatomy of the right colon and implications for right-sided colon surgery. Dis Colon Rectum. 2017;60(3):290–8.

14. Kim NK, Kim YW, Han YD, Cho MS, Hur H, Min BS, et al. Complete mesocolic excision and central vascular ligation for colon cancer: principle, anatomy, surgical technique, and outcomes. Surg Oncol. 2016;25(3):252–62.

15. Alsabilah JF, Razvi SA, Albandar MH, Kim NK. Intraoperative archive of right colonic vascular variability aids central vascular ligation and redefines gastrocolic trunk of Henle variants. Dis Colon Rectum. 2017;60(1):22–9.

16. Lee SJ, Park SC, Kim MJ, Sohn DK, Oh JH. Vascular anatomy in laparoscopic colectomy for right colon cancer. Dis Colon Rectum. 2016;59(8):718–24.

17. Lange JF, Komen N, Akkerman G, Nout E, Horstmanshoff H, Schlesinger F, et al. Riolan's arch: confusing, misnomer, and obsolete. A literature survey of the connection(s) between the superior and inferior mesenteric arteries. Am J Surg. 2007;193(6):742–8.

The Lymphatic Spread of Colon Cancer

Ji Yeon Kim

Abstract

It is essential to have good knowledge of the lymphatic system for the operative treatment of colon cancer, because the lymphatic drainage of the colon is a core subject of colonic oncologic pathology.

This chapter covers the latest progress in our understanding of the anatomy and biology of colonic lymphatics. The anatomy part describes the vascular anatomy, classification and definition of regional lymph nodes, and nodal staging system of the American Joint Committee on Cancer. The lymphatic flow, role of lymphatic system, and mechanism in cancer progression are dealt with over in the field of biology. In addition, some of the ongoing debates such as extramesocolic lymph nodes, skip metastasis, and sentinel lymph nodes are covered along within the biology.

This thorough review of colonic lymphatic system will serve as the basis for effective surgical treatments, which will be discussed elsewhere in this book.

Keywords

Lymphatics · Lymph node · Metastasis

J. Y. Kim
Department of Surgery, Division of Colorectal Surgery, Chungnam National University School of Medicine, Daejeon, South Korea
e-mail: jykim@cnuh.co.kr

21.1 Anatomy of Colon Lymphatics

Having good knowledge of the lymphatic drainage is essential in planning operative treatment for colon cancer. The lymphatic drainage of the colon follows its vascular supply. Therefore, a brief review of the anatomy of the vascular supply and lymphatic drainage of the colon can provide a framework for the discussion of colonic oncologic pathology. Because the colon derives from the midgut and hindgut, its three main arteries include the ileocolic artery and the middle colic artery, both of which arise from the superior mesenteric artery, and the inferior mesenteric artery from the aorta. The branches of these three main arteries create the marginal arcades, which ultimately supply the colon [1].

The superior mesenteric artery supplies the portion of the colon derived from the midgut (cecum, appendix, ascending colon, right two-thirds of the transverse colon), while the inferior mesenteric artery supplies the segments derived from the hindgut (left third of the transverse colon, descending colon, sigmoid, rectum, and upper anal canal). The unnamed branches of these arteries are ramified between the muscle layers of the portion of the colon which they supply and continue to subdivide before ultimately terminating in the circular smooth muscle layers of the bowel wall as branches of the

© Springer Nature Singapore Pte Ltd. 2018
N. K. Kim et al. (eds.), *Surgical Treatment of Colorectal Cancer*,
https://doi.org/10.1007/978-981-10-5143-2_21

appendices epiploicae. The majority of the venous drainage of the colon occurs through the hepatic portal vein via the superior and inferior mesenteric veins, although a small portion of the rectum is drained into the internal iliac vein and the pudendal vein via the middle rectal veins and the inferior rectal veins, respectively [1]. The lymphatic drainage route of the colon largely mirrors that of the arterial circulation, in contrast to most of the anatomy where the lymphatic drainage mirrors the venous circulation. The lymphatic vessels of the cecum as well as those of the ascending and proximal transverse colon drain into the lymph nodes associated with the superior mesenteric artery, while the vessels of the distal transverse and sigmoid colon, along with those from the rectum, drain into the nodes associated with the inferior mesenteric artery [1].

21.1.1 Classification of Colonic Lymph Nodes

The colonic lymph nodes have been conveniently classified into four groups by Jamieson and Dobson [2]: the epicolic, paracolic, intermediate, and main (principal) nodes (Fig. 21.1). Epicolic nodes are minute nodules on the serosal surface of the colon under the peritoneum and in the appendices epiploicae. The epicolic glands are very numerous in young subjects but decrease in number in older patients. They are especially abundant in the sigmoid colon, although they can be found on any part of the large intestine. Paracolic nodes are located on the arcade of medial borders of the ascending and descending colon as well as the mesenteric borders of the transverse and sigmoid colon along the marginal artery. The paracolic nodes are believed to be the

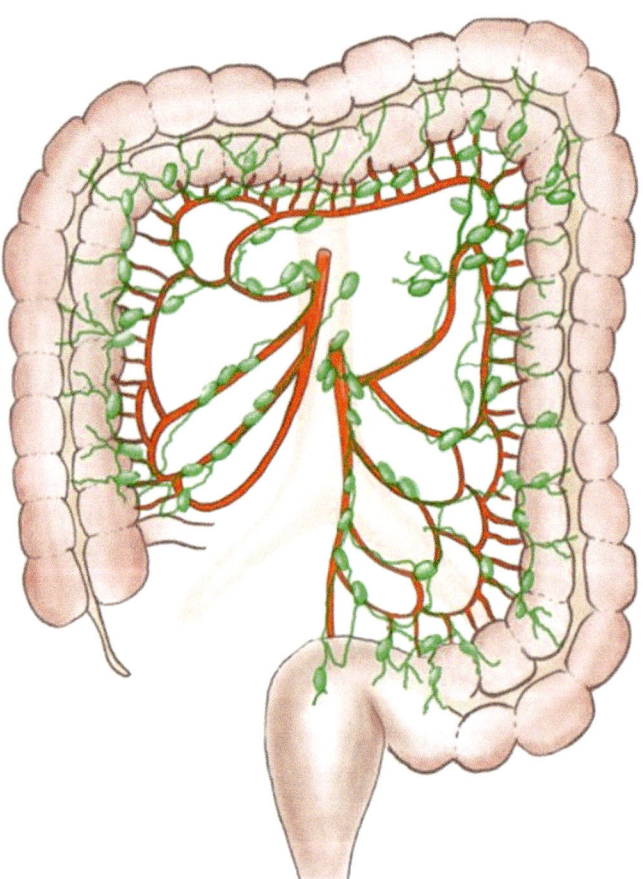

Fig. 21.1 Classification of the lymph node of the colon and rectum (From Sabiston Textbook of Surgery. Ed20. p1322)

most important colonic nodes and considered to have the highest number of filters. Hashiguchi et al. [3] reported that in about 23% of the patients, the epicolic and paracolic lymph node involvement is observed in between 5 and 10 cm from the tumor, while others reported that the epicolic and paracolic lymph node involvement in more than 10 cm from the tumor occurs in only 1–2% of the patients [4, 5]. Intermediate nodes are located along the ileocolic, right colic, middle colic, left colic, sigmoid, and superior rectal arteries [1]. Finally, the main (principal) nodes are populated along the main trunks of the superior and inferior mesenteric arteries and drain into the para-aortic nodes at the origin of these vessels. The lymph then drains to the cisterna chyli via the para-aortic chain of nodes. Colorectal carcinoma staging systems are based on the neoplastic involvement of these various lymph node groups.

The Japanese Society for Cancer of the Colon and Rectum (JSCCR) [6] classified the lymph nodes as shown in Fig. 21.2 and Table 21.1.

21.1.2 N Stage of Colon Cancer

The American Joint Committee on Cancer (AJCC) tumor/node/metastasis (TNM) classification and staging system for colon cancer is the present worldwide staging system. N stage is decided according to the number of regional lymph node metastasis.

NX	Regional lymph nodes cannot be assessed
N0	No regional lymph node metastasis
N1	Metastasis in 1–3 regional lymph nodes
N1a	Metastasis in 1 regional lymph node
N1b	Metastasis in 2–3 regional lymph nodes
N1c	Tumor deposit(s) in the subserosa, mesentery, or nonperitonealized pericolic or perirectal tissues without regional nodal metastasis
N2	Metastasis in 4 or more lymph nodes
N2a	Metastasis in 4–6 regional lymph nodes
N2b	Metastasis in 7 or more regional lymph nodes

Implementation of AJCC 8th Edition Cancer Staging System. American Joint Committee on Cancer. Available at https://cancerstaging.org/About/news/Pages/Implementation-of-AJCC-8th-Edition-Cancer-Staging-System.aspx. Accessed: January 4, 2017

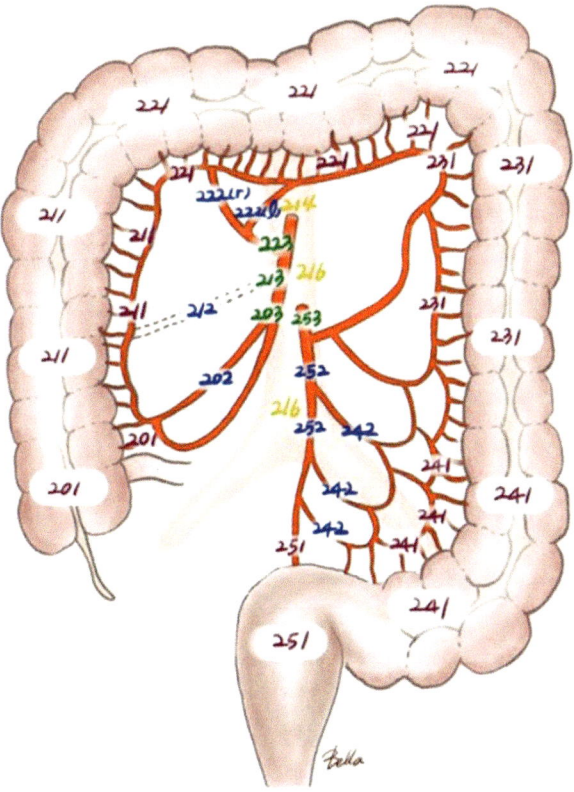

Fig. 21.2 Japanese classification of the lymph node stations. D1–D4 defined by colors: D1 = red; D2 = blue; D3 = green; and D4 = black (Disease of the Colon and Rectum. 2016;59:1209–21, Wolters Kluwer)

Table 21.1 Definitions of locations and dissection of mesocolic lymph nodes

The extent of lymph node dissection (JSCCR, Fig. 21.1)	
D1	Complete dissection of epicolic lymph nodes attached to the colon and paracolic lymph nodes along the marginal artery in the relevant colon segments and no or incomplete dissection along the tumor-supplying arteries
D2	Complete dissection of D1 and intermediate lymph nodes along the tumor-supplying arteries (ileocolic, right colic, middle colic, left colic, sigmoid, or inferior mesenteric arteries from the origin of last sigmoid artery to the origin of the left colic artery)
D3	Complete dissection of D1 to D2 and central lymph nodes, for left-sided tumors along the inferior mesenteric artery between the aorta and the left colic artery, and for right-sided including midtransverse tumors, lymph nodes along the superior mesenteric vein and lateral to the superior mesenteric artery
D4	Complete D1 to D3 and along the aorta and inferior vena cava or superior mesenteric artery/superior mesenteric vein central to the origin of the middle colic artery
Alternative definition of location of lymph node metastases (JSCCR)	
n[1](+)	Lymph node metastases in D1 area, but within 5 cm proximal or distal from the tumor edges
n[2](+)	Lymph node metastases in D1 area >5 cm proximal or distal from the tumor edges or in D2 area
n[3](+)	Lymph node metastases in D3 area
n[4](+)	Lymph node metastases in D4 area (considered distant metastases)

Suffixes + and − added to the D-area designation refer to the status of lymph node metastases reported by the pathologist. Suffixes (p) and (c) added to D2 refer to peripheral and central part of D2, where D2p in some studies is included in the specimen in conventional resections
JSCCR Japanese Society for Cancer of the Colon and Rectum
Disease of the Colon and Rectum. 2016;59:1209–21, Wolters Kluwer

21.1.3 Definition of Regional Lymph Node

A specific definition of regional lymph nodes changes according to the subsite of the primary cancer.

Definitions of regional lymph node groups in anatomic subsites of the colorectum [7]

Cecum: anterior cecal, posterior cecal, ileocolic, right colic
Ascending colon: ileocolic, right colic, middle colic
Hepatic flexure: middle colic, right colic
Transverse colon: middle colic
Splenic flexure: middle colic, left colic, inferior mesenteric
Descending colon: left colic, inferior mesenteric, sigmoid
Sigmoid colon: inferior mesenteric, superior rectal sigmoidal, sigmoid mesenteric
Rectosigmoid colon: perirectal, left colic, sigmoid mesenteric, sigmoidal, inferior mesenteric, superior rectal, middle rectal

Tumor deposits are discrete nodules of adenocarcinoma deposited in pericolonic and perirectal fat. Its presence has been reported as an important prognostic factor [8–12] . Although tumor deposit is founded as various forms associated with surrounding structure including veins, lymphatic vessels, and nerves or it can appear as nodular or scattered in aggregates in pericolic fat [13], it is included in N stage and counts as positive lymph node as abovementioned AJCC system.

21.2 Biology of Lymphatic Spread of Colon Cancer

21.2.1 Lymphatic Spread of Colon Cancer

Lymphatic flow of the colon starts with a network of lymphatic vessels and lymph follicles in the lower part of the lamina propria along the muscularis mucosa but becomes more abundant in the submucosa and the muscle wall [14]. The submucous and subserous layers of the colon have a rich network of lymphatic plexus, which drains into an extramural system of lymph channels and nodes [14]. Any retrograde flow is retarded by the numerous semilunar valves. Although some lymphatic channels exist in the lamina propria above the muscularis mucosa, carcinomas that are confined to the lamina propria are known to be not metastasized. On this basis, the term "invasive carcinoma" is used only when the malignant cells have invaded through the muscularis mucosae [14].

During the infiltration of the superficial part of the submucosa, the lymphogenic spreading is very infrequent, happening in less than 5% of the cases. During the infiltration of the deeper parts of the submucosa and the muscularis propria, the lymphogenic spreading appears in 15–20% of the times and gets even more frequent when the pericolic fat is infiltrated by the tumor [14].

21.2.2 Role of Lymphatic System for Cancer Progression

Lymphatic vasculature and the lymph node have been considered as only a pathway and space for cancer cells to pass and settle traditionally; however, it has been now clear that lymphatics perform many functions for cancer spreading [15]. After Kari et al. reported lymphangiogenesis is used by cancer cells to disseminate [16], many studies have reported that induction of lymphangiogenesis by the tumor facilitates metastatic spread [17–19]. Especially, work from many laboratories has reported that vascular endothelial growth factor-C (VEGF-C) is the main regulator of lymphangiogenesis, and its levels correlate with lymph node metastases [20–24]. Sufficient newly generated lymphatics create more opportunity for tumor cell exit and make more tumor cells to respond lymphatic endothelial cell-derived chemokines and migrate into lymphatics [15]. Recent discoveries reported that lymphatic endothelial cells can also modulate adaptive immune responses and mediate immu-

nosuppression and consequently participate in cancer immunosuppression [25–27].

21.2.3 Mechanism of Lymphatic Metastasis

The mechanisms of lymph node metastasis remain unclear to date. It is considered that preference of tumor cells to enter into the lymphatic system exists; however, it is not known that what kind of specific preference decide tumor cells enter into the lymphatics or blood vessels and survive. VEFG-C-mediated signaling is known to be important for remodeling the microenvironment of the lymph node prior to metastatic cell arrival by stimulating proliferation of lymphatic endothelial cell [28].

The theories on lymphatic spread of epithelial cancer have been explained in two different models, namely, the stepwise model and the parallel spread model. The stepwise model pioneered by Halsted postulates that a nodal metastasis temporally precedes a distant metastasis and the metastatic lymph nodes are regarded as temporary "barriers" or "incubators" for the distant metastasis. Thus, the metastatic lymph nodes will seed cancer cells through lymphatic channels and/or into the systemic circulation [29]. This model is felt somewhat real in the practice. Any efforts to remove a maximum number of involved lymph nodes may prevent further tumor spread and can result in relatively better oncologic outcomes. The concept of complete excision of the mesenteric envelope, so-called complete mesocolic excision (CME),, is based on this model. Proponents of this theory expect that standard adoption of CME will result in improved survival in colon cancer. Hohenberger et al. [30] demonstrated that routine application of CME could result in good oncologic results with 5-year cancer-specific survival rates of 91.4% in stage II and 70.2% in stage III colon cancer. However, the survival benefit of CME approach has not been validated in comparative prospective trials, and therefore it still remains a controversy.

The parallel spread model proposed by Fisher explains that distant metastases occur very early in the natural history of cancer [31]. In the parallel spread model, lymphatic spread is seen as a marker of the biological behavior and its malignant potential. In this perspective, any efforts to remove the lymph nodes as much as possible may not influence the survival outcomes. There are some lines of evidence that support the concept of parallel spread model in colon cancer. Circulating tumor cells in the peripheral blood of colon cancer patients have been found in every stage of the colon cancer [32]. In a recent meta-analysis, molecular detection of tumor cells in regional nodes was found to predict tumor recurrence and worse survival in colon cancer patients with negative lymph node involvement [33]. Genetic analysis also showed a striking disparity between primary colon cancer cells, disseminated tumor cells, and cells populating established metastases, suggesting early dissemination of genetically early stage of clones [34]. In addition, several investigators have shown that metastatic lymph nodes at the root of the mesentery are associated with systemic recurrence and the surgical removal of these nodes is unlikely to affect the survival [35].

Taken together, lymphatic spread of colon cancer is a stochastic rather than a stepwise phenomenon and may occur in the early stage of colon cancer.

21.2.4 Gastrocolic and Splenocolic Ligament Lymph Node Metastases

Lymphatic routes connecting the transverse colon and mesocolon to both the greater omentum and the pancreas have been identified [36]. Several studies [37–40] have reported metastases in the infrapyloric and gastroepiploic lymph nodes. These findings suggest that it is possible to involve lymph nodes along the gastroduodenal artery for tumors located from the distal part of the ascending colon to the proximal part of the splenic flexure. Podesta et al. [41] also reported

the involvement in splenic lymph nodes, in lymph nodes along the pancreatic tail, and in the splenocolic/gastrocolic ligament from tumors in the splenic flexure. This is a result of the embryonic fusion between these structures, and the gastrocolic ligament lymph nodes (infrapyloric and gastroepiploic lymph nodes) are the potential locations for what usually is considered to be extramesocolic lymph nodes, and the tumor tissues in these areas are considered as distant metastases.

Watanabe et al. evaluated lymph flow patterns in splenic flexural colon cancers using laparoscopic real-time indocyanine green fluorescence imaging and suggested that lymph node dissection at the root of the inferior mesenteric vein area is important, and it may be not necessary to ligate both the left branch of the middle colic artery and left colic artery, at least in cases without widespread lymph node metastases [42].

21.2.5 Skip Metastases

A significant proportion of lymph node metastases occur as metastases to central or apical nodes without metastases discovered in the intervening paracolic or intermediate nodes, so-called skip lesions [43–45]. The existence of skip metastases theoretically supports the concept of D3 dissection of complete mesocolic excision to minimize the lymphatic invasion after surgery. However, its true incidence has not been established. The risk of skip metastases in D3 is reported as 18% but seems to be dependent on the methodology of positive lymph nodes detection [39]. Pusztaszeri et al. [46] reported positive lymph nodes between 5 and 10 cm from the tumor edges in 7.8% of 345 patients, and 2% of these were negative lymph nodes in D1 less than 5 cm from the tumor, which shows the occurrence of skip metastases inside D1 (lateral direction). Complete mesocolic excision and extended lymphadenectomy should include these skip lesions, and the advocates of these techniques hypothesize that this is similar to hepatic or other distant metastasectomy in terms of oncological benefit.

21.2.6 Sentinel Lymph Nodes

Although sentinel lymph node biopsy is a standard procedure for treatment of some malignancies as breast cancer or melanoma, its clinical role is controversial in colon cancer. Because undetected metastatic lymph nodes can result in understaging and consequently exclusion from the possible benefit of adjuvant chemotherapy, many research are trying to improve surgical and pathologic technic for more precise diagnosis, including sentinel lymph node mapping. It can have a possibility to detect and resect more malignant lymph node or avoid unnecessary extensive resection [47]. Currently, endoscopic tattooing with near-infrared fluorescence imaging using indocyanine green improved its visibility during laparoscopic resections [48]. Segura et al. reported 14% of upstaging with ex vivo sentinel lymph node mapping with methylene blue staining in the patients staged as N0 by conventional technique [49]. Pouw et al. demonstrate that ex vivo magnetic sentinel lymph node mapping is a feasible technique for use in routine clinical practice, improving nodal staging accuracy of colorectal can-

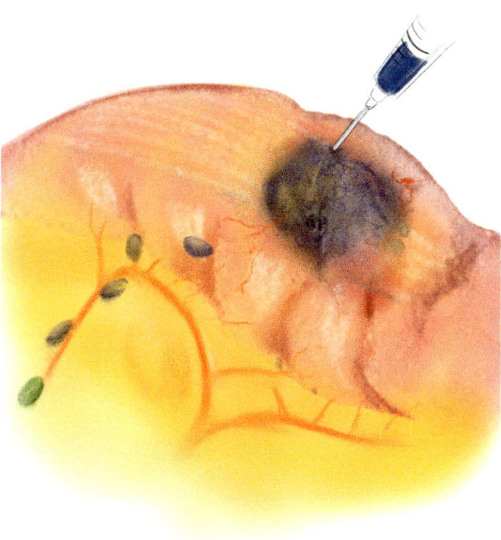

Fig. 21.3 Lymphatic mapping during laparoscopic colon resection. The colon has been delivered extracorporeally through a minilaparotomy incision, and the primary tumor, lymphatic channel, and sentinel lymph node (all stained by the blue dye) can be seen [52]. Reprinted with permission

cer patients [50]. Weixler et al. performed sentinel lymph node mapping with isosulfan blue and indocyanine green and demonstrated a high diagnostic accuracy to detect isolated tumor cells and micrometastases of lymph node for both techniques (Fig. 21.3) [51].

References

1. Healy J, Borley N. In: Standrin S, editor. Gray's anatomy. 39th ed. Edinburgh: Elsevier Churchill Livingstone; 2005. p. 1177–84.
2. Jamieson JK, Dobson JF. The lymphatics of the colon. Proc R Soc Med. 1909;2:149–74.
3. Hashiguchi Y, Hase K, Ueno H, et al. Optimal margins and lymphadenectomy in colonic cancer surgery. Br J Surg. 2011;98:1171–8.
4. Toyota S, Ohta H, Anazawa S. Rationale for extent of lymph node dissection for right colon cancer. Dis Colon Rectum. 1995;38:705–11.
5. Hida J, Yasutomi M, Maruyama T, et al. The extent of lymph node dissection for colon carcinoma: the potential impact on laparoscopic surgery. Cancer. 1997;80:188–92.
6. JSCCR. Japanese Classification of Colorectal Carcinoma. Tokyo: Kanehara; 2010.
7. Compton CC. Colorectal carcinoma: diagnostic, prognostic, and molecular features. Mod Pathol. 2003;16:376–88.
8. Song YX, Gao P, Wang ZN, et al. Can the tumor deposits be counted as metastatic lymph nodes in the UICC TNM staging system for colorectal cancer? PLoS One. 2012;7:e34087.
9. Lin Q, Wei Y, Ren L, et al. Tumor deposit is a poor prognostic indicator in patients who underwent simultaneous resection for synchronous colorectal liver metastases. OncoTargets Ther. 2015;8:233–40.
10. Nagtegaal ID, Tot T, Jayne DG, et al. Lymph nodes, tumor deposits, and TNM: are we getting better? J Clin Oncol. 2011;29:2487–92.
11. Nagtegaal ID, Quirke P. Colorectal tumour deposits in the mesorectum and pericolon; a critical review. Histopathology. 2007;51:141–9.
12. Tateishi S, Arima S, Futami K, et al. A clinicopathological investigation of "tumor nodules" in colorectal cancer. Surg Today. 2005;35:377–84.
13. Puppa G, Sonzogni A, Colombari R, Pelosi G. TNM staging system of colorectal carcinoma: a critical appraisal of challenging issues. Arch Pathol Lab Med. 2010;134:837–52.
14. Fenoglio CM, Kaye GI, Lane N. Distribution of human colonic lymphatics in normal, hyperplastic, and adenomatous tissue. Its relationship to metastasis from small carcinomas in pedunculated adenomas, with two case reports. Gastroenterology. 1973;64:51–66.

15. Podgrabinska S, Skobe M. Role of lymphatic vasculature in regional and distant metastases. Microvasc Res. 2014;95:46–52.

16. Alitalo K, Tammela T, Petrova TV. Lymphangiogenesis in development and human disease. Nature. 2005;438:946–53.

17. Mandriota SJ, Jussila L, Jeltsch M, et al. Vascular endothelial growth factor-C-mediated lymphangiogenesis promotes tumour metastasis. EMBO J. 2001;20:672–82.

18. Skobe M, Hawighorst T, Jackson DG, et al. Induction of tumor lymphangiogenesis by VEGF-C promotes breast cancer metastasis. Nat Med. 2001;7: 192–8.

19. Stacker SA, Caesar C, Baldwin ME, et al. VEGF-D promotes the metastatic spread of tumor cells via the lymphatics. Nat Med. 2001;7:186–91.

20. Brakenhielm E, Burton JB, Johnson M, et al. Modulating metastasis by a lymphangiogenic switch in prostate cancer. Int J Cancer. 2007;121:2153–61.

21. Burton JB, Priceman SJ, Sung JL, et al. Suppression of prostate cancer nodal and systemic metastasis by blockade of the lymphangiogenic axis. Cancer Res. 2008;68:7828–37.

22. Chen Z, Varney ML, Backora MW, et al. Down-regulation of vascular endothelial cell growth factor-C expression using small interfering RNA vectors in mammary tumors inhibits tumor lymphangiogenesis and spontaneous metastasis and enhances survival. Cancer Res. 2005;65:9004–11.

23. He Y, Rajantie I, Pajusola K, et al. Vascular endothelial cell growth factor receptor 3-mediated activation of lymphatic endothelium is crucial for tumor cell entry and spread via lymphatic vessels. Cancer Res. 2005;65:4739–46.

24. Kawakami M, Yanai Y, Hata F, Hirata K. Vascular endothelial growth factor C promotes lymph node metastasis in a rectal cancer orthotopic model. Surg Today. 2005;35:131–8.

25. Girard JP, Moussion C, Forster R. HEVs, lymphatics and homeostatic immune cell trafficking in lymph nodes. Nat Rev Immunol. 2012;12:762–73.

26. Lukacs-Kornek V, Malhotra D, Fletcher AL, et al. Regulated release of nitric oxide by nonhematopoietic stroma controls expansion of the activated T cell pool in lymph nodes. Nat Immunol. 2011;12:1096–104.

27. Podgrabinska S, Kamalu O, Mayer L, et al. Inflamed lymphatic endothelium suppresses dendritic cell maturation and function via Mac-1/ICAM-1-dependent mechanism. J Immunol. 2009;183:1767–79.

28. Pereira ER, Jones D, Jung K, Padera TP. The lymph node microenvironment and its role in the progression of metastatic cancer. Semin Cell Dev Biol. 2015;38:98–105.

29. Klein CA. Parallel progression of primary tumours and metastases. Nat Rev Cancer. 2009;9:302–12.

30. Hohenberger W, Weber K, Matzel K, et al. Standardized surgery for colonic cancer: complete mesocolic excision and central ligation – technical notes and outcome. Color Dis. 2009;11:354–64. discussion 364-355.

31. Fisher B. Biological research in the evolution of cancer surgery: a personal perspective. Cancer Res. 2008;68:10007–20.

32. Torino F, Bonmassar E, Bonmassar L, et al. Circulating tumor cells in colorectal cancer patients. Cancer Treat Rev. 2013;39:759–72.

33. Rahbari NN, Bork U, Motschall E, et al. Molecular detection of tumor cells in regional lymph nodes is associated with disease recurrence and poor survival in node-negative colorectal cancer: a systematic review and meta-analysis. J Clin Oncol. 2012;30: 60–70.

34. Stoecklein NH, Klein CA. Genetic disparity between primary tumours, disseminated tumour cells, and manifest metastasis. Int J Cancer. 2010;126:589–98.

35. Lange MM, Buunen M, van de Velde CJ, Lange JF. Level of arterial ligation in rectal cancer surgery: low tie preferred over high tie. A review. Dis Colon Rectum. 2008;51:1139–45.

36. Stelzner S, Hohenberger W, Weber K, et al. Anatomy of the transverse colon revisited with respect to complete mesocolic excision and possible pathways of aberrant lymphatic tumor spread. Int J Color Dis. 2016;31:377–84.

37. Feng B, Sun J, Ling TL, et al. Laparoscopic complete mesocolic excision (CME) with medial access for right-hemi colon cancer: feasibility and technical strategies. Surg Endosc. 2012;26:3669–75.

38. Feng B, Ling TL, AG L, et al. Completely medial versus hybrid medial approach for laparoscopic complete mesocolic excision in right hemicolon cancer. Surg Endosc. 2014;28:477–83.

39. Perrakis A, Weber K, Merkel S, et al. Lymph node metastasis of carcinomas of transverse colon including flexures. Consideration of the extramesocolic lymph node stations. Int J Color Dis. 2014;29: 1223–9.

40. Bertelsen CA, Bols B, Ingeholm P, et al. Lymph node metastases in the gastrocolic ligament in patients with colon cancer. Dis Colon Rectum. 2014;57:839–45.

41. Podesta A, Scotto G, De Mattei GF, et al. On lymph node excision in malignant neoplasms of the splenocolic fold. Minerva Chir. 1990;45:349–59.

42. Watanabe J, Ota M, Suwa Y, et al. Evaluation of lymph flow patterns in splenic flexural colon cancers using laparoscopic real-time indocyanine green fluorescence imaging. Int J Color Dis. 2017;32:201–7.

43. Yamamoto Y, Takahashi K, Yasuno M, et al. Clinicopathological characteristics of skipping lymph node metastases in patients with colorectal cancer. Jpn J Clin Oncol. 1998;28:378–82.

44. Kim CH, Huh JW, Kim HR, Kim YJ. Prognostic comparison between number and distribution of lymph node metastases in patients with right-sided colon cancer. Ann Surg Oncol. 2014;21:1361–8.

45. Nagasaki T, Akiyoshi T, Fujimoto Y, et al. Prognostic impact of distribution of lymph node metastases in stage III colon cancer. World J Surg. 2015;39:3008–15.

46. Pusztaszeri M, Matter M, Kuonen A, Bouzourene H. Nodal staging in colorectal cancer: should distant lymph nodes be recovered in surgical specimens? Hum Pathol. 2009;40:552–7.

47. Burgdorf SK, Eriksen JR, Gogenur I. Possibly improved treatment of colorectal cancer by sentinel lymph node mapping. Ugeskr Laeger. 2014;176:V07130442.

48. Handgraaf HJ, Boogerd LS, Verbeek FP, et al. Intraoperative fluorescence imaging to localize tumors and sentinel lymph nodes in rectal cancer. Minim Invasive Ther Allied Technol. 2016;25:48–53.

49. Pallares-Segura JL, Balague-Pons C, Dominguez-Agustin N, et al. The role of sentinel lymph node in colon cancer evolution. Cir Esp. 2014;92:670–5.

50. Pouw JJ, Grootendorst MR, Klaase JM, et al. Ex vivo sentinel lymph node mapping in colorectal cancer using a magnetic nanoparticle tracer to improve staging accuracy: a pilot study. Color Dis. 2016;18:1147–53.

51. Weixler B, Rickenbacher A, Raptis DA, et al. Sentinel lymph node mapping with isosulfan blue or indocyanine green in colon cancer shows comparable results and identifies patients with decreased survival: a prospective single-center trial. World J Surg. 2017;41:2378–86.

52. Tsioulias GJ, Wood TF, Spirt M, et al. A novel lymphatic mapping technique to improve localization and staging of early colon cancer during laparoscopic colectomy. Am Surg. 2002;68:561–5.

Part VI

Standard Surgical Concepts and Techniques in Colon Cancer Surgery

Complete Mesocolic Excision and Central Vascular Ligation: History and Outcome

22

Seok-Byung Lim and Jin Cheon Kim

Abstract

Surgical excision with the en-bloc removal of regional lymph nodes is currently the most promising treatment for colon cancer. Complete mesocolic excision (CME) with central vascular ligation (CVL) has recently been introduced in colon cancer surgery as a concept similar to total mesorectal excision (TME) for rectal cancer. This surgical technique involves oncologic resection with careful dissection of the mesocolon along the embryological tissue planes, which results in a colon and mesocolon specimen lined by intact fascial coverage of the tumor and containing all blood vessels, lymphatic vessels, lymph nodes, and surrounding soft tissue that may contain disseminated cancer cells. Subsequent studies have proved the feasibility and safety of the CME with CVL technique in open, laparoscopic, and even robotic surgery for colon cancer. Although the long-term survival benefit of the CME with CVL procedure has not been proven, it should be considered a standard surgical procedure in colon cancer surgery based on the anatomical and oncological backgrounds.

S.-B. Lim • J. C. Kim (✉)
Division of Colon and Rectal Surgery, Department of Surgery, University of Ulsan College of Medicine and Asan Medical Center, Seoul, South Korea
e-mail: sblim@amc.seoul.kr; jckim@amc.seoul.kr

Keywords

Complete mesocolic excision (CME) · Central vascular ligation (CVL) · Outcome

22.1 History of CME and CVL

The complete excision of a colorectal tumor along with the appropriate vascular pedicle and accompanying lymphatic drainage is the cornerstone of the technique for obtaining local control [1]. In fact, TME is a gold standard treatment for rectal cancer. The TME technique is based on the principle that dissection along the mesorectal plane achieves an intact fascial-lined specimen, which possibly contains tumor cells in the blood and lymphatic vessels, lymph nodes, and fascia including the surrounding soft tissues. Several pioneering studies reported total mesocolic excision as a potential determinant of survival following oncological resection. Bokey et al. [2] emphasized that the mobilization of the colon along the anatomic plane is an important principle that influences the outcome; the researcher used a standardized technique for colon cancer resection based on mobilization along the anatomic plane in 1980, and found that survival was improved, after adjusting for other known prognostic factors (shorter overall survival before the introduction of the standardized technique [hazard ratio, 1.5; 95% confidence interval, 1.2–1.8] and significantly shorter colon-cancer-specific survival [hazard ratio, 1.7; 95% confidence interval, 1.3–2.2]).

In 2008, West and Quirke et al. [3] reported the results of a retrospective observational study on the association between pathology grading for colon cancer surgical resection and survival. In that study, 399 resected colon cancer specimens were photographed and graded retrospectively according to the plane of mesocolic dissection: muscularis propria plane (n = 95, 24%), intramesocolic plane (n = 177, 44%), and mesocolic plane (n = 127, 32%). The mean cross-sectional tissue area beyond the muscularis propria was significantly greater with mesocolic plane surgery (mean ± standard deviation, 2181 ± 895 mm^2) as compared to that with intramesocolic (2109 ± 1273 mm^2) and muscularis propria plane (1447 ± 913 mm^2) surgery (p = 0.0003). There was also a significant increase in the distance from the muscularis propria to the mesocolic resection margin with mesocolic plane surgery (44 ± 21 mm) as compared to that with intramesocolic (30 ± 16 mm) and muscularis propria plane (21 ± 12 mm) surgery. The researchers also noted an oncologic advantage of mesocolic plane surgery in patients with stage III cancer (hazard ratio, 0.45; 95% confidence interval 0.24–0.85; p = 0.014); however, in that study, they did not consider the category of mesocolic plane surgery with a high vascular tie adjacent to the aorta as this type of surgery is not routinely performed in Western countries.

Moreover, Hohenberger et al. [4] proposed the concept of CME in conjunction with CVL in 2009. He stated that the mesocolon is covered by visceral and parietal envelopes corresponding to the mesorectum that extend from the mesorectum to the mesocolon. CME involves consequent surgical separation of the visceral fascia layer from the parietal one via sharp dissection. This maneuver enables the complete mobilization of the entire mesocolon, and thus includes the intact visceral fascial layer in the specimen with safe exposure and facilitates the ligation of the supplying vessels at their origin. In that report, the patients with CME had lower 5-year local recurrence rates and better cancer-related 5-year survival rates than those with conventional colectomy (6.5% vs. 3.5% and 82.1% vs. 89.1%,

respectively). Although many authors have reported the outcomes of colon cancer patients undergoing CME with CVL, the CME technique is not commonly implemented due to the anatomical complexity and confusion regarding the fascial structure. Several investigators have recently attempted to determine the actual composition of the multi-layered fascial structure and standardized nomenclature for CME [5].

22.2 Components of CME and CVL

22.2.1 CME

Analogous to the concept of TME in rectal cancer, the concept of CME in colon cancer is based on the presence of a common embryological plane between the mesocolic and mesorectal layers. The embryological plane surrounds the sigmoid and descending colon on the left side up to the pancreas and spleen, and contiguously surrounds the right colon up to the duodenum and pancreatic head. During the embryonal stage, the colon develops within the dorsal mesentery. After a 270-degree counterclockwise rotation of the primitive mid-gut along the axis of the superior mesenteric artery, folding of the dorsal mesentery and contact between the dorsal mesocolon and posterior parietal peritoneum occur. The mesentery of the colon can be separated from the posterior parietal peritoneum at the loose connective plane, termed the Toldt's fascia. Thus, meso-fascial separation or retrofascial separation (Fig. 22.1a, b) [5] offers an integral plane based on which CME can be used to remove lymphatics, vascular tissue, and neural tissue, constituting a complete mesocolic envelope with intact mesentery.

22.2.2 CVL

Lymph node metastasis in colon cancer is known to follow the supplying vessels. CVL, which is similar to D3 extended lymphadenectomy in Eastern countries, may be crucial in removing micrometastatic foci that could possibly be hidden in the central or apical nodes (Fig. 22.2). Although the lymph node yield might not necessarily reflect surgical quality, sufficient removal of the draining

Fig. 22.1 Schematic diagram depicting (**a**) meso-fascial separation and (**b**) retrofascial separation [5] (Published with kind permission of Elsevier and Copyright Clearance Center)

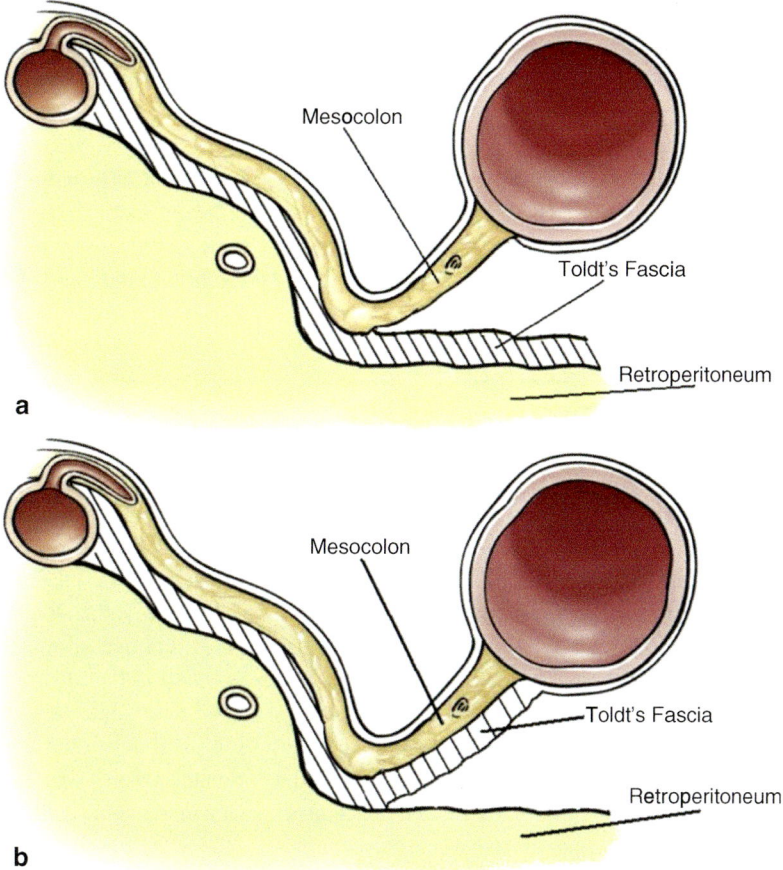

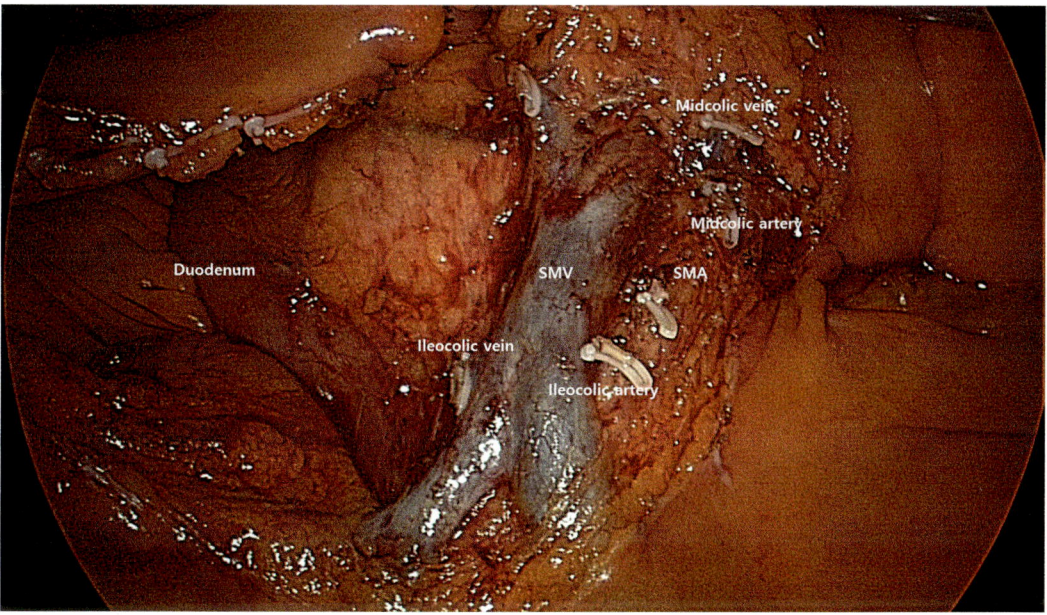

Fig. 22.2 Surgical view after central vascular ligation in a right hemicolectomy. *SMV* superior mesenteric vein, *SMA* superior mesenteric artery

lymph node has demonstrated a survival benefit. The ratio of lymph node metastasis to the total number of harvested lymph nodes has also been reported as a prognostic indicator. As CVL [6] or D3 dissection can obtain greater lymph node yields as compared to conventional surgery, these techniques might be helpful for reducing local or systemic recurrence in a subset of patients with skipped or micrometastatic lymph nodes.

22.3 Adequate Length of the Bowel

Longitudinal spread greater than 10 cm beyond the colon tumor rarely occurs (1–4% in cases with right-sided colon cancer and 0% in case with left-sided colon cancer) [7, 8]. Based on this finding, the general CME technique would favor the 10-cm rule for the proximal and distal bowel margins. The use of adequate proximal and distal margins also ensures that sufficient mesocolon, containing metastatic epicolic and paracolic nodes, is removed. The specific surgical procedure is chosen based on the location of the colon cancer. In the case of cecum or ascending colon cancer, the transverse mesocolon is transected with ligation of the right branch of the middle colic vessels, and the colon is then resected 10 cm from the tumor along with a part of the terminal ileum. For hepatic flexure or proximal transverse colon cancer, the middle colic vessels and the right gastroepiploic vessels are ligated, and the sub-pyloric lymph nodes are removed along with 10–15 cm of the greater omentum [4]. Some authors described their experience with modifications of the classical CME with CVL approach to avoid possible morbidity (without kocherization) or acquire adequate retroperitoneal margin (clearance of the pre-renal soft tissue behind Gerota's fascia for clinical T3 or T4 cancer) [9].

22.4 Outcome of CME and CVL

22.4.1 Pathologic Outcome

In 2010, West, Quirke, and Hohenberger et al. [10] investigated the importance of CME with CVL surgery for colon cancer. They collected 49 CME with CVL specimens from Erlangen, Germany and 40 standard specimens from Leeds, United Kingdom. Tissue morphometry and grading of the plane of surgery were performed and the histopathologic variables were compared. The researchers found that the CME with CVL surgery in Germany removed more tissue, as compared with the standard surgery, in terms of the distance between the tumor and the high vascular tie (median, 131 mm vs. 90 mm; $p < 0.0001$), length of the large bowel (median, 314 mm vs. 206 mm; $P < 0.0001$), and length of the ileum removed (median, 83 mm vs. 63 mm; $p = 0.003$), and area of the mesentery ($19,657$ vs. $11,829$ mm^2; $p < 0.0001$). In addition, CME with CVL surgery was associated with more frequent mesocolic plane resection (92% vs. 40%; $p < 0.0001$) and a greater lymph node yield (median, 30 vs. 18; $p < 0.0001$).

Recently, the Danish Colorectal Cancer Group [11] reported the results of a retrospective, population-based study on 364 CME patients and 1031 non-CME patients. The number of resected lymph nodes in the CME group was significantly greater than that in the non-CME group (mean ± standard deviation, 36.5 ± 15.9 vs. 20.9 ± 10; $p < 0.0001$). Moreover, the percentage of specimens with ≥12 lymph nodes was significantly higher in the CME group than in the non-CME group (89% vs. 99%; $p < 0.0001$).

22.4.2 Oncologic Outcome

The qualified surgical specimen in cancer surgery could be correlated with better long-term oncologic outcomes. Hohenberger et al. [4] reported excellent local 5-year recurrence rates (3.6%) and cancer-related 5-year survival rate (89.1%) after CME surgery in colon cancer. Similarly, West et al. [3] showed a non-stratified 15% 5-year survival benefit of mesocolic plane surgery, in comparison with non-mesocolic resection. Although several studies on CME were reported consecutively in terms of oncological outcome, both using the open and laparoscopic approaches, the results have been controversial. Furthermore, a systematic review of 5246 patients including 34 studies (12 retrospective, 9 prospective, and 13 original articles) in 2015 [12] proposed that CME removes significantly more tissue around the tumor with maximal lymph node clearance as compared to conventional surgery; however, no significant long-term survival benefit was observed. The authors concluded that there is no clear practical benefit for CME, given the limited information on the significant factors (including exclusion criteria, conversion rate of laparoscopic to the open approach in cases of CME, use of adjuvant therapy, histological characteristics, postoperative imaging to assess residual lymph nodes along the superior/inferior mesenteric pedicles, and the length of the residual vessels left in situ) that may influence outcomes.

In contrast, the population-based study by the Danish Colorectal Cancer Group [11] reported that CME surgery is associated with better disease-free survival as compared to conventional resection in patients with stage I–III colon cancer; the authors showed that the 4-year disease-free survival after CME (n = 364) was significantly greater than that following non-CME surgery (n = 1031: 85.8% vs. 75.9%; $p = 0.001$).

A meta-analysis between the open and laparoscopic CME approaches (1 randomized study and seven case-series) in 2016 [13] did not indicate any difference in morbidity or mortality between the approaches. With laparoscopic CME, there was a trend for longer operative time (open vs. laparoscopy: 110–194 min vs. 133–258 min; weighted mean difference, −30.88; 95% confidence interval, −62.38 to 0.61; $p = 0.05$) and shorter length of hospital stay (weighted mean difference, 2.29; 95% confidence interval, −0.39 to 4.98; $p = 0.09$). Moreover, there was no significant difference in overall survival (hazard ratio, 0.85; 95% confidence interval, 0.69–1.06; $p = 0.15$), disease-free survival (hazard ratio, 1.17; 95% confidence interval 0.95–1.44; $p = 0.14$), local recurrence (odd ratio, 1.31; 95% confidence interval, 0.72–2.38; $p = 0.38$), and distant metastases (odd ratio, 0.87; 95% confidence interval, 0.57–1.33; $p = 0.52$).

22.5 Controversies Regarding CME with CVL

There are controversies regarding not only the originality of the principles of CME [14], but also the technical diversity. These procedures were first introduced in 2008–2009 [3, 4], although Asian surgeons had already been performing D2–3 lymphadenectomy for colon cancer based on the location or local invasiveness of the primary tumor [15]. D3 lymphadenectomy for right-sided colon cancer involves the dissection of the paracolic, intermediate, and central (or apical) lymph nodes around the superior mesenteric vessels, equivalent to CVL [16]. A small comparative study [17] attempted to quantitatively measure the surgical specimens obtained from conventional surgery (19 cases) in England, CME with CVL (26 cases) in Germany, and D3 lymph node dissection (60 cases) in Japan, in 2014. The length of the vascular tie to the bowel wall was similar between the CME and D3 specimens ($p = 0.87$), which were both longer than that of the conventional surgery specimens. High rates of mesocolic plane surgery were observed for the CME and D3 specimens (conventional surgery, 47.4%; CME, 88.5%; D3, 71.7%; $p = 0.022$). Thus, it remains unclear whether CME is a novel procedure or whether it is simply a new terminology of a previously practiced technique, and further assessments can differentiate based on the surgical outcome.

Moreover, it is unclear whether a more radical excision, such as CME with CVL, is associated with greater morbidity and mortality. In a systemic review [18], the overall morbidity and 30-day mortality rates of CME with CVL were 19.4% and 3.2%, respectively, similar to those of conventional surgery. However, in the CME series, certain unusual morbidities were also observed, such as chyle leakage, major vascular injury, autonomic nerve injury, and duodenal or ureter injury [19–21].

The lack of an efficient evaluation method for the completeness of CME is another concern. Although a three-grade system (i.e., muscularis propria plane, intramesocolic plane, and mesocolic plane) was introduced in 2008 [3], it has not been universally accepted due to the unclear definition of the mesocolic plane, which has been either designated as the meso-fascial division or the retrofascial division including Toldt's fascia [5]. Furthermore, no long-term survival benefit of CME with CVL for colon cancer has been verified [12].

Conclusion

Despite many controversies, CME with CVL for patients with colon cancer should be carefully considered based on the oncological perspective. This technique achieves a good oncologic outcome with an acceptable morbidity, and is not inferior to conventional surgery. Thus, it appears evident that CME with CVL can be performed without severe technical difficulty and can facilitate accurate anatomical dissection that improves the quality of the resection specimens [22]. A future validation study involving a well-designed clinical trial would strengthen the basis for the suggested routine application of CME with CVL as a standard surgery for colon cancer patients.

References

1. Ruo L, Guillem JG. Surgical management of primary colorectal cancer. Surg Oncol. 1998;7:153–63.
2. Bokey EL, Chapuis PH, Dent OF, Mander BJ, Bissett IP, Newland RC. Surgical technique and survival in patients having a curative resection for colon cancer. Dis Colon Rectum. 2003;46:860–6.
3. West NP, Morris EJ, Rotimi O, Cairns A, Finan PJ, Quirke P. Pathology grading of colon cancer surgical resection and its association with survival: a retrospective observational study. Lancet Oncol. 2008;9:857–65.
4. Hohenberger W, Weber K, Matzel K, Papadopoulos T, Merkel S. Standardized surgery for colonic cancer: complete mesocolic excision and central ligation–technical notes and outcome. Color Dis. 2009;11:354–64.
5. Culligan K, Remzi FH, Soop M, Coffey JC. Review of nomenclature in colonic surgery–proposal of a standardized nomenclature based on mesocolic anatomy. Surgeon. 2013;11:1–5.
6. Gouvas N, Agalianos C, Papaparaskeva K, Perrakis A, Hohenberger W, Xynos E. Surgery along the embryological planes for colon cancer: a systematic review of complete mesocolic excision. Int J Color Dis. 2016;31:1577–94.
7. Morikawa E, Yasutomi M, Shindou K, Matsuda T, Mori N, Hida J, et al. Distribution of metastatic lymph nodes in colorectal cancer by the modified clearing method. Dis Colon Rectum. 1994;37:219–23.
8. Toyota S, Ohta H, Anazawa S. Rationale for extent of lymph node dissection for right colon cancer. Dis Colon Rectum. 1995;38:705–11.
9. Cho MS, Baek SJ, Hur H, Soh Min B, Baik SH, Kyu Kim N. Modified complete mesocolic excision with central vascular ligation for the treatment of right-sided colon cancer: long-term outcomes and prognostic factors. Ann Surg. 2015;261:708–15.
10. West NP, Hohenberger W, Weber K, Perrakis A, Finan PJ, Quirke P. Complete mesocolic excision with central vascular ligation produces an oncologically superior specimen compared with standard surgery for carcinoma of the colon. J Clin Oncol. 2010;28:272–8.
11. Bertelsen CA, Neuenschwander AU, Jansen JE, Wilhelmsen M, Kirkegaard-Klitbo A, Tenma JR, Danish Colorectal Cancer Group, et al. Disease-free survival after complete mesocolic excision compared with conventional colon cancer surgery: a retrospective, population-based study. Lancet Oncol. 2015;16:161–8.
12. Kontovounisios C, Kinross J, Tan E, Brown G, Rasheed S, Tekkis P. Complete mesocolic excision in colorectal cancer: a systematic review. Color Dis. 2015;17:7–16.
13. Athanasiou CD, Markides GA, Kotb A, Jia X, Gonsalves S, Miskovic D. Open compared with laparoscopic complete mesocolic excision with central lymphadenectomy for colon cancer: a systematic review and meta-analysis. Color Dis. 2016;18:O224–35.
14. Hogan AM, Winter DC. Complete mesocolic excision (CME): a "novel" concept? J Surg Oncol. 2009;100(3):182.
15. Watanabe T, Muro K, Ajioka Y, Hashiguchi Y, Ito Y, Saito Y, et al. Japanese Society for Cancer of the colon and Rectum (JSCCR) guidelines 2016 for the treatment of colorectal cancer. Int J Clin Oncol. 2017;20(2):207–39. https://doi.org/10.1007/s10147-017-1101-6.
16. West NP, Kobayashi H, Takahashi K, Perrakis A, Weber K, Hohenberger W, et al. Understanding optimal colonic cancer surgery: comparison of Japanese D3 resection and European complete mesocolic excision with central vascular ligation. J Clin Oncol. 2012;30:1763–9.
17. Kobayashi H, West NP, Takahashi K, Perrakis A, Weber K, Hohenberger W, et al. Quality of surgery for stage III colon cancer: comparison between England, Germany, and Japan. Ann Surg Oncol. 2014;21:S398–404.
18. Killeen S, Mannion M, Devaney A, Winter DC. Complete mesocolic resection and extended lymphadenectomy for colon cancer: a systematic review. Color Dis. 2014;16:577–94.
19. Shin JW, Amar AH, Kim SH, Kwak JM, Baek SJ, Cho JS, et al. Complete mesocolic excision with D3 lymph node dissection in laparoscopic colectomy for stages II and III colon cancer: long-term oncologic outcomes in 168 patients. Tech Coloproctol. 2014;18:795–803.
20. Feng B, Sun J, Ling TL, AG L, Wang ML, Chen XY, et al. Laparoscopic complete mesocolic excision (CME) with medial access for right-hemi colon cancer: feasibility and technical strategies. Surg Endosc. 2012;26:3669–75.
21. Willaert W, Ceelen W. Extent of surgery in cancer of the colon: is more better? World J Gastroenterol. 2015;21:132–8.
22. Bertelsen CA, Bols B, Ingeholm P, Jansen JE, Neuenschwander AU, Vilandt J. Can the quality of colonic surgery be improved by standardization of surgical technique with complete mesocolic excision? Color Dis. 2011;13:1123–9.

Japanese D3 Dissection

23

Hideki Ueno and Kenichi Sugihara

Abstract

The surgical practice for colon cancer in Japan is characterized by stage-based lymphadenectomy, which is standardized based on a long-established anatomical classification of the extent of lymphadenectomy. In the *Japanese Classification of Colorectal Carcinoma*, the anatomical extent of lymphadenectomy is expressed with the D number. The term D3 applies to the type of lymphadenectomy, wherein complete dissection of all three regional lymph node stations (i.e., pericolic, intermediate, and main) is performed. Regarding the optimal extent of bowel resection, the 10-cm rule, or bowel resection at 10 cm from the tumor edge, has long been employed in routine clinical practice. D3 dissection is the standard procedure for cT3 and cT4 colon cancer and for all colon cancers with lymphadenopathy. According to a nationwide survey in Japan, the rate of D3 dissection for stage II and III colorectal cancer patients has increased over time from 58% in 2001 to 75% in 2010; this increase might have been accelerated by the publication of the Japanese guidelines in 2005. Although the literature has often used the terminologies D3 dissection and complete mesocolic excision interchangeably, some important differences should be noted including the extent of bowel resection and treatment of extramesocolic lymph nodes. In 2013, an international prospective cohort study (International Prospective Observational Cohort Study for Optimal Bowel **R**esection **Ex**tent and Central Radicality for Colon Cancer: T-REX study; ClinicalTrials.gov NCT02938481) was launched. Standardization of lymphadenectomy to optimize colon cancer surgery is highly expected in the near future through international initiatives, including the T-REX study.

Keywords

D3 dissection · Complete mesocolic excision (CME) · Japanese Society for Cancer of the Colon and Rectum (JSCCR) · The 10-cm rule International Prospective Observational Cohort Study for Optimal Bowel Resection Extent and Central Radicality for Colon Cancer (T-REX study)

23.1 Introduction

The development and adoption of the concept of total mesorectal excision (TME) surgery for rectal cancer have significantly reduced local recurrence rates and improved survival [1, 2]. Clinical

H. Ueno (✉)
Department of Surgery, National Defense Medical College, Saitama, Japan
e-mail: ueno_surg1@ndmc.ac.jp

K. Sugihara
Tokyo Medical and Dental School, Tokyo, Japan

© Springer Nature Singapore Pte Ltd. 2018
N. K. Kim et al. (eds.), *Surgical Treatment of Colorectal Cancer*,
https://doi.org/10.1007/978-981-10-5143-2_23

evidences on the oncologic benefit of TME have turned surgeons' consciousness to the quality of surgery for colon cancer, and recently, there has been increasing international interest on the extended surgery, including the Japanese D3 dissection and complete mesocolic excision (CME). Recent reports on clinical trials of adjuvant chemotherapy for colorectal cancer show favorable survival results in Japan compared to those in Western countries [3, 4]. Surgical procedure characterized by D3 dissection and pathological practice to meticulously harvest lymph nodes adopted in Japan could be important reasons for this. Complete removal of regional lymph nodes by D3 dissection contributes to decrease cancer recurrence and improve survival by eradicating otherwise undetected tumor cells and by improving accuracy of lymph node evaluation, which contributes to appropriate selection of patients who need adjuvant chemotherapy.

In Japan, it has been well recognized that not all colon cancers require D3 dissection and that the optimal extent of lymphadenectomy varies according to the preoperative and intraoperative tumor stage. The surgical practice for colon cancer in Japan may be characterized by stage-based lymphadenectomy, which is standardized based on a long-established anatomical classification of the extent of lymphadenectomy. Since 1977, the *Japanese Classification of Colorectal Carcinoma*, which is issued by the Japanese Society for Cancer of the Colon and Rectum (JSCCR) and is now on its eighth edition, has consistently played a major role in defining the lymph node stations and the extent of lymphadenectomy to optimize the surgical management of colorectal cancer.

23.2 Classification of Regional Lymph Nodes in Colon Cancer

In the *Japanese Classification of Colorectal Carcinoma*, regional lymph nodes, which are from colonic tumors and are subject to lymphadenectomy, are defined as pericolic, intermediate, and main lymph nodes (Table 23.1, Fig. 23.1).

Table 23.2 shows the incidence of lymph node metastasis according to the national registration in

Table 23.1 Grouping system for regional lymph nodes in colon cancer based on the *Japanese Classification of Colorectal Carcinoma*

LN station	SMA area	IMA area
Pericolic LNs	Along the marginal arteries and vasa recta of the colon	• Along the marginal arteries and vasa recta of the colon • Along the terminal sigmoid artery
Intermediate LNs	Along the colic arteries	• Along the left colic and sigmoid arteries • Along the IMA between the origins of the left colic artery and the terminal sigmoid artery
Main LNs	At the origin of each colic artery	Along the IMA proximal to the origin of the left colic artery

SMA superior mesenteric artery, *IMA* inferior mesenteric artery, *LN* lymph node

Japan (2000–2004, JSCCR). In colon cancer, the incidence of metastasis was highest in the pericolic lymph nodes, followed by the intermediate lymph nodes and the main lymph nodes. Based on literature on D3 lymphadenectomy, main lymph node metastasis was reported to occur in approximately 1–8% [5]. In patients who underwent D3 lymphadenectomy for right-sided colon cancer, the incidence of skip metastasis (i.e., positive main lymph node without involvement of the intermediate nodes) was reported to be 1.6% [6].

The optimal extent of bowel resection is closely associated with how we define regional pericolic lymph nodes, which should be resected because of the risk for metastasis. Currently, there are no standardized international criteria for regional lymph nodes in the pericolic region. As per the tumor-node-metastasis (TNM) classification, all pericolic lymph nodes are treated as regional lymph node with no definition of the extent, on the basis of their clinical implications [7].

In Japan, the 10-cm rule, or bowel resection at 10 cm from the tumor edge, has been employed in routine clinical practice on the assumption that this will ensure that no positive pericolic lymph nodes will remain [8, 9]. In 2006, an additional standard to define regional pericolic lymph nodes that are subject to lymphadenectomy has been introduced by the

Fig. 23.1 Classification of regional lymph nodes of colon cancer

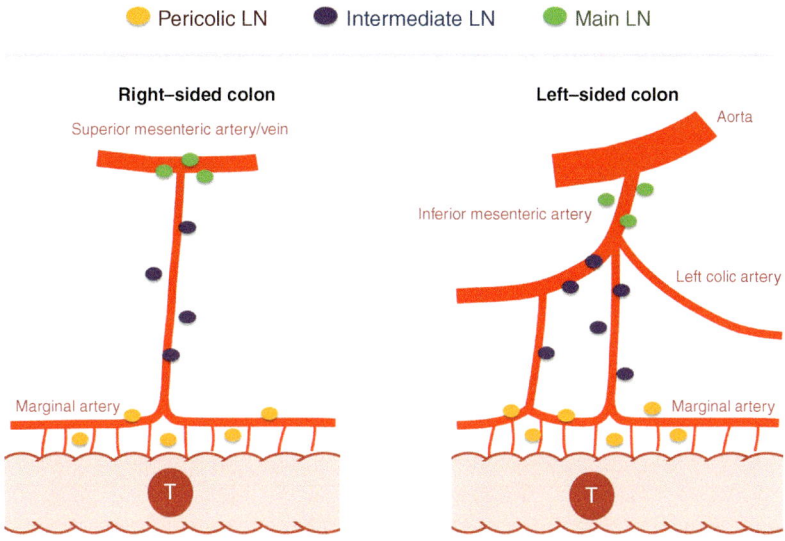

Table 23.2 Incidence of lymph node metastasis according to the lymph node grouping system

Pathologic T stage	No. of patients	Incidence of lymph node metastasis				
		Overall (%)	Most distant lymph node station involved			
			Pericolic (%)	Intermediate (%)	Main (%)	Non-regional (%)
T1	1957	8.6	6.8	1.8	0.0	0.0
T2	1747	20.7	16.3	3.5	0.6	0.3
T3 and T4a	10,696	49.4	30.0	14.1	3.4	2.0
T4b	960	55.4	28.6	14.7	5.5	6.6
Total	15,360	41.4	25.4	11.3	2.8	1.8

National registration in Japan (2000–2004, Japanese Society of the Colon and Rectum)

Japanese Classification of Colorectal Carcinoma as the modified 10-cm rule [10]. By this definition, the distribution of the feeding artery was classified into four types (Fig. 23.2), which determine the regional lymph node area. More specifically, bowel resection at 5 cm from the primary feeding artery was newly employed, with exception of a single case, in which the entrance of the primary feeding artery is located at the primary tumor. If a vascular arcade next to the primary feeding artery enters within 10 cm of the tumor area, it is considered to be the primary feeding artery.

23.3 Concept of the D Number

In the *Japanese Classification of Colorectal Carcinoma*, the anatomical extent of lymphadenectomy is expressed with the D number (Table 23.3, Fig. 23.3) [10]. The term D3 applies to the type of lymphadenectomy, wherein complete dissection of all three regional lymph node stations (i.e., pericolic, intermediate, and main) is performed.

For left-sided colonic cancers, the anatomical landmark (i.e., the left colic artery) that divides the intermediate and main lymph node stations allows surgeons to clearly distinguish between D2 and D3 (Fig. 23.4). On the other hand, for right-sided colon cancers, there is no anatomical structure that serves as a boundary between the intermediate and main lymph node stations (Fig. 23.5). With regard to the distinction between D2 and D3 dissection for right-sided colon cancer, it should be noted that the colic veins are ligated at their origin from the superior mesenteric vein (SMV) in both procedures. During a D3 procedure, the fatty tissue along the axis of the SMV is dissected en bloc in order to achieve complete resection of the main nodes, generally, prior to ligation of the feeding colic artery. A part of the SMA wall may be exposed during a D3 procedure,

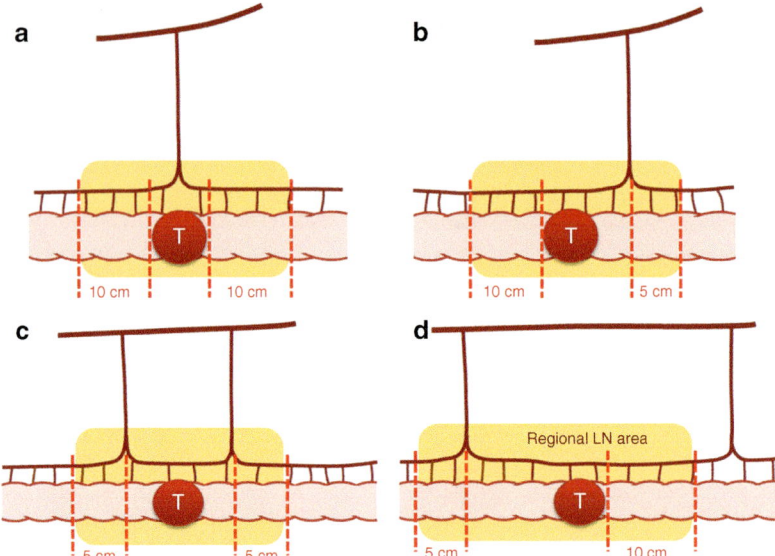

Fig. 23.2 Regional pericolic LNs in colon cancer according to the modified 10-cm rule by the *Japanese Classification of Colorectal Carcinoma*, eighth edition (2012). Under the modified 10-cm rule, the proximal and distal levels of bowel resection are determined according to the distance from the tumor, as well as the location of the primary feeding artery which can classified into four types (**a**–**d**). This rule ensures resection of all pericolic LNs in the regional area, which is highlighted in orange. (**a**) there is a feeding artery in close proximity to the tumor; (**b**) there is only one feeding artery within 10 cm from the tumor; (**c**) there are two feeding arteries within 10 cm from the tumor; (**d**) when there is no feeding artery within 10 cm from the tumor, the artery closest to the tumor is regarded as its feeding artery. *LN* lymph node

Table 23.3 Categories of the extent of lymphadenectomy for colon cancer, defined by the Japanese Society for Cancer of the Colon and Rectum

RX	The extent of lymphadenectomy cannot be assessed
D0	Incomplete dissection of the pericolic lymph nodes
D1	Complete dissection of the pericolic lymph nodes
D2	Compete dissection of the pericolic and intermediate lymph nodes
D3	Compete dissection of all regional lymph nodes

but in general, lymphadenectomy along the SMA is not routine, as long as there is no gross involvement of the main lymph nodes.

23.4 Surgical Indications of D3 Dissection in Japan

Based on the incidence and distribution of positive lymph nodes, the optimal extent of lymphadenectomy is determined according to the preoperative clinical findings and the intraoperative findings regarding the depth of tumor invasion and lymph node status (Fig. 23.6). In Japan, D3 dissection is the standard procedure for cT3 and cT4 colon cancer and for all colon cancers with lymphadenopathy. Considering that approximately 1% of the population has metastasis in the main lymph nodes and that the preoperative diagnostic accuracy for lymph node metastasis is not always satisfactory, the Japanese guidelines allowed surgeons to perform either D2 or D3 dissection for patients with clinical T2 colon cancer [11].

Randomized controlled trials to prove the survival benefit and the clinical value of D3 dissection may be difficult to perform and are currently not available. Based on a prognostic analysis with propensity score that used a prospectively registered, large-scale, multicenter JSCCR database of colon cancer in Japan, D3 dissection was shown to have a significant survival advantage in pT3 and pT4 colon cancer patients, with an estimated hazard ratio for overall survival at 0.8 (95% confidence interval, 0.7 to 0.9) [12]. In

Fig. 23.3 Schema of categorizing the extent of lymphadenectomy for colon cancer

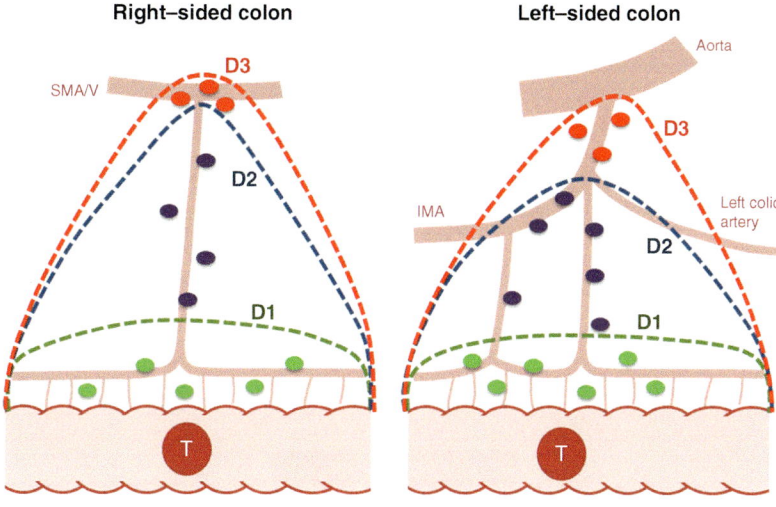

Fig. 23.4 D3 lymphadenectomy for left-sided colon cancer

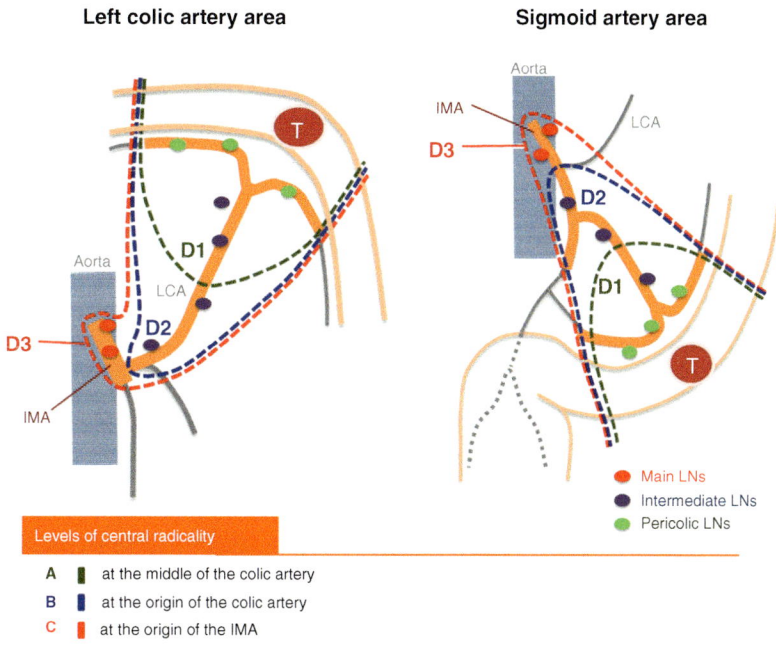

addition, although the prognostic significance of lymphadenectomy is controversial in the setting of metastatic colorectal cancer, a multicenter retrospective study reported that primary tumor resection with D3 dissection may improve survival [13]. On the other hand, a similar analysis using the JSCCR multicenter database failed to prove the prognostic value of D3 dissection in pT2 colon cancer patients [14].

According to a nationwide survey in Japan, the rate of D3 dissection for stage II and III colorectal cancer patients has increased over time from 58% in 2001 to 75% in 2010; this increase might have been accelerated by the publication of the guidelines in 2005 [15].

23.5   Differences Between the Japanese D3 Dissection and CME

The literature has often used the terminologies D3 dissection and CME interchangeably. Although both have similar concepts on the ana-

Fig. 23.5 D3 lymphadenectomy for right-sided colon cancer

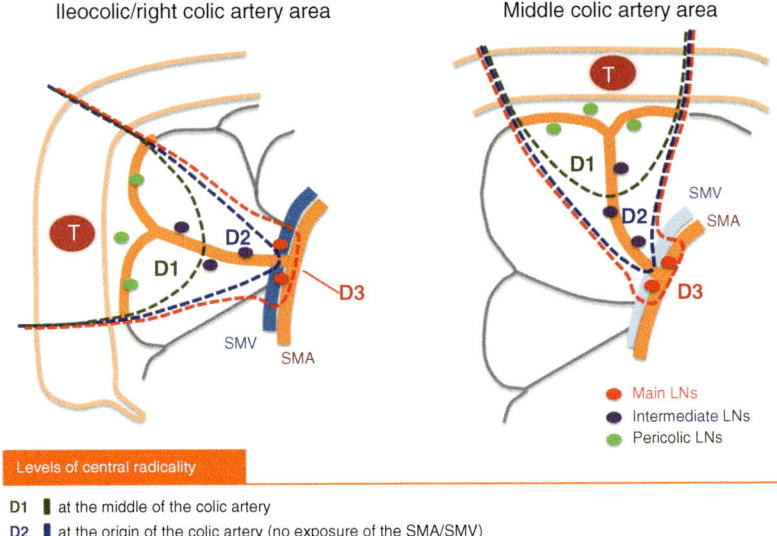

Fig. 23.6 Extent of lymphadenectomy in cStage 0–III colon cancer

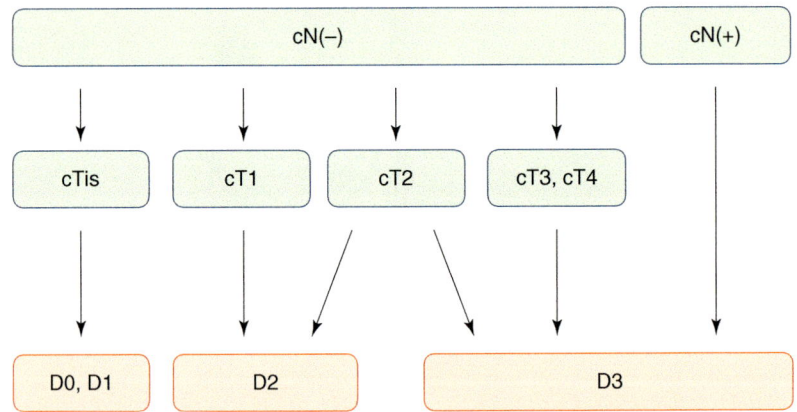

tomic approach to maximize the value of a surgical procedure, some important differences should be noted.

First, sharp anatomic dissection along the embryologic planes with preservation of an intact visceral fascia of the mesocolon is the principal concept of the CME procedure. Needless to say, this concept was introduced based on the popular concept of TME, which involves clear dissection along the fascia propria of the mesorectum, as described by Heald et al. [1, 2] It should be emphasized that the CME procedure requires proximal vascular ligation, but does not specify dissection at the origin of the feeding vessels; therefore, the original article of Hohenberger et al. used the term central vascular ligation

(CVL) together with CME [16]. On the other hand, the concept of the Japanese D3 dissection is removal of all regional lymph node stations depending on the location of the tumor, which includes removal of lymph nodes around the origin of feeding arteries (main nodes).

Second, the difference in the length of the bowel resected between these two procedures should be recognized. In Japan, as previously mentioned, the length of the bowel to be resected is determined based on which pericolic lymph nodes should be regarded as regional. In this regard, the CME technique is more radical because it includes removal of the nearby vascular arcade beyond the 10-cm margin. Consequently, the Japanese D3 specimens were clearly demonstrated to be significantly shorter than the CME specimens, resulting in a smaller amount of mesentery despite an equivalent distance from the high vascular tie to the bowel wall [17].

Note that, under the concept of Japanese D3 dissection, only the primary feeding vessels entering the regional pericolic area are regarded to be important as the resection target. For example, for tumors located at the middle ascending colon or at the hepatic flexure of the colon, the root of the middle colic artery (MCA) is ligated and dissected in a CME procedure; whereas in the D3 dissection procedure, removal of the main lymph nodes with preservation of the MCA and the left branch of the MCA is performed and the right branch of the MCA is ligated at its origin.

Third, central lymphadenectomy is more extended in the original CME than in the Japanese D3 dissection; in other words, dissection of the extramesenteric lymph nodes (i.e., over the head of the pancreas and along the gastroepiploic arcade) is performed during a CME procedure for cancer located at the hepatic flexure of the colon [16, 18]. Considering the potential for extralmesocolic cancer spread via the lymphatic network around the gastrocolic trunk, resection of the infrapyloric and gastroepiploic lymph nodes used to be the routine practice at specialized institutions in Japan. However, pathologically proven metastasis in this area had been rare; consequently, these extramesenteric lymph nodes are not routinely dissected at any Japanese institution today. Similarly, we currently do not perform the Kocher maneuver of mobilizing the duodenum and the pancreatic head to expose the origin of the SMA for tumors that do not invade into the other organs, such as the pancreas or duodenum, as well as for tumors that have massive lymphatic extension beyond the main lymph node area.

23.6 An Ongoing International Prospective Cohort Study

In the Japanese D3 dissection and the CME plus CVL, which are believed to be associated with good surgical outcomes [6, 19], removal of the main nodes is employed. However, whether or not the resection of these main nodes should be included in central radical LN dissection has not been fully confirmed by studies. In addition, we currently have no robust scientific evidence on the appropriate choice of length for bowel resection between the Western-type wide resection and the 10-cm rule adopted in Japan.

In 2013, an international prospective cohort study (International Prospective Observational Cohort Study for Optimal Bowel Resection Extent and Central Radicality for Colon Cancer: T-REX study; ClinicalTrials.gov NCT02938481) was launched. This study aimed to clarify the actual status of metastatic lymph node distribution in colon cancer and to provide robust evidence to establish consensus on the optimal extent of central lymph node dissection and length of bowel resection in colon cancer surgery. Currently, Korea, Germany, Russia, Lithuania, the UK, and Japan are involved in this first international attempt on this field. Morphometric analysis of the international colon cancer specimens [20] was included in this study, and the clinical value of assessment of the quality of surgical specimen will also be disclosed accordingly. Establishment of a consensus on the definition of reginal lymph node and standardization of lymphadenectomy to optimize colon cancer surgery is highly expected in the near future through international initiatives, including the T-REX study.

References

1. Heald RJ, Husband EM, Ryall RDH. The mesorectum in rectal cancer surgery – the clue to pelvic recurrence? Br J Surg. 1982;69:613–6.
2. Heald RJ, Ryall RD. Recurrence and survival after total mesorectal excision for rectal cancer. Lancet. 1986;327:1479–82.
3. Yoshida M, Ishiguro M, Ikejiri K, et al. S-1 as adjuvant chemotherapy for stage III colon cancer: a randomized phase III study (ACTS-CC trial). Ann Oncol. 2014;25:1743–9.
4. Shimada Y, Hamaguchi T, Mizusawa J, et al. Randomised phase III trial of adjuvant chemotherapy with oral uracil and tegafur plus leucovorin versus intravenous fluorouracil and levofolinate in patients with stage III colorectal cancer who have undergone Japanese D2/D3 lymph node dissection: final results of JCOG0205. Eur J Cancer. 2014;50:2231–40.

5. Paquette IM, Madoff RD, Sigurdson ER, et al. Impact of proximal vascular ligation on survival of patients with colon cancer. Ann Surg Oncol. 2016;25:38–45.

6. Kanemitsu Y, Komori K, Kimura K, et al. D3 lymph node dissection in right hemicolectomy with a no-touch isolation technique in patients with colon cancer. Dis Colon Rectum. 2013;56:815–24.

7. Brierley JD, Gospodarowicz MK, Wittekind C, editors. TNM classification of malignant tumours. 8th ed. West Sussex: Wiley; 2017.

8. Hida J, Yasutomi M, Maruyama T, et al. The extent of lymph node dissection for colon carcinoma. The potential impact on laparoscopic surgery. Cancer. 1997;80:188–92.

9. Hashiguchi Y, Hase K, Ueno H, et al. Optimal margins and lymphadenectomy in colonic cancer surgery. Br J Surg. 2011;98:1171–8.

10. Japanese Society for the Cancer of the Colon and Rectum. Japanese classification of colorectal carcinoma (second English edition). Tokyo: Kanehara; 2009.

11. Watanabe T, Muro K, Ajioka Y, et al. Japanese Society for Cancer of the Colon and Rectum (JSCCR) guidelines 2016 for the treatment of colorectal cancer. Int J Clin Oncol. 2017. https://doi.org/10.1007/s10147-017-1101-6. Epub ahead of print.

12. Kotake K, Mizuguchi T, Moritani K, et al. Impact of D3 lymph node dissection on survival for patients with T3 and T4 colon cancer. Int J Color Dis. 2014;29:847–52.

13. Ishihara S, Hayama T, Yamada H, et al. Prognostic impact of primary tumor resection and lymph node dissection in stage IV colorectal cancer with unresectable metastasis: a propensity score analysis in a multicenter retrospective study. Ann Surg Oncol. 2014;21:2949–55.

14. Kotake K, Kobayashi H, Asano M, et al. Influence of extent of lymph node dissection on survival for patients with pT2 colon cancer. Int J Color Dis. 2015;30:813–20.

15. Ishiguro M, Higashi T, Watanabe T, et al. Changes in colorectal cancer care in Japan before and after guideline publication: a nationwide survey about D3 lymph node dissection and adjuvant chemotherapy. J Am Coll Surg. 2014;218:969–77.

16. Hohenberger W, Weber K, Matzel K, et al. Standardized surgery for colonic cancer: complete mesocolic excision and central ligation-technical notes and outcome. Color Dis. 2009;11:354–64.

17. West NP, Kobayashi H, Takahashi K, et al. Understanding optimal colonic cancer surgery: comparison of Japanese D3 resection and European complete mesocolic excision with central vascular ligation. J Clin Oncol. 2012;30:1763–9.

18. Perrakis A, Weber K, Merkel S, et al. Lymph node metastasis of carcionoma of transverse colon including flexures. Consideration of the extramesocolic lymph node stations. Int J Color Dis. 2014;29:1223–9.

19. Bertelsen CA, Neuenschwander AU, Jansen JE, et al. Disease-free survival after complete mesocolic excision compared with conventional colon cancer surgery: a retrospective, population-based study. Lancet Oncol. 2015;16:161–8.

20. West NP, Hohenberger W, Weber K, et al. Complete mesocolic excision with central vascular ligation produces an oncologically superior specimen compared with standard surgery for carcinoma of the colon. J Clin Oncol. 2010;28:272–8.

JCOG0404

24

Yukihide Kanemitsu

Abstract

Although benefits of laparoscopic surgery compared with open surgery have been suggested, the long-term survival of patients undergoing laparoscopic surgery for colon cancer requiring Japanese D3 dissection remains unclear. A randomized controlled trial to establish non-inferiority of laparoscopic surgery to open surgery was conducted. Laparoscopic D3 surgery was not non-inferior to open D3 surgery in terms of overall survival for patients with stage II or III colon cancer. However, because overall survival in both groups was similar and better than expected, laparoscopic D3 surgery could be an acceptable treatment option for patients with stage II or III colon cancer in experienced facilities, so long as considerations are made for patients concerned about the clinical inferiority of laparoscopic surgery.

Keywords

D3 lymph node dissection · Colon cancer · Laparoscopic surgery · Open surgery

Y. Kanemitsu
Department of Colorectal Surgery, National Cancer Centre Hospital, Tokyo, Japan
e-mail: ykanemit@ncc.go.jp

24.1 The Present Is Always Determined by the Past

The establishment of modern surgical medicine is a result of observations and experiments that have accumulated over centuries. The concept of "radical" surgery, termed by Halsted [1], contributed to the field of cancer surgery by using local recurrence as an indicator of incomplete surgery. He considered resection of tissues with recurrence risk without sufficient margins due to cosmetic reasons (i.e., a woman's appearance) to be a "mistaken kindness" [2].

24.2 Theory of Lymph Node Dissection

However, Halsted did not touch on the concept of lymphatic flow, and for colorectal cancer, Miles [3] and Moynihan [4] began the practice of radical surgery in 1908. Miles set the primary goal of rectal resection as lymph node dissection in three directions from the lesion: upward, downward, and laterally. In contrast, Moynihan [4] considered cancer surgery to mean excision of the lymphatic system itself and proposed high ligation of the tumor-feeding artery. As practices based on the understanding of lymph flow, both procedures left major footprints in the history of cancer surgery. Even today, more than 100 years later, Japanese surgeons perform lymph node dissection based on the lymph flow theory.

24.3 Standard of Surgical Treatment for Colorectal Cancer

The standard of surgical treatment for colorectal cancer is colorectal excision with lymph node dissection. In Japan, according to the "Japanese Classification of Colorectal Carcinoma" [5] and "Guidelines for the Treatment of Colorectal Cancer" [6] set forth by the Japanese Society for Cancer of the Colon and Rectum, "D3 lymph node dissection" has been performed as the standard treatment and has demonstrated top-level outcomes on the global scale [7]. This procedure basically involves "*en bloc* resection of the intestinal tract with tumor and the lymph nodes around its lymph flow by surrounding them with the fascia and separating them along the embryonic fascia." Open surgery has been a standard procedure that is performed for colorectal cancer [8].

24.4 Advances Toward Minimization

In recent years, cancer surgery has remarkably advanced, and surgical procedures themselves have advanced toward minimization, as compared with Halsted's procedure. Minimally invasive treatment that reduces physical trauma to the patient's body to the extent possible is widely advocated, and laparoscopic surgery for colorectal cancer is a major example of such treatment. Because laparoscopic surgery enables visualization of microdissection under an enlarged visual field, minimization of abdominal wall damage, and operation in the physiological environment within the body cavity, it has become widespread over the past 25 years as a less harmful procedure.

In the United States and Europe, laparoscopic surgery for colon cancer is accepted as a standard treatment and has some benefits over open surgery including decreased pain, improved postoperative pulmonary function, reduced postoperative ileus, improved incidence of wound infection, faster recovery, and shorter hospital stay. In addition to these short-term outcomes,

long-term outcomes after laparoscopic surgery for colon cancer are comparable to those after open surgery, as demonstrated by several randomized controlled trials (RCTs) [9–14].

Ever since laparoscopic surgery for advanced cancer has been covered by insurance in Japan (i.e., as of 2002), more than 60% of surgeries for advanced colorectal cancer have been performed laparoscopically [15]. In terms of treatment outcomes, several large-scale RCTs in Europe and the United States (COST trial [9, 10], CLASICC trial [11, 12], and COLOR trial [13, 14]) have shown no significant difference in survival and recurrence rates between laparoscopic surgery and open surgery in patients with advanced cancer. These results may have supported the rapid popularization of laparoscopic surgery in Japan. However, these trials were conducted prior to establishment of the current standard procedure in the United States and Europe, i.e., complete mesocolic excision with central vascular ligation. These trials also had several limitations: the proportion of patients with tumors of pathological stage 0–I was high (21–37%); rectal cancer was included in some trials; and the extent of lymph node dissection was not specified [9–14]. In the CLASICC trial [11, 12], which was conducted at 27 facilities and included 32 surgeons in the United Kingdom, 794 patients with colorectal cancer were registered and randomly assigned to either laparoscopic surgery or open surgery at a 2:1 ratio. When Philip Quirke, a British clinical pathologist, randomly extracted 162 resected specimens and analyzed the degree of the previously mentioned CME and CVL using their own scale, 75% underwent D0–D1 surgery, 25% underwent D2, and there were no cases of D3 surgery (personal communication, July 2011).

The D3 dissection technique used in Japan emphasizes anatomical lymph node dissection, defined as the dissection of lymph nodes at the root of the tumor-feeding artery and the longitudinal length of the large intestine to be resected. In contrast, the complete mesocolic excision technique emphasizes preservation of the anatomical planes of surgical resection and central vascular ligation. Although these two concepts differ, the purpose and extent of lymph node dissection are similar. Theoretically, outcomes of the techniques should be equivalent given their same underlying principles [16].

The Japan Clinical Oncology Group (JCOG) 0404 trial was an RCT that aimed to evaluate whether D3 dissection via a laparoscopic route is non-inferior to the same dissection via an open route in terms of overall survival [17]. To overcome the limitations of previous trials, the study population was limited to patients with clinical stage II/III colon cancer. Moreover, a detailed surgical procedure was specified in the protocol. D3 dissection was mandatory in all patients, and additional extended lymph node dissection was allowed if necessary. The short-term outcomes of the trial demonstrated that laparoscopic surgery for colon cancer was more beneficial than open surgery [18].

24.4.1 Short-Term Results of JCOG0404

JCOG0404 began in 2004, which was 10 years later than Europe and the United States. Thirty facilities with experienced and certified surgeons were involved in the trial. Eligibility criteria included the following: patients histopathologically diagnosed with colorectal cancer; tumor located in the cecum, ascending colon, sigmoid colon, or rectosigmoid colon; T3 or T4 without invasion into other organs; lymph node metastasis classified as N0–N2 and M0; tumor size ≤8 cm; and age between 20 and 75 years. Patients were randomly assigned to either the open surgery (OP) group or laparoscopic surgery (LAP) group prior to surgery. When pathological stage III cancer was confirmed by histological examination of resected specimens, adjuvant chemotherapy was administered as three courses of the Roswell Park Memorial Institute 8-week regimen [19] of fluorouracil (500 mg/m^2 by bolus intravenous infusion on days 1, 8, 15, 22, 29, and 36) and leucovorin (250 mg/m^2 by 2 h drip intravenous infusion on days 1, 8, 15, 22, 29, and 36). The primary outcome measure was overall survival (OS), and the number of patients required for the trial was 1050.

Short-term results of the trial were reported at ASCO2012. From October 2004 to March 2009, 1057 patients were assigned to the OP group ($n = 528$) or the LAP group ($n = 529$) (Fig. 24.1; Table 24.1). Twenty-nine patients in the LAP group converted to the OP group (5.4%: technical reasons, 2.3%; indications for open surgery, 2.8%; complications, 0.4%). The 5.4% rate of conversion from LAP to OP was approximately 1/4 of the rates observed in foreign clinical trials [18]. While the amount of bleeding was less in the LAP group compared to the OP group (median, 30 mL vs 85 mL; $p < 0.0001$), operation time was 52 min longer in the LAP group (median, 211 min vs 159 min; $p < 0.0001$; Tables 24.2, 24.3, and 24.4). There was no significant difference between the two groups in the degree of radical dissection, as evaluated by the number of dissected lymph nodes ($p = 0.41$). In the postoperative course, the recovery of gastrointestinal function was faster and the length of hospital stay shorter in the LAP group compared to the OP group ($p < 0.0001$ in both). The incidence of wound-related complications was significantly lower in the LAP group ($p = 0.007$). Moreover, there was no significant difference in the incidence of other complications and in-hospital mortality between the two groups. These results demonstrated that laparoscopic complete mesocolic excision for stage II/III colorectal cancer can be performed safely, with no difference in the degree of radical dissection between laparoscopic and open surgeries. In this trial, quality control using photographs of the surgical field was performed, and results by central evaluation showed that 99% of subjects underwent D3 [20]. At this point, LAP was to be considered a new standard treatment for colorectal cancer if non-inferiority to OS was confirmed in the primary analysis of JCOG0404, which was completed in 2014 [18].

24.4.2 Careful and Fair Evaluation Is Required for a New Procedure

After collecting data from 1057 patients, the trial's final analysis was carried out in August 2014, as follows:

Fig. 24.1 Study design

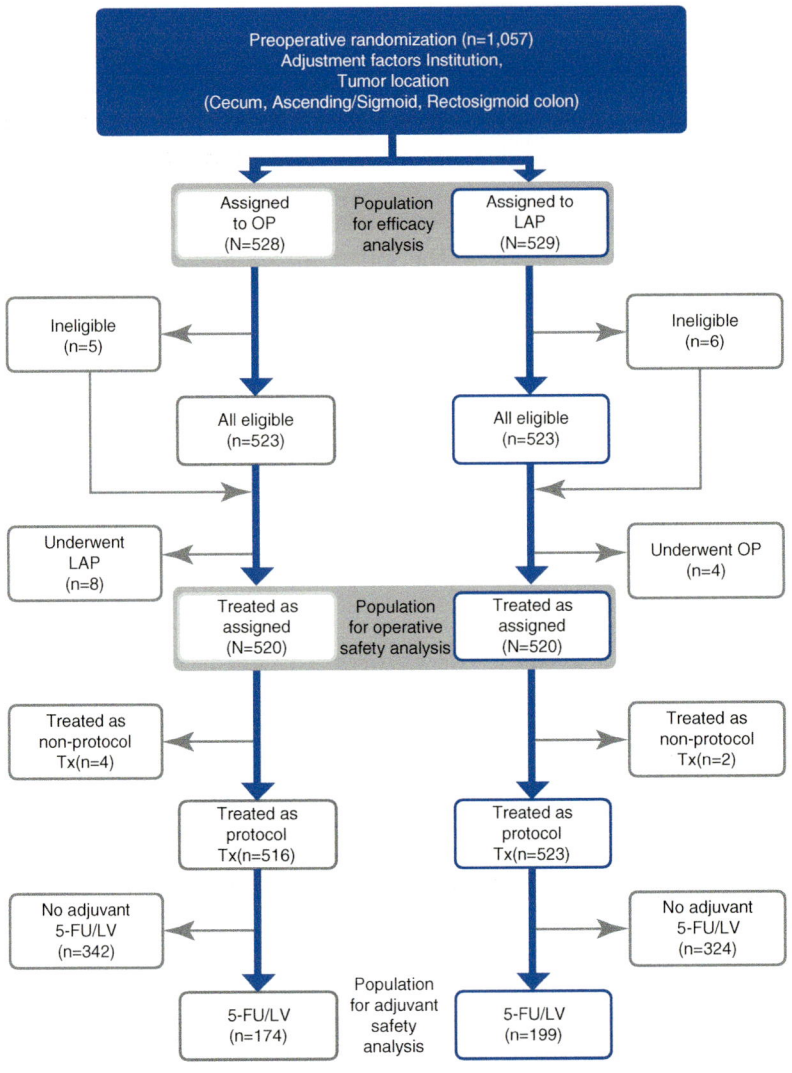

Table 24.1 Patient characteristics (n = 1057)

n		OP (n = 528)	LAP (n = 529)	Total (n = 1057)
Sex	Male	312	282	594
	Female	216	247	463
Age (years)	Median	64	64	64
	Range	33–75	28–75	28–75
Clinical stage	II	366	331	697
	III	160	197	357
	IV	2	1	3
Tumor location	C	55	46	101
	A	100	109	209
	S	236	252	488
	RS	137	122	259

Table 24.2 Operative details

n (%)	OP (n = 528)	LAP (n = 529)	Total (n = 1057)
Type of surgery			
Ileo-cecal resection	54 (10.2)	37 (7.0)	91 (8.6)
Right hemicolectomy	99 (18.8)	111 (21.0)	210 (19.9)
Sigmoidectomy	214 (40.5)	234 (44.2)	448 (42.4)
Anterior resection	154 (29.2)	138 (26.1)	292 (27.6)
Hartmann	1 (0.2)	0 (0)	1 (0.1)
Partial resection	4 (0.8)	7 (1.3)	11 (1.0)
Others	2 (0.4)	2 (0.4)	4 (0.4)
Conversion	–	29 (5.5)	

Table 24.3 Pathological results

n	OP (n = 528)	LAP (n = 529)	Total (n = 1057)
Tumor size (cm)			
Median	4.5	4.3	4.5
Range	1.2–14.0	1.5–9.8	1.2–14.0
Number of harvested lymph nodes			
Median	22	21	22
Range	2–120	2–85	2–120
Pathological stage			
0	4	2	6
I	59	58	117
II	246	222	468
III	203	232	435
IV	15	15	30
Missing[a]	1	0	1

[a]Unresectable disease due to diffuse dissemination

Table 24.4 Late complications (grade 2–4)

	OP (n = 519[a])	LAP (n = 525)	Total (n = 1044)
Overall complications (grade 2–4)	65 (12.5%)	53 (10.1%)	118 (11.3%)
Constipation	31 (6.0%)	23 (4.4%)	54 (5.2%)
Diarrhea	15 (2.9%)	14 (2.7%)	29 (2.8%)
Paralytic ileus	6 (1.2%)	9 (1.7%)	15 (1.4%)
Bowel obstruction of small intestine	16 (3.1%)	11 (2.1%)	27 (2.6%)

[a]1 pt was excluded due to death during hospital stay

- If non-inferiority is not proved …
  Since the null hypothesis "the effectiveness of laparoscopic surgery is inferior to that of open surgery over the non-inferiority margin" cannot be rejected, open surgery will remain the standard procedure.
- If non-inferiority is proved …
  Since the minimal invasiveness assumed with laparoscopic surgery in this study did not significantly differ from expected results [18], laparoscopic surgery will replace open surgery and become the standard procedure.

24.4.3 Primary Results of JCOG0404

Long-term outcomes of the trial were presented at the 2015 Gastrointestinal Cancers Symposium (ASCO-GI 2015) [21]. Two treatment-related deaths occurred in the OP group; one patient died 7 days after surgery (likely due to myocardial infarction), and the other died from febrile neutropenia, pneumonia, diarrhea, and gastrointestinal hemorrhage during postoperative chemotherapy. One patient died during the hospital stay and was therefore excluded from the adverse events analysis. The incidence of grade 2–4 late complications was 11.3% (12.5% in OP, 10.1% in LAP). Late complications included constipation (6.0% in OP, 4.4% in LAP), diarrhea (2.9% in OP, 2.7% in LAP), paralytic ileus (1.2% in OP, 1.7% in LAP), and small bowel obstruction (3.1% in OP, 2.1% in LAP).

Median follow-up for all patients following randomization was 72.8 months (IQR 61.1–72.8). At the time of the last follow-up on March 27, 2014, 128 (12%) of 1057 patients had died (62 (12%) of 528 patients in the OP group and 66 (12%) of 529 patients in the LAP group). Sixty-four patients (36 patients in the OP and 28 patients in the LAP group) were lost to follow-up within 5 years of enrolment. Estimated 5-year overall survival was 90.4% (95% CI, 87.5–92.6) in the OP group and 91.8% (89.1–93.8) in the LAP group. The hazard ratio (HR) for overall survival for LAP versus OP was 1.06 (90% CI, 0.79–1.41; one-sided p for non-inferiority = 0.073; Fig. 24.2); laparoscopic surgery was not non-inferior to open surgery. In a sensitivity analysis of 1045 patients who underwent surgery as assigned, the HR for overall survival for laparoscopic surgery versus open surgery was 1.03 (0.77–1.38, one-sided p for non-inferiority = 0.057). Relapse-free survival is shown in Fig. 24.3; 228 (22%) of the 1057 patients had recurrence or died (111 (21%) of 528 patients in the OP group and 117 (22%) of 529 patients in the LAP group). Five-year relapse-

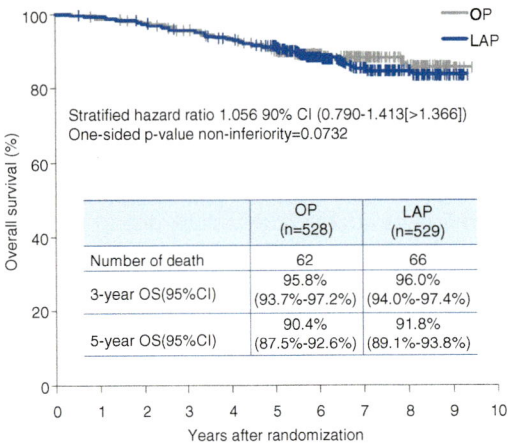

Stratified hazard ratio 1.056 90% CI (0.790-1.413[>1.366])
One-sided p-value non-inferiority=0.0732

	OP (n=528)	LAP (n=529)
Number of death	62	66
3-year OS(95%CI)	95.8% (93.7%-97.2%)	96.0% (94.0%-97.4%)
5-year OS(95%CI)	90.4% (87.5%-92.6%)	91.8% (89.1%-93.8%)

Fig. 24.2 OS

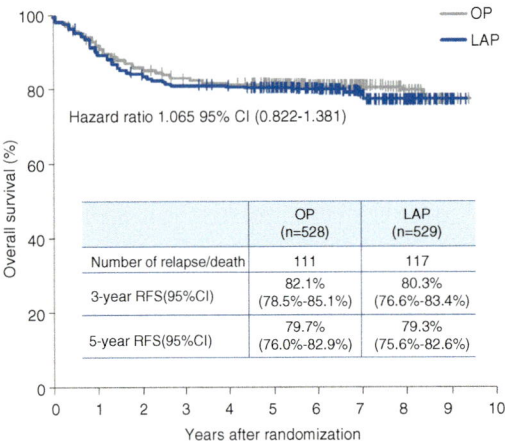

Hazard ratio 1.065 95% CI (0.822-1.381)

	OP (n=528)	LAP (n=529)
Number of relapse/death	111	117
3-year RFS(95%CI)	82.1% (78.5%-85.1%)	80.3% (76.6%-83.4%)
5-year RFS(95%CI)	79.7% (76.0%-82.9%)	79.3% (75.6%-82.6%)

Fig. 24.3 RFS

free survival was 80% (95% CI: 76.0–82.9) in the OP group and 79% (75.6–82.6) in the LAP group. The HR for relapse-free survival for laparoscopic surgery versus open surgery was 1.07 (95% CI: 0.82–1.38). Eighty-nine (17%) of 520 patients in the OP group and 101 (19%) patients in the LAP group experienced recurrence after R0 resection. Of these patients, 39 (44%) in the OP group and 40 (40%) in the LAP group had liver metastasis, 10 (11%) in the OP group and 16 (16%) in the LAP group had peritoneal metastasis, 31 (35%) in the OP group and 33 (33%) in the LAP group had lung metastasis, and 12 (13%) in the OP group and 15 (15%) in the LAP group had lymph node metastasis. Subgroup analyses for overall survival were performed for sex (male

vs female), age (<65 vs ≥65 years), tumor location (cecum, ascending colon, sigmoid colon vs rectosigmoid colon vs upper rectum), clinical stage (II vs III), clinical T stage (cT3 vs cT4), clinical N stage (cN0 vs cN1 vs cN2), and body mass index (BMI; ≤20 vs >20 to 25 vs >25 kg/ m²; Fig. 24.2). Patients with tumors located in the rectosigmoid; who were clinical T4, clinical N2, or had high BMI (>25); and who underwent laparoscopic surgery tended to show worse survival compared to patients in the OP group (Fig. 24.4).

Based on these results, non-inferiority of laparoscopic surgery was not demonstrated for OS in stage II/III colorectal cancer [21]. Potential reasons why non-inferiority could not be proved include (1) biased background factors, (2) protocol deviation, (3) insufficient events, and (4) the possibility that laparoscopic surgery is slightly inferior to open surgery in effectiveness by nature. In the sensitivity analysis performed by the JCOG Data Center, the influence of (1) and (2) was too small to alter the conclusion, but the influence of (3) was significant. In terms of (4), since outcomes in both groups were considerably good with only a slight difference, laparoscopic surgery was considered an acceptable treatment option in experienced facilities, so long as considerations are made for patients concerned about the clinical inferiority of laparoscopic surgery. The numbers of events were insufficient because the treatment outcomes in both groups were more than 10% better than expected and surgery for recurrence and metastasis has advanced further since the trial began 10 years ago.

24.4.4 Patient Factors, Tumor Factors, and Facility Factors to Consider When Performing Laparoscopic Surgery

In the subgroup analysis of patterns of recurrence in JCOG0404, both OS and RFS were significantly lower in the LAP group compared to the OP group in subgroups of patients with pT4, pN2, or BMI >25, after adjusting for patient characteristics. With respect to laparoscopic surgery, manipulations with forceps and pneumoperitoneum during surgery might affect long-term out-

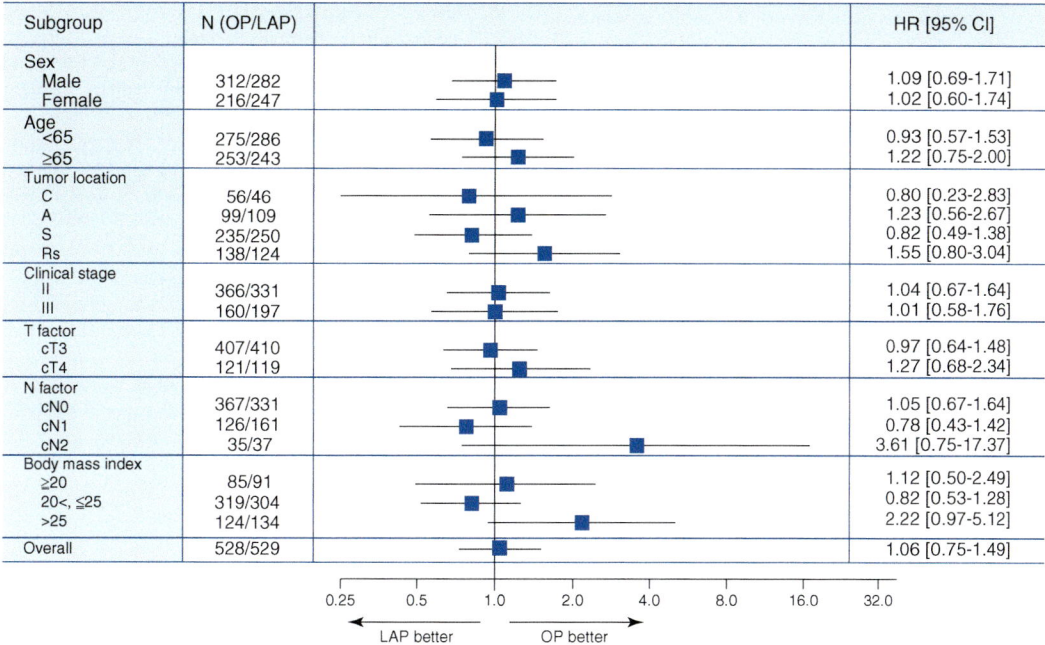

Subgroup	N (OP/LAP)		HR [95% CI]
Sex			
Male	312/282		1.09 [0.69-1.71]
Female	216/247		1.02 [0.60-1.74]
Age			
<65	275/286		0.93 [0.57-1.53]
≥65	253/243		1.22 [0.75-2.00]
Tumor location			
C	56/46		0.80 [0.23-2.83]
A	99/109		1.23 [0.56-2.67]
S	235/250		0.82 [0.49-1.38]
Rs	138/124		1.55 [0.80-3.04]
Clinical stage			
II	366/331		1.04 [0.67-1.64]
III	160/197		1.01 [0.58-1.76]
T factor			
cT3	407/410		0.97 [0.64-1.48]
cT4	121/119		1.27 [0.68-2.34]
N factor			
cN0	367/331		1.05 [0.67-1.64]
cN1	126/161		0.78 [0.43-1.42]
cN2	35/37		3.61 [0.75-17.37]
Body mass index			
≥20	85/91		1.12 [0.50-2.49]
20<, ≤25	319/304		0.82 [0.53-1.28]
>25	124/134		2.22 [0.97-5.12]
Overall	528/529		1.06 [0.75-1.49]

0.25   0.5   1.0   2.0   4.0   8.0   16.0   32.0

← LAP better   OP better →

Fig. 24.4 Subgroup analysis of overall survival

comes, especially in patients with high BMI, advanced clinical node metastasis, and T4 staging [21].

Differences between facilities were evaluated with the mixed effect model using data from JCOG0404, including the facilities as a random effect. After adjusting for age, sex, comorbidity, tumor site, BMI, and clinical stage, differences between facilities were found only in the LAP group for grade 2–4 postoperative early complications. Median incidence rates of grade 2–4 postoperative early complications were 12.7% (range, 12.7–12.7%) in the OP group and 8.8% (range, 4.7–24.0%) in the LAP group, with 69 events and 62 events, respectively. In the effectiveness analysis, there was no significant difference between facilities for 5-year OS in both groups. Median 5-year OS was 92.0% (range, 92.0–92.0) in the OP group and 92.0% (range, 87.9–95.4%) in the LAP group.

On the other hand, for 5-year RFS, there were differences between facilities in the LAP group. Median 5-year RFS was 81.9% (range, 81.9–81.9%) in the OP group and 80.8% (range, 69.8–89.6%) in the LAP group [22].

24.5   Will Open Surgery Survive?

It is currently the age of personalized medicine, and surgical cancer treatment must also be tailored to individual patients. As the number of surgical indications has increased along with remarkable progress in chemotherapy, demands on surgeons have increased. Laparoscopic surgery is an innovative procedure, and there is no doubt that it has brought about major changes in colorectal cancer surgery. Regardless of the results of JCOG0404, advances in laparoscopic surgery will not come to a halt. Since laparoscopic surgery and open surgery are both necessary procedures, neither should be excluded. Rather, surgeons should find ways to integrate both into their treatment plans.

24.6   Future of Colon Cancer Surgery

Although the overall results of JCOG 0404 suggest that open surgery should be the standard treatment for colorectal cancer, laparoscopic surgery should be considered a viable alternative based on the OS and RFS results. The advantages and disadvantages of both procedures should be properly explained to patients prior to surgery. Even if laparoscopic surgery was to replace open surgery and becomes the standard treatment in the future, this may correspond to the "mistaken kindness" described by Halsted [2] without actual clinical benefit of minimal invasiveness. Indeed, there was no actual clinical benefit with respect to minimal invasiveness (55 mL less in bleeding, 1 day shorter length of hospital stay) over the non-inferiority margin (no difference in suture failure/bowel obstruction, approximately 1 h longer operation time, doubled intraoperative organ damage) [21]. After JCOG0404, development of strategies that prioritize patient benefits will be needed, as well as a recognition of the limits of each procedure when considering curative surgery for patients with colon cancer.

References

1. Halsted WSI. The results of operations for the cure of cancer of the breast performed at the Johns Hopkins hospital from June, 1889, to January, 1894. Ann Surg. 1894;20:497–555.
2. Osborne MP. William Stewart Halsted: his life and contributions to surgery. Lancet Oncol. 2007;8:256–65.
3. Miles WE. A method of performing abdomino-perineal excision for carcinoma of the rectum and of the terminal portion of the pelvic colon. Lancet. 1908;172:1812–3.
4. Moynihan BG. The surgical treatment of cancer of the sigmoid flexure and rectum. Surg Gynecol Obstet. 1908;6:4603.
5. Japanese Research Society for Cancer of the Colon and Rectum. Japanese classification of colorectal carcinoma. 2nd English ed. Tokyo: Kanehara Shuppan; 2009.
6. Watanabe T, Itabashi M, Shimada Y, et al. Japanese Society for Cancer of the colon and Rectum. Japanese Society for Cancer of the colon and Rectum (JSCCR) guidelines 2014 for treatment of colorectal cancer. Int J Clin Oncol. 2015;20:207–39.
7. Ishiguro M, Higashi T, Watanabe T, et al. Japanese Society for Cancer of the colon and Rectum guideline committee. Changes in colorectal cancer care in Japan before and after guideline publication: a nationwide survey about D3 lymph node dissection and adjuvant chemotherapy. J Am Coll Surg. 2014;218:969–77.
8. West NP, Kobayashi H, Takahashi K, et al. Understanding optimal colonic cancer surgery: comparison of Japanese D3 resection and European complete mesocolic excision with central vascular ligation. J Clin Oncol. 2012;30:1763–9.
9. Clinical Outmoces of Surgical Therapy Study Group. A comparison of laparoscopically assisted and open colectomy for colon cancer. N Engl J Med. 2004;350:2050–9.
10. Fleshman J, Sargent DJ, Green E, et al. Clinical outcomes of surgical therapy study group. Laparoscopic colectomy for cancer is not inferior to open surgery based on 5-year data from the COST study group trial. Ann Surg. 2007;246:655–62.
11. Veldkamp R, Kuhry E, Hop WC, et al. Colon Cancer laparoscopic or open resection study group (COLOR). Laparoscopic surgery versus open surgery for colon cancer: short-term outcomes of a randomised trial. Lancet Oncol. 2005;6:477–84.
12. Colon Cancer Laparoscopic or Open Resection Study Group, Buunen M, Veldkamp R, et al. Survival after laparoscopic surgery versus open surgery for colon cancer: long-term outcome of a randomised clinical trial. Lancet Oncol. 2009;10:44–52.
13. Guillou PJ, Quirke P, Thorpe H, et al. MRC CLASICC trial group. Short-term endpoints of conventional versus laparoscopic –assisted surgery in patients with colorectal cancer (MRC CLASSIC trial): multicenter, randomized controlled trial. Lancet. 2005;365:1718–26.
14. Green BL, Marshall HC, Collinson F, et al. Long-term follow-up of conventional versus laparoscopically assisted resection in colorectal cancer. Br J Surg. 2013;100:75–82.
15. Kitano S, Yamashita Y, Shiraishi N, et al. 12th nation-wide survey of endoscopic surgery in Japan [in Japanese]. J Jpn Soc Endosc Surg. 2014;19:496–640.
16. Higuchi T, Sugihara K. Complete mesocolic excision (CME) with central vascular ligation (CVL) as standardised surgical technique for colonic cancer: a Japanese multicenter study. Dis Colon Rectum. 2010;53:646.
17. Kitano S, Inomata M, Sato A, et al. Randomized controlled trial to evaluate laparoscopic surgery for colorectal cancer: Japan clinical oncology group study JCOG 0404. Jpn J Clin Oncol. 2005;35: 475–7.
18. Yamamoto S, Inomata M, Katayama H, et al. Short-term surgical outcomes from a randomized controlled trial to evaluate laparoscopic and open D3 dissection for stage II/III colon cancer: Japan clinical oncology group study JCOG 0404. Ann Surg. 2014;260: 23–30.
19. Petrelli N, Douglass HO Jr, Herrera L, et al. The modulation of fluorouracil with leucovorin in metastatic colorectal carcinoma: a prospective randomized phase III trial. Gastrointestinal tumor study group. J Clin Oncol. 1989;7:1419–26.

20. Nakajima K, Inomata M, Akagi T, et al. Quality control by photo documentation for evaluation of laparoscopic and open colectomy with D3 resection for stage II/III colorectal cancer: Japan clinical oncology group study JCOG 0404. Jpn J Clin Oncol. 2014;44:799–806.

21. Kitano S, Inomata M, Mizusawa J, et al. Survival outcomes following laparoscopic versus open D3 dissection for stage II or III colon cancer (JCOG0404): a phase 3, randomised controlled trial. Lancet Gastroenterol Hepatol. 2017;2:261–8.

22. Katayama H, Mizusawa J, Nakamura K, et al. Institutional heterogeneity of survival and morbidity in laparoscopic surgery for colorectal cancer: from the data of a randomized controlled trial comparing open and laparoscopic surgery (JCOG0404). European Cancer Congress (ECC), Vienna, Austria; 25–29 Sep 2015.

Pathologic Assessment and Specimen Quality of Surgery After CME

25

Nobuaki Hoshino, Koya Hida, Takaki Sakurai, and Yoshiharu Sakai

Abstract

Quality of surgery has recently become an important topic in the management of colon cancer. Both en bloc resection and resection of an adequate area of colon and mesocolon are mandatory for high-quality surgery. The quality of surgery is assessed by pathologic evaluation, including morphologic assessment of the plane of dissection, length of colon resected, length of the high tie vascular ligation of the mesenteric artery to the colon, and the number of lymph nodes studied. Morphologic assessment is a qualitative measure of the plane of dissection, and smooth dissection could contribute to good prognosis. The other measures are quantitative and reflect the area of colon and mesocolon resected. Adequate resection area could not only lead to a good prognosis but also enable accurate staging in colon cancer. In this section, we discuss the relationship between quality of surgery and pathologic assessment, highlighting the difference between D3 dissection in Asian countries and complete mesocolic excision (CME) in Western countries. Precise estimation of tumor depth is also considered critical for predicting prognosis in colon cancer. In particular, it is crucial to discriminate a T4 lesion from a T3 lesion, because the former is a potential risk factor for recurrence of disease. However, accurate diagnosis is difficult. We introduce our method of pathologic examination for differentiating these lesions.

Keywords

Complete mesocolic excision · D3 dissection · Pathologic assessment · Specimen quality

25.1 Introduction

Quality of surgery in colon cancer is a topical issue [1]. In Japan, curative resection for colon cancer is performed according to the guideline of the Japanese Society for Cancer of the Colon and Rectum (JSCCR) [2]. The area of the colon and mesocolon to be resected in a horizontal direction is determined by the artery feeding the tumor and the lymphatic networks in the mesocolon. The root of the artery feeding the tumor is removed together with the lymph nodes around the root in a vertical direction. This is the so-called Japanese D3 dissection. In contrast, complete mesocolic excision (CME) has been considered to be important in Western countries since the publication of

N. Hoshino (✉) · K. Hida · Y. Sakai
Department of Surgery, Kyoto University Graduate School of Medicine, Kyoto, Japan
e-mail: hoshinob@kuhp.kyoto-u.ac.jp

T. Sakurai
Department of Diagnostic Pathology, Kyoto University Graduate School of Medicine, Kyoto, Japan

© Springer Nature Singapore Pte Ltd. 2018
N. K. Kim et al. (eds.), *Surgical Treatment of Colorectal Cancer*,
https://doi.org/10.1007/978-981-10-5143-2_25

the results of Hohenberger et al. [3]. The concept of CME includes a morphologically intact meso-colon and adequate resection of the colon and mesocolon. Some retrospective studies in Western countries have reported that the prognosis after CME is better than that after traditional surgery for colon cancer [4, 5]. It is now considered nec-essary to standardize the surgical treatment of colon cancer in Western countries, and Japanese D3 dissection is attracting much attention in this regard because of its promising outcomes [6]. However, the concepts of CME and Japanese D3 dissection differ in that CME entails wider mobi-lization and resection of a longer length of colon. The quality of surgery is assessed by pathologic evaluation. In this section, we compare the patho-logic assessment techniques used and specimen quality between CME and D3 dissection.

25.2 Pathologic Assessment of the Mesocolon

Pathologic assessment of the mesocolon is gener-ally based on four domains: (1) morphologic assess-ment of the plane of dissection, (2) length of colon resected, (3) length of high tie vascular ligation of the mesenteric artery to the colon, and (4) number of lymph nodes studied (NLNS). Morphologic assessment reflects the quality of the surface of the colon and mesocolon dissected, whereas length of colon resected, length of high tie to the colon, and NLNS reflect the area of resected colon and meso-colon. En bloc resection of the colon together with

the mesocolon allows for precise staging of colon cancer and improves prognosis.

25.2.1 Morphologic Assessment of Plane of Dissection

Morphologic assessment of the plane of dissec-tion is classified according to the condition of the dissection surface in a surgical specimen (Fig. 25.1) as follows:

- Mesocolic plane: good-quality surgery, with an intact smooth surface of the mesocolon
- Intramesocolic plane: moderate-quality sur-gery, with disruption that does not reach the muscularis propria in the mesocolon
- Muscularis propria plane: poor-quality sur-gery, with exposure of the muscularis propria

West et al. [7] used the above classification to investigate the association between the plane of dissection and the prognosis in colon cancer according to the MRC CLASICC trial protocol [8], and this classification has since been widely used for assessment of the dissection surface after surgery for colon cancer. West et al. reported that intact smooth plane in the speci-men was associated with good prognosis. A smooth plane of dissection is routinely main-tained in D3 dissection, and postoperative mor-phologic assessment is not common in Japan. Nevertheless, Kobayashi et al. [9] reported no significant difference between D3 dissection and

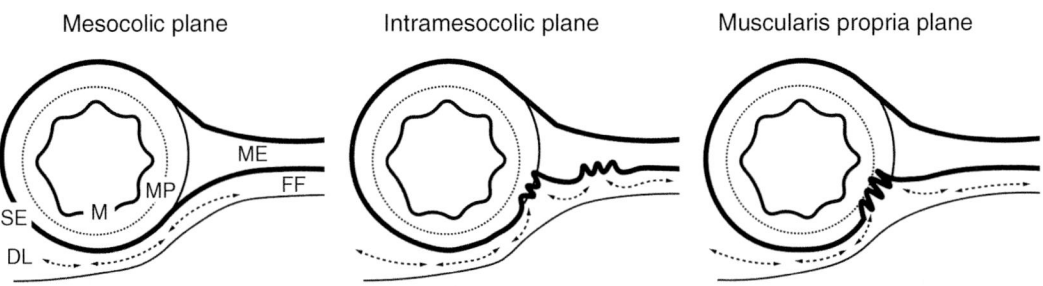

DL:dissection line, FF: fusion fascia, M: mucosa, ME: mesocolon, MP: muscularis propria, SE: serosa

Fig. 25.1 Morphologic classification of the plane of dissection

CME regarding the condition of the plane of dissection of the specimen.

We identified two interesting reports regarding the efficacy of en bloc resection of the mesocolon. Culligan et al. [10] reported abundant lymphatic networks in the mesocolon. However, Gao et al. [11] found no direct lymphatic connections between the mesocolon and the abdominal wall and suggested that the visceral fascia functioned as a barrier to tumor cells. They injected nanocarbon black dye into the subserosal layer around the tumor, and the residue of the dye was found in the mesocolon but not in the abdominal wall that was adjacent to the mesocolon. They also reported that no tumor cells passed through the fascia during an in vitro experiment. These two reports suggest that CME or D3 dissection allows for the complete resection of cancer cells in the mesocolon.

Some problems have been noted in the assessment of the plane of dissection after CME. One problem is that the classification is based on subjective assessment by pathologists. Munkedal et al. [12] reported significant discrepancies in pathologists' grading of the plane of dissection. Another problem is that the good prognosis of surgery in the mesocolic plane was deduced from retrospective studies that were impacted by various confounding factors. A prospective observational study in which detailed classification criteria are defined is needed to determine the impact of morphologic classification on the prognosis.

25.2.2 Length of Colon Resected in a Horizontal Direction

To perform high-quality surgery, it is important that an adequate length of colon is resected so that cancer cells that are floating or spreading in the colon or mesocolon are removed. The area of mesocolon to be resected is estimated from the length of resected colon and the length of the high tie to the colon (Fig. 25.2). An adequate length of resected colon implies an adequate length of resected mesocolon in a horizontal direction. There are reported to be abundant lymphatic net-

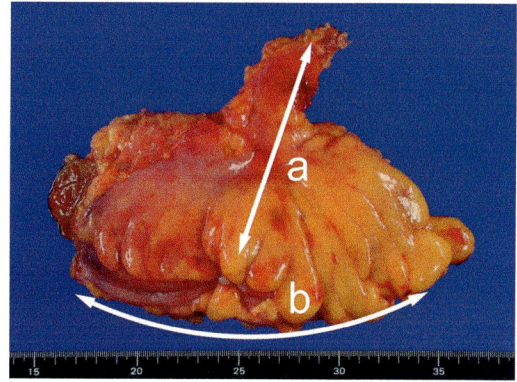

Fig. 25.2 Assessment of the resected area of the mesocolon. (**a**) Length of the high tie to the colon. (**b**) Length of resected colon

works in the mesocolon via which tumor cells can spread; thus, it is mandatory to remove the mesocolon. The "10 cm rule" had been traditionally employed in colon cancer surgery in Japan. This rule suggested that proximal and distal 10 cm of the colon from the tumor should be resected. In the seventh edition of the Japanese Classification of Colorectal Carcinoma, which corresponds to the second edition of the English version [13], the length of colon to be resected is determined by the artery feeding the tumor. The length of resected colon tends to be longer in CME than D3 dissection [9], but there seems to be no definition of the mandatory length of the colon to be resected in CME. Therefore, it is unclear what length of colon needs to be removed to improve survival in both Asian and Western countries. A prospective observational study by the JSCCR is underway to clarify the appropriate length of colon that should be resected (Clinicaltrials.gov identifier, NCT02938481).

25.2.3 Length of the High Tie to the Colon: Resection in a Vertical Direction

In Western countries, the length of the high tie to the colon is used to evaluate the area of the mesocolon to be resected in a vertical direction. However, in D3 dissection, the top of the mesocolon in a vertical direction corresponds to the root of the artery feeding the tumor. Therefore, the length of the colon to be resected is determined by the vascular anatomy and is not routinely measured in Japan. Interestingly, Kobayashi et al. [9] reported that the length of the high tie to the colon in D3 dissection was similar to that in CME.

D3 dissection requires removal of both the root of the feeding artery and the apical lymph nodes. This contributes to not only an accurate evaluation of lymph node metastasis but also a better prognosis. Kawada et al. [14] investigated the prognostic impact of apical lymph node metastasis on cancer-specific death. A combination of apical lymph node metastasis and their prognostic model based on the seventh edition of the TNM classification improved the discriminative ability in the prognosis of stage III colon cancer. Furthermore, Kotake et al. [15] reported a better prognosis in patients who underwent D3 dissection than in those who underwent D2 dissection. Kotake et al. undertook a retrospective propensity-matched analysis of 3425 patients with pT3 or pT4 colon cancer identified in the JSCCR database. In that study, overall survival was significantly improved in patients who underwent D3 dissection (hazard ratio 0.814, 95% confidence interval 0.734–0.904), so D3 dissection is now standard treatment for cT3 or cT4 colon cancer in Japan. A randomized controlled trial comparing the prognosis of D3 dissection (CME plus central vessel ligation) with that of D2 dissection is under way in China [16].

25.2.4 Number of Lymph Nodes Studied

A small NLNS is considered a risk factor for recurrence of colon cancer and poor prognosis. NLNS reflects both the area of resected mesocolon and the accuracy of lymph node assessment. As mentioned earlier, inadequate resection of the colon and mesocolon increases the risk of tumor recurrence because tumor cells may remain in the unresected mesocolon.

The accuracy of lymph node evaluation has been debated for a long time [17]. Inadequate

evaluation of lymph nodes can have a stage migration effect and deprive patients at high risk of the opportunity to receive adjuvant chemotherapy. In Japan, lymph nodes are often retrieved by surgeons from a raw specimen before fixation with formalin, which is different from the lymph node harvesting procedure used in Western countries.

In stage II colon cancer, a small NLNS is considered to be closely associated with a poor prognosis. Caplin et al. [18] reported the impact of a small NLNS on survival in patients with colon cancer and identified an NLNS <6 to be a poor prognostic factor. Since then, various cutoff values have been reported. The American Society of Clinical Oncology recommends that >12 lymph nodes are needed for accurate staging and that adjuvant chemotherapy should be considered in patients with an NLNS <6 [19]. According to the European Society for Medical Oncology, an NLNS <12 is a risk factor for recurrence [20]. As in the JSCCR guideline [2], these recommendations also suggest that an NLNS <12 is a risk factor for disease recurrence.

The lymph node ratio (LNR), that is, the ratio of metastatic lymph nodes to NLNS, is considered a significant prognostic indicator in stage III colon cancer. Berger et al. [21] reported that 5-year overall survival, disease-free survival, and cancer-specific survival were improved by a decrease in the LNR.

Many reports have highlighted an association between a small NLNS/high LNR and a poor prognosis. However, NLNS is reported to be influenced by many clinicopathological factors, including age, sex, obesity, tumor location, surgical method, depth of tumor invasion, differentiation, and examination procedure. Among these factors, most reports have mentioned an association between patient age and NLNS, and the prognostic impact of NLNS may differ between elderly and younger patients [22]. Several cutoff values for NLNS have been proposed, ranging from 6 to 40, and as yet there is no consensus. However, an NLNS <6 is a commonly reported adverse prognostic factor across the studies, and a cutoff value of 12 is representative [19, 20] in stage II colon cancer. Our data, which include

177 patients with stage II colon cancer treated surgically between 2001 and 2008, show a significant difference in relapse-free survival (RFS) and cancer recurrence rates between an NLNS <12 and an NLNS ≥12 (Fig. 25.3). The 5-year recurrence and RFS rates were 0.34 and 0.53, respectively, in patients with an NLNS <12 and 0.08 and 0.81 in those with an NLNS ≥12 (both *P*-values <0.001).

25.3 Pathologic Assessment of Tumor Depth

Precise evaluation of tumor depth is also important for prediction of the prognosis, and it is particularly important to distinguish a T4a lesion from a T3 lesion.

According to the TNM classification, patients with T4a lesions have worse prognosis than those with T3 lesions [23]. The same pattern has also been found in Asian countries [24]. Our data, which include 302 patients with T3 or T4a colon cancer stages I–III treated between 2001 and 2008, revealed a significant difference in RFS ($P = 0.011$) and cancer recurrence ($P = 0.001$) rates between patients with T3 disease and those with T4a disease (Fig. 25.4). Five-year RFS and recurrence rates in patients with T3 disease were 0.74 and 0.17, respectively, and 0.57 and 0.38 in those with T4a disease.

However, it is difficult to diagnose a T3 or T4 lesion accurately. Here we present a patient with T4a sigmoid colon cancer. At our institution, to obtain a precise diagnosis, the tumor is routinely cut by 5 mm, and the resected segments are

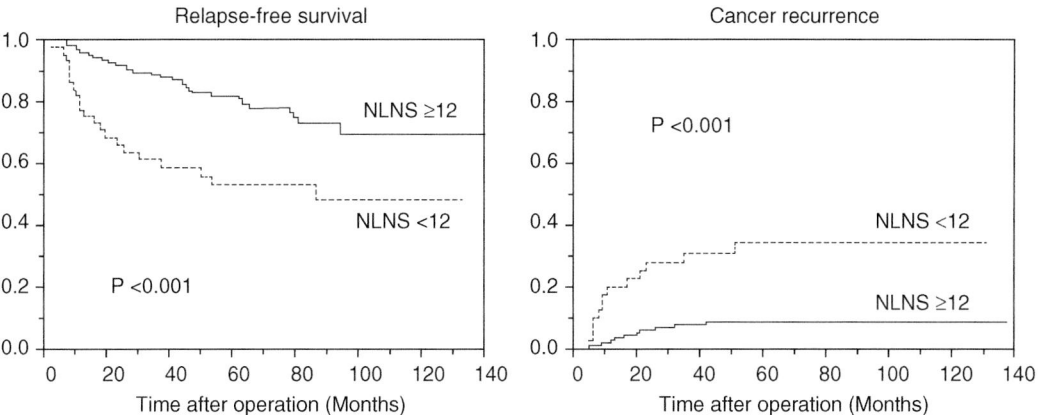

Fig. 25.3 Relapse-free survival and cancer recurrence in patients with an NLNS <12 and an NLNS ≥12

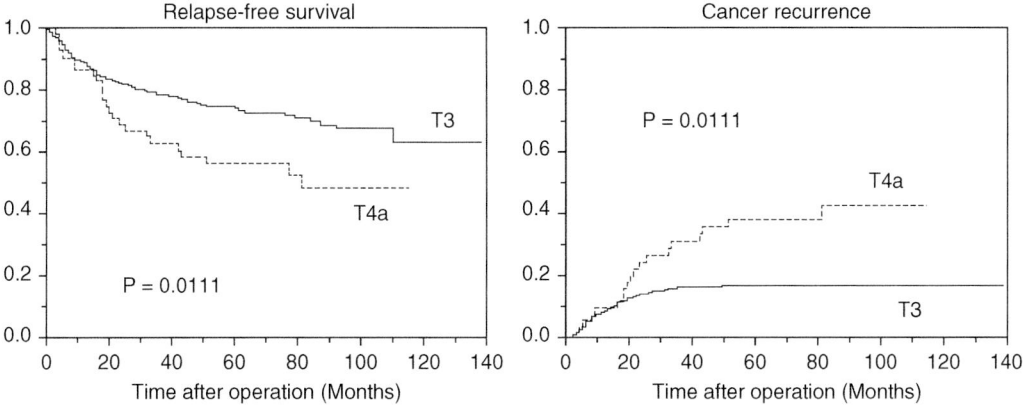

Fig. 25.4 Relapse-free survival and cancer recurrence in patients with T3 and T4a disease

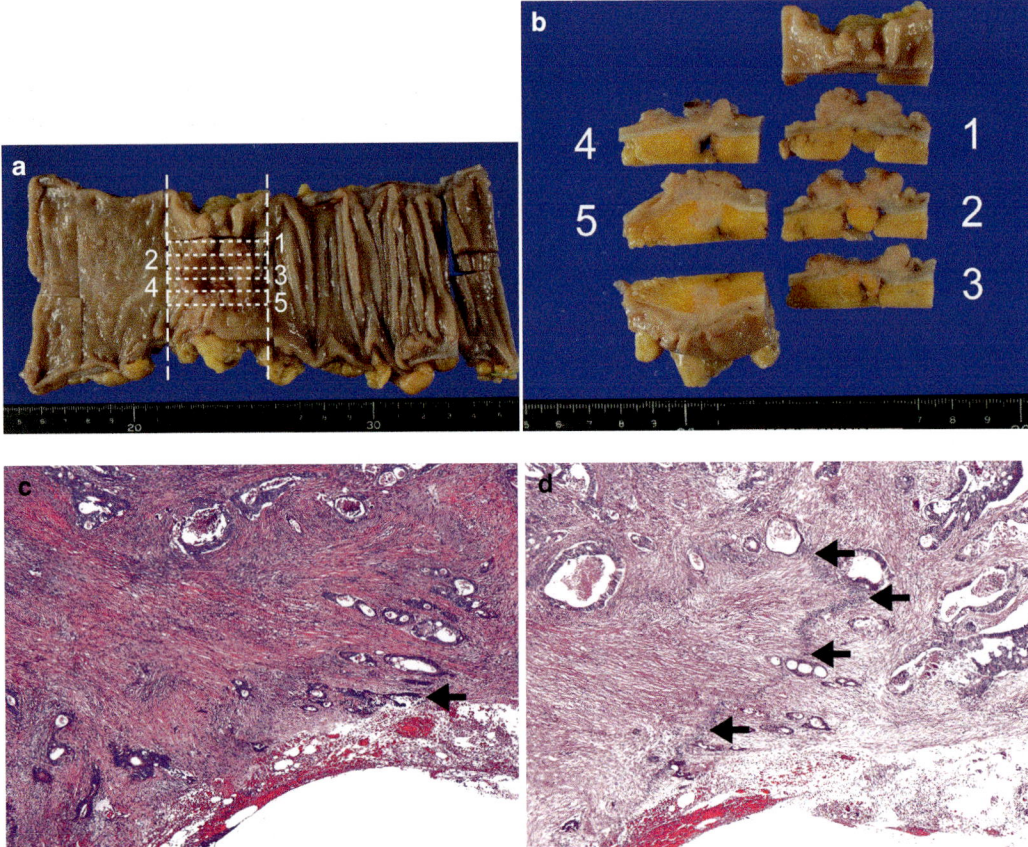

Fig. 25.5 (**a**) The tumor is cut into 5 mm sections. (**b**) The sliced tumor specimens are arranged in sequence and examined macroscopically and then microscopically. (**c**) Tumor cells can be seen to be invading the serosa of the colon (arrow). (**d**) Elastic fibers in the serosa of the colon are clarified by double staining with Victoria blue and hematoxylin-eosin

investigated first macroscopically and then microscopically (Fig. 25.5a–c). In our patient, the tumor can be seen to have invaded the serosa of the colon in the fourth specimen shown in Fig. 25.5b. If there are difficulties in determining the tumor depth, we perform double staining using Victoria blue and hematoxylin-eosin to identify the serosa of the colon. The arrow in Fig. 25.5d indicates stained elastic fibers in the serosa of the colon, confirming that tumor cells have invaded the serosa.

References

1. den Dulk M, van de Velde CJ. Time to focus on the quality of colon-cancer surgery. Lancet Oncol. 2008;9:815–7.

2. Watanabe T, Itabashi M, Shimada Y, Tanaka S, Ito Y, Ajioka Y, et al. Japanese Society for Cancer of the Colon and Rectum (JSCCR) guidelines 2010 for the treatment of colorectal cancer. Int J Clin Oncol. 2012;17:1–29.

3. Hohenberger W, Weber K, Matzel K, Papadopoulos T, Merkel S. Standardized surgery for colonic cancer: complete mesocolic excision and central ligation--technical notes and outcome. Color Dis. 2009;11:354–64.

4. West NP, Hohenberger W, Weber K, Perrakis A, Finan PJ, Quirke P. Complete mesocolic excision with central vascular ligation produces an oncologically superior specimen compared with standard surgery for carcinoma of the colon. J Clin Oncol. 2010;28:272–8.

5. Bertelsen CA, Bols B, Ingeholm P, Jansen JE, Neuenschwander AU, Vilandt J. Can the quality of colonic surgery be improved by standardization of surgical technique with complete mesocolic excision? Color Dis. 2011;13:1123–9.

6. Quirke P, West N. Quality of surgery: has the time come for colon cancer? Lancet Oncol. 2015;16:121–2.

7. West NP, Morris EJ, Rotimi O, Cairns A, Finan PJ, Quirke P. Pathology grading of colon cancer surgical resection and its association with survival: a retrospective observational study. Lancet Oncol. 2008;9:857–65.
8. Guillou PJ, Quirke P, Thorpe H, Walker J, Jayne DG, Smith AM, et al. Short-term endpoints of conventional versus laparoscopic-assisted surgery in patients with colorectal cancer (MRC CLASICC trial): multicentre, randomised controlled trial. Lancet. 2005;365:1718–26.
9. Kobayashi H, West NP, Takahashi K, Perrakis A, Weber K, Hohenberger W, et al. Quality of surgery for stage III colon cancer: comparison between England, Germany, and Japan. Ann Surg Oncol. 2014;21(Suppl 3):S398–404.
10. Culligan K, Sehgal R, Mulligan D, Dunne C, Walsh S, Quondamatteo F, et al. A detailed appraisal of mesocolic lymphangiology--an immunohistochemical and stereological analysis. J Anat. 2014;225:463–72.
11. Gao Z, Ye Y, Zhang W, Shen D, Zhong Y, Jiang K, et al. An anatomical, histopathological, and molecular biological function study of the fascias posterior to the interperitoneal colon and its associated mesocolon: their relevance to colonic surgery. J Anat. 2013;223:123–32.
12. Munkedal DL, Laurberg S, Hagemann-Madsen R, Stribolt KJ, Krag SR, Quirke P, et al. Significant individual variation between pathologists in the evaluation of colon cancer specimens after complete mesocolic excision. Dis Colon Rectum. 2016;59:953–61.
13. Japanese Society for Cancer of the Colon and Rectum. Japanese classification of colorectal carcinoma, 2nd ed. (English). Tokyo: Kanehara; 2009.
14. Kawada H, Kurita N, Nakamura F, Kawamura J, Hasegawa S, Kotake K, et al. Incorporation of apical lymph node status into the seventh edition of the TNM classification improves prediction of prognosis in stage III colonic cancer. Br J Surg. 2014;101:1143–52.
15. Kotake K, Mizuguchi T, Moritani K, Wada O, Ozawa H, Oki I, et al. Impact of D3 lymph node dissection on survival for patients with T3 and T4 colon cancer. Int J Color Dis. 2014;29:847–52.
16. Lu JY, Xu L, Xue HD, Zhou WX, Xu T, Qiu HZ, et al. The radical extent of lymphadenectomy - D2 dissection versus complete mesocolic excision of laparoscopic right colectomy for right-sided colon cancer (RELARC) trial: study protocol for a randomized controlled trial. Trials. 2016;17:582.
17. Hernanz F, Revuelta S, Redondo C, Madrazo C, Castillo J, Gómez-Fleitas M. Colorectal adenocarcinoma: quality of the assessment of lymph node metastases. Dis Colon Rectum. 1994;37:373–6.
18. Caplin S, Cerottini JP, Bosman FT, Constanda MT, Givel JC. For patients with Dukes' B (TNM stage II) colorectal carcinoma, examination of six or fewer lymph nodes is related to poor prognosis. Cancer. 1998;83:666–72.
19. Benson AB 3rd, Schrag D, Somerfield MR, Cohen AM, Figueredo AT, Flynn PJ, et al. American Society of Clinical Oncology recommendations on adjuvant chemotherapy for stage II colon cancer. J Clin Oncol. 2004;22:3408–19.
20. Schmoll HJ, Van Cutsem E, Stein A, Valentini V, Glimelius B, Haustermans K, et al. ESMO consensus guidelines for management of patients with colon and rectal cancer. A personalized approach to clinical decision making. Ann Oncol. 2012;23:2479–516.
21. Berger AC, Sigurdson ER, LeVoyer T, Hanlon A, Mayer RJ, Macdonald JS, et al. Colon cancer survival is associated with decreasing ratio of metastatic to examined lymph nodes. J Clin Oncol. 2005;23:8706–12.
22. Hoshino N, Hasegawa S, Hida K, Kawada K, Sugihara K, Sakai Y. Impact of age on the prognostic value of number of lymph nodes retrieved in patients with stage II colorectal cancer. Int J Color Dis. 2016;31:1307–13.
23. Gunderson LL, Jessup JM, Sargent DJ, Greene FL, Stewart AK. Revised TN categorization for colon cancer based on national survival outcomes data. J Clin Oncol. 2010;28:264–71.
24. Lan YT, Yang SH, Chang SC, Liang WY, Li AF, Wang HS, et al. Analysis of the seventh edition of American Joint Committee on colon cancer staging. Int J Color Dis. 2012;27:657–63.

Laparoscopic Surgery for Colon Cancer: Principles and Pitfalls

26

Jeonghyun Kang and Kang Young Lee

Abstract

Laparoscopic colon cancer resection has been a successful alternative of open surgery, based on accumulated evidence. Postoperative morbidity and mortality were significantly decreased with laparoscopic technique, and oncologic outcome was not inferior to open technique. In the age of complete mesocolic excision, feasibility of laparoscopic technique has been reevaluated, and several technical considerations are under discussion. In Asian countries including Korea, Japan, and China, precise dissection along the embryological plane and central vessel ligation has been regarded as a standard procedure for colon cancer surgery, even in laparoscopic surgery. With the accumulation of experience of laparoscopic complete mesocolic excision, penetration rate of laparoscopic colon cancer surgery in Asian countries is higher than western countries, and quality of colon cancer resection is getting better. In the same time, standardization of procedure is important to improve quality of laparoscopic colon cancer surgery and to educate trainee. In procedure details of laparoscopic colon cancer resection, there are some differences according to anatomical location of colon cancer in the viewpoint of preparation and procedure details.

Keywords

Laparoscopic surgery · Colon cancer · Complete mesocolic excision

26.1 Introduction

Minimally invasive surgical techniques have affected the treatment of colon cancer. The postoperative morbidity and mortality were significantly decreased after the application of the laparoscopic technique [1]. It has been proven that the oncologic outcome of laparoscopic colon cancer surgery was not inferior to that of open surgery [2–5]. The basic principle of laparoscopic colon cancer surgery is not different from open surgery, in regard to making a good surgical view, effective traction and countertraction, fine dissection along the surgical plane, etc. However, it is critical that the factors that differentiate laparoscopic colon cancer surgery from other surgical methods be understood for its success.

26.2 Current Evidence Supporting Laparoscopic Surgery for Colon Cancer

Since the first laparoscopic colectomy was performed in 1991 [6], the laparoscopic technique has often been applied to colon cancer surgeries. In the early period of laparoscopic colon cancer

J. Kang · K. Y. Lee (✉)
Department of Surgery, Yonsei University College of Medicine, Seoul, South Korea
e-mail: KYLEE117@yuhs.ac

© Springer Nature Singapore Pte Ltd. 2018
N. K. Kim et al. (eds.), *Surgical Treatment of Colorectal Cancer*,
https://doi.org/10.1007/978-981-10-5143-2_26

surgery, extra caution for laparoscopic colon cancer surgery was recommended, because the safety of the oncologic outcome was not confirmed. In 2002, the oncologic safety of laparoscopic colon cancer surgery was demonstrated for the first time through a prospective randomized clinical trial in a single institute [7]. Afterwards, the results of several randomized clinical trials followed, which also proved the oncologic safety of laparoscopic colon cancer surgery [2–5, 8].

At the same time, the benefits of laparoscopic colon cancer surgery were demonstrated in short-term outcome. The laparoscopic technique was related to reducing postoperative complications, faster return of bowel motility, reducing postoperative pain, and decreasing the average hospital stay [1, 7, 9–11].

26.3 Specific Consideration: Obstructing Colon Cancer, Combined Resection

The management of obstructing colon cancer is quite challenging, especially in laparoscopic colon surgery. Laparoscopic management options for obstruction colon cancer are not different to open laparotomy. However, it is hard to get working space in laparoscopic surgery because of distended bowel. Limited working space could be resulted in poor oncologic outcome and increased postoperative morbidity [12]. The application of self-expanding stents in obstructed colon as a bridge to surgery could be an alternative option [13–15]. After relieving obstruction, laparoscopic surgery could be performed as like ordinary colon cancer [16]. Application of laparoscopic technique for obstructing colon cancer should be careful not to make additional problem. Patient selection based on the result of treatment for obstruction, preparation, and patient's condition is the key for the success of laparoscopic surgery.

Combined resection for T4 colon cancer is also challenging to apply laparoscopic technique [17, 18]. There are no common criteria to apply laparoscopic technique for combined resection. It depends on surgeon's experience and ability and surgical team's experience. Even in experienced surgical team, intensive preoperative discussion about detailed design for combined resection, reconstruction plan, and real benefit of patient must be needed.

26.4 Feasibility, Technical Consideration in the Era of Complete Mesocolic Excision

The main concept of complete mesocolic excision for colon cancer includes sharp dissection along embryologically developed surgical plane and central vessel ligation [19]. Although feasibility and safety of laparoscopic surgery for colon cancer have already been demonstrated with several clinical trials, technical details and quality of laparoscopic colon cancer surgery were not evaluated thoroughly. In previous studies, the main goal of researches was to prove the non-inferiority of the laparoscopic technique, compared to the open technique. None of the studies included the standardization of the surgical procedure itself. The only inclusion criterion for the successful laparoscopic colon cancer surgery trials referred to above was the surgeon's number of case experiences; there was no evaluation process for the quality of the surgeon's lymph node dissection. In the era of complete mesocolic excision, a reevaluation of the feasibility of the laparoscopic technique for complete mesocolic excision has been raised [20, 21]. The quality of the complete mesocolic excision is recognized as one of the important prognostic factor [22, 23], so the quality of colon cancer resection must be considered in evaluating the effectiveness of laparoscopic colon cancer surgery.

26.4.1 Patients' Position

The way in which the patient was positioned for open surgery was not changed for the laparoscopic procedure. However, in laparoscopic colon cancer resection, the patient should be fixed securely on the table, because the patient's position could be changed during the operation for the sake of the exposure of the target anatomy. The patient's position for laparoscopic colon cancer surgery depends on the anatomical location of the tumor and the operating surgeon's preference. I personally prefer the lithotomy position for all laparoscopic colon cancer surgeries, because it allows for the surgeon to place oneself between the patient's legs.

26.4.2 How to Make Surgical Field

Good exposure of the target anatomy is crucial for a successful operation. In laparoscopic colon cancer surgery, the key component of making the surgical field is removing a small bowel from the surgical field. In left-sided colon cancer surgery, ideally, the root of colonic mesentery from the Treitz ligament to the sacral promontory should be exposed for the central lymph node dissection.

26.4.3 Plane Dissection

The essential component of complete mesocolic excision is a sharp dissection along embryologically developed surgical plane. It is well-demonstrated that a complete excision of lymph nodes bearing mesocolon without the disruption of visceral fascia is a key component to improving the oncologic outcome of colon cancer [19]. At the same time, the preservation of fascia overlying essential retroperitoneal structure is also important lest the ureter and gonadal vessels are injured and to avoid unnecessary bleeding from retroperitoneal structures.

In laparoscopic colon cancer surgery, the basic skill for a sharp plane dissection is exactly the same as with open surgery: effective traction and countertraction and point-by-point sharp dissection. The selection of an instrument for plane dissection is point for consideration in laparoscopic surgery. A monopolar device with hook, spatula, or scissor (hot shear) is one popular instrument for plane dissection. With the development of technology, energy-based devices are adapted for

the plane dissection, generally an ultrasonic energy-based instrument. The adaptation of energy-based devices in laparoscopic colon cancer surgery could reduce chyle leakage, minimize bleeding on dissection plane, and facilitate complete plane dissection [24].

The starting point of the plane dissection is one of the main discussion points in laparoscopic colon cancer surgery, namely, medial-to-lateral dissection, lateral-to-medial dissection, inferior approach, etc. If we keep the oncologic principles, the mode of dissection does not make a difference in the oncologic outcome. However, the standardization of one's own procedure based on an exact understanding of the precise anatomy is crucial for a successful plane dissection. The probability of success should be also considered.

26.4.4 Central Vessel Ligation

Central vessel ligation is another crucial component of complete mesocolic excision for the complete removal of regional lymph nodes, which is an essential part of curative resection of colon cancer. According to the anatomical location of colon cancer, corresponding feeding vessels should be ligated at their origin. For the safety of laparoscopic central vessel ligation, the first step is the complete exposure of the proximal part of the origin of feeding vessels. It is hard to say that complete exposure of proximal part of feeding vessels could improve oncologic outcome in the prophylactic lymph node dissection. However, from a technical viewpoint, the complete exposure of the proximal part and the origin of feeding vessels before the ligation of feeding vessels is important for a safe procedure.

As is the case with the plane dissection, the selection of the instrument for the central vessel ligation could be a discussion point. Dissection with a monopolar hook or spatula and vessel ligation with surgical clips is the traditional way of central vessel ligation. With the development of technology, the application of energy-based devices supports the advance of laparoscopic colon cancer surgery. From a basic technological viewpoint, energy-based devices can be classified into bipolar energy-based devices and ultrasonic energy-based devices. The current energy-based devices can ligate vessels up to 7 mm in diameter without a mechanical clip [25]. This means that all vessels during colon cancer surgery could theoretically be ligated and divided without the application of a surgical clip. Some surgeons do not use surgical clips in their daily practice according to the theoretical guideline, but most colorectal surgeons prefer to apply a surgical clip to the patient's side to minimize the potential risk of bleeding. We should understand the mode of action of advanced instruments; otherwise, unexpected complications may arise.

26.4.5 Keep Blood Flow with Lymph Node Dissection

For the complete regional lymph adenectomy, feeding vessels should be ligated. Feeding vessel ligation at its origin has been regarded as an inevitable procedure for a complete regional lymph adenectomy. However, the potential problem of vessel ligation at its origin is the deterioration of blood flow. From a technical viewpoint, a complete regional lymphadenectomy could be accomplished with the preservation of blood flow. As a solution for the issue of the high ligation of inferior mesenteric artery vs. low ligation, the left colic artery could be preserved after the complete removal of lymph nodes bearing fat tissue around the inferior mesenteric artery. There still is a debate about the safety of this procedure. Potential problem of this technique is concerned about oncologic safety, because lymph nodes bearing tissue could be opened during the procedure. This is an issue to be clarified with further research.

26.5 Laparoscopic Right Hemicolectomy

26.5.1 Position

The patient's position, whether it be the supine or the modified lithotomy position, should be decided according to the placement of the surgical team. The modified lithotomy position offers several options for the surgical team's placement. During laparoscopic right hemicolectomy, the surgeon could be on the patient's left side or between the patient's legs, as is appropriate for each procedure. The mild Trendelenburg position could help the upward shift of omentum and the transverse colon. Additionally left side-tilted position removes the small bowel to the left side abdominal cavity and pelvis, which is helpful for central lymph node dissection on superior mesenteric vessels.

26.5.2 Colon Mobilization

One approach regarding the sequence of colon cancer surgery is the lateral-to-medial approach, which means that colon mobilization is the first step before central vessel ligation. In contrast, in the medial-to-lateral approach, central vessel ligation is the first step of operation, and it involves continued dissection for mobilization of colonic mesentery and right colon. There is no difference in oncologic and operative outcomes.

The preferred way of dissection is the inferior approach as a same concept of lateral-to-medial approach, which means that dissection is started with the mobilization of cecum. Having the cecum and terminal ileum mobilization as the first step of the operation is a relatively good way to identify the surgical plane between the parietal fascia and the colonic mesentery. The appendix or cecum is used for traction by the assistant, and countertraction created with the surgeon's left hand by grasping the parietal peritoneum offers a good surgical view and facilitates the identification of the correct surgical plane (Fig. 26.1). After making a peritoneal incision, precise dissection should be continued up to the duodenum with preservation of the right ureter and the gonadal vessels (Fig. 26.2). The advantage of the inferior-first approach is that the chance of injury to the ureter or the gonadal vessels could be minimized, since those structures are already

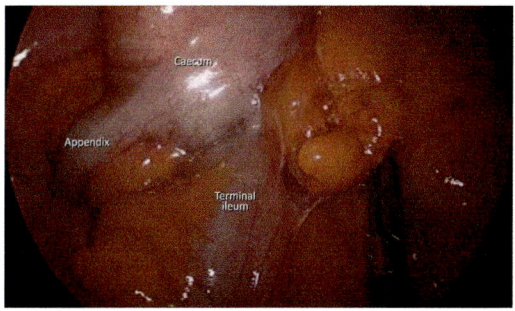

Fig. 26.1 Preparation of the inferior approach. Dissection is started with the mobilization of cecum. The appendix or cecum is used for traction by the assistant, and counter-traction created with the surgeon's left hand by grasping the parietal peritoneum

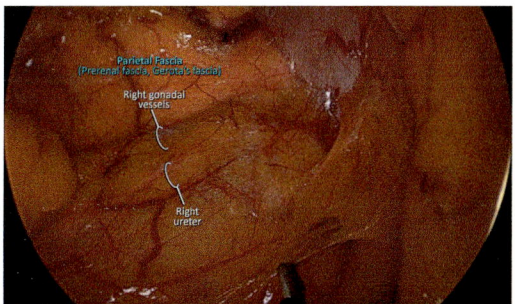

Fig. 26.2 Preservation of the right ureter and the gonadal vessels. The ileum is retracted to a superior direction to expose the mesenteric attachments to the retroperitoneum; the right ureter and the gonadal vessels are visualized

separated from the colonic mesentery before the vascular dissection. Also, it has been my experience that the time spent to identify the exact surgical place can be reduced.

26.5.3 Central Vessel Ligation

In laparoscopic right hemicolectomy, the ileocolic vascular pedicle is an anatomical landmark to start vascular dissection. Traction to right, inferior direction created by the assistant could help the identification of the location of the ileocolic and superior mesenteric vessels. If the cecum and its mesentery are mobilized before vascular dissection, the identification of the ileocolic vessels becomes easier. In laparoscopic surgery, having an anatomical landmark—not only for the identification of vascular anatomy, but also for the

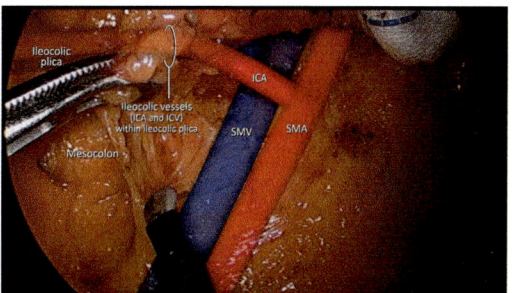

Fig. 26.3 Lymphadenectomy of the ileocolic pedicle. The ileocolic artery (ICA) is branching from the superior mesenteric artery (SMA)

whole procedure—is important to keep track of the right direction of the dissection and to minimize the chances of making a mistake. My personal preference for the surgeon's location for a central lymph node dissection is between the patient's legs, with an image to continue the dissection heading to the falciform ligament.

The first step of central vessel ligation is the complete exposure of the superior mesenteric vein and the origin of corresponding vessels. For the safety of central vessel ligation, ligation of a vessel surrounded by fat tissues should be avoided. After making a peritoneal incision along an imaginary line of the superior mesenteric vein, a layer-by-layer dissection is needed to identify the superior mesenteric vein. Vascular dissection is focused on the right side of the superior mesenteric vein, because there is no consensus on lymph node dissection on the superior mesenteric artery from the viewpoint of complete regional lymph adenectomy and its oncologic outcomes. The origin of the ileocolic artery and vein is identified on the right border of the superior mesenteric vein, and both vessels are ligated and divided safely (Fig. 26.3). Further dissection on the superior mesenteric vessels and the mid-colic artery is identified. In case of hepatic flexure cancer, lymph node dissection around the origin of the mid-colic artery is important from the viewpoint of complete regional lymph adenectomy. However, we don't have to ligate the mid-colic artery at its origin as a routine procedure. Considering the resection margin and central lymphatic drainage, only the right branch of mid-colic artery can be ligated (Fig. 26.4).

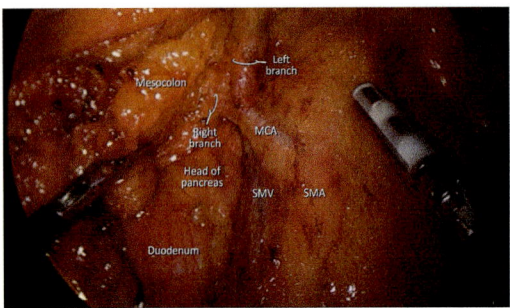

Fig. 26.4 Identification of right and left branches of the middle colic vessels. The middle colic pedicle is lifted anteriorly using two points of retraction

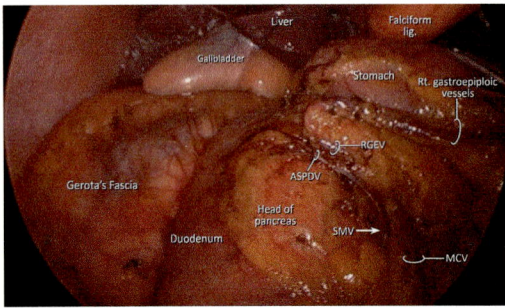

Fig. 26.5 Identification of right gastroepiploic vessels for guide to dividing the gastrocolic ligament. The right gastroepiploic vein (RGEV) along the surface of the pancreas must be preserved. *ASPDV* anterior superior pancreatic duodenal vein, *SMV* superior mesenteric vein, *MCV* middle colic vein

The division of gastrocolic ligament is a controversial topic. There is ongoing debate about dissection along the right gastroepiploic vessels and their origin. So far, there is no concrete evidence to support lymph node dissection along the right gastroepiploic vessels. However, they could be a good guide to dividing the gastrocolic ligament (Fig. 26.5).

26.5.4 Specimen Extraction

After the completion of the dissection, the specimen is extracted, and anastomosis is performed. By the extension of supra-umbilical camera port wound, the specimen could be extracted, and extracorporeal anastomosis is performed in the conventional way. In case of extracorporeal anas-

tomosis, extra caution is needed to prevent rotation of terminal ileum mesentery. For that reason, some surgeon prefers intracorporeal anastomosis, but this technique could be applied after overcoming learning curve of procedure.

26.6 Laparoscopic Sigmoid Colectomy

26.6.1 Position

The steep Trendelenburg and right-sided tilt position is the first step to remove the small bowel from the pelvic and surgical field. For the patient's safety, a chest belt to fix the patient on the table could be useful. The complete exposure of the surgical field is crucial for ensuring the quality of the surgery. For the sigmoid colectomy, the exposure of the anatomy from the Treitz ligament to the sacral promontory is needed. A technical tip for making the surgical field is to have an image to flip over the small bowel over its axis, instead of focusing on the small bowel itself. By focusing on the small bowel mesentery, the whole small bowel could be moved to the right side of the abdominal cavity. In addition, surgical gauze could give us extra help for the exposure. When surgical gauze is applied for exposure, it should be applied on the small bowel itself, not on a mesentery, for effective exposure.

26.6.2 Mobilization of Colon

Again, the sequence of operation is a traditional point of contention. The effectiveness of the lateral-to-medial approach versus the medial-to-lateral approach for colon cancer resection is the debated issue.

The preferred way of dissection is lateral approach. The lateral approach is more convenient, because gravity can provide natural traction in a right-sided position. The sigmoid colon itself could be used as a retractor to remove the small bowel in the case of obstruction or morbid obese patients. The mobilization of the colon was started with the detachment of the natural adhesion of the sigmoid colon from the left lateral abdominal wall. The sigmoid-descending junction is the preferred site to identify the embryological plane, because it is a relatively easy point to develop the surgical plane. When the correct surgical plane is developed, the dissection can be continued along the surgical plane between Gerota's fascia and the descending colon (Fig. 26.6). Splenic flexure mobilization is an optional procedure to undergo after the consideration of the bowel length for the anastomosis after the resection of cancer. In case of a splenic flexure mobilization, a precise dissection along the embryological plane is also important to access the lesser sac (Fig. 26.7). A natural fusion among the colon, the omentum, and Gerota's fascia occurred, but there is a lot of variation in the degree of fusion and the placement of the colon. The splenic flexure mobilization is a consecutive procedure of the mobilization of the descending colon from Gerota's fascia. Through a

precise dissection along the embryological plane, the omentum's adhesion to the colon is certainly noticed ahead of splenic flexure. From this point, the omentum should be detached from the colon, and then we can access the lesser sac naturally. A complete mobilization of the splenic flexure can be achieved through the division of the colonic mesentery from the inferior border of pancreas and the detachment of the omentum from the distal transverse colon.

26.6.3 Central Vessel Ligation

Central vessel ligation is one of the essential components of a complete mesocolic excision. Making a peritoneal incision on the medial side of the sigmoid attachment on the retroperitoneal structure is the first step of a central vessel ligation. Two preferred sites of starting a medial dissection are the medial part of the inferior mesenteric vein by the Treitz ligament and the sacral promontory area. After the assistant lifts up the inferior mesenteric vein, a peritoneal incision between the inferior mesenteric vein and the Treitz ligament is made, and precise dissection is continued along the avascular space, which is a dissection plane between the colonic mesentery and Gerota's fascia. Further dissection eventually connects it to the previous dissection area.

The sacral promontory area is also a good place to start medical dissection. After the assistant lifts up the sigmoid colon mesentery, a peritoneal incision is made with countertraction with the surgeon's left hand. If a peritoneal incision was made on the right point, air insufflation under the peritoneum would be noticed. After that, further dissection can continue along the developed space by means of air infiltration. Before the perivascular dissection, a complete mobilization of inferior mesenteric artery pedicle is essential for the complete removal of lymph nodes bearing tissue and for the patient's safety. Dissection in the space between the interior mesenteric artery and the aorta is quite tricky, because it is hard to identify the exact surgical plane and lymphatic vessels, and nerve fibers around the aorta are running up along the inferior mesenteric artery.

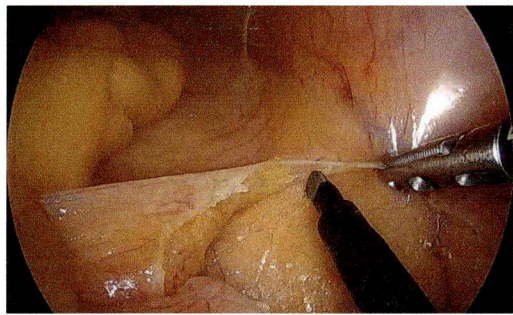

Fig. 26.6 Lateral dissection between Gerota's fascia and the descending colon. The white line of Toldt is incised, and the dissection begun in the avascular plane between the mesocolon and retroperitoneum

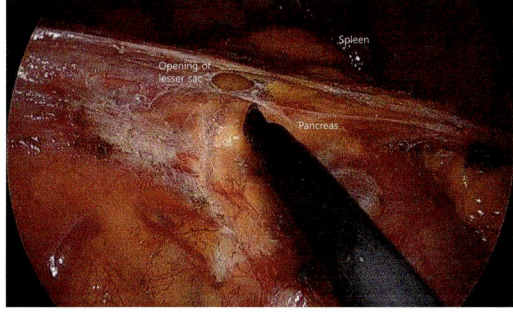

Fig. 26.7 Splenic flexure mobilization. Accessing the lesser sac after dissection of a natural fusion among the colon, the omentum and Gerota's fascia

In sigmoid colon cancer surgery, the level of inferior mesenteric artery ligation is a point of contention regarding high ligation versus low ligation, as is the case with rectal cancer surgery. High ligation means the ligation of the inferior mesenteric artery at the bifurcation level from the aorta. The main idea of high ligation is for complete regional lymphadenectomy [26]. In contrast, low ligation refers to ligating the artery after the bifurcation of the left colic artery from the inferior mesenteric artery. The idea of low ligation is based on the data which showed no statistically significant difference according to the level of artery ligation and the effort to keep the blood flow to left colic artery to improve the perfusion on the proximal bowel of anastomosis [27]; even the traditional concept of low ligation does not remove lymph nodes bearing tissue around the inferior mesenteric artery.

However, low ligation can be performed after the complete removal of lymph nodes bearing tissue around the inferior mesenteric artery. After the mobilization of the vascular pedicle of the inferior mesenteric artery, perivascular dissection is started on the bifurcation level of the left colic artery and continued to the origin of the inferior mesenteric artery. With further dissection, all named vessels—inferior mesenteric artery, left colic artery, sigmoid artery, and inferior mesenteric vein—are identified. Then the sigmoid artery and the inferior mesenteric vein are ligated and divided, preserving the left colic artery completely removing the regional lymph nodes bearing fat tissue (Fig. 26.8). Vascular ligation after

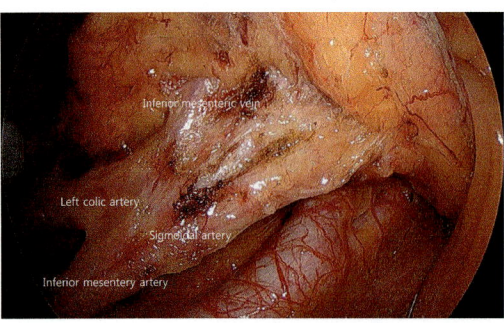

Fig. 26.8 Blood vessels of left colon. *IMA* inferior mesenteric artery, *IMV* inferior mesenteric vein, *SA* sigmoidal artery

the complete dissection of lymph nodes bearing tissue also has the benefit of secure ligation of each vessel and the minimization of the possibility of an accident caused by a vascular anomaly on the left colic artery.

26.6.4 Specimen Extraction

Generally, after cutting the distal colon of cancer with a laparoscopic linear stapler, a specimen is extracted for the removal of cancer and for the preparation of anastomosis. The extraction site can be decided according to the surgeon's preference. The Pfannenstiel incision for specimen extraction has several benefits from the viewpoint of cosmesis and technical issues. The incidence of incisional hernia is low after a Pfannenstiel incision, compared to a midline incision. Also, after the removal of tumor in the sigmoid colon, end-to-end anastomosis can be performed under direct vision. Accordingly, operation time can be reduced, since we don't have to make a pneumoperitoneum again for anastomosis.

26.7   Laparoscopic Left Hemicolectomy

26.7.1 Position

The Trendelenburg and right-sided tilt position is helpful to remove the small bowel from surgical field. As like sigmoid colon cancer surgery, the exposure of the mesentery from the Treitz ligament to the sacral promontory is essential.

26.7.2 Mobilization of the Colon

For left hemicolectomy, the complete mobilization of the splenic flexure is an essential step. Even in the case of splenic flexure cancer, the whole descending colon should be mobilized to procure enough length for anastomosis. The mobilization of descending colon is exactly the same procedure as in sigmoid colon cancer surgery. However, on the splenic flexure, the resection margin of the omentum should be considered. After getting into the lesser sac, the omentum is divided considering the resection margin.

26.7.3 Central Vessel Ligation

It is hard to discuss the central vessel ligation of splenic flexure cancer, because there is no consensus yet. Extent of lymph node dissection is a matter for further research.

References

1. Ohtani H, Tamamori Y, Arimoto Y, Nishiguchi Y, Maeda K, Hirakawa K. A meta-analysis of the short- and long-term results of randomized controlled trials that compared laparoscopy-assisted and open colectomy for colon cancer. J Cancer. 2012;3:49–57. https://doi.org/10.7150/jca.3621.
2. Guillou PJ, Quirke P, Thorpe H, Walker J, Jayne DG, Smith AM, et al. Short-term endpoints of conventional versus laparoscopic-assisted surgery in patients with colorectal cancer (MRC CLASICC trial): multicentre, randomised controlled trial. Lancet. 2005;365(9472):1718–26. https://doi.org/10.1016/s0140-6736(05)66545-2.
3. Hewett PJ, Allardyce RA, Bagshaw PF, Frampton CM, Frizelle FA, Rieger NA, et al. Short-term outcomes of the Australasian randomized clinical study comparing laparoscopic and conventional open surgical treatments for colon cancer: the ALCCaS trial. Ann Surg. 2008;248(5):728–38. https://doi.org/10.1097/SLA.0b013e31818b7595.
4. Nelson H, Sargent DJ, Wieand HS, Fleshman J, Anvari M, Stryker SJ, et al. A comparison of laparoscopically assisted and open colectomy for colon cancer. N Engl J Med. 2004;350(20):2050–9. https://doi.org/10.1056/NEJMoa032651.
5. Veldkamp R, Kuhry E, Hop WC, Jeekel J, Kazemier G, Bonjer HJ, et al. Laparoscopic surgery versus open surgery for colon cancer: short-term outcomes of a randomised trial. Lancet Oncol. 2005;6(7):477–84. https://doi.org/10.1016/s1470-2045(05)70221-7.
6. Cooperman AM, Katz V, Zimmon D, Botero G. Laparoscopic colon resection: a case report. J Laparoendosc Surg. 1991;1(4):221–4.
7. Lacy AM, Garcia-Valdecasas JC, Delgado S, Castells A, Taura P, Pique JM, et al. Laparoscopy-assisted colectomy versus open colectomy for treatment of non-metastatic colon cancer: a randomised trial. Lancet. 2002;359(9325):2224–9. https://doi.org/10.1016/s0140-6736(02)09290-5.
8. Hazebroek EJ. COLOR: a randomized clinical trial comparing laparoscopic and open resection for colon cancer. Surg Endosc. 2002;16(6):949–53. https://doi.org/10.1007/s00464-001-8165-z.
9. Milsom JW, Bohm B, Hammerhofer KA, Fazio V, Steiger E, Elson P. A prospective, randomized trial comparing laparoscopic versus conventional techniques in colorectal cancer surgery: a preliminary report. J Am Coll Surg. 1998;187(1):46–54. discussion 54-5.
10. Schwenk W, Kehlet H. Meta-analysis of short-term outcomes after laparoscopic resection for colorectal cancer (Br J Surg 2004; 91: 1111-1124). Br J Surg. 2004;91(12):1653–4. https://doi.org/10.1002/bjs.4895.
11. Yamamoto S, Inomata M, Katayama H, Mizusawa J, Etoh T, Konishi F, et al. Short-term surgical outcomes from a randomized controlled trial to evaluate laparoscopic and open D3 dissection for stage II/III colon cancer: Japan Clinical Oncology Group Study JCOG 0404. Ann Surg. 2014;260(1):23–30. https://doi.org/10.1097/sla.0000000000000499.
12. Cortet M, Grimault A, Cheynel N, Lepage C, Bouvier AM, Faivre J. Patterns of recurrence of obstructing colon cancers after surgery for cure: a population-based study. Color Dis. 2013;15(9):1100–6. https://doi.org/10.1111/codi.12268.
13. Gianotti L, Tamini N, Nespoli L, Rota M, Bolzonaro E, Frego R, et al. A prospective evaluation of short-term and long-term results from colonic stenting for palliation or as a bridge to elective operation versus immediate surgery for large-bowel obstruction. Surg Endosc. 2013;27(3):832–42. https://doi.org/10.1007/s00464-012-2520-0.
14. Huang X, Lv B, Zhang S, Meng L. Preoperative colonic stents versus emergency surgery for acute left-sided malignant colonic obstruction: a meta-analysis. J Gastrointest Surg. 2014;18(3):584–91. https://doi.org/10.1007/s11605-013-2344-9.
15. Kim JS, Hur H, Min BS, Sohn SK, Cho CH, Kim NK. Oncologic outcomes of self-expanding metallic stent insertion as a bridge to surgery in the management of left-sided colon cancer obstruction: comparison with nonobstructing elective surgery. World J Surg. 2009;33(6):1281–6. https://doi.org/10.1007/s00268-009-0007-5.
16. Stipa F, Pigazzi A, Bascone B, Cimitan A, Villotti G, Burza A, et al. Management of obstructive colorectal cancer with endoscopic stenting followed by single-stage surgery: open or laparoscopic resection? Surg Endosc. 2008;22(6):1477–81. https://doi.org/10.1007/s00464-007-9654-5.
17. Kim IY, Kim BR, Kim YW. The short-term and oncologic outcomes of laparoscopic versus open surgery for T4 colon cancer. Surg Endosc. 2016;30(4):1508–18. https://doi.org/10.1007/s00464-015-4364-x.
18. Shukla PJ, Trencheva K, Merchant C, Maggiori L, Michelassi F, Sonoda T, et al. Laparoscopic resection of t4 colon cancers: is it feasible? Dis Colon Rectum. 2015;58(1):25–31. https://doi.org/10.1097/dcr.0000000000000220.

19. Hohenberger W, Weber K, Matzel K, Papadopoulos T, Merkel S. Standardized surgery for colonic cancer: complete mesocolic excision and central ligation--technical notes and outcome. Color Dis. 2009;11(4):354–364.; discussion 364-5. https://doi.org/10.1111/j.1463-1318.2008.01735.x.

20. Adamina M, Manwaring ML, Park KJ, Delaney CP. Laparoscopic complete mesocolic excision for right colon cancer. Surg Endosc. 2012;26(10):2976–80. https://doi.org/10.1007/s00464-012-2294-4.

21. Kang J, Kim IK, Kang SI, Sohn SK, Lee KY. Laparoscopic right hemicolectomy with complete mesocolic excision. Surg Endosc. 2014;28(9):2747–51. https://doi.org/10.1007/s00464-014-3521-y.

22. Galizia G, Lieto E, De Vita F, Ferraraccio F, Zamboli A, Mabilia A, et al. Is complete mesocolic excision with central vascular ligation safe and effective in the surgical treatment of right-sided colon cancers? A prospective study. Int J Color Dis. 2014;29(1):89–97. https://doi.org/10.1007/s00384-013-1766-x.

23. West NP, Kobayashi H, Takahashi K, Perrakis A, Weber K, Hohenberger W, et al. Understanding optimal colonic cancer surgery: comparison of Japanese D3 resection and European complete mesocolic excision with central vascular ligation. J Clin Oncol. 2012;30(15):1763–9. https://doi.org/10.1200/jco.2011.38.3992.

24. Campagnacci R, de Sanctis A, Baldarelli M, Rimini M, Lezoche G, Guerrieri M. Electrothermal bipolar vessel sealing device vs. ultrasonic coagulating shears in laparoscopic colectomies: a comparative study. Surg Endosc. 2007;21(9):1526–31. https://doi.org/10.1007/s00464-006-9143-2.

25. Janssen PF, Brolmann HA, Huirne JA. Effectiveness of electrothermal bipolar vessel-sealing devices versus other electrothermal and ultrasonic devices for abdominal surgical hemostasis: a systematic review. Surg Endosc. 2012;26(10):2892–901. https://doi.org/10.1007/s00464-012-2276-6.

26. Kanemitsu Y, Hirai T, Komori K, Kato T. Survival benefit of high ligation of the inferior mesenteric artery in sigmoid colon or rectal cancer surgery. Br J Surg. 2006;93(5):609–15. https://doi.org/10.1002/bjs.5327.

27. Sekimoto M, Takemasa I, Mizushima T, Ikeda M, Yamamoto H, Doki Y, et al. Laparoscopic lymph node dissection around the inferior mesenteric artery with preservation of the left colic artery. Surg Endosc. 2011;25(3):861–6. https://doi.org/10.1007/s00464-010-1284-7.

Robotic Surgery for Colon Cancer: Principles and Pitfalls

27

Jianmin Xu, Ye Wei, Dexiang Zhu, and Qingyang Feng

Abstract

Robotic surgical systems are developed to overcome the inherent limitations of traditional laparoscopic surgery, with stable camera of three-dimensional imaging, improved ergonomics, tremor elimination, ambidextrous capability, motion scaling, and flexible instruments. Several trials have showed that robotic surgery is safe and comparable, but not superior to standard laparoscopic approaches, with higher cost and longer time. Standard surgical procedures are needed for robotic colon resections. Recently several prototypes have been developed to address the current problems. And single-incision robotic surgery and natural orifice transluminal endoscopic surgery are under development now.

Keywords

Robotic colon surgery · Advantages Indications · Perioperative preparation Surgical procedures

J. Xu (✉) • Y. Wei • D. Zhu • Q. Feng
Colorectal Cancer Center, Zhongshan Hospital, Fudan University, Shanghai, China
e-mail: xujmin@aliyun.com;
xu.jianmin1@zs-hospital.sh.cn

27.1 Development of Robotic Colon Surgery

Minimally invasive colon surgery has developed over the past three decades. Jacobs et al. firstly reported laparoscopic colectomy in 1991 [1]. Since then, several large trials have been conducted to compare laparoscopic colectomy with open colectomy. The COST, COLOR, MRC CLASICC, LAPKON II, and ALCCaS trials have demonstrated that laparoscopic resection results in improved short-term patient-oriented outcomes and equivalent oncologic outcomes versus the open approach [2–4]. Therefore, laparoscopic colectomy is recommended on National Comprehensive Cancer Network (NCCN) guideline and Chinese Colorectal Cancer Guideline. However, only 55.4% of elective colon resection are laparoscopic operation in the USA [5]. The common reasons include technically demanding surgeons, few standard procedures, poor ergonomics and inability in narrow surgical space, and obese abdominal cavity.

So robotic surgical systems are developed to overcome the inherent limitations of traditional laparoscopic surgery, providing assistance to the surgeon with improvements to perception, processing, and action [6]. So far, the da Vinci robotic system (Intuitive Surgical Inc., Sunnyvale, CA, USA), approved by the Food and Drug Administration in 2000, is the most widely used robotic surgical model. Weber et al.

firstly performed robotic-assisted colectomies with da Vinci robotic system in 2001 [7]. And then several studies on robotic colon surgery have been published and shown that robotic colon resection can be performed safely and successfully, with favorable short-term postoperative and oncologic outcomes. Robotic systems have the potential to address some of the limitations of laparoscopy by providing enhanced visualization and great precision, while associated with longer operative times and higher costs than laparoscopic colectomy [8].

27.2 Advantages of Robotic Surgical System

The da Vinci Si surgical system consists of three integrated components, an ergonomics surgeon console, a patient cart with four interactive robotic arms, and a video tower housing the dedicated system processors and the high-definition three-dimensional (3D) vision system (https://www.davincisurgerycommunity.com/). The video tower displays high-definition 3D vision for a true perception of depth during surgery, increasing the surgeon's confidence as a result of the superior view of the tissue plains and the critical anatomy. The patient cart is composed of multiple components including one camera arm and three robotic arms. The robotic arms are designed with unique wristed architecture providing 7 degrees of freedom, a range of motion greater than even the human wrist. The system enables the surgeon to perform dextrous in very deliberate motion control of the instruments to enable very precise dissection and reconstructed surgical tasks. Sitting at the surgeon console, surgeons can control the movements of the patient cart precisely and seamlessly, avoiding long standing during surgery and reducing physiological fatigue [9, 10]. Moreover, the master controllers provide tremor filtration to stabilize the surgical procedure.

A meta-analysis of eight studies showed that robotic total mesorectal excision had fewer genitourinary complications, lower rates of positive circumferential margins, and a measurement of pathological success, and other outcomes were equal to those of traditional laparoscopic surgery, and so robotic technology has been maturely applied to rectal resection in the narrow deep pelvic anatomy with tight boundaries and close proximity to pelvic nerves [11]. Robotic colectomy is still developing. Several meta-analyses showed that, compared with conventional laparoscopic right colectomy, robotic right colectomy was associated with reduced estimated blood losses, reduced postoperative complications, longer operative times, and a significantly faster recovery of bowel function, without a proved enhanced oncological accuracy to date [12, 13]. In terms of oncologic parameters, lymph node detection rate and positive surgical margin rate in the robotic group were similar to those in the laparoscopic group. To date, long-term survival outcomes after robotic right colectomy have not been reported yet. And the data of robotic left colectomy is few. Robotic left colectomy had similar perioperative and oncologic outcomes with increased operative times, which need further evaluation [14]. So the Society of American Gastrointestinal and Endoscopic Surgeons (SAGES) consider that da Vinci surgical system is safe and comparable, but not superior to standard laparoscopic approaches, with higher cost, and current data are limited [15].

27.3 Indications and Contraindications for Robotic Colon Surgery

The indications of robotic colon surgery are similar to those of conventional laparoscopic surgery. The contraindications are as follows: general anesthesia intolerance, e.g., patients with severely insufficient heart, lung, or liver function; severe coagulation disorder; pregnancy; extensive abdominal or pelvic metastasis which is difficult to dissect with a robotic system; tumor obstruction with obvious distention; tumor perforation with acute peritonitis; difficult to puncture due to extensive abdominal adhesion; moribund condition, massive ascites, intra-abdominal hemorrhage, or shock; and severe obesity, with a body mass index (BMI) >40 kg/m^2 (extended puncture device and surgical instruments in the robotic surgical system are unavailable now).

27.4   Perioperative Preparation

Patient preparation includes bowel preparation and prophylactic administration of antibiotics during anesthesia induction. General anesthesia with endotracheal intubation is adopted during the operation, and a urethral catheter is indwelled; nasogastric tube can be placed as well when necessary. Other preoperative preparations are similar to those for conventional surgery.

The robotic arms interface with its specifically designed supporting components, and the laparoscopic instruments can also be used by assistants in surgery. The robotic arms can selectively hold different instruments: hot shears (monopolar curved scissors), electrocautery, harmonic scalpel, fenestrated grasper, fenestrated bipolar forceps, Maryland bipolar forceps, grasping retractor, and so on. Laparoscopic instruments used by the assistant include laparoscopic bowel forceps, scissors, suction irrigation sets, 5 mm Ligasure V, Hemo-lock clip applier, and linear cut stapler. The instruments for extracorporeal anastomosis are the surgical incision protector and circular stapler. Sterile drapes for robotic arms are needed.

Robotic system preparation include a system power-on self-test. Ensure that all robotic instruments are present and the system is in good conditions. In particular, check if the arm motion is flexible, the wrist and instrument movement is not restricted, and the scissors and forceps are normal. Install the sterile drapes for the robotic system. Once the light from the illuminator is delivered to the endoscope, set the white balance, adjust the focus, and calibrate the camera. After that, heat the endoscope (not beyond 55 °C) to avoid fogging. Arrange equipment around and above the operating table and properly fix equipment power transmission lines to avoid affecting the motion of the robotic arms. If the robotic arms collide during the procedure, reposition them. The surgeon can adjust the

height and tilt of the stereo viewer and move the armrest up and down by controlling the console screen.

27.5   Surgical Procedures for Robotic Colon Resections [16]

27.5.1 Robotic Sigmoid Resection

27.5.1.1   Surgical Position
The herringbone position or the modified lithotomy position is used for radical resection of sigmoid cancer. After the patient is secured, the operating table is turned to the Trendelenburg position with the right side inclined downward. The patient's left leg is placed downward to avoid colliding with the robotic arms.

27.5.1.2   Trocar Number and Location
Usually, four to five trocars are placed for the surgery: one for the camera (Trocar C), three for the robotic arms (Trocars R1, R2, and R3), and one for the assistant (Trocar A). If splenic flexure is mobilized during the surgery, Trocar R4 should be used instead of Trocar R2 for the robotic arms. Details are shown in Fig. 27.1.

Trocar C: 12 mm in diameter, placed 3–4 cm to the upper right of the umbilicus.

Trocar R1: 8 mm in diameter, placed at the McBurney's point (one-third of the distance from the right anterior superior iliac spine to the umbilicus).

Trocar R2: 8 mm in diameter, placed at the intersection of the left mid-clavicular line and the horizontal line through Trocar C.

Trocar R3: 8 mm in diameter, placed at the intersection of the left anterior axillary line and the horizontal line through Trocar C. This trocar is always used to help mobilize the lower rectum.

Trocar R4: 8 mm in diameter, placed 3–4 cm below the xiphoid process, in the middle of the anterior midline and the right mid-clavicular line. This trocar is used to mobilize splenic flexure.

Trocar A: 5 mm or 12 mm in diameter, placed at the intersection of the vertical line through the

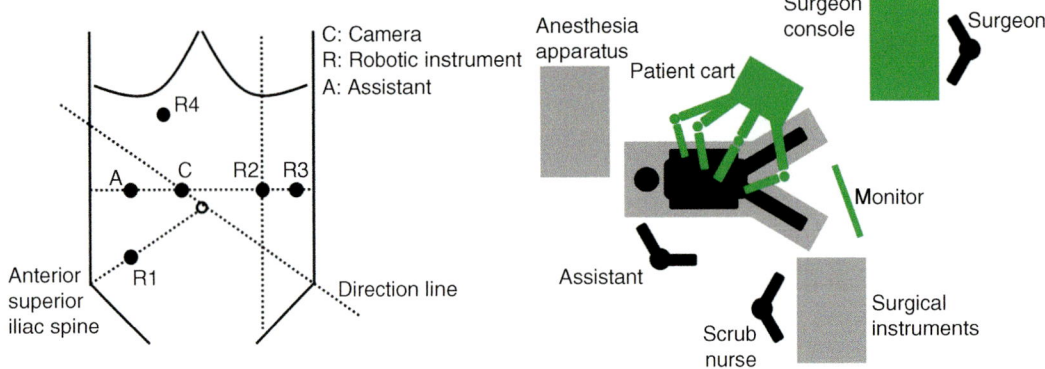

Fig. 27.1 Trocar location and operating room setup for robotic sigmoid resection

McBurney's point and the horizontal line through Trocar C.

The location of Trocar C is relatively fixed. The locations of other trocars could be adjusted according to the tumor site, the patient's body shape, and the surgeon's operating habits, although the operating center should be fixed to the tumor. The adjacent trocars should be 8–10 cm from each other to avoid collisions of robotic arms. All measurements should be based on the tension after the pneumoperitoneum. Trocars R1, R2, and/or R3 are used to mobilize the rectum, and trocars R1, R4, and/or R3 are used to mobilize splenic flexure.

27.5.1.3　Abdominal Exploration

After establishing pneumoperitoneum at a pressure of 8–15 mmHg, the camera on either the laparoscope or the surgical robot can be used for abdominal exploration. If tissue adhesions are found to interfere with the trocar puncture, laparoscopic instruments should be used to release them. Before the Robotic system is connected, the patient's position should be adjusted to ensure sufficient exposure of the operative field.

27.5.1.4　Robotic System Connections

The patient cart is placed on the left side of the patient, with the direction line through the left anterior superior iliac spine, trocar C, and the center column of the patient cart (Fig. 27.1). All robotic arms should surround the operating center: the camera arm is located in the middle,

and the instrument arms on the sides, with joints fully extended outward to avoid collisions. The digital pattern on the instrument arms should face straight ahead. When connecting robotic arms with trocars, movements should be gentle to avoid pulling up the trocars. After the robotic arms are fixed, neither the patient nor the operating table should be moved again.

27.5.1.5　Surgical Procedure

Exposure of the operative field: The medial-to-lateral approach is recommended for the surgery. To improve the exposure of operative field, the uterus could be suspended in female patients, and the bladder could be suspended in male patients. With Trocar A, the assistant moves the small intestine and greater omentum to the right upper abdominal cavity. The mesenteric junction of the rectosigmoid and posterior peritoneum is tilted upward and outward to identify the abdominal aortic bifurcation.

Division of vessels: A mesenteric window is opened just at the sacral promontory plane. The inferior mesenteric vessels are dissected through the space between the visceral and parietal peritoneum (Toldt's space) and ligated at their origin points using Hemo-locks. Lymph nodes are also swept clearly.

Mobilization of the side peritoneum: The sigmoid is tilted rightward, and the Toldt's space is dissected. The left ureter should be exposed and safeguarded during the mobilization.

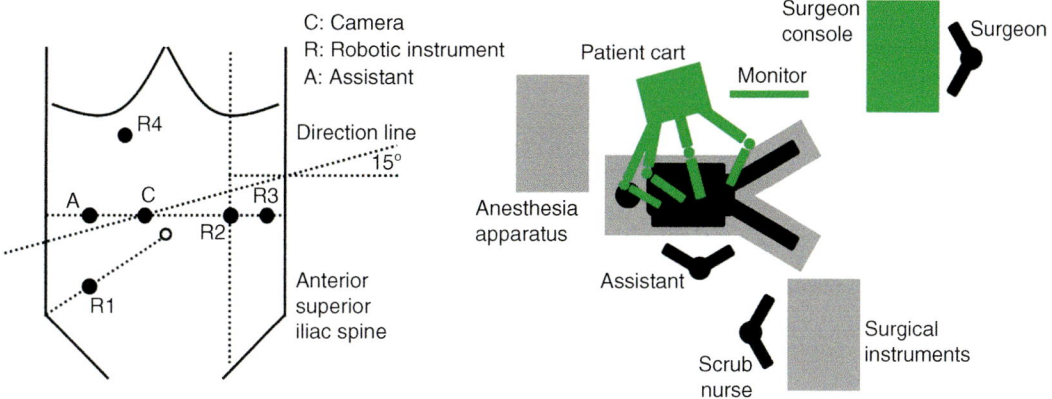

Fig. 27.2 Trocar location and operating room setup for splenic flexure mobilization in robotic sigmoid resection

Mobilization of splenic flexure: First, the robotic arms should be removed. Then, the patient cart should be replaced beside the left shoulder of the patient, with the direction line through Trocar C and at an angle of 15° from the horizontal line (Fig. 27.2). The surgical robotic system should also be reconnected. Trocars R1 and R4 are used to mobilize splenic flexure. For patients with short sigmoid as confirmed in preoperative evaluation, splenic flexure can be mobilized before the rectosigmoid. In addition, mobilization of splenic flexure could also be conducted with conventional laparoscopic instruments, which called hybrid technique.

Mobilization of the descending and sigmoid colon: The descending and sigmoid colon is mobilized along the prerenal fascia on the surface of the ureter. The nerve plexus should be safeguarded during the mobilization. The mesocolon is cut according to the proximal resection margin.

Mobilization of the rectum: The rectum is mobilized in a circular route, following the principles of total mesorectal excision. The mobilization starts from the posterior rectum wall and gradually extends to the lateral sides; the anterior rectum wall is dissected last. For patients with contracted pelvis, lateral sides can also be dissected after the posterior and anterior wall. Trocar R3 is always used to help tilt the rectum. The tension of the arms should be controlled to avoid soft tissue avulsion. The tumor

site will determine whether to open the peritoneal reflection and the length of the mobilized rectum.

Division of the distal mural margin: The distal mural margin can be dissected using electric scissors and hook or ultrasonic energy instruments. The margin should be more than 2 cm below the inferior edge of the tumor.

Anastomosis: Extracorporeal or intracorporeal anastomosis should be selected according to the tumor site and the patient's body shape. In extracorporeal anastomosis, the incision is made in the left lower abdomen. The bowel with the tumor is pulled out for anastomosis under direct vision. A reinforcement suture can be made if necessary. In intracorporeal anastomosis, the tumor is removed from a small incision in the left lower abdomen or an enlarged puncture incision. A purse-string suture is placed in the proximal resection margin, and the anvil is tied around the margin of the colon. Then, the proximal colon along with the anvil is returned to the abdomen. The incision is closed, and the pneumoperitoneum is reestablished. The circular stapler is inserted through the anus, and the anastomosis is made under visualization of the surgical Robotic system. For small tumors, the affected bowel can be pulled out from the anus to remove the tumor. The anvil is tied to the proximal resection margin and is returned through the anus. The anastomosis is made under visualization of the surgical Robotic system and is checked for any leaks by air or methylene blue perfusion. A reinforcement suture can be made under visualization of the surgical Robotic system if necessary.

Incision closure: To close the pelvic peritoneum, the pneumoperitoneum should be reestablished, and the surgical Robotic system should also be reconnected. The abdominal cavity is irrigated with normal saline or distilled water and drained adequately. Then, all incisions are closed.

27.5.2 Robotic Left Hemicolectomy

27.5.2.1 Surgical Position

The herringbone position or the modified lithotomy position is used for the surgery. After the patient is secured, the operating table is turned to the reverse Trendelenburg position with the right side inclined downward. The patient's left leg is placed downward to avoid collision with the robotic arms.

27.5.2.2 Trocar Number and Location

Usually, five trocars are placed for the surgery: one for the camera (Trocar C), three for the robotic arms (Trocars R1, R2, and R3), and one for the assistant (Trocar A). Details are shown in Fig. 27.3.

Trocar C: 12 mm in diameter, placed 3–4 cm to the upper right of the umbilicus.

Trocar R1: 8 mm in diameter, placed at the McBurney's point (one-third of the distance from the right anterior superior iliac spine to the umbilicus).

Trocar R2: 8 mm in diameter, placed at the right side of the anterior midline, 3–4 cm below the xiphoid process. Ensure that it is placed above the transverse colon.

Trocar R3: 8 mm in diameter, placed on the anterior midline 3–4 cm above the symphysis pubis.

Trocar A: 5 mm or 12 mm in diameter, placed outside the right midclavicular line in the middle of Trocar C and Trocar R2.

The location of Trocar C is relatively fixed; the locations of other trocars could be adjusted according to the tumor site, the patient's body shape, and the surgeon's operating habits. The operating center should be fixed to the tumor. The adjacent trocars should be 8–10 cm from each other to avoid collisions of the robotic arms. All measurements should be based on the tension after the pneumoperitoneum.

27.5.2.3 Abdominal Exploration

The same procedures apply as those in Sect. 27.5.1.3.

27.5.2.4 Robotic System Connections

The patient cart is placed beside the left shoulder of the patient, with the direction line through Trocar C and the center column of the cart at an angle of 15° from the horizontal line (Fig. 27.3). Other considerations are the same as those in Sect. 27.5.1.4.

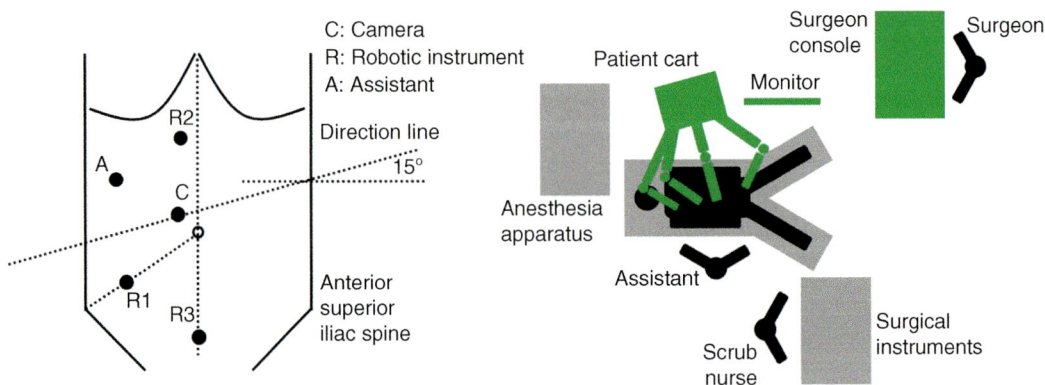

Fig. 27.3 Trocar location and operating room setup for robotic left hemicolectomy

27.5.2.5   Surgical Procedure

Exposure of the operative field: The medial-to-lateral approach is recommended. Through Trocar A, an assistant moves the small intestine and greater omentum to the right abdominal cavity. The mesenteric junction of the descending and sigmoid colon is tilted upward and outward, and the junction of the sigmoid colon and rectum is tilted downward and outward to identify the abdominal aortic bifurcation.

Division of vessels: A mesenteric window is opened just at the sacral promontory plane. The first and second branches of the sigmoid vessels and the left colic vessels are dissected through the Toldt's space along the inferior mesenteric vessels. The vessels are ligated at their origin points from the inferior mesenteric vessels, using Hemo-locks. Lymph nodes are also swept clearly.

Mobilization of the descending colon: From the left side of the inferior mesenteric vein, the descending colon is mobilized through the Toldt's space between the mesocolon and the left prerenal fascia. Mobilization is from up to down, or from up to down and from inner to outside, on the surface of the left spermatic or ovarian vessels and the left ureter.

Mobilization of splenic flexure: Splenic flexure is mobilized through the Toldt's space inward and upward. The left branch of middle colic artery is ligated, and the left gastrocolic and splenocolic ligaments are dissected to fully mobilize splenic flexure.

Mobilization of the sigmoid colon and upper rectum: The descending and sigmoid colon are fully mobilized through the Toldt's space; the upper rectum can also be mobilized if necessary. The length of resected bowel is decided, and the affected bowel is dissected.

Anastomosis: The affected bowel is pulled out through a left rectus incision to remove the tumor. An alternative is side-to-side or end-to-side anastomosis of the transverse and sigmoid colon.

Incision closure: The abdominal cavity is irrigated with normal saline or distilled water and drained adequately. Then, all incisions are closed.

27.5.3 Robotic Right Hemicolectomy

27.5.3.1   Surgical Position

Supine position is used for radical resection. The patient should be set close to the cranial side of the operating table, and the anterior superior spine should be higher than the middle plane. After the patient is secured, the operating table is turned to the Trendelenburg position with an angle of 15–30° and left side downward with an angle of 10–15°.

27.5.3.2   Trocar Number and Location

Usually, five trocars are placed in the surgery: one for the camera (Trocar C), three for the robotic arms (Trocars R1, R2, and R3), and one for the assistant (Trocar A). Details are shown in Fig. 27.4.

Trocar C: 12 mm in diameter, placed 3–4 cm to the lower left of the umbilicus.

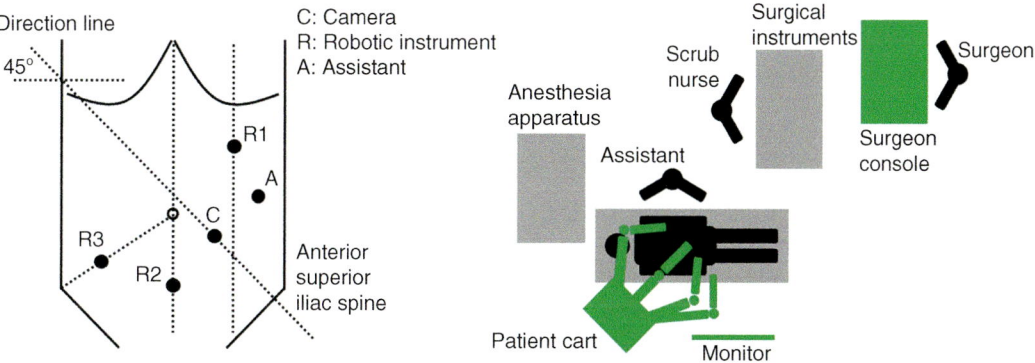

Fig. 27.4 Trocar location and operating room setup for robotic right hemicolectomy

Trocar R1: 8 mm in diameter, placed on the left midclavicular line, 7–8 cm below the costal margin.

Trocar R2: 8 mm in diameter, placed on the anterior midline, 6–8 cm above the symphysis pubis.

Trocar R3: 8 mm in diameter, placed at the McBurney's point (one-third of the distance from the right anterior superior iliac spine to the umbilicus).

Trocar A: 5 mm or 12 mm in diameter, placed outside the left midclavicular line, 6–8 cm below Trocar R1, and more than 8 cm away from Trocar C.

The location of Trocar C is relatively fixed. The locations of other trocars could be adjusted according to the tumor site, the patient's body shape, and the surgeon's operating habits. The operating center should be fixed to the tumor. The adjacent trocars should be 8–10 cm away from each other, avoiding collisions of robotic arms. All measurement should be based on the tension after pneumoperitoneum.

27.5.3.3   Abdominal Exploration
The same as Sect. 27.5.1.3.

27.5.3.4   Robotic System Connections
The patient cart is placed beside the right shoulder of the patient, with the direction line through Trocar C and the center column of the patient cart, with an angle of 45° from the horizontal line (Fig. 27.4). There should be enough space beside the patient's hip to avoid collision with robotic arms when mobilizing the hepatic flexure. Other considerations are the same as Sect. 27.5.1.4.

27.5.3.5   Surgical Procedure
Exposure of the operative field: The medial-to-lateral approach is recommended. With Trocar A, the assistant moves the small intestine to the left abdomen and lifts the right mesocolon to expose the junction of ileocolic artery and superior mesenteric vein.

Division of vessels: Dissection is performed upward along the superior mesenteric vessels to divide each branch and sweep the lymph nodes. Hemo-locks are used to ligate the ileocolic vessels, right colic vessels, and the right branch of

middle colic vessels. For tumors located at or near the hepatic flexure which need expanded surgery, the right gastroepiploic vessels are also ligated at the inferior edge of pancreas.

Mobilization of the ascending colon: From the right side of the superior mesenteric vein, the ascending colon is mobilized through the Toldt's space between the mesocolon and right prerenal fascia. Mobilization is performed from downside to upside, from inner to outside, on the surface of the right spermatic or ovarian vessels, right ureter pancreas, and duodenum.

Mobilization of hepatic flexure: Gastrocolic ligament is opened to mobilize hepatic flexure rightward. The right gastroepiploic vessels and corresponding lymph nodes should be swept if the tumor locates at or near hepatic flexure. More than 10 cm length of greater omentum should be dissected and cut off.

Mobilization of the side peritoneum: From the ileocecal junction, the right-sided peritoneum is mobilized upward and converged with hepatic flexure.

Anastomosis: The mesentery of the colon and small intestine is mobilized till resection margin. The bowel is resected according to the tumor site. Intracorporeal anastomosis and extracorporeal anastomosis with assistant incision are both feasible. In intracorporeal anastomosis, the terminal ileum is get close to the colon. Linear stapler is used for a side-to-side anastomosis. Then another linear stapler is used to cut off the specimen.

The affected bowel is pulled out through the left rectus incision to remove the tumor. It is alternative to make side-to-side or end-to-side anastomosis of ileal and transverse colon. Circular stapler can also be used for end-to-side anastomosis.

Incision closure: The abdominal cavity is irrigated with normal saline or distilled water and drained adequately. Then, all incisions are closed.

27.6   Robotic Multiple Organ Resection

Local invasion and distant metastasis are common in patients with colorectal cancer, and thus, multiple organ resection is an important measure for radical resection of colorectal cancer. Robotic surgery is also applicable in combination resection, although it should only be performed by experienced surgeons after a multidisciplinary team consultation [17]. For locally advanced colorectal cancer with invasion of adjacent organs, robotic surgery can be performed to resect the organs without withdrawing and refixing the robotic arms. This type of surgery can also be applied in synchronous resection of colorectal cancer with distant metastases such as liver or lung metastases that need re-punching and re-docking after one lesion being resected. Additionally, during the resections of different lesions, the same ports should be used when possible to minimize trauma. Robotic liver resection has been demonstrated to be safe and effective, but the long-term effects of synchronous resection of colorectal cancer and liver metastasis lesions remain to be evaluated [18].

27.7   Perioperative Morbidity and Mechanical Fault

Complications of robotic surgery are mostly similar to those of conventional laparoscopic surgery, while some unique. Intraoperative complications include puncture vascular and bowel injury, complications associated with pneumoperitoneum, intraoperative bleeding related to vascular injury, injury of adjacent organs, complications related to anastomosis and enterostomy, failure or inflexibility of the arms, tissues embedded into the conjunction of operative devices, and rupture of hot shear holster, and target anatomy is unreachable. Postoperative complications include anastomotic leakage, intestinal obstruction, urinary and sexual dysfunction, trocar and stoma hernia, and chyle leakage. Robotic surgery has some risks related to robotic surgical systems, especially for remote surgeries. Accurate control depends on the connecting data quality between the surgeon console and the robot in the operation room. Instruments and electrical equipment are all vulnerable, and the robotic surgical system is also no exception.

Error handling is an important component of robotic surgical safety. Faults in the robotic system during surgery can generally be categorized as recoverable and non-recoverable fault. With a recoverable fault, the indicator lighter on the robotic arm will glow yellow, and the system will trigger an alarm sound. Following instructions on the screen, operation room staff can resolve the fault and continue the procedure. When a non-recoverable fault occurs, the indicator lighter on the robotic arm will glow red, and the system will trigger the alarm. Operation room staff needs to record the error number on the screen to share it with customer service, and then restart the system. Some non-recoverable faults can be solved this way, and the surgical procedure can go on. However, when a severe fault occurs that cannot be resolved by restarting the system repeatedly, it is necessary to remove the robotic surgical system, convert to laparoscopic or open surgery, and have a maintenance engineer come and repair the system. There is an emergency brake button on the main console. Do not touch it unless the situation is an emergency.

27.8   Postoperative Therapy

Closely observe the changes in respiration, body temperature, drainage volume and character, urine volume and color, incision recovery, and so on. Notice whether there is hypercapnia, bleeding in the abdominal cavity, anastomotic bleeding, anastomotic fistula or infection, and so on.

Give proper nutrition support, turn over and pat the back, help with expectoration and reducing phlegm, prophylactically use antibiotics, and exercise urination function early. Early ambulation prevents deep venous thrombosis. Bowel movements resume significantly earlier in patients who undergo robotic surgery, and their oral intake could be resumed earlier according to their conditions.

27.9   Future of Robotic Surgical System

The da Vinci robotic system provided several advantages over traditional laparoscopic surgery, including stable camera of 3D imaging, improved ergonomics, tremor elimination, ambidextrous capability, motion scaling, and instruments with multiple degrees of freedom (https://www.davincisurgerycommunity.com/). There are, however, several drawbacks of da Vinci robotic systems. The frequent criticism about current da Vinci system is the absence of tactile feedback, which can lead to unexpected damages of tissue and organ. Another main concern is the high financial cost, which associated with initial outlay and maintenance of surgical system and purchasing disposable equipment. The other potential disadvantages include prolonged operative time, bulky with cumbersome robotic arms, and the relatively limited number of compatible instruments and equipment.

Several prototypes have been developed to address the current problems. The Telelap Alf-X system by Sofar (Milan, Italy) is the first system to incorporate haptic feedback technology, which allows the surgeon to feel the instrument in their hands, sense the force applied, and palpate the texture of the tissues [19]. Micro Hand S robot system (Changsha, China) also has succeeded in accomplishing the first operations of clinical use, which have solved some existing drawbacks [20].

In recent years, single-incision robotic surgery and natural orifice transluminal endoscopic surgery (NOTES) are developed to further minimize incision-related complications and improve cosmetic outcomes [21]. By combining laparo-endoscopic single-site surgery techniques with the da Vinci robotic platform, single-incision robotic colectomy is a safe and feasible procedure in terms of perioperative outcomes [22]. And Titan's SPORT (single port orifice robotic technology) surgical system (Titan Medical Inc., Canada) is another single-incision robotic platform, including a 3D vision system, articulating instruments, and a surgeon console, is still under development, and has been tested only in experimental setting so far [23]. In addition, several snakelike robots are currently under development because of flexible architecture and multiple degrees of freedom [24]. In the near future, the combination of robotic surgery and real-time image guidance, or the additional lymph node information that near-infrared fluorescence provides, will gain more popularity.

References

1. Jacobs M, Verdeja JC, Goldstein HS. Minimally invasive colon resection (laparoscopic colectomy). Surg Laparosc Endosc. 1991;1(3):144–50.
2. Koopmann MC, Heise CP. Laparoscopic and minimally invasive resection of malignant colorectal disease. Surg Clin North Am. 2008;88(5):1047–72. https://doi.org/10.1016/j.suc.2008.05.009.
3. Blackmore AE, Wong MT, Tang CL. Evolution of laparoscopy in colorectal surgery: an evidence-based review. World J Gastroenterol. 2014;20(17):4926–33. https://doi.org/10.3748/wjg.v20.i17.4926.
4. Millo P, Rispoli C, Rocco N, Contul RB, Fabozzi M, Grivon M, et al. Laparoscopic surgery for colon cancer. Ann Gastroenterol. 2013;26(3):198–203.
5. Moghadamyeghaneh Z, Carmichael JC, Mills S, Pigazzi A, Nguyen NT, Stamos MJ. Variations in laparoscopic colectomy utilization in the United States. Dis Colon Rectum. 2015;58(10):950–6. https://doi.org/10.1097/DCR.0000000000000448.
6. Roy S, Evans C. Overview of robotic colorectal surgery: current and future practical developments. World J Gastrointest Surg. 2016;8(2):143–50. https://doi.org/10.4240/wjgs.v8.i2.143.
7. Weber PA, Merola S, Wasielewski A, Ballantyne GH. Telerobotic-assisted laparoscopic right and sigmoid colectomies for benign disease. Dis Colon Rectum. 2002;45(12):1689–1694., 1695-6. https://doi.org/10.1097/01.DCR.0000037657.78153.A8.
8. Pappou EP, Weiser MR. Robotic colonic resection. J Surg Oncol. 2015;112(3):315–20. https://doi.org/10.1002/jso.23953.
9. Butler KA, Kapetanakis VE, Smith BE, Sanjak M, Verheijde JL, Chang YH, et al. Surgeon fatigue and postural stability: is robotic better than laparoscopic surgery? J Laparoendosc Adv Surg Tech A. 2013;23(4):343–6. https://doi.org/10.1089/lap.2012.0531.
10. Hubert N, Gilles M, Desbrosses K, Meyer JP, Felblinger J, Hubert J. Ergonomic assessment of the surgeon's physical workload during standard and robotic assisted laparoscopic procedures. Int J Med Robot. 2013;9(2):142–7. https://doi.org/10.1002/rcs.1489.
11. Xiong B, Ma L, Huang W, Zhao Q, Cheng Y, Liu J. Robotic versus laparoscopic total mesorectal excision for rectal cancer: a meta-analysis of eight studies. J Gastrointest Surg. 2015;19(3):516–26. https://doi.org/10.1007/s11605-014-2697-8.
12. Xu H, Li J, Sun Y, Li Z, Zhen Y, Wang B, et al. Robotic versus laparoscopic right colectomy: a meta-analysis. World J Surg Oncol. 2014;12:274. https://doi.org/10.1186/1477-7819-12-274.

13. Rondelli F, Balzarotti R, Villa F, Guerra A, Avenia N, Mariani E, et al. Is robot-assisted laparoscopic right colectomy more effective than the conventional laparoscopic procedure? A meta-analysis of short-term outcomes. Int J Surg. 2015;18:75–82. https://doi.org/10.1016/j.ijsu.2015.04.044.

14. Lim DR, Min BS, Kim MS, Alasari S, Kim G, Hur H, et al. Robotic versus laparoscopic anterior resection of sigmoid colon cancer: comparative study of long-term oncologic outcomes. Surg Endosc. 2013;27(4):1379–85. https://doi.org/10.1007/s00464-012-2619-3.

15. Tsuda S, Oleynikov D, Gould J, Azagury D, Sandler B, Hutter M, et al. SAGES TAVAC safety and effectiveness analysis: da Vinci (R) Surgical System (Intuitive Surgical, Sunnyvale, CA). Surg Endosc. 2015;29(10):2873–84. https://doi.org/10.1007/s00464-015-4428-y.

16. Xu J, Qin X. Expert consensus on robotic surgery for colorectal cancer (2015 edition). Chin J Cancer. 2016;35:23. https://doi.org/10.1186/s40880-016-0085-3.

17. Xu JM, Wei Y, Wang XY, Fan H, Chang WJ, Ren L, et al. Robot-assisted one-stage resection of rectal cancer with liver and lung metastases. World J Gastroenterol. 2015;21(9):2848–53. https://doi.org/10.3748/wjg.v21.i9.2848.

18. Montalti R, Berardi G, Patriti A, Vivarelli M, Troisi RI. Outcomes of robotic vs laparoscopic hepatectomy: a systematic review and meta-analysis. World J Gastroenterol. 2015;21(27):8441–51. https://doi.org/10.3748/wjg.v21.i27.8441.

19. Gidaro S, Altobelli E, Falavolti C, Bove AM, Ruiz EM, Stark M, et al. Vesicourethral anastomosis using a novel telesurgical system with haptic sensation, the Telelap Alf-X: a pilot study. Surg Technol Int. 2014;24:35–40.

20. Yi B, Wang G, Li J, Jiang J, Son Z, Su H, et al. The first clinical use of domestically produced Chinese minimally invasive surgical robot system "Micro Hand S". Surg Endosc. 2016;30(6):2649–55. https://doi.org/10.1007/s00464-015-4506-1.

21. Weaver A, Steele S. Robotics in colorectal surgery. F1000Res. 2016;5:2373. https://doi.org/10.12688/f1000research.9389.1.

22. Juo YY, Luka S, Obias V. Single-incision robotic colectomy (SIRC): current status and future directions. J Surg Oncol. 2015;112(3):321–5. https://doi.org/10.1002/jso.23935.

23. Whealon M, Vinci A, Pigazzi A. Future of minimally invasive colorectal surgery. Clin Colon Rectal Surg. 2016;29(3):221–31. https://doi.org/10.1055/s-0036-1584499.

24. Mahvash M, Zenati M. Toward a hybrid snake robot for single-port surgery. Conf Proc IEEE Eng Med Biol Soc. 2011;2011:5372–5. https://doi.org/10.1109/IEMBS.2011.6091329.

Part VII

Safety and Future of Minimal Invasive Surgery for Colorectal Cancer

Safe Bowel Anastomosis in Minimal Invasive Surgery for Colorectal Cancer

28

Cheng-Jen Ma and Jaw-Yuan Wang

Abstract

The minimal invasive surgery for colorectal cancer is considered a safe procedure with evolutions of preoperative preparation, antibiotic prophylaxis, surgical technique, surgical devices, and postoperative management in the last decades. It should take notes in details of techniques performed, devices selected, and conditions of bowel where an anastomosis is made and new technology to facilitate making an anastomosis that may help to reduce the occurrence of anastomotic complications, such as bleeding, leakage and dehiscence, stenosis, and fistula which are harmful for patients and have negative impacts on surgical as well as oncological outcomes.

Keywords

Anastomosis · Minimal invasive surgery Colorectal cancer

C.-J. Ma (✉) • J.-Y. Wang
Kaohsiung Medical University and Hospital,
Kaohsiung, Taiwan
e-mail: kmu880402@gmail.com;
jayuwa@cc.kmu.edu.tw

28.1 Introduction

Owing to the evolutions of preoperative preparation, antibiotic prophylaxis, surgical technique, surgical devices, and postoperative management in the last decades, the surgery for colorectal cancer is considered a safe procedure [1]. Meanwhile, the laparoscopic surgery for colorectal cancer demonstrates better short-term outcomes, oncologic safety, and equivalent long-term outcomes of open surgery [2]. After the first report of robotic colorectal surgery in 2001 by Cadière et al. [3], who performed transanal resections for three patients, surgical robotics are gaining emerging application in managing the colorectal cancer. Robotic colorectal surgery provides favorable results with less blood loss, lower conversion and complication rates, and satisfactory lymph nodes harvested, whereas operation time is relatively longer [4]. Nonetheless, anastomotic complications, like bleeding, leakage, dehiscence, stricture, and fistula, still occur in the comparable incidences of open surgery or laparoscopic surgery.

28.2 Bleeding from an Anastomosis

Most bleeding from an anastomosis is self-limited that stops spontaneously within 24 hours and doesn't need blood transfusion or

© Springer Nature Singapore Pte Ltd. 2018
N. K. Kim et al. (eds.), *Surgical Treatment of Colorectal Cancer*,
https://doi.org/10.1007/978-981-10-5143-2_28

intervention. It may present as dark blood in the first several bowel movements. However, bleeding can occasionally result in hemodynamic instability that needs blood transfusion and endoscopic, angiographic, or even surgical intervention to cease bleeding.

The reported rate of bleeding in a meta-analysis by Neutzling et al. is 4.2%, and there is no significant association between the risk of bleeding and the methods of stapled or hand-sewn anastomoses [5]. The blood supply of the bowel and the rectum comes from the feeding vessels in the mesentery, and involvement of mesentery in an anastomosis may lead to bleeding. Therefore, mesentery should be adequately cleared, and any bleeding during this step should be stopped by suture ligation, which opposed to electrocauterization is more reliable, before hand-sewn anastomosis. While making stapled anastomosis, it should be noticed that each limb of stapler is placed at the antimesenteric sides to prevent mesentery involved in it. Lastly, suture should be tight enough, and the gap of sutures should be appropriate (approximate 3 mm) to secure the suture line. Staple height should be adjusted according to the thickness of the bowel wall where anastomosis is constructed. If staple height is not high enough, bleeding may occur.

28.3   Leakage and Dehiscence

The leak rates of colorectal surgery depend on the level of the anastomoses, which below the peritoneal reflection (or extraperitoneal) are greater than those above the peritoneal reflection (or intraperitoneal) (6.6% versus 1.5%; overall 2.4%) [6]. Extraperitoneal anastomoses are lack of peritoneum, which has ability to absorb accumulation of fluid within the dependent dead space of pelvis and has innervations for patients to present peritoneal signs that reflect anastomotic leakage. As the consequence, colorectal anastomoses, which are mostly extraperitoneal, are most risky and most obscure for leakage.

Although mechanical bowel preparation is considered an important factor in preventing complications after colorectal surgery, it has been

questioned nowadays with advances in surgical techniques, administration of prophylactic antibiotics, and quality of patient care [7]. However, it must be cautioned that the presence of stool in the rectum while doing colorectal anastomosis with stapler may result in burst of rectal stump or other problems that lead to failure of anastomosis.

Circulation at the cutting edges, where the anastomosis is made, is always a crucial factor. Blood supply not only provides oxygen, nutrients, and immune components but also cells that are essential for healing of an anastomosis. In the case of rectal cancer, in which high ligation of inferior mesentery artery (IMA) proximal to the left colic artery is a part of the procedure, circulation of the proximal end of the colon depends on the marginal artery from the middle colic artery. It may be crucial when the marginal artery is stenotic with inadequate blood supply, especially in the elderly or in patients with cardiorespiratory comorbidity. In addition, relative ischemia of the rectal remnant after total mesorectal excision (TME) is also a factor because its blood supply only relies on the inferior hemorrhoidal vessels.

Tension is another factor that should be considered. Tension between a colorectal anastomosis not only compromises circulation to the anastomosis, worsening the critical situation of blood supply mentioned above, but also creates a shearing force that may result in rupture of an anastomosis. Male gender and obesity with narrow pelvis increase the difficulty and complexity of rectal resection and are technically challenging that associate with significant higher rates of leakage of ultralow anastomoses less than 5 cm from the anal verge [8, 9]. In the end, the mechanical strength of the anastomosis is essential to make a watertight and airtight anastomosis free from leakage, no matter by hand-sewn or by staplers.

28.3.1 Advanced Methods to Prevent Leakage

Since the circulation plays a significant role in anastomotic leakage, it is important to optimize the perfusion of the resection margin. Technique of high dissection of the IMA to harvest pathologically satisfactory lymph nodes and low ligation of the IMA to preserve the left colic artery that feeds the proximal side of a colorectal anastomosis demonstrated favorable short-term clinical outcomes [10]. Although this study lacks long-term results with limited case number enrolled regarding anastomotic leakage, it needs more large-scale randomized clinical trial, and theoretically high dissection and low ligation technique may reduce rates of leakage of colorectal anastomoses of rectal cancer, especially for rectal cancer patients following neoadjuvant concurrent chemoradiotherapy.

Fluorescence imaging along with venous injection of indocyanine green is a novel technology to visualize the perfusion of the transaction line ready for forming an anastomosis intraoperatively during left-sided robotic colorectal cancer surgery in that hypoperfusion is a major factor of anastomotic leakage mentioned above. The use of indocyanine green fluorescence imaging allows surgeons to decide where is the point with optimal blood perfusion for transection to construct an anastomosis. A retrospective case-control study of robotic rectal cancer surgery reported that revision of the proximal colon transection point was made in three patients (19%), but no revision was done for distal rectal stump in all patients, and the rate of anastomotic leakage was significantly lower in the indocyanine green fluorescence imaging group (6%) than in the control group (18%) [11].

Tension between an anastomosis should be prevented, and adequate mobilization of colon during colorectal cancer surgery to release tension is a significant step that can't be avoided to prevent anastomotic leakage. Watertight and airtight anastomosis is the basic request for a surgeon undergoing colorectal surgery; nonetheless, the gap of sutures (approximate 3 mm) and the staple height (that is too low) should be considered to prevent interfering in microcirculation of the anastomosis. Additionally, low staple height opposed to the tissue thickness may cause anastomotic bursting.

Staple line reinforcement may have positive impact on the anastomotic leakage; however, it remains controversial and inconclusive as no powerful data could demonstrate it. The application of fibrin glue over an anastomosis theoretically forms a barrier to seal the gaps of sutures or staples and to protect the anastomosis from leakage, especially the extraperitoneal anastomosis, where there is no coverage of the peritoneum or the omentum. A retrospective case-control study conducted by Kim et al. revealed that the use of fibrin glue was an independent factor of preventing anastomotic leakage in sphincter-preserving surgery for rectal cancer, without oncologic advantages [12]. Various types of buttressing materials, including non-, semi-, and absorbable, provide a neutralization plate for an anastomosis to release the tension between the both sides of the anastomosis; seal the gaps of the suture or the staple line of the anastomosis; increase the bursting pressure, which is the internal pressure exerted on the anastomoses right before failure will occur; and thus reduce tearing of tissues, bleeding, and leakage [13]. Staple or suture line reinforcement with buttressing materials in gastrointestinal surgery is well known, but there is no promising evidence of its application in colorectal surgery.

28.3.2 Defensive Methods to Predict Leakage

Defensive methods cannot prevent but predict anastomotic leakage. Laser Doppler flowmetry is a method to assess blood flow to the colon and the rectum. Blood flow was measured at the proximal colon side, the anastomotic site, and the distal rectal stump before and after mobilizing, dividing, and anastomosing the colon and the rectum. The magnitude of reduction of perfusion to the rectal stump significantly correlated with anastomotic leakage, of which mean rectal stump flow reduction was 6.2% in patients without leak versus 16% in patients with anastomotic leak [14].

Intraoperative dye test examines watertight and airtight of a colorectal anastomosis that provides an objective evidence of anastomotic leakage. This examination helps surgeons make decisions to reinforce the anastomosis with additional suture and/or to create a defunctioning colostomy to prevent development of serious complications resulting from leakage and to decrease incidence of anastomotic leaks in patients undergoing resection for rectal cancer [15].

To drain or not to drain the extraperitoneal anastomoses after rectal cancer surgery is an issue of controversy. A large observational prospective study of 978 patients demonstrated that anastomotic leakage with drains increased significantly in patients receiving low anterior resection for rectal cancer [16]. On the other hand, a recent randomized clinical trial (GRECCAR 5) found that a pelvic drain for extraperitoneal anastomoses after rectal cancer surgery had no significant benefits in clinical outcomes between the two study groups no matter the rate of pelvic sepsis, surgical morbidity, the rate of reoperation, the rate of stoma closure, or the length of hospital stay [17]. Nevertheless, considering neoadjuvant concurrent chemoradiotherapy and TME for middle and lower third rectal cancer, which have resulted in higher rate of sphincter preservation but higher rate of anastomotic leakage and pelvic sepsis on the other hand, a pelvic drain not only eliminates accumulation of fluid within this dead space where there is no peritoneum to absorb it, avoids potential contamination of pelvic fluid after TME, but also detects anastomotic leakage, whereas there are no innervations after TME in the pelvis to present pain and peritoneal signs that may obscure anastomotic leakage.

Diverting, protective, or defunctioning stomas do not decrease the rate of anastomotic leakage but minimize the severity and sequelae of leakage and decrease the rate of reoperation as the result. In any situation where possibility of anastomotic leakage is encountered during operation, creating a loop colostomy or ileostomy may be beneficial. In addition, we recently found that early closure of defunctioning stoma increases complications related to stoma closure after concurrent chemoradiotherapy and low anterior resection in patients with rectal cancer [18].

28.4 Anastomotic Stenosis

Clinical presentation of anastomotic stenosis is partial or total bowel obstruction at the level of anastomosis. Anastomotic stenosis may be the sequels of anastomotic ischemia, leakage, or dehiscence mentioned at the former section. Other factors, such as inflammation, radiation [19], recurrence of malignancy, and stapled method of anastomosis constructed [20], are also contributory to anastomotic stenosis. Stenosis occurs more likely with stapled colorectal anastomosis when compared to hand-sewn method (8% versus 2%) [5], but there is no significant difference between stapled and hand-sewn methods with ileocolic anastomoses [21]. This is because of not only relative small caliber of left-sided colon and relative formed fecal materials but also lack of peritoneum coverage within the pelvic cavity. The incidence of stenosis of colorectal anastomoses is greater in male than in female gender as well, and it reflects more technical difficulties of surgery in narrow pelvic space [22]. Sometimes the diameter of the proximal colon is too small to do an end-to-end colorectal anastomosis, and a side-to-end colorectal anastomosis is an ideal option to prevent anastomotic stenosis.

28.5 Fistula

Different types of fistulas can develop between the anastomosis and the skin, genitourinary tract, presacral space, and vagina. It can be, similar to the anastomotic stenosis, the sequels of anastomotic ischemia, leakage, or dehiscence and can be an early complication of inadvertent inclusion of the posterior vaginal wall, even mistaken placement of staple within the vagina during making an anastomosis. It can also result from additional excision of adjacent organ in en bloc resection for locally advanced colorectal cancer, especially within the pelvic cavity, such as the bladder, vagina, uterus, fallopian tube, ovary, ureter, and urethra. Because of the anatomic relationships, the lower in the pelvic space the cancer is, the higher the rate of fistula occurs. Preoperative neoadjuvant radial therapy is another risk factor for fistulae [23].

Conclusions

The safety of colorectal surgery for patients with colorectal cancer improves recently with the improvements of preoperative preparation, antibiotic prophylaxis, surgical technique, surgical devices, perioperative nutrition support, and postoperative management. A certain percentage of anastomotic complications remain encountered, including bleeding, leakage or dehiscence, stenosis, and fistula. The application of technology and techniques to optimize anastomoses is practical and clinically useful in minimally invasive surgery for colorectal cancer to minimize anastomotic complications as well as to enhance short-term and long-term outcomes of these patients.

References

1. Paun BC, Cassie S, MacLean AR, Dixon E, Buie WD. Postoperative complications following surgery for rectal cancer. Ann Surg. 2010;251:807–18.
2. Biondi A, Grosso G, Mistretta A, Marventano S, Toscano C, Drago F, et al. Laparoscopic vs. open approach for colorectal cancer: evolution over time of minimal invasive surgery. BMC Surg. 2013;13(Suppl 2):S12.
3. Cadiere GB, Himpens J, Germay O, Izizaw R, Degueldre M, Vandromme J, et al. Feasibility of robotic laparoscopic surgery: 146 cases. World J Surg. 2001;25:1467–77.
4. Papanikolaou IG. Robotic surgery for colorectal cancer: systematic review of the literature. Surg Laparosc Endosc Percutan Tech. 2014;24:478–83.
5. Neutzling CB, Lustosa SA, Proenca IM, da Silva EM, Matos D. Stapled versus handsewn methods for colorectal anastomosis surgery. Cochrane Database Syst Rev. 2012:CD003144.
6. Platell C, Barwood N, Dorfmann G, Makin G. The incidence of anastomotic leaks in patients undergoing colorectal surgery. Color Dis. 2007;9:71–9.
7. Slim K, Vicaut E, Panis Y, Chipponi J. Meta-analysis of randomized clinical trials of colorectal surgery with or without mechanical bowel preparation. Br J Surg. 2004;91:1125–30.
8. Law WI, Chu KW, Ho JW, Chan CW. Risk factors for anastomotic leakage after low anterior resection with total mesorectal excision. Am J Surg. 2000;179:92–6.
9. Rullier E, Laurent C, Garrelon JL, Michel P, Saric J, Parneix M. Risk factors for anastomotic leakage after resection of rectal cancer. Br J Surg. 1998;85:355–8.
10. Huang CW, Yeh YS, WC S, Tsai HL, Choy TK, Huang MY, et al. Robotic surgery with high dissection and low ligation technique for consecutive patients with rectal cancer following preoperative concurrent chemoradiotherapy. Int J Color Dis. 2016;31:1169–77.
11. Jafari MD, Lee KH, Halabi WJ, Mills SD, Carmichael JC, Stamos MJ, et al. The use of indocyanine green fluorescence to assess anastomotic perfusion during robotic assisted laparoscopic rectal surgery. Surg Endosc. 2013;27(8):3003.
12. Kim HJ, Huh JW, Kim HR, Kim YJ. Oncologic impact of anastomotic leakage in rectal cancer surgery according to the use of fibrin glue: case-control study using propensity score matching method. Am J Surg. 2014;207(6):840.
13. Yo LS, Consten EC, Quarles van Ufford HM, Gooszen HG, Gagner M. Buttressing of the staple line in gastrointestinal anastomoses: overview of new technology designed to reduce perioperative complications. Dig Surg. 2006;23:283–91.
14. Vignali A, Gianotti L, Braga M, Radaelli G, Malvezzi L, Di Carlo V. Altered microperfusion at the rectal stump is predictive for rectal anastomotic leak. Dis Colon Rectum. 2000;43:76–82.
15. Chen CW, Chen MJ, Yeh YS, Tsai HL, Chang YT, Wang JY. Intraoperative anastomotic dye test significantly decreases incidence of anastomotic leaks in patients undergoing resection for rectal cancer. Tech Coloproctol. 2013;17:579–83.
16. Yeh CY, Changchien CR, Wang JY, Chen JS, Chen HH, Chiang JM, et al. Pelvic drainage and other risk factors for leakage after elective anterior resection in rectal cancer patients: a prospective study of 978 patients. Ann Surg. 2005;241:9–13.
17. Denost Q, Rouanet P, Faucheron JL, Panis Y, Meunier B, Cotte E, et al. To drain or not to drain infraperitoneal anastomosis after rectal excision for cancer: the GRECCAR 5 randomized trial. Ann Surg. 2017;265:474–80.
18. Yin TC, Tsai HL, Yang PF, Su WC, Ma CJ, Huang CW, et al. Early closure of defunctioning stoma increases complications related to stoma closure after concurrent chemoradiotherapy and low anterior resection in patients with rectal cancer. World J Surg Oncol. 2017;15:80.
19. Luchtefeld MA, Milsom JW, Senagore A, Surrell JA, Mazier WP. Colorectal anastomotic stenosis. Results of a survey of the ASCRS membership. Dis Colon Rectum. 1989;32:733–6.
20. MacRae HM, McLeod RS. Handsewn vs. stapled anastomoses in colon and rectal surgery: a meta-analysis. Dis Colon Rectum. 1998;41:180–9.
21. Choy PY, Bissett IP, Docherty JG, Parry BR, Merrie AE. Stapled versus handsewn methods for ileocolic anastomoses. Cochrane Database Syst Rev. 2007:CD004320.

22. Bannura GC, Cumsille MA, Barrera AE, Contreras JP, Melo CL, Soto DC. Predictive factors of stenosis after stapled colorectal anastomosis: prospective analysis of 179 consecutive patients. World J Surg. 2004;28:921–5.

23. Matthiessen P, Hansson L, Sjodahl R, Rutegard J. Anastomotic-vaginal fistula (AVF) after anterior resection of the rectum for cancer--occurrence and risk factors. Color Dis. 2010;12:351–7.

Future Perspectives in Robotic Colorectal Surgery

29

Andee Dzulkarnaen Zakaria, James Wei Tatt Toh, and Seon-Hahn Kim

Abstract

The revolution of robotic colorectal surgery has caused a tremendous increase in its adoption, and the number of patients undergoing these procedures has grown quickly worldwide, including in Asia. Since the original concept of "master and slave," robotic technology has maximized capabilities far beyond human limits, namely extra robotic arms controlled by the operating surgeon, wrist-like articulation, magnified three dimensional visualization with high-definition and depth perception with the use of an ergonomic and stable stereo-optic camera. The advantage of robotic surgery is maximized in confined spaces—in colorectal surgery, this is in the domain of low rectal cancers, for which robotic surgery can help to achieve good oncological and functional outcomes and improve the ease of surgery for the surgeon. New advances in technology integration of hardware, software, and design architectures, such as nanorobotic technology, hybrid augmented virtual reality, artificial intelligence, and concepts yet to be realized, may synergize and enhance robotic colorectal surgery in the future. Robotic surgical systems have the potential to optimize the surgical management of, and enhance survival and functional outcomes in, patients with low rectal cancer.

Keywords

Robotic · Colorectal surgery · Future
Advanced · Minimal invasive surgery · MIS

A. D. Zakaria
Colorectal Division, Korea University Anam Hospital, Seoul, South Korea

Korea University College of Medicine, Seoul, South Korea

Department of Surgery, School of Medical Sciences, Universiti Sains Malaysia, Kubang Kerian, Kelantan, Malaysia

J. W. T. Toh
Colorectal Division, Korea University Anam Hospital, Seoul, South Korea

Korea University College of Medicine, Seoul, South Korea

Colorectal Division, Department of Surgery, Westmead Hospital, Sydney, NSW, Australia

S.-H. Kim (✉)
Colorectal Division, Korea University Anam Hospital, Seoul, South Korea

Korea University College of Medicine, Seoul, South Korea
e-mail: drkimsh@korea.ac.kr

29.1 Robotic Colorectal Surgery: Past, Present, and Future

"Study the past if you would define the future..."
Confucius

© Springer Nature Singapore Pte Ltd. 2018
N. K. Kim et al. (eds.), *Surgical Treatment of Colorectal Cancer*,
https://doi.org/10.1007/978-981-10-5143-2_29

29.1.1 History of Robotic Surgery

The word *robot* (pronounced /ˈrəʊbɒt/) originated from *robota* ("forced labor") first used by Karel Čapek in the Czech play "Rossum's Universal Robots" in 1920 (Fig. 29.1). It is defined by the *Oxford English Dictionary* as a machine, especially one programmable by computer, that is capable of carrying out a complex series of actions automatically [1]. In the realm

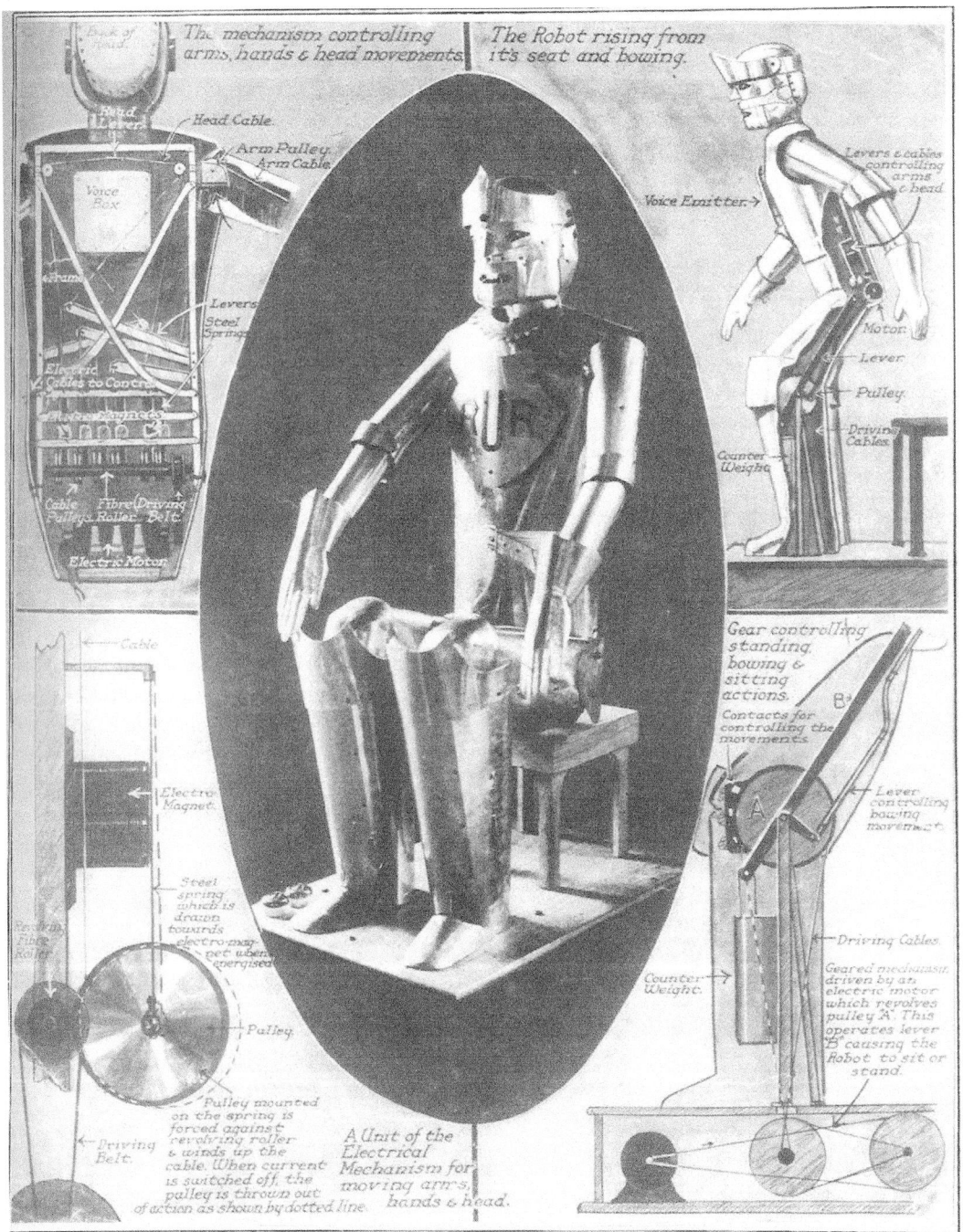

Fig. 29.1 "Rossum's Universal Robots" in 1920

of science fiction, a robot machine resembles a human being and is able to replicate automatically certain human movements and functions. An external control device may be used to guide it, or the control may be embedded within it in order to take on human form. The computer systems to control their precision and movements, haptic and tactile sensory feedback, and information processing in imaging (ultrahigh-dimensional depth perception) are fully robotic [2].

On the other hand, robotic surgery, computer-assisted surgery, or robotically assisted surgery refers to robotic systems used to aid in surgical procedures. Robotically assisted surgery was developed with the main objective to overcome the limitations of preexisting minimally invasive surgical procedures and to enhance the capabilities of surgeons performing conventional open surgery.

29.1.2 Timeline of Robotic Colorectal Surgery Worldwide

Arthrobot was developed to assist in surgery and was used for the first time in Vancouver in 1983; it was invented by team of biomedical physics engineers and engineering students—namely, Dr. James McEwen, Geof Auchinleck, and Dr. Brian Day [3]. It was used in more than 60 arthroscopic surgical procedures over a period of 12 months, and National Geographic featured the device in *The Robotics Revolution* in 1985. A surgical scrub nurse robot, which handed over operative instruments upon voice commands, and a medical laboratory robotic arm were also created around this time. In the same year, the Unimation Puma 200 (initial version) and 560 (its successor) were used to place a needle to biopsy the brain using computed tomography stereotactic guidance, with the technology improving accurate positioning [4]. In 1992, PROBOT, developed at Imperial College London, was used by Dr. Senthil Nathan to perform prostatic surgery at Guy's and St Thomas' Hospital, London. This procedure was regarded as the first purely robotic surgical procedure in the world. PROBOT was specifically designed for transurethral resection of the prostate [5]. ROBODOC, designed by Integrated

Surgical Systems (working closely with IBM) to assist in hip replacement surgeries, was the first surgical robot approved by the U.S. Food and Drug Administration (FDA) that same year [6].

This heralded the modern era of robotic systems, which was started by SRI International and Intuitive Surgical, with the introduction of the da Vinci Surgical System and Computer Motion with the automated endoscopic system for optimal positioning and the ZEUS robotic surgical system [7]. Robert E. Michler performed the first robotic procedure with the ZEUS robotic system at The Ohio State University Medical Center in Columbus [8]. The ZEUS system was also used to perform the Lindbergh operation, which was a cholecystectomy performed remotely in September 2001 [9]. The FDA approved the automated endoscopic system for optimal positioning system for clinical use as a robotic camera holder, whereas the ZEUS system was limited for use only as a surgical assistant in 1994.

The da Vinci robotic system (Intuitive Surgical Inc., Sunnyvale, CA) was the first robotic system approved by the FDA in 2001 for intra-abdominal surgery in the United States [10]. Since then, the da Vinci system has been widely used worldwide for robotic colorectal surgeries. Initial case reports by Weber et al. [11] reported three robotic right and sigmoid colectomies for benign disease using the da Vinci robotic system in 2002. In 2003, Delaney et al. [12] demonstrated the feasibility and safety of the da Vinci system compared with standard laparoscopic approaches, although their patient cohort was small. This was followed by studies by D'Annibale et al. [13] in 2004, reporting 53 robotic colorectal surgeries, including 22 cases of malignant colorectal disease. These earlier studies of robotic colorectal surgery suggested operative and postoperative results similar to those of standard laparoscopic techniques.

In 2006, Pigazzi et al. [14] reported the feasibility and safety of robotic total mesorectal excision for rectal cancer. The study showed similar results between robotic and laparoscopic low anterior resection with total mesorectal excision and autonomic nerve preservation. Rawlings et al. [15], reporting the outcomes of 17 robotic right hemicolectomies and 13 robotic anterior resections, similarly showed that it was technically feasible to use the da Vinci system. In 2007, the same group showed similar results between robotic and laparoscopic colectomies [16], a finding supported by Hellan et al. [17], who reported six robotic total mesorectal cases compared with conventional laparoscopic surgeries, and included a series of 39 consecutive unselected patients with primary rectal cancer in 2007. In 2008, Spinoglio et al. [18] reported that robotic colon surgery was also feasible and safe, but a longer operating time was required.

29.1.3 Timeline of Robotic Colorectal Surgery in Asia

The first report of robotic colorectal surgery in the literature from an Asian region was by Baik et al. [19], who reported robotic total mesorectal excision for a patient with rectal cancer in June 2006. Again, feasibility, safety, and oncological outcomes similar to those of laparoscopic surgery were achieved. Ng et al. [20] described the first case of robotic abdominoperineal resection in Hong Kong and China in August 2006. In 2008, Baik et al. [21] reported simultaneous robotic total mesorectal excision and total abdominal hysterectomy for rectal cancer and uterine myoma.

Baik et al. [22] performed the first prospective randomized trial comparing robotic low anterior resection and laparoscopic low anterior resection. The objective of their study was to compare the short-term results between robotic and laparoscopic tumor-specific mesorectal excision for patients with rectal cancer using the da Vinci Surgical System and conventional laparoscopy. The researchers recruited 18 patients for each arm of the study. The study showed that tumor-specific mesorectal excision was safely and effectively performed using the da Vinci Surgical System, and the perioperative outcomes were acceptable. In 2009, Choi et al. [23] reported 50 consecutive patients who underwent fully robotic single docking in lower anterior resection; this technique was first developed in Asia. Since then, many publications have emerged from Asia, including reports, systematic reviews, and trials of robotic colorectal surgery.

29.2 Current Scenario of Robotic Colorectal Surgery

"The more brilliant the lightning, the quicker it disappears . . ." Avicenna

29.2.1 West Meets East

Robotic surgery for urologic surgery, general laparoscopic surgery, gynecologic laparoscopic surgery, and general thoracoscopic and thoracoscopic-related cardiovascular procedures was approved by the FDA in 2000 [24]. Case selection, case planning, and technical expertise is important in robotic colorectal surgery. Preoperative planning is essential by staging through the use of magnetic resonance imaging, endoscopic ultrasound, and computed tomography, and gaining technical expertise and overcoming the learning curve are crucial.

Throughout the years, robotic surgery has brought surgeons from the West and East together, with experts in their fields meeting to discuss and share ideas and techniques. The same occurred for minimally invasive laparoscopic surgery, which reported short-term benefits such as reducing postoperative morbidity—including pain, length of stay, earlier return of bowel function, and better cosmesis for patients, without detrimental effects on oncological outcomes—with many landmarks trial including CLASSIC [25], COLOR I [26], COLOR II [27], ROLARR [28], and ACOSOG-Z6051 [29].

Robotic surgery addressed the few shortcomings in laparoscopic surgery—the two-dimensional views, limited dexterity with rigid instruments, fixed instrument tips with 4 degrees of freedom, and an inability of the surgeon to hold two instruments and control the camera at the same time. On the other hand, the da Vinci Robotic Surgical System offers stereo-optic three-dimensional imaging with a stable, self-controlling camera and an operating platform with four articulating instruments with 7 degrees of freedom, motion scaling, tremor-free movements, and ergonomic comfort.

The potential benefits of robotic colectomy compared with conventional laparoscopic colectomy may include less blood loss [30, 31], quicker return of bowel function [30, 32], a lower rate of complications [30, 33, 34], and shorter hospital length of stay [30, 33]. In low anterior resection, the advantage of robotic surgery may be a better view in confined spaces associated with less bleeding [35, 36], reduced pain [35, 37], shorter hospital length of stay [35, 38], improved cancer margins [39, 40], decreased rate of conversion to open surgery [39, 41–43], and quicker return to a normal diet [35, 41].

Approximately 3 million patients worldwide have benefited from the da Vinci robotic technology. While technically feasible and safe, the oncologic and functional outcomes of robotic colorectal surgery over conventional laparoscopic surgery are still a matter of debate. Furthermore, a consensus on robotic technique has not been achieved. Technical variations include techniques of docking the robotic arms, placing ports and trocars, and ergonomics to avoid clashing between robotics arms.

In China in 2015, an expert consensus on robotic surgery for colorectal cancer designed a comprehensive protocol [44]. Other recommendations exist, such as those by Morelli et al. [45] Even though equivalent results between robotic and laparoscopic surgery have been reported overall [46–48], the quality of total mesorectal excision, circumferential margin positivity, and actuarial survival data reported in meta-analyses and systematic reviews have varied between studies, and the level of evidence is inconclusive.

Recent evidence of long-term oncologic survival and recurrence suggested that robotic total mesorectal excision for rectal cancer showed better survival than laparoscopic total mesorectal excision. Robotic surgery was a good prognostic factor for overall survival and cancer-specific survival, suggesting that potential oncologic benefits may be obtained by experienced robotic colorectal surgeons [49].

The benefit of robotic colorectal surgery for extensive pelvic surgery and nononcological cases is unclear. It has been reported that pelvic exenteration with the da Vinci robotic system is feasible for locally advanced rectal cancer [50] and for benign diverticular disease combined with natural orifice specimen extraction [51].

29.2.2 Future Challenges

Concerns have been raised regarding the revolution of robotic technology. With robotic technology replacing human effort in various tasks and roles, technological unemployment (the loss of jobs caused by technological change) is possible. For centuries, experts have predicted that machines would make human workers obsolete and increase unemployment [52, 53]. A recent example of this involved the Taiwanese technology company Foxconn; in July 2011, Foxconn announced a 3-year plan to replace workers with more robots. Foxconn's plan to increase the number of robots from thousands to millions over a 3-year period [54] may herald a new era of technological unemployment. Lawyers have speculated that an increased prevalence of robots in the workplace could lead to the need to revise redundancy laws [55].

Another major concern with robotic technology is occupational safety and health implications. A discussion paper drawn up by the European Agency for Safety and Health at Work highlighted how the spread of robotics presents both opportunities and challenges for occupational safety and health [56]. Michio Kaku [57], a theoretical physicist and author of the Japanese national bestselling book *Physics of the Future: How Science Will Shape Human Destiny and Our Daily Lives by the Year 2100*, predicted that by 2100 that most jobs will be replaced by robotic technology, particularly repetitive, production, and commodity-based jobs. Occupations that engage in intellectual capitalism, creativity, imagination, leadership, analysis, humor, common sense, screen-/scriptwriting, and scientific endeavors will be resilient against the technological revolution [57].

The da Vinci Surgical System is the only robotic system approved by the FDA that is currently being used for surgical procedures. The main barrier to its use at most institutions has been financial limitations [24]. A significant learning curve also is associated with its use. Critics of robotic surgery argue that, within the domain of colorectal surgery, the literature has not shown a significant difference in outcomes between robotic and traditional laparoscopic surgeries [58]. The literature has also demonstrated a lack of benefit for robotically performed hysterectomies.

Furthermore, the da Vinci system uses proprietary software that cannot be modified by physicians, thereby limiting the freedom to modify the operating system [59]. Concerns also exist regarding the use of robotic technology without sufficient training and supervision [60]. Technical safety reports have indicated that stray electrical currents may be released from inappropriate parts of the surgical tips used by the system. However, stray currents may also occur in nonrobotic laparoscopic procedures [61].

Timothy Lenoir claimed that in the "heroic age of medicine," the view of the surgeon as a hero for his intuitive knowledge of human anatomy and his well-crafted techniques in repairing vital body systems will dissolve the creative freedoms of the surgeon. Lenoir argues that the da Vinci's three-dimensional console and robotic arms create a mediating form of action called medialization, in which internal knowledge of images and routes within the body become external knowledge mapped into simplistic computer coding [62].

It is believed that, as technology improves, cooperation between robots and humans will reach completely new standards [63, 64], with the line between human and robot challenged by artificial intelligence. Human common sense, intellectuality, emotionality, and sensibility will be matched by robotic intelligence and precision.

29.3 The Future of Robotic Colorectal Surgery

"The true sign of intelligence is not knowledge but imagination." Albert Einstein

29.3.1 Innovation and Technology

The future is *now*—either ongoing or new ideas that bring surgery forward to the next level. The best way to predict the future is to create and postulate it; as opponents of robotics say, it is difficult to predict the future. To rise above criticism and opponents' comments, collaborations between manufacturers and end users, namely the robotic colorectal surgeon, have to grow and evolve to achieve a better healthcare environment in healthy conditions. With the benefits of robotic surgery still unclear, early adopters have paved the way forward. Innovators have shown resilience, moving forward with the technology despite criticism and opposition due to a lack of evidence. The same issues arise with most new technologies, but perhaps because of its cost, a higher burden of proof has been set for robotic surgery. Despite its limited availability, its cost, and the learning curve, the revolution of robotic technology has shown promise in specialized centers, but it has also been met with significant barriers and scrutiny, particularly from those not trained in robotic surgery. Long-term results from randomized multicenter trials (COLRAR [www.clinical trials.gov identifier NCT01423214) and ROLARR (identifier NCT01196000) are eagerly awaited. Current ongoing trials or potential innovations and technologies research future thinking and planning for the coming era of robotics colorectal surgery that will enhance and bring its to next level.

Platforms that use robotic surgical systems to minimize surgical incisions include robotic single port or site surgery, Robotic NOTES, transanal robotics, endorobotics; these will maximize the benefits of minimal invasive and scarless surgery. However, technology of augmented hand or multichannel working interchangeable hands in one single port/arms yet minimal manipulations and nearly no touch tumor bearing will be achieved. New commercial players interested under trials and researchers and commercial bio medical companies. And yet the revolution of automation concepts such as auto-robotic or auto-driven, autopilot robotic surgery system like drone surgeon or self-driven from automotive and production industries' can be colloborated with future robotics colorectal system.

Imaging and visualization aspects in robotic surgical systems also need to be modified and upgraded. The concepts of multimodal imaging and imaging-guided surgery, real-time anatomy identification such as Firefly™ fluorescent imaging, near-infrared fluorescence, and indocyanine green perfusion are current available but may need to be more widely available and have more evidence on their use. Augmented vision and virtual reality technology may be the next step to enhance these visualizations. Furthermore, Artis Zeego by Siemens Healthcare is nicknamed "the future of flexible"; this unique robotic technology is used mainly in intervention radiology and applies flexibility to execute tasks, support the cutting edge, and use space and resources. The concept of augmented and automated eye from image digitalization such as ultra-laser vision, which postulates capabilities beyond those of the human eye in terms of identifying shades of colors, matching prints, and completing missing pieces. Last but not least, advancements from artificial intelligence technology, hybrid imaging, real-time virtual reality, or therapeutic devices may benefit those listed above.

With regard to information behind the sciences of advanced intelligence and strategy, navigation systems may be a new concept to be embarked on in robotic colorectal surgery; this may involve navigation camera systems in planning, simulation, and guidance before surgery and even during the intraoperative period. Ideas include topographical anatomical landmark mapping and marking by fusing with augmented reality, such as volume and surface renderings, virtual modeling, adjacent borders, and segmentation of organs and related adjacent organs. Information-integrated computer surgery also may give promising hope for the future.

Collaboration and integration, such as collaboration with endoscopy technology with endolu-

minal or transluminal endorobotic endoscopic mucosal resection and endoscopic submucosal dissection, needs more exploration in this field. Collaborations between multidisciplinary fields such as intensive medicine and interventional radiology, even beyond the operating theater, can provide better care to patients. Verb Surgical Inc. recently announced that the company demonstrated its first digital surgery prototype to its collaboration partners at Ethicon Endo-Surgery, Inc., part of the Johnson & Johnson Medical Devices Companies, and Verily Life Sciences (formerly Google Life Sciences), and to senior leadership from Johnson & Johnson and Alphabet Inc. The digital surgery platform includes all elements of the company's five technology pillars: robotics, visualization, advanced instrumentation, data analytics, and connectivity. A few prototypes were tested and ideas sparked, such as "Supercirujano" Steel Hands and Scott Huennekens's (president and CEO of Verb Surgical) vision of next-generation robotic surgery under Verb Surgery 4.0. It is new concept of "digital surgery" includes data and imaging integration into a surgical robot and improved decision making through artificial intelligence technology.

Others miscellaneous future concepts and ideas that need to be explored include haptic and tactile sensations in cognitive technology used in robotic colorectal surgery; this demands soft-tissue differentiation, the careful manipulation of tissues, and suturing for the surgeon at the console. The TELELAP ALFX is a surgical robot that offers haptic feedback by exerting forces on the surgeon's hands; this requires a complex system of processors and actuators to achieve adequate fidelity and is therefore inherently complex [65]. Furthermore, gross tactile information and sensation in minimal access surgery have been developed and tested in order to locate arteries and detect blood flow, and, for example, in identifying the inferior mesenteric artery, as with the Tact Array (Pressure Profile Systems) [66].

Originating from the idea of the landmark Lindbergh operation, the ideas of tele-surgery and tele-health are based on tele-tap technology that surgery across border may be benefited to colloborate with robotic surgery. In this nano-technology era, integration of ideas such as nanorobotics, nanoparticles, nanomaterials, nanogenomics, nanomolecular, and nanotechnology are related and give promising results, with many loopholes and space still to explore. Currently, the usage of smart stapler feedback analysis already on the market and in practice that analyzes tissue perfusion and measures thickness and tension can provide almost none or zero stapler leaks. In the future, our hope is that it can further can measure perianastomosis perfusion and determine an anastomosis leakage rate. Maybe auto-extending or customized length and thickness of a universal stapler would be available in the future. To date, the use of Endowrist One gives good results and shows sustainable performance in equivalent minimal thermal spread and means burst pressure can be better tested in three arteries, namely the splenic, mesentery, and renal arteries [67]. Leonard et al. [68] sparked the idea about smart tissue anastomosis robotic (STAR) as a proof of concept for a vision-guided robotic system featuring an actuated laparoscopic suturing tool capable of executing running sutures from image-based commands and measurement of the surface contour of anastomoses between bowels.

29.3.2 Ideal Robotic Surgical System: Robotic Intelligence

Currently available robotic surgical systems are extremely expensive to purchase and maintain in a noncompetitive market. A bulky robotic "slave" with four arms and many wires require a spacious operating room setup. The surgery is not completely robotic and not fully under autonomous control of the surgeon, even though all the safety, feasibility, and surgical outcomes, such as economic costs, survival, complication, and results analysis, can, based on evidence and practical use, be achieved. The concept of personalized surgery with precision skills is good to be adapted rather than tools or appliances.

Ideally, a "humanoid" robot can be imagined as having smooth movements, being friendly to all humankind and nature, having a sleek appearance, and performing smart interactions with its "master," performing beyond human ability, sensibility, and capability yet fulfilling all the criteria of original surgical procedures and objectives indefinitely. In addition to making sure robotic surgery is the ideal and ultimate concept, the operator or robotic surgeon has to ready and synchronize updated surgical skills and be technically ready with new innovations and technologies, with cost-effectiveness that can progress and evolve over time. Smart collaboration and cooperation with other new groups, either medical (e.g., biomedical engineering, radiology, immunology, pathology, oncology, genetics) or nonmedical (such as software engineering, artificial intelligence, biomedical architecture) will open new diversity in robotic surgery beyond the current imagination. Here, the sky is the limit.

Hence, we can imagine that the ideal robotic system will be mounted from above, sleek, and small; have multiple stable arms; couple with hybrid imaging such as radiography, computed tomography, or magnetic resonance imaging without docking; and assist intraoperatively by offering a totally single and superpowered robotic colorectal approach. In addition, the surgeon's console should be dynamic yet confined to a cart; we suggest that it be more spacious without engaging the head, and allow full hand-motion control, as if virtually doing the surgical procedure in real time while receiving haptic and tactile sensations. The process includes perceiving, analyzing, understanding, and judging information before performing and executing actions. For periplanning, training, or simulated robotic surgery, virtual exact images exist of organs and all the surrounding adjacent organs involved, with interaction showing cautions during surgery. The use of next-generation energy, tools, and staplers with intelligence capabilities is needed to complete these state-of-the-art surgeries. The efficacy versus invasiveness between patients and robotic surgeon comfort zone should become a common endpoint for both. We also postulate the idea of future surgery as information-integrated computerized surgery that combines robotics, imaging, and artificial intelligence (Fig. 29.2),

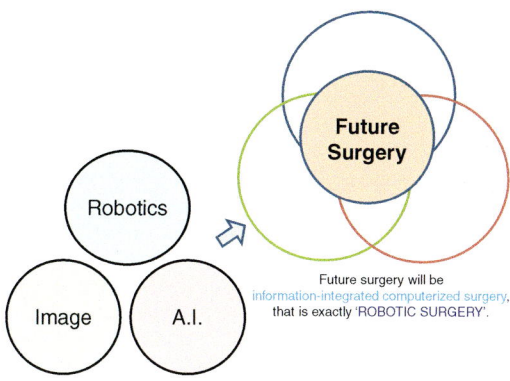

Fig. 29.2 Future surgery concepts

allowing an autonomous robotic surgeon more dominance and control at all times, with zero error; it will be highly competent and produce efficient teamwork to offer the best management to all patients. Perhaps sipping coffee and listening to a favorite playlist of songs while doing robotic colorectal surgery is an idea for surgeons to relax, and could allow them to take brief breaks during surgery outside the operation theater. Last, in whatever we achieve as the ideal concept for a robotic surgery system in the future, the main important objective of our ancient Hippocratic oath is "First do no harm" (*Primum non nocere*), and this needs to be a pillar in all medical practice.

29.4 Training in Privileging and Credentialing in Robotic Colorectal Surgery

"A journey of a thousand miles begins with a single step." Laozi

First, every surgeon must be competent enough to master and command the robotics system before apply to patient practices. The steep learning curve from simulations to the real world also involves from robotic surgeon to be, assistant and supporting staff in order to master and command the robotic surgical systems. Training is needed to gain privileges and be credentialed to perform robotic colorectal surgery in order to certify and recognize this delicate procedure. The concepts of learning, unlearning, and

relearning form a cycle to maintain, translate, and transfer knowledge and education from person to person. Similar concepts apply to experts in highly specialized robotic colorectal surgery in order to standardize and maintain certain protocols and safety when handling this highly technical apparatus. In addition, different steep curve of learning has to be achieved in view of the number of cases and proper handling and techniques of robotic colorectal surgery. Currently, apprenticeships, fellowships, or proctorships are offered by various centers in view of having no certified training center available. Experts on robotic colorectal surgical teams have to set up proper and standard syllabi to recognize and acknowledge privileging and credentialing for robotic colorectal surgery trainees around the world and particularly in Asian regions. Much has been said about validating the acquisition of practical skills through distance learning processes, but the questions is whether any consensus or best practices are available now. To answer this, continuing medical education, process audits by higher authorities, plus determining patient outcomes, benefits, and practices via evidence-based medicine, such as publications, international conferences, and summit meetings of experts, are good starting points for these novel ideas and practices. Job descriptions, job automation, and risk assessments of robotic colorectal surgeons need to be considered before they are credited as robotic surgeons.

Pitfalls of these ideas include the possibility of a single commercial company in control of the market and the high cost to be trained and certified; we may need to think before we embark on these ideas. However, we believe that the advantages outweigh the disadvantages for these ideas. In the future, we hypothesize that trainees will be able to do their training at their own center and, with the advance of robotic surgery, be monitored by a supervisor virtually, across continents, if necessary. Ideas of free trade among the robotic community will give opportunities to developing countries to have similar chances to advance in the era of robotic surgery. This is all only the beginning of the journey. Let medicine reach to all, beyond boundaries, as we own the future . . .

References

1. Definition of 'robot'. Oxford English Dictionary.
2. Robotics. Oxford Dictionaries. Retrieved 27 February 2017.
3. Medical Post 23:1985.
4. Kwoh YS, Hou J, Jonckheere EA, Hayall S. A robot with improved absolute positioning accuracy for CT guided stereotactic brain surgery. IEEE Trans Biomed Eng. 1988;35(2):153–61.
5. Lanfranco AR, Castellanos AE, Desai JP, Meyers WC. Robotic surgery. Ann Surg. 2004;239(1):14–21.
6. ROBODOC: surgical robot success story.
7. Meadows M. Computer-assisted surgery: an update. FDA Consumer magazine. Food and Drug Administration. Archived from the original on 1 Mar 2009.
8. McConnell PI, Schneeberger EW, Michler RE. History and development of robotic cardiac surgery. Probl Gen Surg. 2003;20(2):20–30.
9. Linbergh operation – IRCAD/EITS Laparoscopic Center.
10. Ballantyne GH, Merola P, Weber A, Wasielewski A. Robotic solutions to the pitfalls of laparoscopic colectomy. Osp Ital Chir. 2001;7:405–12.
11. Weber PA, Merola S, Wasielewski A, Ballantyne GH. Telerobotic-assisted laparoscopic right and sigmoid colectomies for benign disease. Dis Colon Rectum. 2002;45:1689–94. discussion 1695-6.
12. Delaney CP, Lynch AG, Senagore AJ, Fazio VW. Comparison of robotically performed and traditional laparoscopic colorectal surgery. Dis Colon Rectum. 2003;46:1633–9.
13. D'Annibale A, Morpurgo E, Fiscon V, Trevisan P, Sovernigo G, Orsini C, et al. Robotic and laparosocpic surgery for treatment of colorectal disease. Dis Colon Rectum. 2004;47:2162–8.
14. Pigazzi A, Ellenhorn JD, Ballantyne GH, Paz IB. Robotic-assisted laparoscopic low anterior resection with total mesorectal excision for rectal cancer. Surg Endosc. 2006;20:1521–5.
15. Rawlings AL, Woodland JH, Crawford DL. Telerobotic surgery for right and sigmoid colectomies: 30 consecutive cases. Surg Endosc. 2006;20:1713–8.
16. Rawlings AL, Woodland JH, Vegunta RK, Crawford DL. Robotic versus laparoscopic colectomy. Surg Endosc. 2007;21:1701–8.
17. Hellan M, Anderson C, Ellenhorn JD, Paz B, Pigazzi A. Short-term outcomes after robotic-assisted total mesorectal excision for rectal cancer. Ann Surg Oncol. 2007;14:3168–73.
18. Spinoglio G, Summa M, Priora F, Quarati R, Testa S. Robotic colorectal surgery: first 50 cases experience. Dis Colon Rectum. 2008;51:1627–32.
19. Baik SH, Kang CM, Lee WJ, Kim NK, Sohn SK, Chi HS, et al. Robotic total mesorectal excision for the treatment of rectal cancer. J Robot Surg. 2007;1:99–102.
20. Ng SS, Lee JF, Yiu RY, Li JC, Hon SS. Telerobotic-assisted laparoscopic abdominoperineal resection for low rectal cancer: report of the first case in Hong Kong and China with an updated literature review. World J Gastroenterol. 2007;13:2514–8.
21. Baik SH, Kim YT, Ko YT, Kang CM, Lee WJ, Kim NK, et al. Simultaneous robotic total mesorectal excision and total abdominal hysterectomy for rectal cancer and uterine myoma. Int J Color Dis. 2008;23:207–8.
22. Baik SH, Ko YT, Kang CM, Lee WJ, Kim NK, Sohn SK, et al. Robotic tumor-specific mesorectal excision of rectal cancer: short-term outcome of a pilot randomized trial. Surg Endosc. 2008;22:1601–8.
23. Choi DJ, Kim SH, Lee PJM, Kim J, Woo SW. Single stage totally robotic dissection for rectal cancer surgery: technique and short-term outcome in 50 consecutive patients. Dis Colon Rectum. 2009;52(11):1824–30.
24. The slow rise of the robot surgeon. MIT Technology Review. 24 Mar 2010.
25. Jayne DG, Guillou PJ, Thorpe H, Quirke P, Copeland J, Smith AM, Heath RM, Brown JM, UK MRC CLASICC Trial Group. Randomized trial of laparoscopic-assisted resection of colorectal carcinoma: 3-year results of the UK MRC CLASICC Trial Group. J Clin Oncol. 2007;25(21):3061–8.
26. COLOR Study Group. COLOR: a randomized clinical trial comparing laparoscopic and open resection for colon cancer. Dig Surg. 2000;17(6):617–22.
27. van der Pas MH, Haglind E, Cuesta MA, Fürst A, Lacy AM, Hop WC, Bonjer HJ, COlorectal cancer Laparoscopic or Open Resection II (COLOR II) Study Group. Laparoscopic versus open surgery for rectal cancer (COLOR II): short-term outcomes of a randomised, phase 3 trial. Lancet Oncol. 2013;14(3):210–8.
28. Collinson FJ, Jayne DG, Pigazzi A, Tsang C, Barrie JM, Edlin R, Garbett C, Guillou P, Holloway I, Howard H, et al. An international, multicentre, prospective, randomised, controlled, unblinded, parallel-group trial of robotic-assisted versus standard laparoscopic surgery for the curative treatment of rectal cancer. Int J Color Dis. 2012;27:233–41.
29. Nandakumar G, Fleshman JW. Laparoscopy for rectal cancer. Surg Oncol Clin N Am. 2010;19:793–802.
30. Chang Y, Wang J, Chang D. A meta-analysis of robotic versus laparoscopic colectomy. J Surg Res. 2015;195(2):465–74.
31. Rondelli F, Balzarotti R, Villa F, et al. Is robot-assisted laparoscopic right colectomy more effective than the conventional laparoscopic procedure? A meta-analysis of short-term outcomes. Int J Surg. 2015;18:75–82.
32. Zarak A, Castillo A, Kichler K, de la Cruz L, Tamariz L, Kaza S. Robotic versus laparoscopic surgery for colonic disease: a meta-analysis of postoperative variables. Surg Endosc. 2015;29(6):1341–7.
33. Altieri M, Yang J, Telem D, et al. Robotic approaches may offer benefit in colorectal procedures, more

controversial in other areas: a review of 168,248 cases. Surg Endosc. 2015;30(3):925–33.

34. Lorenzon L, Bini F, Balducci G, Ferri M, Salvi P, Marinozzi F. Laparoscopic versus robotic-assisted colectomy and rectal resection: a systematic review and meta-analysis. Int J Color Dis. 2015;31(2):161–73.

35. Kang J, Yoon KJ, Min BS, Hur H, Baik SH, Kim NK, Lee KY. The impact of robotic surgery for mid and low rectal cancer: a case-matched analysis of 3-arm comparison – open, laparoscopic, and robotic surgery. Ann Surg. 2013;257(1):95–101.

36. deSouza AL, Prasad LM, Ricci J, Park JJ, Marecik SJ, Zimmern A, Blumetti J, Abcarian H. A comparison of open and robotic total mesorectal excision for rectal adenocarcinoma. Dis Colon Rectum. 2011;54(3):275–82.

37. Park JS, Choi GS, Lim KH, Jang YS, Jun SH. S052: a comparison of robot-assisted, laparoscopic, and open surgery in the treatment of rectal cancer. Surg Endosc. 2011;25(1):240–8.

38. Ghezzi TL, Luca F, Valvo M, Corleta OC, Zuccaro M, Cenciarelli S, Biffi R. Robotic versus open total mesorectal excision for rectal cancer: comparative study of short- and long-term outcomes. Eur J Surg Oncol. 2014;40:1072. https://doi.org/10.1016/j.ejso.2014.02.235.

39. D'Annibale A, Pernazza G, Monsellato I, Pende V, Lucandri G, Mazzocchi P, Alfano G. Total mesorectal excision: a comparison of oncological and functional outcomes between robotic and laparoscopic surgery for rectal cancer. Surg Endosc. 2013;27(6):1887–95.

40. Xiong B, Ma L, Zhang C, Cheng Y. Robotic versus laparoscopic total mesorectal excision for rectal cancer: a meta-analysis. J Surg Res. 2014;188(2):404–14.

41. Baik SH, Kwon HY, Kim JS, Hur H, Sohn SK, Cho CH, Kim H. Robotic versus laparoscopic low anterior resection of rectal cancer: short-term outcome of a prospective comparative study. Ann Surg Oncol. 2009;16(6):1480–7.

42. Speicher PJ, Englum BR, Ganapathi AM, Nussbaum DP, Mantyh CR, Migaly J. Robotic low anterior resection for rectal cancer: a national perspective on short-term oncologic outcomes. Ann Surg. 2015;262:1040.

43. Liao G, Zhao Z, Lin S, Li R, Yuan Y, Du S, Chen J, Deng H. Robotic-assisted versus laparoscopic colorectal surgery: a meta-analysis of four randomized controlled trials. World J Surg Oncol. 2014;12:122.

44. Xu J, Qin X. Expert consensus on robotic surgery for colorectal cancer (2015 edition). Chin J Cancer. 2016;35:23.

45. Morelli L, Guadagni S, Di Franco G, et al. Int J Color Dis. 2015;30:1281.

46. Lim DR, Min BS, Kim MS, Alasari S, Kim G, Hur H, Baik SH, Lee KY, Kim NK. Robotic versus laparoscopic anterior resection of sigmoid colon cancer: comparative study of long-term oncologic outcomes. Surg Endosc. 2013;27:1379–85.

47. Cho MS, Baek SJ, Hur H, Min BS, Baik SH, Lee KY, Kim NK. Short and long-term outcomes of robotic versus laparoscopic total mesorectal excision for rectal cancer: a case-matched retrospective study. Medicine. 2015;94(11):e522.

48. Park EJ, Cho MS, Baek SJ, Hur H, Min BS, Baik SH, Lee KY, Kim NK. Long-term oncologic outcomes of robotic low anterior resection for rectal cancer: a comparative study with laparoscopic surgery. Ann Surg. 2015;261(1):129–37.

49. Kim J, Baek SJ, Kang DW, Roh YE, Lee JW, Kwak HD, Kwak JM, Kim SH. Robotic resection is a good prognostic factor in rectal cancer compared with laparoscopic resection: long-term survival analysis using propensity score matching. Dis Colon Rectum. 2017;60(3):266–73.

50. Shin JW, Kim J, Kwak JM, Hara M, Cheon J, Kang SH, Kang SG, Stevenson AR, Coughlin G, Kim SH. First report: robotic pelvic exenteration for locally advanced rectal cancer. Color Dis. 2014;16(1):O9–14.

51. Robotic Sigmoid Colectomy with NOSE Jesse M Cheney, cst, csfa October 2016. The Surgical Technologist.

52. A future without jobs? Two views of the changing work force. The New York Times. 9 Mar 2016.

53. Jump up. Thompson, Derek. A World Without Work.

54. Yan (30 July 2011). Foxconn to replace workers with 1 million robots in 3 years. Xinhua News Agency.

55. Judgment day - employment law and robots in the workplace.

56. Focal Points Seminar on review articles in the future of work - Safety and health at work - EU-OSHA.

57. Michio Kaku, Physics of the future: Future of Medicine, How science will shape human destiny and our daily lives by the year 2100.

58. Prepping robots to perform surgery. New York Times. 4 May 2008.

59. Babbage Science and Technology (18 Jan 2012). Surgical robots: the kindness of strangers. The Economist.

60. Salesmen in the surgical suite. New York Times. 25 Mar 2013.

61. Patients scarred after robotic surgery. CNBC. 19 Apr 2013.

62. Lenoir T. In: Thurtle P, editor. Semiotic flesh: information and the human body. Seattle, WA: University of Washington Press; 2002. p. 28–51.

63. Draft standard for intelligent assist devices — Personnel Safety Requirements.

64. ISO/TS 15066:2016 - Robots and robotic devices -- Collaborative robots.

65. Gidaro S, Buscarini M, Ruiz E, Stark M, Labruzzo A. Telelap Alf-X: a novel telesurgical system for the 21st century. Surg Technol Int. 2012;22:20–5.

66. Hamed A, Tang SC, Ren H, Squires A, Payne C, Masamune K, Tang G, Mohammadpour J, Tse ZTH. Advances in haptics, tactile sensing, and manipulation for robot-assisted minimally invasive surgery, non-invasive surgery, and diagnosis. J Robot. 2012;2012:1.

67. Data on file. Intuitive surgical. 2012.

68. Leonard S, Wu KL, Kim Y, Krieger A, Kim PC. Smart tissue anastomosis robot (STAR): a vision-guided robotics system for laparoscopic suturing. IEEE Trans Biomed Eng. 2014;61(4):1305–17.

Part VIII

Current Status of Adjuvant Treatment

The Role of Systemic Chemotherapy in Colorectal Cancer

30

Hiroyuki Uetake, Shinichi Yamauchi, and Kenichi Sugihara

Abstract

In recent decades, treatment for metastatic colorectal cancer (mCRC) has remarkably progressed with the advent of biological agents. Under such circumstances, it becomes a key issue which biological agent is a preferred treatment, especially for first-line treatment of mCRC patients with RAS wild-type tumor. For unresectable diseases, preferred treatment depends on the treatment goal; patients should be treated to seek for maximum shrinkage or treatment duration. If the former, anti-EGFR mab might be a preferred option in terms of depth of response. If the latter, bevacizumab might be preferred in terms of maintenance therapy. For potentially resectable diseases, such as liver-limited diseases, a similar strategy for treatment can be recommended. There are several types of liver metastases (LM). If LM is bulky and unresectable, a tumor shrinkage is needed so that LM can be converted to be resectable. If LM is disseminated and unresectable, a pathological effect is needed to prevent recurrence after liver resection. If the former, anti-EGFR mab might be preferred, and if the latter, bevacizumab might be better, considering the characteristics of biological agents.

Postoperative adjuvant chemotherapy is performed after curative resection for colorectal cancer to prevent recurrence and improve patients' prognosis. Because therapeutic outcomes for colorectal cancer are better in Japan than in other countries, adjuvant chemotherapy tailored to be optimal for individual patients should be introduced based on not only evidence from overseas but also the results of Japanese clinical trials. Attention is focusing on biomarkers for identifying high-risk patients who require adjuvant chemotherapy.

Keywords

Oxaliplatin · Irinotecan · Biological agent Tumor shrinkage · Maintenance therapy Conversion therapy · Adjuvant chemotherapy Biomarker

H. Uetake (✉) • S. Yamauchi • K. Sugihara
Graduate School, Tokyo Medical and Dental University, Tokyo, Japan
e-mail: h-uetake.srg2@tmd.ac.jp

30.1 Introduction

Great strides have been made in the treatment of cancer due to the development of novel chemotherapeutic agents and multidrug combination therapies as well as advances in supportive

© Springer Nature Singapore Pte Ltd. 2018
N. K. Kim et al. (eds.), *Surgical Treatment of Colorectal Cancer*,
https://doi.org/10.1007/978-981-10-5143-2_30

care, all of which have resulted in better response rates and improvements in survival. To restrict the growth and spread of cancer cells, the targets of traditional anticancer agents include DNA or RNA activity, the multicomponent machineries of cancer cells, and microtubules. The most rapid developments in recent years, however, have been molecular targeted therapies, which are small molecules or antibodies that exert their antitumor effects by targeting specific molecules in cancer cells. This type of therapy may cause less harm to normal cells and have fewer side effects than other types of cancer treatment. Although traditional cytotoxic chemotherapy remains the treatment of choice for many malignancies, targeted therapies are now a component of treatment for many cancer types including breast, colorectal, lung, and pancreatic cancers.

The development of effective anticancer agents has not only prolonged survival in patients but has also made unresectable lesions treatable with surgery ("conversion chemotherapy"), which has been suggested to improve patients' prognosis. Although the therapeutic efficacy of chemotherapy for unresectable advanced or recurrent colorectal cancer is improving, it remains the case that patients can recover with chemotherapy alone. Recurrence occurs at a fixed rate after curative resection of the primary lesion, but postoperative adjuvant chemotherapy has been shown to reduce the recurrence rate. Thus, postoperative adjuvant chemotherapy is an important treatment that reportedly increases the rate of cure after surgery. Combination chemotherapy regimens including oxaliplatin-based therapies, which are effective adjuvant chemotherapies in Europe and the United States, also cause a high incidence of adverse events and should only be used in appropriate patient groups. Studies are now underway on the different uses of oral anticancer agents and indications for adjuvant chemotherapy in patients with stage II cancer, including personalized therapy with a biomarker-based approach.

30.2 Chemotherapy for Unresectable Advanced or Recurrent Colorectal Cancer

30.2.1 Multidrug Combination Therapies

The most well-known multidrug combination regimens are fluorouracil (5-FU)/leucovorin (LV) and oxaliplatin (FOLFOX) and 5-FU/LV plus irinotecan (FOLFIRI). Regimens in which the 5-FU/LV component of the multidrug combination therapy has been replaced by the oral anticancer agents capecitabine or S1 include capecitabine and oxaliplatin (CapOX), capecitabine and irinotecan (CapeIRI), S-1 and oxaliplatin (SOX), and S-1 and irinotecan (IRIS). CapOx has comparable efficacy to FOLFOX4 as first-line therapy [1], and IRIS has comparable efficacy to FOLFIRI as second-line therapy [2]. However, although multidrug combination therapies are highly effective, they are also more likely to cause adverse events. The National Comprehensive Cancer Network (27 centers in the United States) Clinical Practice Guidelines in Oncology [3] states that the first step in treating unresectable colorectal cancer is to determine whether the patient could be a candidate for intensive therapy; if this is not the case, monotherapy with a regimen such as 5-FU/LV is recommended.

30.2.2 Therapeutic Efficacy of Molecular Targeted Drugs

The molecular targeted cancer drugs currently used for the treatment of unresectable recurrent colorectal cancer are bevacizumab, cetuximab, and panitumumab; ramucirumab and regorafenib are also used as second- and third-line therapies, respectively. Bevacizumab is a humanized monoclonal antibody directed against vascular endothelial growth factor and is thus an angiogenesis inhibitor. Its combined use in first-line therapy with irinotecan, leucovorin, plus fluoro-uracil (IFL) [4], FOLFOX, or CapOX [1] has additional therapeutic effects. Cetuximab and panitumumab are antibodies that target the epithelial growth factor receptors (EGFRs), which are found on the cell surface. Cetuximab is a chimeric monoclonal antibody, and panitumumab is a fully human monoclonal antibody. The results of clinical trials have shown that anti-EGFR antibodies are not effective against tumors with the *KRAS* mutation [5] and, as such, are currently only used in patients with wild-type *KRAS* [6]. Cetuximab in combination therapy was initially found to exert therapeutic effects as second-line and subsequent therapies, but its use in first-line therapy was later shown to have additional effects to that of FOLFIRI in the CRYSTAL (Cetuximab Combined With Irinotecan in First-line Therapy for Metastatic Colorectal Cancer) study [7]. Panitumumab was also shown to exert additional effects when used in combination with FOLFOX as first-line therapy [8], with FOLFIRI as second-line therapy [9], and as third-line monotherapy [10].

30.2.3 Different Uses of Molecular Targeted Drugs: Oxaliplatin-Based First-Line Therapies

Compared with combination therapies including bevacizumab, those containing anti-EGFR antibodies are said to be more effective in shrinking tumors, but the difference between their response rates remains unclear [11]. However, combination therapies including anti-EGFR antibodies are superior in terms of depth of response (DpR) [12]. The DpR of combination therapies including anti-EGFR antibodies is 48.9% or 50.9% for FOLFIRI plus cetuximab, 65% for FOLFOX plus panitumumab, and 57.9% for FOLFOX plus cetuximab, compared with 44.4% for FOLFOX plus bevacizumab, 32.3% or 37.8% for FOLFIRI plus bevacizumab, 43.5% for SOX plus bevacizumab, and 43.4% for FOLFOXIRI plus bevacizumab [13–15]. Bevacizumab exerts additional effects when used in combination with 5-FU monotherapy [16]. Because bevacizumab exerts additional effects when used in combination with 5-FU monotherapy, it may also extend the effect of maintenance therapy even after the discontinuation of oxaliplatin in combination therapy. The response rates of combination therapies including bevacizumab and anti-EGFR agents are almost equivalent, and when the therapeutic goal is to reduce tumor size by 30% and then prolong overall survival with maintenance therapy, bevacizumab combination therapy is also indicated for patients with wild-type *KRAS*. For patients in whom the goal is to reduce tumor size by 50% or 60% rather than by only 30%, combination therapy with anti-EGFR antibodies is recommended, as they have superior DpR (Fig. 30.1). The European Society for Medical Oncology consensus guidelines were revised in 2016 [17]. These establish

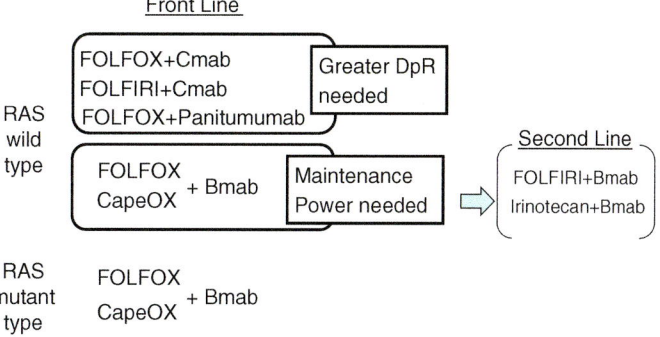

Fig. 30.1 Treatment strategy for advanced colorectal cancer

separate therapeutic goals of cytoreduction and disease control and suggest different regimens for combination therapy including antibodies in patients who are able to undergo intensive chemotherapy. An easy way to view this classification may be to view cytoreduction as prioritizing DpR and disease control as prioritizing maintenance capacity.

30.3 Chemotherapy for Colorectal Cancer Liver Metastasis

In the Japanese Classification of Colorectal Carcinoma, liver metastasis is classified as H1, H2, or 3H depending on its severity, and its grade is further defined in combination with the severity of lymph node and distant metastases [18]. H1 is classified as ≤4 metastatic liver lesions of a maximum diameter ≤5 cm, H2 as all cases other than those classified as H1 or H3, and H3 is classified as ≥5 metastatic liver lesions of a maximum diameter >5 cm.

30.3.1 Post-hepatectomy Adjuvant Chemotherapy

The therapeutic outcomes described above make it clear that chemotherapeutic intervention in some form is required for all H stages of colorectal cancer liver metastasis. Although post-hepatectomy adjuvant chemotherapy is effective, clinical trials of hepatic artery infusion (with the aim of suppressing residual liver recurrence, which is the most common outcome after hepatectomy) and regimens such as 5-FU/LV have not led to any significant differences in survival, suggesting that this therapy may be insufficiently intensive. It is also possible that microscopic liver metastases cannot be controlled at the 5-FU/LV level or that the dose intensity of chemotherapy may not be maintained after hepatectomy. The JCOG0603 Study of 12 cycles of mFOLFOX6 as post-hepatectomy adjuvant chemotherapy is currently underway in Japan to investigate the value of adjuvant chemotherapy with a multidrug regimen.

30.3.2 Perioperative Chemotherapy

Because postoperative adjuvant chemotherapy in the resection of colorectal cancer liver metastases has not been shown to be of value, the use of perioperative or pre- and postoperative chemotherapy to control microscopic metastases is regarded as crucial. Sorbye et al. [19] reported that six preoperative and six postoperative cycles of FOLFOX4 therapy for patients with resectable colorectal cancer liver metastases prolonged survival compared with surgical treatment alone. Preoperative chemotherapy with an intensive regimen such as FOLFOX is highly effective in shrinking tumors, and when regimens with a high incidence of adverse events are used, it may be possible to maintain adequate dose intensity by dividing their administration between the preoperative (when liver function is well maintained) and postoperative periods. Given that the main aim of preoperative chemotherapy in resectable cases is to prolong survival or achieve a cure by means of the combination of chemotherapy and surgery, it may be possible to suppress recurrence by maintaining adequate dose intensity with regimens similar to Sorbye's perioperative chemotherapy (Fig. 30.2) [20, 21]. Identifying the best agents and dosing methods to achieve this goal is a matter for further investigation. Conversion therapy, in which unresectable colorectal cancer liver metastases are treated with chemotherapy and shrunk to the point at which surgery can be performed, has been the subject of recent attention. Adam et al. [22] found that a 5-year survival of 33% was achieved by the resection of hepatic metastases that had become resectable after chemotherapy, compared to the 5% 5-year survival rate for patients who did not undergo resection. Based on these data, the standard treatment is currently to

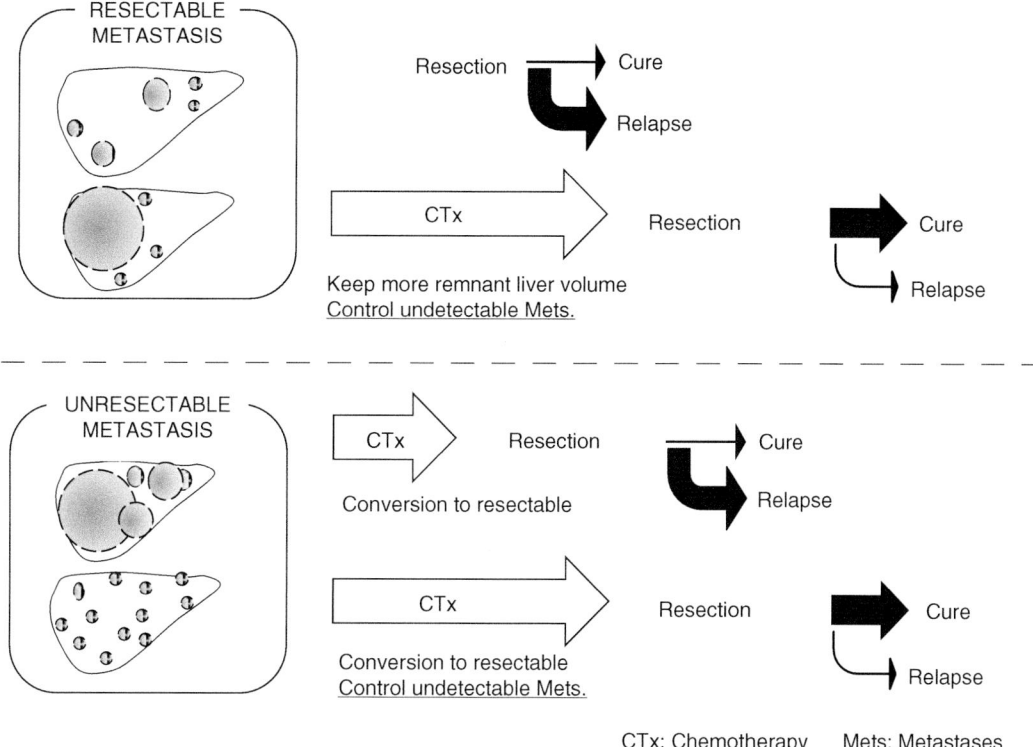

Fig. 30.2 Aim of preoperative chemotherapy for liver-limited metastasis. *CTx* chemotherapy, *Mets* metastases

perform hepatectomy in patients with unresectable colorectal cancer liver metastases that have become resectable as a result of chemotherapy, rather than aiming for conversion.

30.3.3 Cetuximab Combination Therapy

The CELIM Study was a phase II randomized trial of the response to cetuximab plus FOLFOX6 or cetuximab plus FOLFIRI and the resection rate of hepatic lesions after treatment of 111 colorectal cancer patients with unresectable liver metastases [23]. The response rates were 68% for the FOLFOX6 arm and 57% for the FOLFIRI arm, and good conversion rates were achieved, with R0 resection performed in 38% of patients in the FOLFOX6 arm and 30% of those in the FOLFIRI arm.

30.3.4 Bevacizumab Combination Therapy

Wong et al. [24] reported that a 40% (12/30) conversion rate was achieved with the use of capecitabine, oxaliplatin, and bevacizumab combination therapy. The authors reported the results of a multicenter joint phase II clinical trial (TRICC-0808) of preoperative therapy with bevacizumab plus mFOLFOX6 for patients with stage H2 or H3 colorectal cancer liver metastases [25]. The efficacy analysis was done in 45 patients, in whom 26 had unresectable cancer. The response rate to chemotherapy was 46.2%, and the disease control rate was 92.4%. Six patients underwent hepatectomy after six cycles of preoperative chemotherapy (23.1% conversion rate during the protocol treatment). Five patients underwent hepatectomy after the protocol treatment, including three who underwent

Fig. 30.3 Number of liver metastases detected before chemotherapy, after chemotherapy, and intraoperatively. *CTx* chemotherapy

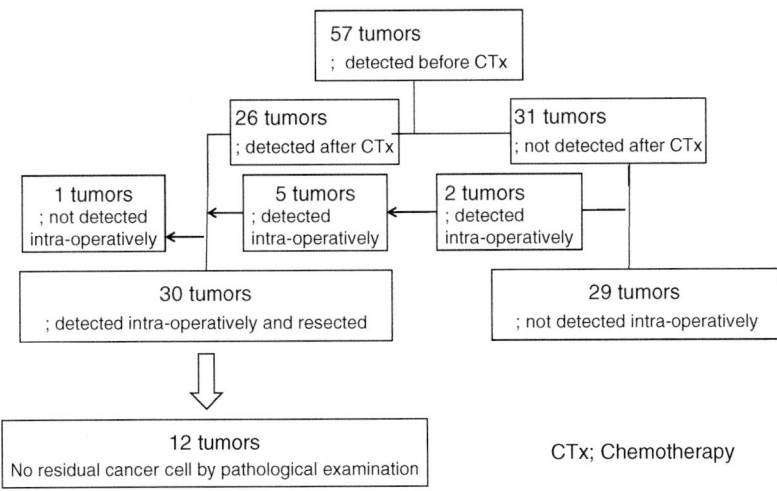

CTx; Chemotherapy

hepatectomy after continued treatment with bevacizumab plus mFOLFOX6, resulting in a total conversion rate after bevacizumab plus mFOLFOX6 therapy of 34.6% (9/26). Figure 30.3 shows the therapeutic outcomes of preoperative bevacizumab plus mFOLFOX6 therapy for patients in our department with colorectal cancer liver metastases [21, 26]. Bevacizumab plus mFOLFOX6 therapy was used to treat 45 patients with H2 or H3 liver metastases, and the response rate was 71%; 12 of these patients had a single liver metastasis, of whom 11 responded to treatment (92% response rate) and 4 subsequently underwent hepatectomy (33% conversion rate). Together with another four patients with resectable liver metastases who also underwent preoperative chemotherapy, hepatectomy was performed in eight patients. A total of 57 metastatic lesions were present before chemotherapy (1–14 lesions per patient, median, 7.5 lesions). After chemotherapy, angiographic computed tomography visualized 26 lesions, with an additional 5 lesions visualized by intraoperative contrast-enhanced ultrasonography. Then 30 lesions were excised, excluding 1 lesion that was not discovered intraoperatively; pathological tests did not identify cancer cells in 12 of the resected 30 lesions (40%).

Combination therapy including bevacizumab has strong pathological antitumor effects on liver metastatic lesions, and the pathological response rate is positively correlated with survival [27–30]. The resection of liver metastatic lesions as a result of conversion chemotherapy improves prognosis for patients with unresectable colorectal cancer liver metastases and is thus a promising treatment strategy. As described above, studies suggest that a good conversion rate may be achieved by using molecular targeted therapeutic drugs and by keeping in mind the possibility of post-chemotherapy resection when assessing patients. Because achieving a cure and prolonging survival are the important goals of conversion therapy, it may be necessary to take into consideration the results of recurrence and survival from clinical trials when determining the appropriate regimens for conversion therapy. Chemotherapy can be expected to not only shrink tumors but also to control micrometastases. It will be important for future clinical trials to take into account the different types of liver metastases when deciding how to use antibodies with the aim of prolonging survival, for example, by treating large nodular metastases with anti-EGFR antibodies, which are superior in their ability to shrink tumors [6], and by treating tiny scattered nodules with bevacizumab.

30.4 Adjuvant Chemotherapy for Colorectal Cancer

The prognosis for resectable colorectal cancer is improved, and radical resection appropriate to the stage of colorectal cancer offers a high cure rate. Once an unresectable recurrence develops, however, cure is difficult to achieve even if several different treatment modalities are used, including chemotherapy. The goal of postoperative adjuvant chemotherapy is to prevent recurrence after radical surgery and improve prognosis, and the drugs and regimens used in actual treatment are those that have been shown to decrease the recurrence rate, have a positive effect on survival, and have been confirmed as safe in randomized, controlled trials (RCTs) [31].

30.4.1 The Transformation of Postoperative Adjuvant Chemotherapy and Its Current Status

30.4.1.1 Recommended Treatments in Europe and North America (Table 30.1)

Several clinical trials of postoperative adjuvant chemotherapy for colon cancer were carried out in Europe and North America during the 1980s and 1990s, and these demonstrated the value of adjuvant chemotherapy with 5-FU over surgery alone [32–35]. In the 1990s, after the additional effect of levofolinate (LV) and the superiority of 5-FU/LV compared with 5-FU/levamisole (LEV) had also been established, 5-FU/LV became established as the standard treatment [36]. Further clinical trials of the form of administration of fluoropyrimidines led to the currently recommended method of administration of 5-FU/LV, and the oral agents tegafur-uracil (UFT)/LV and capecitabine were also shown to be effective [37, 38]. Moving into the 2000s, multiple drug therapies were found to be effective, and the efficacy of adjuvant chemotherapy with oxaliplatin was demonstrated in the National Surgical Adjuvant Breast and Bowel Project (NSABP) C-07 and the Multicenter International Study of Oxaliplatin/5-Fluorouracil/Leucovorin in the Adjuvant Treatment of Colon Cancer (MOSAIC) trials, both of which addressed stage II and III colorectal cancer [39, 40]. The capecitabine plus oxaliplatin (XELOXA) trial also showed that capecitabine plus oxaliplatin (CapeOX) is effective for stage III patients [41]. However, the Cancer and Leukemia Group B (CALGB) 89803

and Pan-European Trials in Adjuvant Colon Cancer (PETACC)-3 trials, which verified the additional effect of irinotecan, did not show that adjuvant chemotherapy was valuable [42, 43].

After the combined use of molecular targeted drugs in systemic chemotherapy was shown to be valuable in the treatment of unresectable advanced or recurrent colorectal cancer, the NSABP C-08, AVANT (bevacizumab plus oxaliplatin-based chemotherapy as adjuvant treatment for colon cancer) and North Central Cancer Treatment Group (NCCTG) intergroup N0147 clinical trials were performed in the expectation that these drugs would also provide an additional effect in adjuvant chemotherapy, but neither bevacizumab nor cetuximab was found to be effective as part of adjuvant chemotherapy [44–46].

The United States National Comprehensive Cancer Network (NCCN) guidelines (version 1, 2017) state that the recommended postoperative adjuvant chemotherapy regimens for stage III colon cancer are (1) FOLFOX (oxaliplatin and an infusional regimen of 5-FU/LV) or CapeOX, (2) FLOX (oxaliplatin and a weekly Roswell Park regimen of bolus 5-FU/LV), and (3) capecitabine or 5-FU/LV. For stage II colon cancer, for patients with a low risk of recurrence, the recommended treatments are (1) observation and (2) capecitabine or 5-FU, and for those at high risk of recurrence, the recommended treatments are (1) capecitabine or 5-FU/LV; (2) FOLFOX, CapeOX, or FLOX; and (3) observation [3] (Fig. 30.4). Moreover, they state that "a survival benefit has not been demonstrated for addition of oxaliplatin to 5-FU/leucovorin in stage II colon cancer. FOLFOX is reasonable for stage II patients with multiple high-risk factors and is not good- or average-risk patients with stage II colon cancer." They also say that "A benefit for the addition of oxaliplatin to 5-FU/leucovorin in older has not been proven."

The NCCN guidelines also set out recommended regimens for adjuvant chemotherapy for rectal cancer in accordance with clinical staging in the same way as for colon cancer, but in Europe and North America, the use of preoperative adjuvant therapy that includes radiotherapy is common, and since this proportion differs from that in Japanese clinical practice, treatment should be

Table 30.1 Major overseas clinical trials

	Name of trial	Year of publication	Test group vs. control group	Stage	Number of patients	DFS		p value	OS		p value
Value of 5-FU, etc.	Intergroup-0035 [2]	1990	5-FU/LV vs. surgery only	III	304	63%	3.5 year	0.0064	71%	3.5 year	0.0064
					315	47%			55%		
	Francini et al. [3]	1994	5-FU/LV vs. surgery only	II/III	116	74%	5 year	0.0044	79%	5 year	0.0044
					118	59%			65%		
	IMPACT [4]	1995	5-FU/LV vs. surgery only	II/III	736	71%	3.5 year	<0.0001	83%	3 year	0.029
					757	62%			78%		
	NCCTG [5]	1997	5-FU/LV vs. surgery only	II/III	158	74%	5 year	<0.01	74%	5 year	0.02
					151	58%			63%		
	NSABP C-04 [6]	1999	5-FU/LV vs. 5-FU/LEV vs. 5-FU/LV/LEV	II/III	691	65%	5 year	0.04	74%	5 year	0.07
					696	60%		0.13	70%		0.11
					691	64%			73%		
Comparison with oral fluoropyrimidines	NSABP C-06 [7]	2006	UFT/LV vs. 5-FU/LV	II/III	805	67%	5 year	0.96	78.5%	5 year	0.45
					803	68.2%			78.7%		
	X-ACT [8]	2005	Capecitabine vs. 5-FU/LV	III	1004	60.8%	5 year	<0.0001	71.4%	5 year	<0.0001
					983	56.7%			68.4%		
Combination therapy with oxaliplatin	NSABP C-07 [9]	2007	FLOX vs. 5-FU/LV	II/III	1209	69.4%	5 year	0.002	77.7%	6 year	0.06
					1200	64.2%			73.5%		
	MOSAIC [10]	2009	FOLFOX4 vs. 5-FU/LV	II/III	1123	73.3%	5 year	0.003	78.5%	6 year	0.046
					1123	67.4%			76.0%		
	XELOXA [11]	2015	XELOX vs. 5-FU/LV	III	944	63%	7 year	0.004	73%	7 year	0.04
					942	56%			67%		

Category	Trial	Year	Regimen	Stage	n	%		p	%		p
Combination therapy with irinotecan	CALGB 89803 [12]	2007	IFL vs. 5-FU/LV	III	635	61.1%	5 year	0.84	68%	5 year	0.74
					629	59%			71%		
	PETACC-3 [13]	2009	FOLFIRI vs. 5-FU/LV	II/III	1050	56.7%	5 year	0.106	73.6%	5 year	0.094
					1044	54.3%			71.3%		
Combination therapy with molecular targeted drugs	NSABP C-08 [14]	2013	mFOLFOX6 +bevacizumab vs. mFOLFOX6	II/III	1334	77.9%	3 year	0.35	82.5%	5 year	0.56
					1338	75.1%			80.7%		
	AVANT [15]	2012	FOLFOX4 vs. FOLFOX4 +bevacizumab vs. XELOX +bevacizumab	High risk II/ III	955	76%	3 year	*	85%	5 year	+
					960	73%		**	81%		++
					952	75%			82%		
	NCCTG intergroup N0147 [16]	2012	mFOLFOX6 +cetuximab vs. mFOLFOX6	III (Data on the right are wild-type *KRAS*)	954	71.5%	3 year	0.08	85.6%	3 year	0.15
					909	74.6%			87.3%		

*p = 0.07, **p = 0.44, +p = 0.02, ++p = 0.21

Fig. 30.4 Comparison of recommended treatments according to Japanese and US guidelines

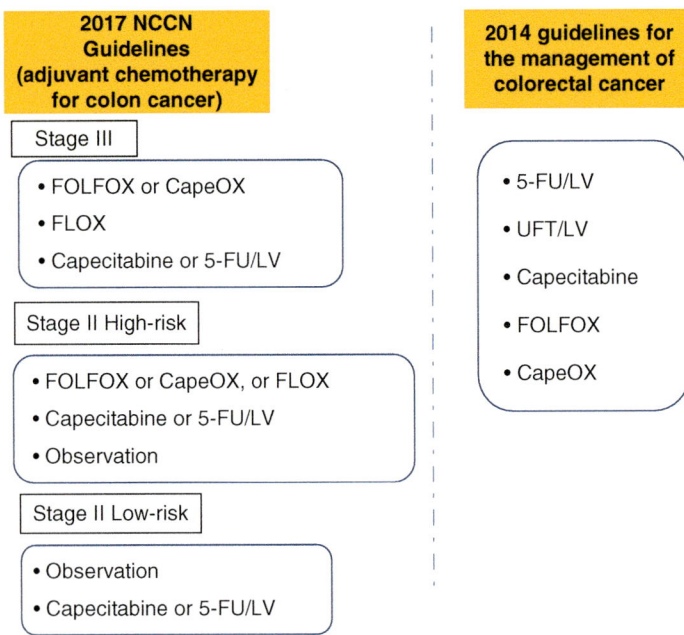

2017 NCCN Guidelines (adjuvant chemotherapy for colon cancer)

Stage III

- FOLFOX or CapeOX
- FLOX
- Capecitabine or 5-FU/LV

Stage II High-risk

- FOLFOX or CapeOX, or FLOX
- Capecitabine or 5-FU/LV
- Observation

Stage II Low-risk

- Observation
- Capecitabine or 5-FU/LV

2014 guidelines for the management of colorectal cancer

- 5-FU/LV
- UFT/LV
- Capecitabine
- FOLFOX
- CapeOX

determined on the basis of the results of Japanese RCTs, while making reference to evidence from Europe and North America.

30.4.1.2 Indications for Adjuvant Chemotherapy and Recommended Treatments in Japan (Table 30.2)

According to the guidelines for the management of colorectal cancer, the indications for postoperative adjuvant chemotherapy comprise (1) stage III colorectal cancer that has undergone R0 resection, (2) preservation of major organ function, (3) performance status (PS) 0–1, (4) recovery from postoperative complications, (5) consent appropriately obtained, and (6) no serious complications [31]. Turning to evidence from Japan, meta-analyses have shown that postoperative adjuvant chemotherapy with an oral 5-FU-based regimen for stage III colorectal cancer patients significantly reduces recurrence and mortality rates compared with surgery alone [47, 48]. In the NSASCC trial, oral UFT monotherapy was shown to be of use as adjuvant chemotherapy for stage III rectal cancer [49]. In the JCOG0205 trial, which compared bolus 5-F/LV and oral UFT/LV, the oral regimen was found to be

noninferior in terms of 3-year disease-free survival (DFS), the primary endpoint [50]. That trial differed from the NSABP C-06 trial in that it addressed adjuvant therapy for Japanese patients who had undergone surgery in a Japanese institution, and all subjects were stage III. In the NSABP C-06 trial, although bolus administration and oral administration of 5-FU were equally effective in preventing recurrence, 5-year overall survival (OS) was 69.6% in the NSABP C-06 trial, but far higher, at 87.5%, in the JCOG0205 trial. This survival rate exceeds the survival rate for stage III patients treated with adjuvant chemotherapy including oxaliplatin in Europe and North America [39–41]. In light of this evidence, the guidelines for the management of colorectal cancer list (1) 5-FU/LV, (2) UFT/LV, (3) capecitabine, (4) FOLFOX, and (5) CapeOX as the standard treatments for postoperative adjuvant chemotherapy in Japan [31] (Fig. 30.2).

The ACTS-CC and JCOG0910 trials have been performed in Japan as comparative trials of oral anticancer agents for stage III colon cancer (including rectosigmoid (RS) cancer) [51, 52]. The ACTS-RC trial also addressed rectal cancer [23]. The ACTS-CC trial demonstrated the non-inferiority of S-1 compared with UFT/LV as

Table 30.2 Major clinical trials in Japan

Name of trial	Year of publication	Test group vs. control group	Stage	Number of patients	DFS		p value	OS		p value
NSASCC [20]	2006	UFT vs. surgery only	III (rectal cancer)	139	78%	3 year	0.0014	91%	3 year	0.0048
				135	60%			81%		
JCOG0205 [21]	2014	UFT/LV vs. 5-FU/LV	III (excluding Rb)	546	77.8%	3 year	0.0236 (noninferiority)	87.5%	5 year	–
				546	79.3%			88.4%		
ACTS-CC [22]	2014	S-1 vs. UFT/LV	III (including RS)	758	75.5%	3 year	<0.0001 (noninferiority)	93.6%	3 year	0.36
				760	72.5%			92.7%		
JCOG0910 (CAPS) [23]	2015	S-1 vs. capecitabine	III (excluding Rb)	782	77.9%	3 year	0.46 (noninferiority)	–	–	–
				782	82%			–		
ACTS-RC [24]	2016	S-1 vs. UFT	II/III (rectal cancer)	479	66.4%	5 year	0.016	82%	5 year	0.54
				480	61.7%			80.2%		
ACT-CC02 [25]	In progress	SOX vs. UFT/LV	IIIb (excluding Rb)	966 patients enrolled	–		–	–		–
ACURA [27]	2016	UFT vs. surgery only	II	985	80.2%	5 year	0.31	94.5%	5 year	0.69
				997	78.4%			94.3%		
JCOG0603 [28]	In progress	mFOLFOX6 vs. surgery only	After curative liver metastasis resection	300 patients enrollment planned	–		–	–		–

adjuvant chemotherapy for stage III colon cancer (including RS cancer) (hazard ratio (HR) 0.85, $p = 0.1003$). However, the JCOG0910 trial failed to demonstrate the noninferiority of S-1 compared with capecitabine. The ACTS-RC trial was an RCT that demonstrated the superiority of S-1 compared with UFT monotherapy as adjuvant chemotherapy for stage II/III rectal cancer and showed that recurrence-free survival (RFS) was superior for S-1 compared with UFT (HR 0.77, $p = 0.0165$) [53]. The results are still awaited of the ACTS-CC02 trial, which has completed patient enrollment as an RCT to verify the superiority of SOX therapy compared with UFT/LV as adjuvant chemotherapy for stage IIIb colorectal cancer (excluding Rb rectal cancer) [54].

30.4.2 Postoperative Adjuvant Chemotherapy for Stage II Colorectal Cancer

Although 5-year survival for stage II colorectal cancer is comparatively good at 84%, recurrence occurs in approximately 13% of patients. According to the guidelines for the management of colorectal cancer, "The value of postoperative adjuvant chemotherapy for stage II colorectal cancer has yet to be established, and it is not recommended that adjuvant chemotherapy be performed uniformly for all stage II colorectal cancers." However, they also state that "The strategy of targeting the subgroup of stage II cancers with poor prognosis to receive adjuvant chemotherapy can at this point be regarded as a reasonable choice," and demonstrating the necessity of adjuvant chemotherapy for patients at high risk of recurrence is an urgent task. The clinicopathological high-risk factors mentioned in the NCCN and European Society for Medical Oncology (ESMO) guidelines include stage T4, perforation, intestinal obstruction, vascular invasion, poorly differentiated adenocarcinoma, undifferentiated carcinoma, and fewer than 12 lymph nodes dissected. Microsatellite instability and loss of heterozygosity at chromosome18q have been reported to constitute molecular biological biomarkers of high-risk groups, but opinions on these are not uniform. In Japan, the SACURA trial, an RCT comparing no postoperative treatment with postoperative adjuvant chemotherapy with UFT (for 1 year) for stage II colorectal cancer patients, enrolled 2024 patients in 270 facilities [55]. The results did not show the superiority of UFT (HR 0.91, $p = 0.31$), and since this trial included an additional pathological and molecular biomarker study to investigate prognostic factors and factors predicting response to UFT by means of tests such as genetic screening of resected specimens, its results are attracting attention.

30.4.3 Adjuvant Chemotherapy After Distant Metastatic Resection (Curative B Resection)

Surgical resection is the standard treatment for resectable distant metastases in the liver, lungs, or elsewhere, but the post-resection recurrence rate is high, at 50–70%. Some form of chemotherapy after metastatic resection is therefore required, but the current guidelines on the management of colorectal cancer state that, since the safety and efficacy of postoperative adjuvant chemotherapy after resection have yet to be established, it should preferably be undertaken as part of a clinical trial. The JCOG0603 trial of 12 cycles of mFOLFOX6 therapy as adjuvant chemotherapy after hepatectomy is currently underway in Japan, investigating the value of adjuvant chemotherapy with combination therapy including oxaliplatin [56].

30.4.4 Postoperative Adjuvant Chemotherapy for Elderly Patients with Colorectal Cancer

Subgroup analyses in overseas RCTs have focused on the efficacy of adjuvant chemotherapy for elderly colorectal cancer patients [57]. Among these analyses, the results of a subgroup analysis in the MOSAIC trial [40] showed that FOLFOX4 therapy did not provide any additional effect compared to 5-FU/LV therapy for stage II colorectal cancer patients aged 70–75 years.

References

1. Cassidy J, Clarke S, Díaz-Rubio E, Scheithauer W, Figer A, Wong R, et al. XELOX vs FOLFOX-4 as first-line therapy for metastatic colorectal cancer: NO16966 updated results. Br J Cancer. 2011;105:58–64. https://doi.org/10.1038/bjc.2011.201.
2. Muro K, Boku N, Shimada Y, Tsuji A, Sameshima S, Baba H, et al. Irinotecan plus S-1 (IRIS) versus fluorouracil and folinic acid plus irinotecan (FOLFIRI) as second-line chemotherapy for metastatic colorectal cancer: a randomised phase 2/3 non-inferiority study (FIRIS study). Lancet Oncol. 2010;11:853–60. https://doi.org/10.1016/S1470-2045(10)70181-9.
3. NCCN web site. http://www.nccn.org/. Accessed 30 Jan 2017.
4. Hurwitz H, Fehrenbacher L, Novotny W, Cartwright T, Hainsworth J, Heim W, et al. Bevacizumab plus irinotecan, fluorouracil, and leucovorin for metastatic colorectal cancer. N Engl J Med. 2004;350:2335–42.
5. Karapetis CS, Khambata-Ford S, Jonker DJ, O'Callaghan CJ, Tu D, Tebbutt NC, et al. K-ras mutations and benefit from cetuximab in advanced colorectal cancer. N Engl J Med. 2008;359:1757–65. https://doi.org/10.1056/NEJMoa0804385.
6. Douillard JY, Siena S, Peeters M, Koukakis R, Terwey JH, Tabernero J. Impact of early tumour shrinkage and resection on outcomes in patients with wild-type RAS metastatic colorectal cancer. Eur J Cancer. 2015;51:1231–42. https://doi.org/10.1016/j.ejca.2015.03.026.
7. Van Cutsem E, Köhne CH, Hitre E, Zaluski J, Chang Chien CR, Makhson A, et al. Cetuximab and chemotherapy as initial treatment for metastatic colorectal cancer. N Engl J Med. 2009;360:1408–17. https://doi.org/10.1056/NEJMoa0805019.
8. Douillard JY, Siena S, Cassidy J, Tabernero J, Burkes R, Barugel M, et al. Randomized, phase III trial of panitumumab with infusional fluorouracil, leucovorin, and oxaliplatin (FOLFOX4) versus FOLFOX4 alone as first-line treatment in patients with previously untreated metastatic colorectal cancer: PRIME study. J Clin Oncol. 2010;28:4697–705. https://doi.org/10.1200/JCO.2009.27.4860.
9. Peeters M, Price TJ, Cervantes A, Sobrero AF, Ducreux M, Hotko Y, André T, et al. Randomized, phase III trial of panitumumab with infusional fluorouracil, leucovorin, and irinotecan (FOLFIRI) compared with FOLFIRI alone as second-line treatment in patients with metastatic colorectal cancer. J Clin Oncol. 2010;28:4706–13. https://doi.org/10.1200/JCO.2009.27.6055.
10. Van Cutsem E, Peeters M, Siena S, Humblet Y, Hendlisz A, Neyns B, et al. Open-label phase III trial of panitumumab plus best supportive care compared with best supportive care alone with chemotherapy-refractory metastatic colorectal cancer. J Clin Oncol. 2007;25:1658–64.
11. Heinemann V, Rivera F, O'Neil BH, Stintzing S, Koukakis R, Terwey JH, et al. A study-level meta-analysis of efficacy data from head-to-head first-line trials of epidermal growth factor receptor inhibitors versus bevacizumab in patients with RAS wild-type metastatic colorectal cancer. Eur J Cancer. 2016;67:11–20. https://doi.org/10.1016/j.ejca.2016.07.019.
12. Mansmann UR, Laubender RP. Methodologic diligence is needed to define and validate tumor-size response metrics to predict overall survival in first-line metastatic colorectal cancer. J Clin Oncol. 2013;31:4373–4. https://doi.org/10.1200/JCO.2013.51.2954.
13. Nakamura M, Yamada Y, Takahari D, Matsumoto H, Baba H, Yoshida K, et al. Updated results of the SOFT study: a randomized phase III trial of S-1/oxaliplatin (SOX) plus bevacizumab versus 5-FU/l-LV/oxaliplatin (mFOLFOX6) plus bevacizumab in patients with metastatic colorectal cancer (mCRC). J Clin Oncol. 2014; 32:5s (Suppl): abstr 3586.
14. Stintzing S, Modest DP, Fischer von Weikersthal L, Decker T, Kiani A, et al. Independent radiological evaluation of objective response, early tumor shrinkage, and depth of response in FIRE-3 (AIO KRK-0306) in the final as evaluable population. Ann Oncol. 2014;25:v1–v41. https://doi.org/10.1093/annonc/mdu438.9.
15. Cremolini C, Loupakis F, Lonardi S, Trenta P, Antoniotti C, Masi G, et al. Early tumor shrinkage (ETS) and deepness of response (DoR) to predict progression-free, postprogression, and overall survival: results from the phase III TRIBE trial. J Clin Oncol. 2014;32(Suppl 3):abstr 521.
16. Tebbutt NC, et al. Capecitabine, bevacizumab, and mitomycin in first-line treatment of metastatic colorectal cancer: results of the Australasian Gastrointestinal Trials Group Randomized Phase III MAX Study. J Clin Oncol. 2010;28:3191–8. https://doi.org/10.1200/JCO.2009.27.7723.
17. Van Cutsem E, Cervantes A, Adam R, Sobrero A, Van Krieken JH, Aderka D, et al. ESMO consensus guidelines for the management of patients with metastatic colorectal cancer. Ann Oncol. 2016;27:1386–422. https://doi.org/10.1093/annonc/mdw235.
18. Japanese classification of colorectal carcinoma. Kanehara, Tokyo. 2009.
19. Sorbye H, Mauer M, Gruenberger T, Glimelius B, Poston GJ, Schlag PM, et al. Perioperative chemotherapy with FOLFOX4 and surgery versus surgery alone for resectable liver metastases from colorectal cancer (EORTC Intergroup trial 40983): a randomised controlled trial. Lancet. 2008;371:1007–16. https://doi.org/10.1016/S0140-6736(08)60455-9.
20. Sugihara K, Uetake H. Therapeutic strategies for hepatic metastasis of colorectal cancer; 2011 update. J Hepatobiliary Pancreat Sci. 2012;19:523–7. https://doi.org/10.1007/s00534-012-0524-8.
21. Uetake H, Tanaka S, Ishikawa T, Sugihara K, Arii S. Fate of metastatic foci after chemotherapy and

usefulness of contrast-enhanced intraoperative ultrasonography to detect minute hepatic lesions. J Hepatobiliary Pancreat Sci. 2012;19:509–14. https://doi.org/10.1007/s00534-012-0510-1.

22. Adam R, Delvart V, Pascal G, Valeanu A, Castaing D, Azoulay D, et al. Rescue surgery for unresectable colorectal liver metastases downstaged by chemotherapy: a model to predict long-term survival. Ann Surg. 2004;240:644–57.

23. Folprecht G, Gruenberger T, MD Bechstein WO, Raab HR, Lordick F, Hartmann JT, Lang H, Frilling A, Stoehlmacher J, Weitz J, Konopke R, Stroszczynski C, Liersch T, Ockert D, Herrmann T, Goekkurt E, Parisi F, Köhne CH. Tumour response and secondary resectability of colorectal liver metastases following neoadjuvant chemotherapy with cetuximab: the CELIM randomised phase 2 trial. Lancet Oncol. 2010;11:38–47. https://doi.org/10.1016/S1470-2045(09)70330-4.

24. Wong R, Cunningham D, Barbachano Y, Saffery C, Valle J, Hickish T, et al. A multicentre study of capecitabine, oxaliplatin plus bevacizumab as perioperative treatment of patients with poor-risk colorectal liver-only metastases not selected for upfront resection. Ann Oncol. 2011;22:2042–8. https://doi.org/10.1093/annonc/mdq714.

25. Uetake H, Yasuno M, Ishiguro M, Kameoka S, Shimada Y, Takahashi K, et al. A multicenter phase II trial of mFOLFOX6 plus bevacizumab to treat liver-only metastases of colorectal cancer that are unsuitable for upfront resection (TRICC0808). Ann Surg Oncol. 2015;22:908–15. https://doi.org/10.1245/s10434-014-4094-7.

26. Uetake H. High pathological CR rate and low recurrence rate was observed in liver metastasis of colorectal cancer after preoperative bevacizumab plus FOLFOX therapy. Cancer Res. 2011;71(8 Supplement):3218.

27. Klinger M, Tamandl D, Eipeldauer S, Hacker S, Herberger B, Kaczirek K, et al. Bevacizumab improves pathological response of colorectal cancer liver metastases treated with XELOX/FOLFOX. Ann Surg Oncol. 2010;17:2059–65. https://doi.org/10.1245/s10434-010-0972-9.

28. Ribero D, Wang H, Donadon M, Zorzi D, Thomas MB, Eng C, et al. Bevacizumab improves pathologic response and protects against hepatic injury in patients treated with oxaliplatin-based chemotherapy for colorectal liver metastases. Cancer. 2007;110:2761–7.

29. Blazer DG 3rd, Kishi Y, Maru DM, Kopetz S, Chun YS, Overman MJ, et al. Pathologic response to preoperative chemotherapy: a new outcome end point after resection of hepatic colorectal metastases. J Clin Oncol. 2008;26:5344–51. https://doi.org/10.1200/JCO.2008.17.5299.

30. Duffy A, Shia J, Huitzil-Melendez FD, Fong Y, O'Reilly EM. Pathologic complete response to neoadjuvant FOLFOX in combination with bevacizumab in unresectable metastatic colorectal carcinoma. Clin Colorectal Cancer. 2008;7:140–3. https://doi.org/10.3816/CCC.2008.n.019.

31. JSCCR. Guidelines 2016 for the treatment of colorectal cancer.

32. Moertel CG, Fleming TR, Macdonald JS, Haller DG, Laurie JA, Goodman PJ, et al. Levamisole and fluorouracil for adjuvant therapy of resected colon carcinoma. N Engl J Med. 1990;322:352–8.

33. Francini G, Petrioli R, Lorenzini L, Mancini S, Armenio S, Tanzini G, et al. Folinic acid and 5-fluorouracil as adjuvant chemotherapy in colon cancer. Gastroenterology. 1994;106:899–906.

34. Efficacy of adjuvant fluorouracil and folinic acid in colon cancer. International Multicentre Pooled Analysis of Colon Cancer Trials (IMPACT) investigators. Lancet. 1995;345:939–44.

35. O'Connell MJ, Mailliard JA, Kahn MJ, Macdonald JS, Haller DG, Mayer RJ, et al. Controlled trial of fluorouracil and low-dose leucovorin given for 6 months as postoperative adjuvant therapy for colon cancer. J Clin Oncol. 1997;15:246–50.

36. Wolmark N, Rockette H, Mamounas E, Jones J, Wieand S, Wickerham DL, et al. Clinical trial to assess the relative efficacy of fluorouracil and leucovorin, fluorouracil and levamisole, and fluorouracil, leucovorin, and levamisole in patients with Dukes' B and C carcinoma of the colon: results from National Surgical Adjuvant Breast and Bowel Project C-04. J Clin Oncol. 1999;17:3553–9.

37. Lembersky BC, Wieand HS, Petrelli NJ, O'Connell MJ, Colangelo LH, Smith RE, et al. Oral uracil and tegafur plus leucovorin compared with intravenous fluorouracil and leucovorin in stage II and III carcinoma of the colon: results from National Surgical Adjuvant Breast and Bowel Project Protocol C-06. J Clin Oncol. 2006;24:2059–64.

38. Twelves C, Wong A, Nowacki MP, Abt M, Burris H 3rd, Carrato A, et al. Capecitabine as adjuvant treatment for stage III colon cancer. N Engl J Med. 2005;352:2696–704.

39. Kuebler JP, Wieand HS, O'Connell MJ, Smith RE, Colangelo LH, Yothers G, Petrelli NJ, Findlay MP, Seay TE, Atkins JN, Zapas JL, Goodwin JW, Fehrenbacher L, Ramanathan RK, Conley BA, Flynn PJ, Soori G, Colman LK, Levine EA, Lanier KS, Wolmark N. Oxaliplatin combined with weekly bolus fluorouracil and leucovorin as surgical adjuvant chemotherapy for stage II and III colon cancer: results from NSABP C-07. J Clin Oncol. 2007;25:2198–204.

40. André T, Boni C, Navarro M, Tabernero J, Hickish T, Topham C, et al. Improved overall survival with oxaliplatin, fluorouracil, and leucovorin as adjuvant treatment in stage II or III colon cancer in the MOSAIC trial. J Clin Oncol. 2009;27:3109–16.

41. Schmoll HJ, Tabernero J, Maroun J, de Braud F, Price T, Van Cutsem E, et al. Capecitabine plus oxaliplatin compared with fluorouracil/folinic acid as adjuvant therapy for stage III colon cancer: final results of the NO16968 randomized controlled phase III trial. J Clin Oncol. 2015;33:3733–40.

42. Saltz LB, Niedzwiecki D, Hollis D, Goldberg RM, Hantel A, Thomas JP, et al. Irinotecan fluorouracil

plus leucovorin is not superior to fluorouracil plus leucovorin alone as adjuvant treatment for stage III colon cancer: results of CALGB 89803. J Clin Oncol. 2007;25:3456–61.

43. Van Cutsem E, Labianca R, Bodoky G, Barone C, Aranda E, Nordlinger B, et al. Randomized phase III trial comparing biweekly infusional fluorouracil/leucovorin alone or with irinotecan in the adjuvant treatment of stage III colon cancer: PETACC-3. J Clin Oncol. 2009;27:3117–25.

44. Allegra CJ, Yothers G, O'Connell MJ, Sharif S, Petrelli NJ, Lopa SH, et al. Bevacizumab in stage II-III colon cancer: 5-year update of the National Surgical Adjuvant Breast and Bowel Project C-08 trial. J Clin Oncol. 2013;31:359–64.

45. de Gramont A, Van Custem E, Schmoll HJ, Tabernero J, Clarke S, Moore MJ, et al. Bevacizumab plus oxaliplatin-based chemotherapy as adjuvant treatment for colon cancer (AVANT): a phase 3 randomised controlled trial. Lancet Oncol. 2012;13:1225–33.

46. Alberts SR, Sargent DJ, Nair S, Mahoney MR, Mooney M, Thibodeau SN, et al. Effect of oxaliplatin, fluorouracil, and leucovorin with or without cetuximab on survival among patients with resected stage III colon cancer: a randomized trial. JAMA. 2012;307:1383–93.

47. Sakamoto J, Hamada C, Kodaira S, Nakazato H, Ohashi Y. Adjuvant therapy with oral fluoropyrimidine as main chemotherapeutic agents after curative resection for colorectal cancer. Individual patients data meta-analysis of randomized trial. Jpn J Clin Oncol. 1999;29:78–86.

48. Meta-Analysis Group of the Japanese Society for Cancer of the Colon and Rectum and the Meta-Analysis Group in Cancer. Efficacy of oral adjuvant therapy after resection of colorectal cancer: 5-year result from three randomized trials. J Clin Oncol. 2004;22:484–92.

49. Akasu T, Moriya Y, Ohashi Y, Yoshida S, Shirao K, Kodaira S, National Surgical Adjuvant Study of Colorectal Cancer. Adjuvant chemotherapy with uracil-tegafur for pathological stage III rectal cancer after mesorectal excision with selective lateral pelvic lymphadenectomy: a multicenter randomized controlled trial. Jpn J Clin Oncol. 2006;36:237–44.

50. Shimada Y, Hamaguchi T, Mizusawa J, Saito N, Kanemitsu Y, Takiguchi N, et al. Randomised phase III trial of adjuvant chemotherapy with oral uracil and tegafur plus leucovorin versus intravenous fluorouracil and levofolinate in patients with stage III colorectal cancer who have undergone Japanese D2/D3 lymph node dissection: Final results of JCOG0205. Eur J Cancer. 2014;50:2231–40.

51. Yoshida M, Ishiguro M, Ikejiri K, Mochizuki I, Nakamoto Y, Kinugasa Y, et al. S-1 as adjuvant chemotherapy for stage III colon cancer: a randomized phase III study (ACTS-CC trial). Ann Oncol. 2014;25:1743–9.

52. Hamaguchi T, Shimada Y, Mizusawa J, Kinugasa Y, Kanemitsu Y, Ohue M, et al. Randomized phase III study of adjuvant chemotherapy with S-1 versus capecitabine in patients with stage III colon cancer (CC): results of Japan Clinical Oncology Group study (JCOG0910). ASCO, 2015, abst#3512.

53. Oki E, Murata A, Yoshida K, Maeda K, Ikejiri K, Munemoto Y, Sasaki K, et al. A randomized phase III trial comparing S-1 versus UFT as adjuvant chemotherapy for stage II/III rectal cancer (JFMC35-C1: ACTS-RC). Ann Oncol. 2016;27:1266–72.

54. Takiuchi H, Tomita N, Boku N, Watanabe T, Kotake K, Itabashi M, et al. Preplanned initial safety analysis of ACTS-CC 02 trial: a large randomized phase III trial of SOX versus UFT/LV as adjuvant chemotherapy for high-risk stage III colon cancer. 2012 Gastrointestinal Cancers Symposium, abst#572.

55. Kajiwara Y, Ishiguro M, Teramukai S, Matsuda C, Fujii S, Kinugasa Y, et al. A randomized phase III trial of 1-year adjuvant chemotherapy with oral tegafur-uracil (UFT) vs. surgery alone in stage II colon cancer: SACURA trial. ASCO 2016, abst#3617.

56. Kanemitsu Y, Kato T, Shimizu Y, Inaba Y, Shimada Y, Nakamura K, et al. A randomized phase II/III trial comparing hepatectomy followed by mFOLFOX6 with hepatectomy alone as treatment for liver metastasis from colorectal cancer: Japan Clinical Oncology Group Study JCOG0603. Jpn J Clin Oncol. 2009;39:406–9.

57. Tournigand C, André T, Bonnetain F, Chibaudel B, Lledo G, Hickish T, et al. Adjuvant therapy with fluorouracil and oxaliplatin in stage II and elderly patients (between ages 70 and 75 years) with colon cancer: subgroup analyses of the multicenter international study of oxaliplatin, fluorouracil, and leucovorin in the adjuvant treatment of colon cancer trial. J Clin Oncol. 2012;30:3353–60.

Recent Update on the Role of Radiation Therapy in Colorectal Cancer

Woong Sub Koom

Abstract

In recent decades, the improvements in surgical techniques, imaging modalities, chemotherapy regimens, and radiotherapy have resulted in survival improvement. In the current guideline, preoperative long-course chemoradiotherapy or short-course radiotherapy is the standard treatment for locally advanced rectal cancer. On the other hand, various treatment schemes have been conducted for further improvement of clinical outcomes for patients with stage II or III rectal cancer. Novel clinical trials have concept for more effective systemic treatments, risk-adapted radiotherapy, and the increased awareness of quality of life. The induction chemotherapy followed by preoperative chemoradiotherapy or consolidation chemotherapy after preoperative chemoradiotherapy has been conducted to investigate a reducing systemic metastasis. The omission of radiotherapy has been addressed as a risk-adaptation concept for selected patients with response to neoadjuvant chemotherapy as well as low-risk local recurrence. In terms of quality of life, minimal or omitted surgery following complete response to preoperative chemoradiotherapy has been challenged. Here, the current status for novel multimodal approaches for rectal cancer is discussed.

Keywords

Short-course radiotherapy · Long-course chemoradiotherapy · Risk-adaptive radiotherapy · Total neoadjuvant therapy · Nonoperative management

31.1 Introduction

Currently, either preoperative long-course chemoradiotherapy or short-course radiotherapy is the standard of care for patients with stage II or III rectal cancer. The improved surgical technique and preoperative (chemo)radiotherapy achieved excellent local control less than 5–10%. But this improvement did not translate into improvement in disease-free and overall survival rates. Distant metastases of 30% are still predominant failure patterns. So, same style neoadjuvant approaches in all stage II or III patients have been questioned. Preoperative (chemo)radiotherapy is overtreatment for the patient with low risk of local recurrence after TME alone. On the other hand, advanced strategies are required to improve control of systemic recurrence while maintaining local control rate. Recently, total neoadjuvant

W. S. Koom
Department of Radiation Oncology, Yonsei
University College of Medicine, Seoul, South Korea
e-mail: mdgold@yuhs.ac

© Springer Nature Singapore Pte Ltd. 2018
N. K. Kim et al. (eds.), *Surgical Treatment of Colorectal Cancer*,
https://doi.org/10.1007/978-981-10-5143-2_31

therapy (TNT) approach, which is induction or consolidation chemotherapy before or after chemoradiotherapy, has been conducted increasingly. In terms of quality of life, a "watch-and-wait" nonoperative management (NOM) approach has been pursued to preserve sphincter function in the patients achieving a pathologic complete response to preoperative chemoradiotherapy. First of all, patient selection based on the risk stratification is the most important step to modify multimodal approaches. Further developments for accurate imaging techniques, genetic biomarkers, and clinicopathological features are warranted to select the patients and apply most appropriate treatment approaches.

31.2 Evolution of Preoperative Approaches

31.2.1 Preoperative Radiotherapy

Surgical techniques have evolved significantly for the last decades so that the likelihood of complete cure is increasing. However, sizable portion of patients are at risk of both local recurrence and distant metastasis even after complete surgical resection, and continued efforts to improve initial local control have been accompanied [1–3]. Having colostomy permanently in some patients which deteriorates the patient's quality of life afterward is another major issue. In this context, an erstwhile treatment approach has focused on the ability of surgery to secure plane and adjuvant treatment to control nearby tumor cells, while reducing the use of colostomy, particularly in distal tumors. Above all among various anticancer therapies, a number of data have emerged indicating that radiation therapy is the essential component of the treatment for rectal cancer. The first well-known success story of integrating radiation therapy with surgical resection was in the postoperative clinical setting and then confirmed in the preoperative clinical setting [4–12].

Most of these trials had shown that radiotherapy was successfully utilized to reduce local recurrence rates, but this benefit did translate little into improvements in disease-free survival or overall survival. Firstly, the Swedish Rectal Cancer Trial, which randomly assigned 1168 patients with resectable disease either to short-course preoperative radiotherapy followed by surgery or surgery alone, demonstrated the improved survival in the preoperative radiotherapy arm [13]. Unfortunately, this survival benefit was not replicated in other trials, and considerable rates of RT-related late toxicities were reported in this trial [13, 14]. The Dutch Colorectal Cancer Group trial was organized to reproduce the merit of preoperative short-course radiotherapy, which was clearly shown in the Swedish trial, in the era of the advanced surgical technique (total mesorectal excision (TME)) [15, 16]. The validity of the statement from the Swedish Rectal Cancer Trial was confirmed in the TME era, in terms of local control but not survival aspects.

31.2.1.1 Swedish Rectal Cancer Trial

The schedule of 5 Gy × 5 fractions was first established as the standard short-course radiotherapy in the preoperative setting of rectal cancer ever since the Swedish Rectal Cancer Trial was published. This short-course radiation schedule (25 Gy in 5 fractions in 5 consecutive days) was determined to have a similar biologically equivalent dose with conventional radiation schedule of 45 Gy in 25 fractions in 5 weeks, despite the stark difference in the real physical dose delivered. After a median follow-up of 5 years, the Swedish trial showed that adding short-course radiotherapy before surgery reduced the risk of local recurrence from 27% to 11% ($P < 0.001$), thus leading to improved 5-year overall survival and disease-free survival. This benefit was seen regardless of Dukes' stage. Overall in-hospital mortality risk was not increased in patients with short-course radiotherapy and surgery when compared to those with surgery alone but increased in patients who received radiotherapy with low-quality technique. Long-term result after a median follow-up of 13 years confirmed the value of initial findings [17]. Again, local recurrence rate was decreased from 26% to 9% ($P < 0.001$), and overall survival was increased from 30% to 38%

($P < 0.001$) by adding short-course regimen of preoperative radiotherapy. This benefit was seen at all tumor heights except in the patients with tumors located greater than 10 cm from the anal verge.

31.2.1.2 Dutch Rectal Cancer Trial

Total mesorectal excision (TME) has become a standard surgical approach as it significantly improved the local control ability [18]. As such, a concern had grown that the benefit of short-course radiation in the Swedish Rectal Cancer Trial might have been due to the higher risk of local failure after suboptimal excision and thus would not show a similar effect in the clinical setting of TME. The Dutch Colorectal Cancer Group initiated to investigate the impact of short-course radiotherapy followed by TME surgery within 1 week for resectable rectal cancer [15]. This Dutch TME trial failed to demonstrate an significant improvement in overall survival for irradiated group than nonirradiated group, but did show a significant difference in local failure, with 10-year rate of local recurrence of 5% vs. 11% in the preoperative short-course arm vs. surgery alone arm, respectively, after 12 years of follow-up ($P < 0.001$) [16]. Unplanned subset analysis revealed that a significant improvement in 10-year overall survival was observed in patients with the stage III disease who had negative circumferential resection margin (CRM), with 10-year rate of overall survival of 50% vs. 40%, respectively. Toxicities, such as bowel frequency, fecal incontinence, anal blood loss, and mucus discharge, were reported to be higher in the preoperative radiotherapy group than in the surgery alone group [19].

31.2.1.3 MRC CR07 Trial

The short-course preoperative treatment was reinforced by the MRC CR07 trial [20]. A total of 1350 patients with operable rectal cancer were randomized to two arms: short-course preoperative radiotherapy with 25 Gy in 5 fractions or selective postoperative chemoradiotherapy with daily 1.8 Gy in 25 fractions and concomitant chemotherapy for patients with involved CRM. Patients with neoadjuvant radiotherapy showed a decrease in the relative risk of local recurrence by 61%.

31.2.2 Preoperative Chemoradiotherapy

It is obvious that the combination of radiotherapy and surgery reduces the rate of local recurrence. However, no studies have confirmed that radiotherapy improves the patient survival seen in the Swedish trial [13, 14]. Therefore, 5-FU-based chemotherapy was combined with radiotherapy through several phase III trials to improve pathologic and clinical outcome. According to the meta-analysis which included FFCD-9203 [21], EORTC-22921 [22], and four other studies [23–26], reduced local recurrence rates were yielded by the addition of chemotherapy to neoadjuvant radiotherapy in the locally advanced rectal cancer with odds ratio of 0.56 (95% CI, 0.42–0.75)) [27]. Therefore, now, a standard treatment approach in the treatment of locally advanced rectal cancer is adding chemotherapy to conventional fractionated radiotherapy, primarily based on that chemoradiotherapy enhanced the local control and improved the pathologic complete remission rates [28].

Postoperative chemoradiotherapy after rectal cancer resection was considered to be the standard of care for stage II/III rectal cancer, based mainly on evidence from trials of colon cancer. As evidence for the effects of preoperative chemoradiotherapy on pathologic complete remission and local tumor control increased, several questions emerged as follows: (1) the optimal sequence of adding chemoradiotherapy in relation to resection and (2) the best radiosensitizing or systemic agent to be combined with radiation. Some studies had examined the preoperative and postoperative chemoradiotherapy in order to determine the optimal timing of chemoradiotherapy in relation to surgical resection. The German Rectal Cancer Study Group trial was the landmark study which was published in 2004 [29]. This trial enrolled 823 patients with cT3/4 or N+ disease to randomize into either preoperative or postoperative chemoradiotherapy group.

At a median 46-month follow-up, a significant reduction of local recurrence was observed in the preoperative chemoradiotherapy compared to postoperative chemoradiotherapy (6% vs. 13%; $P = 0.006$). The difference persisted even after 11 years of follow-up [30].

31.3 Short-Course Radiotherapy vs. Long-Course Chemoradiotherapy

Both preoperative short-course radiotherapy and long-course chemoradiotherapy are the standards of care for high-risk rectal cancer in terms of effective local control and low morbidity [28]. Preoperative short-course radiotherapy is a preferred in some European countries. However, in the United States, stage II or III rectal cancer is generally treated with preoperative long-course chemoradiotherapy [31]. Short-course radiotherapy consisted of 25 Gy in 5 fractions in 1 week followed by surgery within 1 week. Long-course chemoradiotherapy consisted of 50.4 Gy in 1.8 Gy per fraction over 5–6 weeks concurrent with infusional 5-FU or oral capecitabine followed by surgery in 4–6 weeks [32]. The advantage of short-course radiotherapy is simplicity, good compliance, patient convenience, and cost benefit, whereas long-course chemoradiotherapy has the advantage of the superior downsizing of the tumor thus increasing the chance of sphincter preservation. Also, smaller radiation fractions per fraction may be less late radiation toxicity compared with 5 Gy per fraction of short-course radiotherapy [32].

The Polish Colorectal Study Group conducted prospective randomized clinical trial to compare preoperative short-course radiotherapy to long-course chemoradiotherapy directly [24, 33]. A total of 316 patients with resectable T3-4 rectal carcinoma without tumor infiltration of the anal sphincter and a lesion accessible to digital rectal examination were randomly assigned to receive short-course radiotherapy or long-course chemoradiotherapy. Digital rectal exam is a major role to evaluate eligibility, whereas MRI was not applied. Adjuvant chemotherapy was not mandatory. Although significant downsizing was achieved in long-course chemoradiotherapy, the primary end point, a 15% improvement in sphincter preservation, was not obtained (short course 61%, long course 58%; P = 0.57). Long-course chemoradiotherapy improved both pathologic complete response rates (16.1% vs. 0.7%) and negative CRM rates (95.6% vs. 87.1%). But these positive results did not translate into a significant difference in overall survival, relapse-free survival, or local recurrence between groups. Crude incidence of local recurrence was similar but relatively high in long-course chemoradiotherapy (short course 9.0%, long course 14.2%; $P = 0.17$). No significant difference in late toxicity, quality of life, anorectal function, and sexual functioning were detected between two groups.

More recently, the Trans-Tasman Radiation Oncology Group (TROG) in Australia and New Zealand reported results of a randomized trial comparing short-course radiotherapy and long-course chemoradiotherapy for patients with only T3 localized rectal cancer using ultrasound or MRI [26]. This study showed more modernized evaluation program and homogeneous patient group. Also, adjuvant chemotherapy was delivered for 6 months in short-course group or 4 months in long-course group. A total of 326 patients were randomly assigned to each group. The 3-year local recurrence rates were 7.5% for short-course group and 4.4% for long-course group. This small difference of 3.1% was not significant ($P = 0.24$) and failed to meet the primary end point of 10% difference between two groups (a difference in 3-year local recurrence rate of 15% in short course vs. 5% in long-course). Noteworthy difference of local recurrence in distal rectal cancer was observed. In 79 patients with distal rectal cancer, 6 of 48 patients on short-course group and 1 of 31 patients on long-course group experienced local recurrence. As expected, a higher rate of pathologic complete remission (15% vs. 1%) was achieved with long-course chemoradiotherapy, but no difference in 5-year disease-free survival or overall survival rate was observed. The late toxicity and quality of life were similar in two groups. Even in much higher pathologic complete response rate in the long-course group, the abdominoperineal resection rates were similar in short course and long course. Possible reasons for failing to reduce the abdominoperineal resection rate were insufficient downsizing, concerns about residual microscopic disease even after a good clinical response, and the surgical practice of basing clinical decisions on the pretreatment distal margin rather than the perioperative clinical response to radiotherapy [32].

Both polish and TROG trials were underpowered to detect modest but clinically significant differences in long-term outcomes. It therefore remains unclear which neoadjuvant strategy is superior [34]. The Berlin Rectal Cancer Trial was commenced in 2004 and has closed to recruitment [35]. A total of 760 patients with T2N+ or T3 disease were randomized to receive either short-course radiotherapy or 5-FU-based chemoradiotherapy followed by total mesorectal excision surgery. Adjuvant chemotherapy was prespecified. Total mesorectal excision quality was independently documented by the surgeon and the pathologist. Hypothesis of the study was that chemoradiotherapy is superior to short-course radiotherapy in terms of local recurrence after 5 years. Its result is pending, and this may help answer the question regarding the optimal preoperative strategy. Given current evidence, both short-course radiotherapy and long-course chemoradiotherapy are safe and effective in terms of local control and toxicity. Preferred strategy has been depending on countries and physicians until now [34]. But long-course chemoradiotherapy is preferred for distal rectal tumors, high-risk T3 and all T4 tumors, and tumors that are borderline candidates for sphincter preservation [34].

31.4 Risk Stratification of Rectal Cancer

Both neoadjuvant short-course radiotherapy and long-course chemoradiotherapy reduce the risk of local recurrence compared with surgery alone, but neoadjuvant radiotherapy has not shown survival benefit [36]. Based on current evidence, these monolithic neoadjuvant approaches with 5-FU- or capecitabine-based long-course chemoradiotherapy or short-course radiotherapy to all patients with TNM stage II/III rectal cancer need to be questioned [37]. Some surgeons are of the opinion that they can achieve a good local control rate without preoperative RT, provided that a high-quality surgery is performed [31]. Several groups have recently explored omitting radiotherapy when MRI suggests the tumor is easily resectable and the mesorectal fascia is not threatened regardless of nodal stage. This omission is associated with the local recurrence rates of <5% [38–42].

Outcomes of rectal cancer vary significantly according to the stage of disease and several prognostic factors. Risk stratification and individualized treatment have been suggested for stage II/III rectal cancer. In a pooled analysis of survival and relapse rates in five North American phase III trials receiving postoperative therapy for rectal cancer, 5-year overall survival rates for T3N0, T3N1, and T3N2 were 75%, 60%, and 44%, respectively [43]. In another population-based analysis, the 5-year overall survival rates were 64%, 52.4%, and 37.5% for N0, N1, and N2 disease, respectively [44]. Patients were separated into four risk groups by TN stage: low risk (T1/2N0), intermediate risk (T1/2N1, T3N0), moderately high risk (T1/2N2, T3N1, T4N0), and high risk (T3N2, T4N1/2) [28]. In addition to TN stage, several poor risk factors of primary rectal cancer have been reported including depth of extramural spread, the distance from the anal verge, the circumferential location, the distance of the tumors from the mesorectal fascia, and the involvement of extramural vessels [38]. All established pathological risk factors can be identified by MRI preoperatively [36]. The MERCURY trial evaluated the extramural depth of tumor spread, defined as the distance between muscularis propria and the tumor. This study found that it was feasible to determine prognosis with a true measurement of the distance of extramural tumor spread by high-resolution MRI [31, 45]. There are many conflicts for treatment of T3 rectal tumor. T3 tumors are heterogeneous group from tumors that barely extend beyond the lamina muscularis propria to those that extend to or invade the mesorectal fascia [36]. Based on the extent of extramural spread, T3 tumors showed different survival rate. Tumors with extramural spread ≤5 mm had a 5-year survival of 83.4% compared with those tumors >5 mm, which had a 5-year overall survival rate of 54.1% ($p < 0.0001$) [46]. In the MERCURY study, patients with safe mesorectal fascia margins and T2/T3 tumors of <5 mm extramural spread on high-resolution MRI had good prognosis; 5-year disease-free survival and overall survival rates were 85% and 68% with surgery alone [39]. Patients with low-lying tumors requiring abdominoperineal resection have adverse outcomes. In a pooled analysis of five European randomized controlled trials for rectal cancer, local recurrence, cancer-specific survival, and overall survival rates were significantly worse in those patients who underwent abdominoperineal resection [47]. The Second St. Gallen European Organisation for Research and Treatment of Cancer Gastrointestinal Cancer Conference asked "Do T3 rectal cancers always need radiotherapy?" Omitting radiotherapy would offer the benefit of improved wound healing, less frequent anastomotic leaks, avoidance of long-term radiation toxicity, and a smaller risk of secondary malignancies [38]. For easily resectable cancers of the mid-rectum with no detectable lymph node metastases (cT3 cN0), 71% of panelists did not feel combination treatment was required for all patients, but 25% did, albeit there was some debate as to the definition of "easily resectable," which may be defined as tumors with <5 mm infiltration depth into the mesorectal fat and at least 1 mm distance from the mesorectal fascia. In contrast, for cT3 cN0 low rectal cancer, 66% voted that short-course radiotherapy or long-course chemoradiotherapy is necessary [38]. The most main risk factor for a local recurrence after rectal cancer surgery is the surgical plane. In the CR07 and NCIC-CTGCO16 trials, both an uninvolved circumferential resection margin, which was defined as tumor at a minimum distance of 1 mm from the circumferential resection margin on pathology, and a superior surgical plane, were associated with low local

recurrence rates [48, 49]. In the long-term results from MERCURY study, only those patients with a predicted MRI margin of ≤1 mm between tumor and mesorectal fascia had significantly higher rates of local recurrence compared with those with predicted MRI margin of >5 mm [36, 50]. In the Second St. Gallen European Organisation for Research and Treatment of Cancer Gastrointestinal Cancer Conference, a large majority of panelists believe chemoradiotherapy to be required when MRI shows a "threatened or breached circumferential resection margin," or in cancers which require surgical resection beyond the conventional total mesorectal excision and in clinically unresectable cancers [38]. Another factor influencing the risk on local recurrence is the extramural venous invasion. The extramural venous invasion has been shown to be associated with development of liver metastases as well as local recurrence in rectal cancer [51, 52].

On the basis of MRI staging, Dewdney A et al. categorized rectal cancer into three prognostic groups according to stage, the predicted relationship of the tumor to the circumferential resection margin, lymph node status, the degree of extramural spread, and the presence of extramural venous invasion enabling patient selection for preoperative treatment (Table 31.1) [36].

They suggested that those patients with low-risk rectal cancer can undergo surgery alone with favorable long-term outcomes sparing them from radiation-induced long-term toxicities. Those

Table 31.1 Prognostic classification of rectal cancer based on pretreatment staging magnetic resonance imaging

Risk features	Low risk	Moderate risk	High risk
Extramural spread	≤5 mm	>5 mm	>5 mm
Nodal status	N0	N1–2	N2
Circumferential resection margin	Not at risk	Not at risk	At risk
Position of tumor	High	Low or high	Low
Extramural venous invasion	Absent	Present	Present

patients with high-risk disease will need to be evaluated for intensified preoperative regimens to reduce distant failures and improve survival [36]. Future developments will be warranted to aim at identifying and selecting patients for their most appropriate treatment alternatives. Thus, clinicopathological and molecular features as well as accurate imaging and response monitoring during treatment will take an integrative part in the multimodality management of rectal cancer patients [37].

31.5 Total Neoadjuvant Therapy (TNT) Approach

The improved surgical techniques and neoadjuvant chemoradiotherapy have markedly decreased the rates of local recurrence for locally advanced rectal cancer. However, distant metastatic disease remains the most significant cause of death for these patients [53]. Therefore these patients will need to be evaluated for intensified treatment approach to reduce distant failures and improve survival. One could hypothesize that administering chemotherapy at an earlier point might treat micrometastases, thereby reducing the incidence of distant recurrence. This is the rationale for moving full systemic chemotherapy treatment forward to an earlier point in the rectal cancer treatment algorithm [28]. Although systemic therapy delivery to the neoadjuvant strategy may be associated with its own caveats, such as selection of radioresistant clones, induction of accelerated repopulation, and possibly reduced compliance to chemoradiotherapy, it may have the promise to improve compliance rates, reduce toxicity, and decrease distant relapse rates resulting from administering systemic chemotherapy with sufficient dose and intensity [37, 53]. Such a rationale makes the strategy called "total neoadjuvant therapy (TNT) approach " incorporating both chemotherapy and chemoradiotherapy in the neoadjuvant setting, and recently, multiple prospective trials have reported on the use of TNT for patients with locally advanced rectal cancer [37, 53].

Ludmir EB et al. clearly described several promising benefits of delivering chemotherapy in the neoadjuvant setting compared with adjuvant chemotherapy. Whereas postoperative complications and treatment-related toxicities limited adjuvant chemotherapy compliance, neoadjuvant chemotherapy allows for greater treatment compliance and reduces overall toxicity rates. Furthermore, earlier delivery of full-dose, systemic therapy to eliminate micrometastatic disease has the potential to decrease the risk of disease progression during treatment and improve disease-related outcomes. Others have noted that positioning surgery as the final step in the treatment algorithm for locally advanced rectal cancer could allow for earlier reversal of a diverting stoma postoperatively [54]. TNT also gives rise to increasing rates of tumor regression and downstaging resulting in further increasing complete (R0) resection rates. Conversely, a major disadvantage is that the delay in definitive surgery could allow for local disease progression, particularly in those patients who do not respond to TNT. In terms of surgical compliance or complication, TNT may decrease the performance status of patients who undergo planned surgical resection and/or potentially increase surgical complication rates [53].

31.5.1 Delayed Surgery and Consolidation Chemotherapy After Preoperative Chemoradiotherapy

The most commonly used time interval between completion of preoperative chemoradiotherapy and surgical resection has traditionally been 4–6 weeks. However, the response to chemoradiotherapy for rectal cancer is time-dependent, and maximal local tumor regression may well take longer than the standard 6 weeks to surgery. During this prolonged interval between chemoradiotherapy and surgery, adding consolidation chemotherapy can give rise to not only allow more time to regress tumor before surgery but also provide effective systemic treatment early to reduce the risk of developing systemic disease [37].

The Timing of Rectal Cancer Response to Chemoradiation Consortium in the United States conducted a prospective, multi-institutional phase II trial to test effect of adding mFOLFOX6 after neoadjuvant chemoradiotherapy in locally advanced rectal cancer [55]. The patients were assigned to four groups to receive chemoradiotherapy (with concurrent 5-FU) followed by mFOLFOX6 and then surgical resection. Patients in group 1 had total mesorectal excision 6–8 weeks after chemoradiation. Patients in groups 2–4 received two, four, or six cycles of mFOLFOX6, respectively, during the waiting period before surgery (performed 11, 15, and 19 weeks, respectively, after completion of chemoradiotherapy). Treatment compliance with neoadjuvant chemotherapy was tolerable with about 80% of patients completing all prescribed neoadjuvant chemotherapy cycles. Furthermore, the postoperative complication rates did not increase in spite of adding more chemotherapy cycles. The pathologic complete remission rates increased significantly with increasing cycles of FOLFOX between chemoradiotherapy and total mesorectal excision (18% in group 1, 25% in group 2, 30% in group 3, and 38% in group 4). This approach has now been tested in a randomized phase II study in Germany (CAO/ARO/AIO-12) as well as in the randomized phase III RAPIDO trial for short-course radiotherapy [37, 56].

The Polish Colorectal Study Group conducted a randomized phase III trial to assess the role of consolidation neoadjuvant chemotherapy between radiotherapy and surgery. The patients with fixed cT3 or cT4 cancer were randomized to receive either short-course radiotherapy (25Gy in 5 fractions) followed by three cycles of FOLFOX or long-course chemoradiotherapy (50.4 Gy over 5 weeks) with concurrent FOLFOX6. About 12 weeks' interval from radiotherapy to surgery was similar in both arms. Preoperative treatment acute toxicity was lower in short-course radiotherapy with consolidation than long-course chemoradiotherapy. Also, compliance with

oxaliplatin delivery favored the short-course radiotherapy with neoadjuvant chemotherapy over the long-course chemoradiotherapy (72% vs. 64%). There were no differences in the R0 resection (primary end point), pathologic complete response rate, local control, or disease-free survival rates between the treatment arms. Nevertheless, an improved overall survival favors the 5 × 5 Gy schedule with consolidation chemotherapy [57].

31.5.2 Induction Chemotherapy Followed by Chemoradiotherapy and then Surgery

The Spanish Grupo Cancer de Recto 3 (GCR-3) phase II trial compared conventional preoperative chemoradiotherapy and adjuvant chemotherapy with induction chemotherapy before chemoradiotherapy. Patients with T3–T4 and/or N+ disease were randomized to receive four cycles of capecitabine/oxaliplatin (CAPOX) either before neoadjuvant chemoradiotherapy (induction chemotherapy) or after surgery (adjuvant chemotherapy). There were no significant differences between the two arms in pathologic complete remission and disease-free survival rates, 5-year cumulative incidence of local relapse, incidence of distant metastases, or overall survival. The induction chemotherapy had both markedly improved chemotherapy compliance and low-grade ≥3 toxicity [58, 59].

Marechal et al. in Brussels [60] conducted a randomized phase II trial to compare standard therapy (preoperative 5-FU-based chemoradiotherapy followed by surgery) with induction FOLFOX, followed by chemoradiotherapy, and then surgery. The primary endpoint was the rate of ypT0/1N0 achievement. Fifty seven patients were randomly assigned. On planned interim analysis, the ypT0/1N0 rates were no different between two arms. So, the study was deemed futile and prematurely closed.

Thus, there is no clear evidence that the implementation of induction chemotherapy prior to chemoradiotherapy did improve outcomes [28]. Whether or not the improvement in applicability and dose density of induction chemotherapy will ultimately translate into improved disease-free survival will have to be tested in a larger phase III trial [37]. Currently there is an ongoing randomized phase III trial (the French PRODIGE 23 trial) that is randomly assigning 460 patients with locally advanced rectal cancer to either receive induction chemotherapy with FOLFIRINOX (5-FU, leucovorin, irinotecan, and oxaliplatin), followed by preoperative chemoradiotherapy (arm 1), or to receive preoperative chemoradiotherapy alone (arm 2) [28] (Table 31.2).

31.6 "Watch-and-Wait" Nonoperative Management (NOM) Approaches

Surgery has been the cornerstone of curative treatment for rectal cancer, but it is associated with perioperative complications, including vascular injury, bleeding, infection, wound complications, and/or ureteral injury. Furthermore, long-term effects such as anorectal, urinary, and/or sexual dysfunction have been associated with surgery [34, 61]. For some patients with distal rectal cancer, the psychosocial morbidity of a permanent colostomy has been serious problem for their quality of life [62, 63]. The achievement of pathologic complete response after neoadjuvant chemoradiotherapy occurs in 10–38% of rectal cancer [64], and subsequent local recurrence in these patients is rare [65]. Also, pathologic complete response is associated with improved overall survival and disease-free survival in comparison to partial responders or nonresponders [66–68]. Good prognosis in this cohort is possibly explained as a more favorable tumor biologic profile [66]. Given the potential surgical morbidity and good prognosis of pathologic complete response, several investigators have suggested a subset of patients experiencing a pathologic complete response may not benefit from surgery [34]. The potential clinical advantage of nonoperative management (NOM) is to avoid the complications associated with surgery.

A NOM is reasonable for elderly patients and for those with significant medical comorbidities. Another interest is the perceived reduction in quality of life with a permanent stoma in the patient with low-lying tumor who had clinically had pathologic complete response after neoadjuvant chemoradiotherapy [69].

Investigators from the University of Sao Paulo were the first to pioneer the selective nonoperative management (NOM) approach for patients with potentially resectable rectal cancer who experience a clinically complete response to chemoradiotherapy [37]. In early report, Habr-Gama et al. reported overall long-term results of stage 0 rectal cancer following neoadjuvant chemoradiotherapy and compared long-term results between operative and nonoperative treatment [70]. After 8 weeks from completion of chemoradiotherapy, patients were reevaluated by an experienced colorectal surgeon to assess tumor response using the same pretreatment clinical, endoscopic, and radiologic parameters. During proctoscopy, biopsies were obtained for pathologic examination. The presence of any significant residual ulcer or positive biopsies performed during proctoscopy was considered incomplete clinical response. Patients without any abnormality during tumor response assessment were considered to have complete clinical response. Patients deemed to have a clinical complete response were referred to monthly follow-up visits for repeat physical and digital rectal examination, proctoscopy, biopsies, and serum CEA levels. Patients in this group were carefully advised that initial tumor remission could be temporary, and, therefore, a strict follow-up adherence was mandatory. Abdominal and pelvic CT scans and chest radiographs were repeated every 6 months during the first year. Patients with sustained complete tumor regression for at least 12 months were considered stage 0. In an updated series published in 2006, they described the outcomes of 361 patients with distal, resectable cT2–4 and/or cN+ rectal cancer treated with neoadjuvant chemoradiotherapy (50.4 Gy plus 5-FU/leucovorin) [70, 71]. Patients with complete clinical response were not immediately operated on and were closely followed. One hundred

Table 31.2 Total neoadjuvant therapy (TNT) approach studies assessing neoadjuvant chemotherapy (either consolidation or induction chemotherapy)

	Design	No.	CRT regimen	NAC regimen	Adjuvant therapy	Compliance	Postoperative complication rate, %	pCR rate, %	R0 resection rate, %	DFS (3-year), %	OS (3-year), %
Consolidation chemotherapy											
Garcia-Aguila [55]	Phase II nonrandomized four-arm	259	CRT (w/5-FU)	None	mFOLFOX6 (8 cycles) recommended, but not mandatory	NR	15 (Grade ≥3)	18	98	NR	NR
			CRT (w/5-FU)	mFOLFOX6 (2 cycles)		82% completed NAC	6 (Grade ≥3)	25	100		
			CRT (w/5-FU)	mFOLFOX6 (4 cycles)		81% completed NAC	4 (Grade ≥3)	30	96		
			CRT (w/5-FU)	mFOLFOX6 (6 cycles)		77% completed NAC	9 (Grade ≥3)	38	100		
Bujko (Polish II trial) [57]	Phase III randomized two-arm	515	RT (5 × 5Gy)	FOLFOX4 (3 cycles)	Not reported; left to treating physician discretion	63% completed both RT and NAC; 72% oxaliplatin compliance	29 (all complications)	16	77	53	73
			CRT (w/5-FU/leucovorin/oxaliplatin)	None		66% completed CRT; 64% oxaliplatin compliance.	25 (all complications)	12	71	52	65
Induction chemotherapy											
GCR-3 [58, 59]	Phase II randomized two-arm	108	CAPOX (four cycles)	CRT (w/CAPOX)	None	94% completed NAC; 85% completed RT.	51 (all grades)	14	86	64	74
			None	CRT (w/CAPOX)	CAPOX (4 cycles)	57% completed adjuvant ChT; 80% completed RT.	45 (all grades)	13	87	62	77
Marechal [60]	Phase II randomized two-arm	57	mFOLFOX6 (two cycles)	CRT (w/5-FU)	Not reported; left to treating physician discretion	96% completed both NAC and CRT	25 (all complications)	25	96	NR	NR
			None	CRT (w/5-FU)		97% completed CRT.	31 (all complications)	28	86	NR	NR

This table was cited from Ludmir et al. [53]

5-FU 5-fluorouracil, *Cape* capecitabine, *CAPOX* capecitabine/oxaliplatin, *ChT* chemotherapy, *CRT* chemoradiotherapy, *DFS* disease-free survival, *FOLFOX6* 5-fluorouracil, leucovorin, and oxaliplatin, *GCR-3* Spanish Rectal Cancer Group Study 3, *Gy* gray, *mFOLFOX6* modified FOLFOX6, *NAC* neoadjuvant chemotherapy, *NR* not reported, *OS* overall survival, *pCR* pathologic complete response, *R0* microscopically clear resection, *RT* radiotherapy twenty-two patients were considered to have complete clinical response after the first tumor response assessment. Of these, only 99 patients sustained complete clinical response for at least 12 months and were considered stage c0 (27.4%) and managed nonoperatively. At a mean follow-up of 60 months, this cohort experienced 13 (13%) recurrences. Of these, five (5%) recurrences were endorectal, seven (7%) systemic, and one (1%) combined. All five isolated endorectal recurrences were salvaged. The 5-year overall survival and disease-free survival rates were 93% and 85%, respectively. A NOM after complete clinical response following neoadjuvant chemoradiotherapy may be safe and associated with good survival rates in a highly selected group of patients with sustained clinical complete response >12 months after chemoradiotherapy.

In a recent prospective study, this group used a more intense chemoradiotherapy regimen of 54 Gy in 32 fractions with three concurrent cycles of 5-FU/leucovorin every 21 days, followed by three further cycles of consolidation chemotherapy before response assessment 9 weeks after completion of chemoradiotherapy [72]. Forty-seven (68%) patients had initial complete clinical response. Of these, eight developed local regrowth within the first 12 months of follow-up (17%). Thirty-nine sustained complete clinical response at a median follow-up of 56 months (57%). An additional four patients (10%) developed late local recurrences (>12 months of follow-up). Overall, 35 (50%) patients never underwent surgery due to sustained clinical complete response.

Researchers in the Netherlands [73] initiated a prospective study of a "watch-and-wait" nonoperative management aiming to replicate the results from Sao Paulo with high-resolution MRI. At 6–8 weeks after neoadjuvant chemoradiotherapy, reevaluation was performed using digital rectal examination, MRI, and endoscopy with biopsies. A clinical complete response was defined as no residual tumor on MRI, no residual tumor at endoscopy with negative biopsies from the tumor location, and no palpable tumor by digital rectal examination. Only 21 of the 192 (11%) patients had evidence of clinical complete

response. Of these one patient developed endoluminal recurrence, and successfully was treated with salvage surgery. The other 20 patients remained alive without disease. In the comparison to 20 patients with pathologic complete response after radical surgery, The 2-year disease-free survival (89% vs. 93%) and overall survival rates (100% vs. 91%) were similar for the clinical complete response and pathologic complete response patients. But patients treated with NOM had less toxicity and better bowel function. More comprehensive evaluation using MRI than Habr-Gama et al.'s study resulted in low rate of clinical complete response rate.

The recent Oncological Outcome after Clinical Complete Response in Patients with Rectal Cancer (OnCoRe) project in the United Kingdom attempted to provide the safety of the NOM by comparing oncological outcomes between patients managed by watch and wait who achieved a clinical complete response and those who had surgical resection after chemoradiotherapy [74]. Using propensity-score matching (including T stage, age, and performance status), 109 patients underwent the watch-and-wait approach, while the other 109 patients underwent radical surgery. No differences in 3-year non-regrowth disease-free survival were noted between watch and wait and surgical resection (88% vs. 78%, $p = 0.043$). Similarly, no difference in 3-year overall survival was noted (96% vs. 87%, $p = 0.024$). However, patients in the watch-and-wait group had significantly better 3-year colostomy-free survival than those who underwent surgical resection (74% vs. 47%, $p < 0.0001$).

There are potential pitfalls for NOM. A discrepancy between clinical complete response and pathologic complete response is problematic to extrapolate the favorable results of patients with a pathologic complete response to those with a clinical complete response. Although local salvage therapy may be successful for most of regrowing disease, regrowth partly was associated with systemic metastases [75]. In addition, there is no clear evidence to predict an unfavorable biology. Further study of radiographic and biologic predictors including genetic expression profiles of clinical complete response and pathologic complete response may ultimately facilitate improved selection of patients eligible for NOM [69]. At present, NOM approach could be useful to very select patients with distal tumors who will have a poor functional outcome and psychosocial morbidity of a permanent stoma after surgery [31].

References

1. Galandiuk S, Wieand HS, Moertel CG, Cha SS, Fitzgibbons RJ Jr, Pemberton JH, et al. Patterns of recurrence after curative resection of carcinoma of the colon and rectum. Surg Gynecol Obstet. 1992;174(1):27–32.
2. Minsky BD, Mies C, Recht A, Rich TA, Chaffey JT. Resectable adenocarcinoma of the rectosigmoid and rectum. I. Patterns of failure and survival. Cancer. 1988;61(7):1408–16.
3. Phillips RK, Hittinger R, Blesovsky L, Fry JS, Fielding LP. Local recurrence following 'curative' surgery for large bowel cancer: I. The overall picture. Br J Surg. 1984;71(1):12–6.
4. Gastrointestinal Tumor Study Group. Prolongation of the disease-free interval in surgically treated rectal carcinoma. N Engl J Med. 1985;312(23): 1465–72.
5. Balslev I, Pedersen M, Teglbjaerg PS, Hanberg-Soerensen F, Bone J, Jacobsen NO, et al. Postoperative radiotherapy in Dukes' B and C carcinoma of the rectum and rectosigmoid. A randomized multicenter study. Cancer. 1986;58(1):22–8.
6. Douglass HO Jr, Moertel CG, Mayer RJ, Thomas PR, Lindblad AS, Mittleman A, et al. Survival after postoperative combination treatment of rectal cancer. N Engl J Med. 1986;315(20):1294–5.
7. Fisher B, Wolmark N, Rockette H, Redmond C, Deutsch M, Wickerham DL, et al. Postoperative adjuvant chemotherapy or radiation therapy for rectal cancer: results from NSABP protocol R-01. J Natl Cancer Inst. 1988;80(1):21–9.
8. Gerard A, Buyse M, Nordlinger B, Loygue J, Pene F, Kempf P, et al. Preoperative radiotherapy as adjuvant treatment in rectal cancer. Final results of a randomized study of the European Organization for Research and Treatment of Cancer (EORTC). Ann Surg. 1988;208(5):606–14.
9. Higgins GA, Humphrey EW, Dwight RW, Roswit B, Lee LE Jr, Keehn RJ. Preoperative radiation and surgery for cancer of the rectum. Veterans Administration Surgical Oncology Group Trial II. Cancer. 1986;58(2):352–9.
10. Rider WD, Palmer JA, Mahoney LJ, Robertson CT. Preoperative irradiation in operable cancer of the rectum: report of the Toronto trial. Can J Surg. 1977;20(4):335–8.
11. Roswit B, Higgins GA, Keehn RJ. Preoperative irradiation for carcinoma of the rectum and rectosigmoid colon: report of a National Veterans Administration randomized study. Cancer. 1975;35(6):1597–602.
12. Wassif SB, Langenhorst BG, Hop WCJ. The contribution of preoperative radiotherapy in the management of borderline operability rectal cance. In: Jones SE, Salmon SE, editors. Adjuvant therapy of cancer II. New York: Grune & Stratton; 1979. p. 613–20.
13. Cedermark B, Dahlberg M, Glimelius B, Pahlman L, Rutqvist LE, Wilking N. Improved survival with preoperative radiotherapy in resectable rectal cancer. N Engl J Med. 1997;336(14):980–7.
14. Birgisson H, Pahlman L, Gunnarsson U, Glimelius B. Adverse effects of preoperative radiation therapy for rectal cancer: long-term follow-up of the Swedish Rectal Cancer Trial. J Clin Oncol. 2005;23(34):8697–705.
15. Kapiteijn E, Marijnen CA, Nagtegaal ID, Putter H, Steup WH, Wiggers T, et al. Preoperative radiotherapy combined with total mesorectal excision for resectable rectal cancer. N Engl J Med. 2001;345(9):638–46.
16. van Gijn W, Marijnen CA, Nagtegaal ID, Kranenbarg EM, Putter H, Wiggers T, et al. Preoperative radiotherapy combined with total mesorectal excision for resectable rectal cancer: 12-year follow-up of the multicentre, randomised controlled TME trial. Lancet Oncol. 2011;12(6):575–82.
17. Folkesson J, Birgisson H, Pahlman L, Cedermark B, Glimelius B, Gunnarsson U. Swedish rectal cancer trial: long lasting benefits from radiotherapy on survival and local recurrence rate. J Clin Oncol. 2005;23(24):5644–50.
18. MacFarlane JK, Ryall RD, Heald RJ. Mesorectal excision for rectal cancer. Lancet (Lond, Engl). 1993;341(8843):457–60.
19. Peeters KC, van de Velde CJ, Leer JW, Martijn H, Junggeburt JM, Kranenbarg EK, et al. Late side effects of short-course preoperative radiotherapy combined with total mesorectal excision for rectal cancer: increased bowel dysfunction in irradiated patients – a Dutch colorectal cancer group study. J Clin Oncol. 2005;23(25):6199–206.
20. Sebag-Montefiore D, Stephens RJ, Steele R, Monson J, Grieve R, Khanna S, et al. Preoperative radiotherapy versus selective postoperative chemoradiotherapy in patients with rectal cancer (MRC CR07 and NCIC-CTG C016): a multicentre, randomised trial. Lancet (Lond, Engl). 2009;373(9666):811–20.
21. Gerard JP, Conroy T, Bonnetain F, Bouche O, Chapet O, Closon-Dejardin MT, et al. Preoperative radiotherapy with or without concurrent fluorouracil and leucovorin in T3-4 rectal cancers: results of FFCD 9203. J Clin Oncol. 2006;24(28):4620–5.
22. Bosset JF, Calais G, Mineur L, Maingon P, Stojanovic-Rundic S, Bensadoun RJ, et al. Fluorouracil-based adjuvant chemotherapy after preoperative chemoradiotherapy in rectal cancer: long-term results of

the EORTC 22921 randomised study. Lancet Oncol. 2014;15(2):184–90.

23. Boulis-Wassif S, Gerard A, Loygue J, Camelot D, Buyse M, Duez N. Final results of a randomized trial on the treatment of rectal cancer with preoperative radiotherapy alone or in combination with 5-fluorouracil, followed by radical surgery. Trial of the European Organization on Research and Treatment of Cancer Gastrointestinal Tract Cancer Cooperative Group. Cancer. 1984;53(9):1811–8.

24. Bujko K, Nowacki MP, Nasierowska-Guttmejer A, Michalski W, Bebenek M, Kryj M. Long-term results of a randomized trial comparing preoperative short-course radiotherapy with preoperative conventionally fractionated chemoradiation for rectal cancer. Br J Surg. 2006;93(10):1215–23.

25. Latkauskas T, Pauzas H, Gineikiene I, Janciauskiene R, Juozaityte E, Saladzinskas Z, et al. Initial results of a randomized controlled trial comparing clinical and pathological downstaging of rectal cancer after preoperative short-course radiotherapy or long-term chemoradiotherapy, both with delayed surgery. Colorectal Dis. 2012;14(3):294–8.

26. Ngan SY, Burmeister B, Fisher RJ, Solomon M, Goldstein D, Joseph D, et al. Randomized trial of short-course radiotherapy versus long-course chemoradiation comparing rates of local recurrence in patients with T3 rectal cancer: Trans-Tasman Radiation Oncology Group trial 01.04. J Clin Oncol. 2012;30(31):3827–33.

27. McCarthy K, Pearson K, Fulton R, Hewitt J. Preoperative chemoradiation for non-metastatic locally advanced rectal cancer. Cochrane Database Syst Rev. 2012;12:Cd008368.

28. Salem ME, Hartley M, Unger K, Marshall JL. Neoadjuvant combined-modality therapy for locally advanced rectal cancer and its future directions. Oncology (Williston Park, NY). 2016;30(6):546–62.

29. Sauer R, Becker H, Hohenberger W, Rodel C, Wittekind C, Fietkau R, et al. Preoperative versus postoperative chemoradiotherapy for rectal cancer. N Engl J Med. 2004;351(17):1731–40.

30. Sauer R, Liersch T, Merkel S, Fietkau R, Hohenberger W, Hess C, et al. Preoperative versus postoperative chemoradiotherapy for locally advanced rectal cancer: results of the German CAO/ARO/AIO-94 randomized phase III trial after a median follow-up of 11 years. J Clin Oncol. 2012;30(16):1926–33.

31. Artac M, Korkmaz L, El-Rayes B, Philip PA. An update on the multimodality of localized rectal cancer. Crit Rev Oncol Hematol. 2016;108:23–32.

32. Ngan SY. Preoperative treatment of locally advanced rectal cancer: assets and drawbacks of short course and long course in clinical practice. Semin Radiat Oncol. 2016;26(3):186–92.

33. Bujko K, Nowacki MP, Nasierowska-Guttmejer A, Michalski W, Bebenek M, Pudelko M, et al. Sphincter preservation following preoperative radiotherapy for rectal cancer: report of a randomised trial comparing short-term radiotherapy vs. conventionally fractionated radiochemotherapy. Radiother Oncol. 2004;72(1):15–24.

34. Lee M, Gibbs P, Wong R. Multidisciplinary management of locally advanced rectal cancer – an evolving landscape? Clin Colorectal Cancer. 2015;14(4):251–61.

35. Siegel R, Burock S, Wernecke KD, Kretzschmar A, Dietel M, Loy V, et al. Preoperative short-course radiotherapy versus combined radiochemotherapy in locally advanced rectal cancer: a multi-centre prospectively randomised study of the Berlin Cancer Society. BMC Cancer. 2009;9:50.

36. Dewdney A, Cunningham D, Chau I. Selecting patients with locally advanced rectal cancer for neoadjuvant treatment strategies. Oncologist. 2013;18(7):833–42.

37. Rodel C, Hofheinz R, Fokas E. Rectal cancer: neoadjuvant chemoradiotherapy. Best Pract Res Clin Gastroenterol. 2016;30(4):629–39.

38. Lutz MP, Zalcberg JR, Glynne-Jones R, Ruers T, Ducreux M, Arnold D, et al. Second St. Gallen European Organisation for Research and Treatment of Cancer Gastrointestinal Cancer Conference: consensus recommendations on controversial issues in the primary treatment of rectal cancer. Eur J Cancer (Oxford, Engl: 1990). 2016;63:11–24.

39. Taylor FG, Quirke P, Heald RJ, Moran B, Blomqvist L, Swift I, et al. Preoperative high-resolution magnetic resonance imaging can identify good prognosis stage I, II, and III rectal cancer best managed by surgery alone: a prospective, multicenter, European study. Ann Surg. 2011;253(4):711–9.

40. Frasson M, Garcia-Granero E, Roda D, Flor-Lorente B, Rosello S, Esclapez P, et al. Preoperative chemoradiation may not always be needed for patients with T3 and T2N+ rectal cancer. Cancer. 2011;117(14):3118–25.

41. Mathis KL, Larson DW, Dozois EJ, Cima RR, Huebner M, Haddock MG, et al. Outcomes following surgery without radiotherapy for rectal cancer. Br J Surg. 2012;99(1):137–43.

42. Marinello FG, Frasson M, Baguena G, Flor-Lorente B, Cervantes A, Rosello S, et al. Selective approach for upper rectal cancer treatment: total mesorectal excision and preoperative chemoradiation are seldom necessary. Dis Colon Rectum. 2015;58(6):556–65.

43. Gunderson LL, Sargent DJ, Tepper JE, Wolmark N, O'Connell MJ, Begovic M, et al. Impact of T and N stage and treatment on survival and relapse in adjuvant rectal cancer: a pooled analysis. J Clin Oncol. 2004;22(10):1785–96.

44. Gunderson LL, Jessup JM, Sargent DJ, Greene FL, Stewart A. Revised tumor and node categorization for rectal cancer based on surveillance, epidemiology, and end results and rectal pooled analysis outcomes. J Clin Oncol. 2010;28(2):256–63.

45. Fowler JM, Beagley CE, Blomqvist L, Brown G, Daniels IR, Heald RJ, Moran BJ, Norman AR, Peppercorn PD, Quirke P, Sebag-Montefiore D. Extramural depth of tumor invasion at thin-section

MR in patients with rectal cancer: results of the MERCURY study. Radiology. 2007;243(1):132–9.

46. Merkel S, Mansmann U, Siassi M, Papadopoulos T, Hohenberger W, Hermanek P. The prognostic inhomogeneity in pT3 rectal carcinomas. Int J Color Dis. 2001;16(5):298–304.

47. den Dulk M, Putter H, Collette L, Marijnen CA, Folkesson J, Bosset JF, et al. The abdominoperineal resection itself is associated with an adverse outcome: the European experience based on a pooled analysis of five European randomised clinical trials on rectal cancer. Eur J Cancer (Oxford, Engl: 1990). 2009;45(7):1175–83.

48. Quirke P, Steele R, Monson J, Grieve R, Khanna S, Couture J, et al. Effect of the plane of surgery achieved on local recurrence in patients with operable rectal cancer: a prospective study using data from the MRC CR07 and NCIC-CTG C016 randomised clinical trial. Lancet (Lond, Engl). 2009;373(9666):821–8.

49. Joye I, Haustermans K. Which patients with rectal cancer do not need radiotherapy? Semin Radiat Oncol. 2016;26(3):199–204.

50. Taylor FG, Quirke P, Heald RJ, Moran B, Blomqvist L, Swift I, et al. One millimetre is the safe cutoff for magnetic resonance imaging prediction of surgical margin status in rectal cancer. Br J Surg. 2011;98(6):872–9.

51. Dresen RC, Peters EE, Rutten HJ, Nieuwenhuijzen GA, Demeyere TB, van den Brule AJ, et al. Local recurrence in rectal cancer can be predicted by histopathological factors. Eur J Surg Oncol. 2009;35(10):1071–7.

52. Ouchi K, Sugawara T, Ono H, Fujiya T, Kamiyama Y, Kakugawa Y, et al. Histologic features and clinical significance of venous invasion in colorectal carcinoma with hepatic metastasis. Cancer. 1996;78(11):2313–7.

53. Ludmir EB, Palta M, Willett CG, Czito BG. Total neoadjuvant therapy for rectal cancer: an emerging option. Cancer. 2017;123(9):1497–506.

54. Gollins S, Sebag-Montefiore D. Neoadjuvant treatment strategies for locally advanced rectal cancer. Clin Oncol. 2016;28(2):146–51.

55. Garcia-Aguilar J, Chow OS, Smith DD, Marcet JE, Cataldo PA, Varma MG, et al. Effect of adding mFOLFOX6 after neoadjuvant chemoradiation in locally advanced rectal cancer: a multicentre, phase 2 trial. Lancet Oncol. 2015;16(8):957–66.

56. Nilsson PJ, van Etten B, Hospers GA, Pahlman L, van de Velde CJ, Beets-Tan RG, et al. Short-course radiotherapy followed by neo-adjuvant chemotherapy in locally advanced rectal cancer – the RAPIDO trial. BMC Cancer. 2013;13:279.

57. Bujko K, Wyrwicz L, Rutkowski A, Malinowska M, Pietrzak L, Krynski J, et al. Long-course oxaliplatin-based preoperative chemoradiation versus 5 x 5 Gy and consolidation chemotherapy for cT4 or fixed cT3 rectal cancer: results of a randomized phase III study. Ann Oncol. 2016;27(5):834–42.

58. Fernandez-Martos C, Pericay C, Aparicio J, Salud A, Safont M, Massuti B, et al. Phase II, randomized study of concomitant chemoradiotherapy followed by surgery and adjuvant capecitabine plus oxaliplatin (CAPOX) compared with induction CAPOX followed by concomitant chemoradiotherapy and surgery in magnetic resonance imaging-defined, locally advanced rectal cancer: Grupo cancer de recto 3 study. J Clin Oncol. 2010;28(5):859–65.

59. Fernandez-Martos C, Garcia-Albeniz X, Pericay C, Maurel J, Aparicio J, Montagut C, et al. Chemoradiation, surgery and adjuvant chemotherapy versus induction chemotherapy followed by chemoradiation and surgery: long-term results of the Spanish GCR-3 phase II randomized trialdagger. Ann Oncol. 2015;26(8):1722–8.

60. Marechal R, Vos B, Polus M, Delaunoit T, Peeters M, Demetter P, et al. Short course chemotherapy followed by concomitant chemoradiotherapy and surgery in locally advanced rectal cancer: a randomized multicentric phase II study. Ann Oncol. 2012;23(6):1525–30.

61. Goodman KA. Definitive chemoradiotherapy ("Watch-and-Wait" approach). Semin Radiat Oncol. 2016;26(3):205–10.

62. Hendren SK, O'Connor BI, Liu M, Asano T, Cohen Z, Swallow CJ, et al. Prevalence of male and female sexual dysfunction is high following surgery for rectal cancer. Ann Surg. 2005;242(2):212–23.

63. Paun BC, Cassie S, MacLean AR, Dixon E, Buie WD. Postoperative complications following surgery for rectal cancer. Ann Surg. 2010;251(5):807–18.

64. Glynne-Jones R, Hughes R. Critical appraisal of the 'wait and see' approach in rectal cancer for clinical complete responders after chemoradiation. Br J Surg. 2012;99(7):897–909.

65. Capirci C, Valentini V, Cionini L, De Paoli A, Rodel C, Glynne-Jones R, et al. Prognostic value of pathologic complete response after neoadjuvant therapy in locally advanced rectal cancer: long-term analysis of 566 ypCR patients. Int J Radiat Oncol Biol Phys. 2008;72(1):99–107.

66. Maas M, Nelemans PJ, Valentini V, Das P, Rodel C, Kuo LJ, et al. Long-term outcome in patients with a pathological complete response after chemoradiation for rectal cancer: a pooled analysis of individual patient data. Lancet Oncol. 2010;11(9):835–44.

67. Zorcolo L, Rosman AS, Restivo A, Pisano M, Nigri GR, Fancellu A, et al. Complete pathologic response after combined modality treatment for rectal cancer and long-term survival: a meta-analysis. Ann Surg Oncol. 2012;19(9):2822–32.

68. Martin ST, Heneghan HM, Winter DC. Systematic review and meta-analysis of outcomes following pathological complete response to neoadjuvant chemoradiotherapy for rectal cancer. Br J Surg. 2012;99(7):918–28.

69. Torok JA, Palta M, Willett CG, Czito BG. Nonoperative management of rectal cancer. Cancer. 2016;122(1):34–41.

70. Habr-Gama A, Perez RO, Nadalin W, Sabbaga J, Ribeiro U Jr, Silva e Sousa AH Jr, et al. Operative versus nonoperative treatment for stage 0 distal rectal cancer following chemoradiation therapy: long-term results. Ann Surg. 2004;240(4):711–7. discussion 7-8.

71. Habr-Gama A, Perez RO, Proscurshim I, Campos FG, Nadalin W, Kiss D, et al. Patterns of failure and survival for nonoperative treatment of stage c0 distal rectal cancer following neoadjuvant chemoradiation therapy. J Gastrointest Surg. 2006;10(10):1319–28. discussion 28-9.

72. Habr-Gama A, Sabbaga J, Gama-Rodrigues J, Sao Juliao GP, Proscurshim I, Bailao Aguilar P, et al. Watch and wait approach following extended neoadjuvant chemoradiation for distal rectal cancer: are we getting closer to anal cancer management? Dis Colon Rectum. 2013;56(10):1109–17.

73. Maas M, Beets-Tan RG, Lambregts DM, Lammering G, Nelemans PJ, Engelen SM, et al. Wait-and-see policy for clinical complete responders after chemoradiation for rectal cancer. J Clin Oncol. 2011;29(35):4633–40.

74. Renehan AG, Malcomson L, Emsley R, Gollins S, Maw A, Myint AS, et al. Watch-and-wait approach versus surgical resection after chemoradiotherapy for patients with rectal cancer (the OnCoRe project): a propensity-score matched cohort analysis. Lancet Oncol. 2016;17(2):174–83.

75. Habr-Gama A, Gama-Rodrigues J, Sao Juliao GP, Proscurshim I, Sabbagh C, Lynn PB, et al. Local recurrence after complete clinical response and watch and wait in rectal cancer after neoadjuvant chemoradiation: impact of salvage therapy on local disease control. Int J Radiat Oncol Biol Phys. 2014;88(4):822–8.

Part IX

Integrated Approach for Optimal Treatment of Stage IV and Recurrent Colorectal Cancer

Peritoneal Metastasis

32

Hideaki Yano

Abstract

Colorectal peritoneal metastasis (CPM) used to be generally considered a systemic and fatal condition; however, it has been growingly accepted that CPM can still be a local disease rather than a systemic disease as analogous to liver or lung metastasis.

Cytoreductive surgery (CRS) combined with hyperthermic intraperitoneal chemotherapy (HIPEC) is now considered an optimal treatment for CPM with accumulating evidence. There is a good reason that CRS+HIPEC, widely accepted as a standard of care for pseudomyxoma peritonei (PMP), could be a viable option for CPM given a similarity between CPM and PMP.

Recent years have also seen that modern systemic chemotherapy with or without molecular targeted agents can be effective for CPM. It is possible that neoadjuvant or adjuvant chemotherapy combined with CRS+HIPEC could further improve outcomes.

Patient selection, utilising modern images and increasingly laparoscopy, is crucial. Particularly, diagnostic laparoscopy is likely to play a significant role in predicting the likelihood of achieving complete cytoreduction and assessing the peritoneal cancer index (PCI) score.

Keywords

Colorectal peritoneal metastasis · Cytoreductive surgery · Peritonectomy · HIPEC

32.1 Introduction

It is well established that in a certain number of patients with colorectal liver or lung metastasis cure can be achieved by metastasectomy. Likewise, some cases with colorectal peritoneal metastasis (CPM) may present as local spread rather than systemic spread and may be amenable to cure by surgical resection.

It can be safely said that the treatment that has the most evidence and is therefore believed to be optimal for CPM is cytoreductive surgery (CRS) in the form of peritonectomy combined with hyperthermic intraperitoneal chemotherapy (HIPEC) [1].

CRS+HIPEC has already been established as a standard of care for pseudomyxoma peritonei (PMP) [2] and is now considered the most reliable treatment for CPM considering the similarity between PMP and CPM.

H. Yano
Division of Colorectal Surgery, Department of Surgery, National Center for Global Health and Medicine, Tokyo, Japan
e-mail: yano-tky@umin.ac.jp

© Springer Nature Singapore Pte Ltd. 2018
N. K. Kim et al. (eds.), *Surgical Treatment of Colorectal Cancer*,
https://doi.org/10.1007/978-981-10-5143-2_32

32.2 Conventional Treatment of Synchronous Colorectal Peritoneal Metastasis

According to the Japanese national colorectal cancer registry that accumulated 25,612 cases between 2000 and 2004, the incidence of peritoneal metastasis at the time of diagnosis/surgery (synchronous peritoneal metastasis) was 4.5%, second most to liver metastasis (10.9%), followed by lung metastasis (2.4%) [3].

The majority of colorectal cancers with synchronous peritoneal metastasis presents with symptoms, such as bleeding or obstruction. Therefore, resection of primary cancers is justified unless the patients are too unfit or there are anatomical limitations, e.g. (a) ascending or transverse colon cancer where the primary tumours or metastatic nodes massively invade the duodenum or pancreas, (b) rectosigmoid or rectal cancers that massively invades the bladder or prostate, etc.

Possible clinical scenarios would be (a) peritoneal involvement was suspected on preoperative CT or PET scans and extensive peritoneal involvement was confirmed on surgery where the primary tumour was removed to palliate symptoms (bleeding, obstruction, etc.) unless too unfit or extensive local spread, otherwise only bypass or stoma was fashioned; or (b) limited to moderate peritoneal involvement was established unexpectedly only on surgery where both primary and peritoneal tumours were removed (R1) or only primary tumours were removed (R2). And then systemic chemotherapy would be given postoperatively (as adjuvant if R1) wherever possible.

Potential problems in those scenarios in relation to CRS+HIPEC would be (a) systemic chemotherapy is considered to be less effective for peritoneal metastasis than for liver or lung metastasis; (b) the rate of 'curative' resection, and the possibility of achieving cure, is extremely low and could be improved by CRS+HIPEC; (c) it is possible that the resection of primary tumours in the presence of macroscopic peritoneal deposits could induce the implantation of tumour cells onto the newly created raw surfaces; and (d) the increasing use of laparoscopic or robotic surgery could be detrimental to the diagnosis and treatment of peritoneal metastasis because of misdiagnosis of small peritoneal nodules or inadequate dissection as a result of its limited operative views.

Therefore, new treatment strategies could be more judicious which include (a) delayed and scheduled CRS+HIPEC where the primary tumour is deliberately left in situ with either stenting or stoma formation and definitive CRS+HIPEC is performed following 3–6 months of systemic ± intraperitoneal chemotherapy; (b) upfront HIPEC where HIPEC is given at the time of surgery provided R1 surgery is achieved; or (c) second-look HIPEC where a second-look laparotomy is performed after 6–12 months of initial surgery where CRS+HIPEC is performed if peritoneal disease is found or otherwise HIPEC only.

32.3 Conventional Treatment of Metachronous Colorectal Peritoneal Metastasis

Amongst all the differences between peritoneal and other distant metastases/recurrences is the difficulty of radiological imaging studies. By utilising CT, MRI and PET, the diagnosis can be made fairly easily and, moreover, even its surgical resectability can now be predicted quite accurately in liver or lung metastasis, which strikes a sharp contrast to peritoneal metastasis. As a result, metachronous CPM tend to be detected at a later stage.

In order to achieve early discovery and early intervention, the identification of high-risk patients who will be likely to develop peritoneal recurrence and the proactive use of diagnostic laparoscopy are crucial with a caveat that it might be controversial whether early discovery will actually lead to better survival as is the case with liver or lung metastasis.

32.4 Systemic Chemotherapy

Although various novel agents have been introduced and have proven to be effective for the management of metastatic colorectal cancer, evidence is lacking in the efficacy of modern chemotherapy regimens including FOLFOX and FOLFIRI in combination with molecular-targeted agents such as cetuximab, panitumumab and bevacizumab in patients with CPM. None of the large-scale clinical trials that evaluated modern systemic chemotherapy have reported response or survival specific to patients with CPM. It is likely that because such trials recruit only patients with evaluable lesions where reliable measurements of tumour size are available on X-ray, CT or MRI, patients with CPM are usually excluded. Hence, limited evidence is available on the response and survival associated with systemic chemotherapy for patients with CPM.

CPM has generally been considered to carry poorer prognosis compared to liver or lung metastasis. Franko et al. analysed 2095 patients with metastatic colorectal cancer who were recruited in a large-scale clinical trial. They found the median survival time of 12.7 months in patients with CPM which was significantly shorter than 17.6 months in patients without CPM [4].

32.5 Surgical Treatment

A surgical approach combining CRS and HIPEC is gaining acceptance in the oncologic community as a treatment option for patients with CPM. This treatment was first described by Spratt et al. in 1980 [5] before being further developed by Paul Sugarbaker of the Washington Cancer Institute in the 1900s [6].

This procedure involves stripping of the diseased peritoneum (peritonectomy) with multiple visceral resections, performed with an aim of achieving macroscopic tumour removal. Then, prior to any intestinal anastomosis, a heated chemotherapeutic agent is administered and perfused in the abdomen for a certain period of time to chemically sterilise all peritoneal surfaces (usually mitomycin C or oxaliplatin for 30–60 min at the temperature of 41–43 °C). HIPEC allows a high local concentration of a cytotoxic drug with minimal systemic adverse effect thereby aiming to achieve microscopic

tumour removal. Hyperthermia has been demonstrated to have a synergistic effect with chemotherapy and thus enhance the cytotoxicity of the drug [7].

To reiterate, the rationale behind CRS+HIPEC for CPM revolves around (a) the analogy between CPM and PMP and (b) the higher surgical curability of colorectal cancer in general than any other gastrointestinal malignancies.

Factors that preclude CRS+HIPEC generally include gross involvement of the (a) small bowel and its mesentery; (b) retroperitoneum, particularly ureters; and (c) hepatoduodenal ligament and porta hepatis.

In recent years, there has been accumulating evidence of the efficacy and safety of CRS+HIPEC for CPM. In summary, it is increasingly known that (a) CRS+HIPEC can confer 5-year survival of 30–40% in selected patients, (b) better survival is achieved in patients with less peritoneal involvement, (c) CRS+HIPEC is associated with 12% of morbidity and with less than 1% of mortality in experienced teams and (d) favourable outcomes continue to be reported globally [1].

Recent major studies reporting outcomes of CRS+HIPEC are summarised in Table 32.1. The median survival of patients undergoing CRS+HIPEC was 33 (range, 22–63) months. The median 1-, 2-, 3- and 5-year survival rates were 85% (range, 70–94%), 65% (range, 45–81%), 46% (range, 44–62%) and 40% (29–51%), respectively [8–16]. In highly selected patients with limited CPM, the median survival may be as high as 63 months and 5-year survival as high as 51% as reported by Elias et al. [13].

Much has been learnt from these clinical trials, with the development of staging systems in the form of preoperative/intraoperative scoring to aid selection in order to improve outcomes. Completeness of cytoreduction and the extent of CPM are universally the most important prognostic factors. Peritoneal cancer index (PCI, range 0–39) is the most widely spread scoring system (Fig. 32.1) to describe the extent of CPM, which not only predicts the likelihood of complete cytoreduction but also is a strong prognosticator in patients with a complete cytoreduction. The

Table 32.1 CRS+HIPEC for colorectal peritoneal metastasis

Principal investigators	Reference number	Year of publication	Countries	Period of accrual	Number of patients	Median survival time (months)	1-year survival (%)	2-year survival (%)	3-year survival (%)	5-year survival (%)
Zoetmulder	8	2003	Netherlands	1998–2001	39	22	70	45	–	–
Verwaal	9	2005	Netherlands	1995–2003	59	43	94	–	56	43
Msika	10	2007	France	1996–2006	30	38	–	72	–	44
Bartlett	11	2008	USA	2001–2007	36	–	85	–	45	–
Levine	12	2008	USA	1992–2005	30	41	–	–	62	36
Elias	13	2009	France	1998–2003	48	63	–	81	–	51
Morris	14	2009	Australia	1997–2008	54	33	87	70	44	–
Elias	15	2010	French multicentre	1990–2007	439	33	85	60	45	29
Cavaliere	16	2011	Italian multicentre	1995–2007	124	25	83	50	–	–

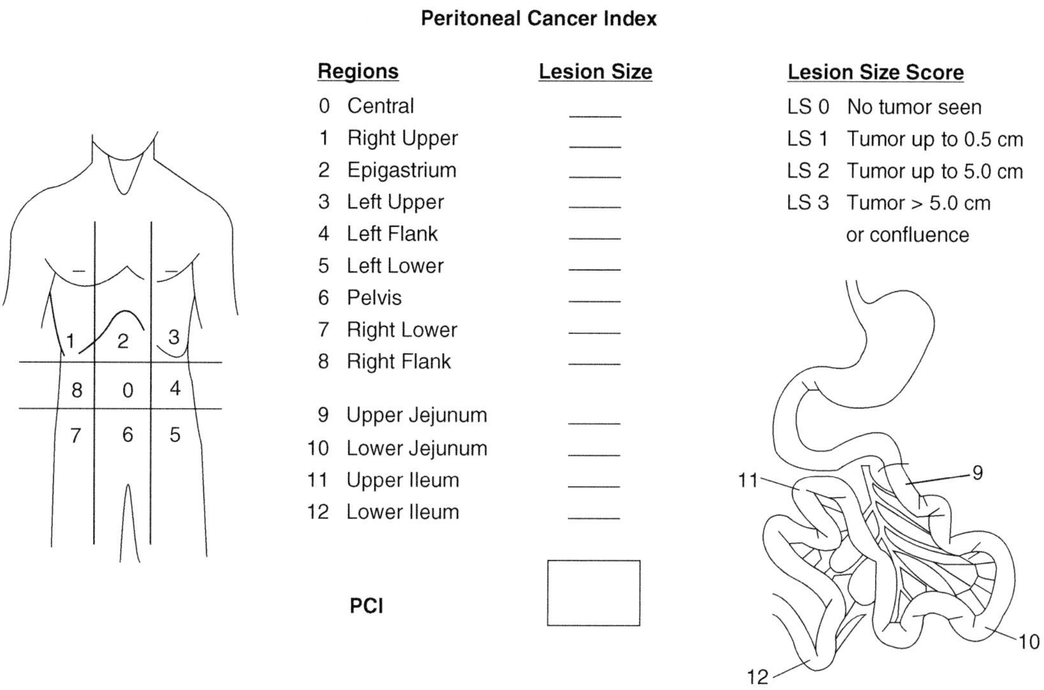

Peritoneal Cancer Index

Regions	Lesion Size	Lesion Size Score
0 Central	____	LS 0 No tumor seen
1 Right Upper	____	LS 1 Tumor up to 0.5 cm
2 Epigastrium	____	LS 2 Tumor up to 5.0 cm
3 Left Upper	____	LS 3 Tumor > 5.0 cm
4 Left Flank	____	or confluence
5 Left Lower	____	
6 Pelvis	____	
7 Right Lower	____	
8 Right Flank	____	
9 Upper Jejunum	____	
10 Lower Jejunum	____	
11 Upper Ileum	____	
12 Lower Ileum	____	

PCI

Fig. 32.1 Peritoneal cancer index (PCI)

5-year survival ranged from 44% in patients with a low PCI (<6), 22% in patients with a PCI [7–12] to 7% in patients with a high PCI (>19) [15]. Currently, a PCI >20 should be considered as a contraindication for CRS+HIPEC.

The combination of major surgery and HIPEC in patients with CPM carries significant morbidity (16–65%) and mortality (0–16%) [17]. Perioperative complications include intraabdominal haemorrhage, anastomotic leak or fistula, respiratory failure, venous thromboembolism and haematological toxicity associated with HIPEC occurs in 8–31% [18]. A learning curve exists in this major operation, and according to the most recent reports, the mortality is less than 1% in experienced hands.

With the accumulating evidence including a randomised controlled trial [8], a few multi-institutional registries [19] and innumerable case series, the efficacy of CRS+HIPEC for CPM is described in a number of national guidelines. The Netherlands, France, Germany, Spain, the UK, Norway, Korea and Italy have all clearly stated that selected patients should be treated at experienced centres. The National Institute of Care and Excellence (NICE), UK, states in its guidance (IPG 331) that current evidence on the efficacy of cytoreduction surgery (CRS) followed by hyperthermic intraoperative peritoneal chemotherapy (HIPEC) for peritoneal carcinomatosis shows some improvement in survival for selected patients with colorectal metastases, but evidence is limited for other types of cancer. It also states that the evidence on safety shows significant risks of morbidity and mortality which need to be balanced against the perceived benefit for each patient and that, therefore, this procedure should only be used with special arrangements for clinical governance, consent and audit or research [20].

32.6 Multimodal Treatment

It is logically reasonable to try to combine the novel chemotherapy and the aggressive surgery, namely, CRS+HIPEC. In the recent COMBATAC trial, after the primary cancers are removed by laparotomy or laparoscopy, the patients are given

3–6 months of chemotherapy and undergo CRS+HIPEC followed by postoperative chemotherapy [21].

32.7 Second-Look HIPEC

A further emerging concept is 'second-look' at 6–12 months for patients at high risk of CPM based on perforated primary tumours (T4), resected Krukenberg ovarian metastases or resected localised peritoneal disease at the primary operation. Forty-one high-risk patients had systemic chemotherapy and underwent second-look laparotomy at 6–12 months after primary surgery [22]. Low-volume resectable peritoneal metastases were present in 23 patients (56%), who subsequently underwent CRS+HIPEC; and no macroscopic disease was present in the remaining 18 patients (44%), who underwent HIPEC alone [22].

These promising results led to the prospective multicentre trial ProphyloCHIP, in which patients at high risk of CPM after resection of primary tumour and who are receiving standard oxaliplatin-based adjuvant chemotherapy will be randomised to surveillance alone or systematic exploratory laparotomy plus HIPEC. The primary outcome measure is the 3-year disease-free survival, and the secondary outcome measures are the 3- and 5-year overall survivals.

32.8 Prophylactic/Adjuvant/ Upfront HIPEC

Prophylactic/adjuvant/upfront HIPEC may be appropriate for some of the patients who are at high risk of CPM after initial surgery. At institutions where HIPEC is available at the time of primary colorectal cancer resection, the primary resection is augmented intraoperatively by complete cytoreductive surgery. Not only the bowel resection but also greater and lesser omentectomy and oophorectomy in women are required. Prior to the intestinal reconstruction, HIPEC is administered. After HIPEC, the bowel anastomosis is performed and the abdomen is closed.

These patients then receive intensive adjuvant chemotherapy.

It is thought that the intraoperative chemotherapy combined with a primary colon cancer resection is of very low morbidity and carries no mortality. Patients who might benefit from upfront HIPEC include those with a tumour perforation (T4), a positive peritoneal cytology, adjacent organ involvement or fistula formation and rupture of the primary cancer during the resection.

A couple of trial are ongoing in the Netherlands, Spain and Italy.

Conclusion

Recent results suggest that judicious selection of patients (e.g. PCI <20) for CRS+HIPEC is crucial and CRS+HIPEC is likely to be superior to the current best systemic chemotherapy. Integrated treatment strategy combining systemic chemotherapy and CRS+HIPEC appears to be most effective.

As we await the results of ongoing trials, we must continue to commit to future trials that will contribute to the body of evidence to support CRS+HIPEC. A neoadjuvant trial by the German group to investigate the role of preoperative systemic chemotherapy prior to CRS+HIPEC will allow us to determine if neoadjuvant chemotherapy may facilitate cytoreductive surgery by downstaging the peritoneal disease burden and thereby improve survival. In addition, the role of prophylactic HIPEC for patients at high risk of CPM requires to be elucidated.

References

1. Sugarbaker PH, Ryan DP. Cytoreductive surgery plus hyperthermic perioperative chemotherapy to treat peritoneal metastases from colorectal cancer: standard of care or an experimental approach? Lancet Oncol. 2012;13(8):362–9.
2. Sugarbaker PH. New standard of care for appendiceal epithelial neoplasms and pseudomyxoma peritonei syndrome? Lancet Oncol. 2006;7(1):69–76.
3. Watanabe T, Muro K, Ajioka Y, et al. Japanese Society for Cancer of the Colon and Rectum (JSCCR) guidelines 2016 for the treatment of colorectal cancer. Int

J Clin Oncol. 2017. doi: https://doi.org/10.1007/s10147-017-1101-6. [Epub ahead of print].

4. Franko J, Shi Q, Goldman CD, et al. Treatment of colorectal peritoneal carcinomatosis with systemic chemotherapy: a pooled analysis of north central cancer treatment group phase III trials N9741 and N9841. J Clin Oncol. 2012;30:263–7.

5. Spratt JS, Adcock RA, Muscovin M, Sherrill W, McKeown J. Clinical delivery system for intraperitoneal hyperthermic chemotherapy. Cancer Res. 1980;40:256–26.

6. Sugarbaker PH. Peritonectomy procedures. Ann Surg. 1995;221:29–42.

7. van de Vaart PJ, van der Vange N, Zoetmulder FA, et al. Intraperitoneal cisplatin with regional hyperthermia in advanced ovarian cancer: Pharmacokinetics and cisplatin-DNA adduct formation in patients and ovarian cancer cell lines. Eur J Cancer. 34(1):148–54, 199.

8. Verwaal VJ, van Ruth S, de Bree E, et al. Randomized trial of cytoreduction and hyperthermic intraperitoneal chemotherapy versus systemic chemotherapy and palliative surgery in patients with peritoneal carcinomatosis of colorectal cancer. J Clin Oncol. 2003;21(20):3737–43.

9. Verwaal VJ, van Ruth S, Witkamp A, et al. Long-term survival of peritoneal carcinomatosis of colorectal origin. Ann Surg Oncol. 2005;12(1):65–71.

10. Kianmanesh R, Scaringi S, Sabate JM, et al. Iterative cytoreductive surgery associated with hyperthermic intraperitoneal chemotherapy for treatment of peritoneal carcinomatosis of colorectal origin with or without liver metastases. Ann Surg. 2007;245(4):597–603.

11. Franko J, Gusani NJ, Holtzman MP, et al. Multivisceral resection does not affect morbidity and survival after cytoreductive surgery and chemoperfusion for carcinomatosis from colorectal cancer. Ann Surg Oncol. 2008;15(11):3065–72.

12. Shen P, Thai K, Stewart JH, et al. Peritoneal surface disease from colorectal cancer: comparison with the hepatic metastases surgical paradigm in optimally resected patients. Ann Surg Oncol. 2008;15(12):3422–32.

13. Elias D, Lefevre JH, Chevalier J, et al. Complete cytoreductive surgery plus intraperitoneal chemohyperthermia with oxaliplatin for peritoneal carcinomatosis of colorectal origin. J Clin Oncol. 2009;27(5):681–5.

14. Chua TC, Yan TD, Ng KM, Zhao J, et al. Significance of lymph node metastasis in patients with colorectal cancer peritoneal carcinomatosis. World J Surg. 2009;33(7):1488–94.

15. Elias D, Gilly F, Boutitie F, et al. Peritoneal colorectal carcinomatosis treated with surgery and perioperative intraperitoneal chemotherapy: retrospective analysis of 523 patients from a multicentric french study. J Clin Oncol. 2010;28(1):63–8.

16. Cavaliere F, De Simone M, Virzi S, et al. Prognostic factors and oncologic outcome in 146 patients with colorectal peritoneal carcinomatosis treated with cytoreductive surgery combined with hyperthermic intraperitoneal chemotherapy: Italian multicenter study S.I.T.I.L.O. Eur J Surg Oncol. 2011;37(2):148–54.

17. Younan R, Kusamura S, Baratti D, et al. Morbidity, toxicity, and mortality classification systems in the local regional treatment of peritoneal surface malignancy. J Surg Oncol. 2008;98(4):253–7.

18. Chua TC, Yan TD, Saxena A, et al. Should the treatment of peritoneal carcinomatosis by cytoreductive surgery and hyperthermic intraperitoneal chemotherapy still be regarded as a highly morbid procedure?: a systematic review of morbidity and mortality. Ann Surg. 2009;249(6):900–7.

19. Glehen O, Kwiatkowski F, Sugarbaker PH, et al. Cytoreductive surgery combined with perioperative intraperitoneal chemotherapy for the management of peritoneal carcinomatosis from colorectal cancer: a multi-institutional study. J Clin Oncol. 2004;22(16):3284–92.

20. IPG331. Cytoreduction surgery followed by hyperthermic intraoperative peritoneal chemotherapy for peritoneal carcinomatosis. NICE Guidance. National Institute for Health and Care Excellence. http://www.nice.org.uk/guidance/ipg331.

21. Glockzin G, Rochon J, Arnold D, et al. A prospective multicenter phase II study evaluating multimodality treatment of patients with peritoneal carcinomatosis arising from appendiceal and colorectal cancer: the COMBATAC trial. BMC Cancer. 2013;13:67. https://doi.org/10.1186/1471-2407-13-67.

22. Elias D, Honore C, Dumont F, Ducreux M, Boige V, Malka D, et al. Results of systematic second look surgery plus HIPEC in asymptomatic patients presenting a high risk of developing colorectal peritoneal carcinomatosis. Ann Surg. 2011;254:289–93.

Hepatic Metastasis

33

Albert Chan

Abstract

Colorectal cancer is the third most common cancer in the world. About 30–50% of the patients with colorectal cancer would develop liver metastasis in the course of their illness. About one-third of the metastatic liver lesions (CRM) are considered to be resectable, and long-term cure is not infrequently observed. Advances in the surgical management of CRM have certainly improved the chance of resection in recent years. While the selection criteria for open resection is becoming well established in most centers globally, the introduction of laparoscopy to liver resection has shown to be safe and feasible in many recent reported series. The controversy around the optimal approach for synchronous CRM remains unresolved, but the inception of laparoscopic liver surgery has favored the approach with simultaneous resections, especially when left lateral sectionectomy or other minor liver resections are required. On the other hand, various approaches have been proposed to improve the resectability rate for bilobar CRM. A two-stage hepatectomy was associated with a 5-year overall survival rate of up to 30–40%. Alternatively, the recently popular-ized ALPPS procedure conferred a 2-year overall survival rate of over 50%. For unre-sectable bilobar CRM, liver transplantation has been proposed to be an effective treatment under stringent selection criteria that, in turn, offered a 5-year overall survival rate up to 60%. A randomized control trial to compare its efficacy with resection is currently under-way, and the outcome of this study will be of significance to ascertain its role in the surgical management of CRM.

Keywords

Hepatectomy · ALPPS · Laparoscopy · Liver transplantation · Colorectal liver metastasis

33.1 Introduction

Colorectal cancer is the third most common cancer in the world. It is expected that 30–50% of the patients with colorectal cancer would develop liver metastasis in the course of their illness [1, 2]. Among them, 25–31% of patients with metastatic liver tumors were considered to be resectable [3], and long-term survival was not infrequently achievable [4, 5]. It is for this reason that colorectal liver metastasis, even though was regarded as a stage IV disease, is no longer considered to be unsalvageable and every effort should be made to increase the chance for

A. Chan
Department of Surgery, The University of Hong Kong, Queen Mary Hospital, Hong Kong, China
e-mail: acchan@hku.hk

© Springer Nature Singapore Pte Ltd. 2018
N. K. Kim et al. (eds.), *Surgical Treatment of Colorectal Cancer*,
https://doi.org/10.1007/978-981-10-5143-2_33

resection in this patient. The current chapter will offer an update on the latest development in the surgical management of colorectal liver metastasis.

33.2 Indications for Resections

Careful preoperative planning is mandatory to ensure a safe outcome for major liver resection in colorectal liver metastasis, especially for patients after preoperative chemotherapy due to the potential hepatotoxicity of the chemotherapeutic agents. Performance of indocyanine green clearance test and volumetric evaluation of the future liver remnant by either computed tomography or magnetic resonance imaging are becoming routine tests for preoperative liver function assessment in many Asian centers. The objective of resection is to achieve complete tumor clearance with a negative resection margin. Margin involvement has been recognized as an important factor to affect survival. A recent study from Johns Hopkins Hospital showed that the 5-year overall survivals after resection of liver metastasis with a negative margin were significantly better than those with positive margins (54.9% vs. 36.2%, $p = 0.005$) [6]. In another study by Jung et al., a positive resection margin was attributable to early recurrence and deaths within 6 months after surgery [7].

The criteria for major liver resection, i.e., more than two Couinaud's segments are as follows:

- Future liver remnant volume: more than 30% standard liver volume or more than 40% standard liver volume if preoperative chemotherapy was given
- Serum platelet count $\geq 100 \times 10^9$/L
- Indocyanine green clearance rate $\leq 17\%$ at 15 min
- Normal liver function or Child's A cirrhosis

Unlike resection for hepatocellular carcinoma when anatomical resection is favored due to the mode of tumor spread via the portal circulation, it remained debatable if the same principle is applied to colorectal liver metastasis. In a recent meta-analysis that involved 2505 patients in 12 studies with colorectal liver metastasis undergoing resections, no difference in survival was observed between parenchymal-sparing resection and anatomical resections with a 5-year overall survival of 44.7% and 44.6%, respectively ($p = 0.97$) [8]. From the oncological perspective, as far as a R0 resection is achieved either by parenchymal-sparing or anatomical resection, overall survival is not significantly affected, but the chance for repeated resection would be higher for parenchymal-sparing resection if second intrahepatic recurrence was developed [9].

33.3 Laparoscopic Liver Resection

With the recent advances in visualization technology (Fig. 33.1) and hemostatic devices for minimally invasive surgery, there has been a substantial increase in the number of laparoscopic liver resections performed globally [10, 11]. When compared with open resections, laparoscopic approach was associated with less blood loss and shorter hospital stay (Fig. 33.2), with similar oncological outcome with respect to margin status, disease-free as well as overall survival [12–14]. In the recent Morioka consensus statement, minor wedge resection and left lateral sectionectomy via laparoscopic approach has been accepted as the standard of practice [15]. In fact, complete laparoscopic resection for both primary colorectal cancer and synchronous liver metastasis in one operation has been recently shown to be feasible with low postoperative morbidity rate and reduced hospital stay. Left lateral sectionectomy is being reported as the most common type of resection (about 70% of all cases) performed so far [16, 17]. With cumulative experience in advanced laparoscopic liver resection, simultaneous total laparoscopic major liver resection with colorectal resection will very much likely become an area of clinical interest in the near future. Factors favorable for laparoscopic major hepatectomy include:

- Future liver remnant $\geq 40\%$ standard liver volume
- Single, long ipsilateral portal vein

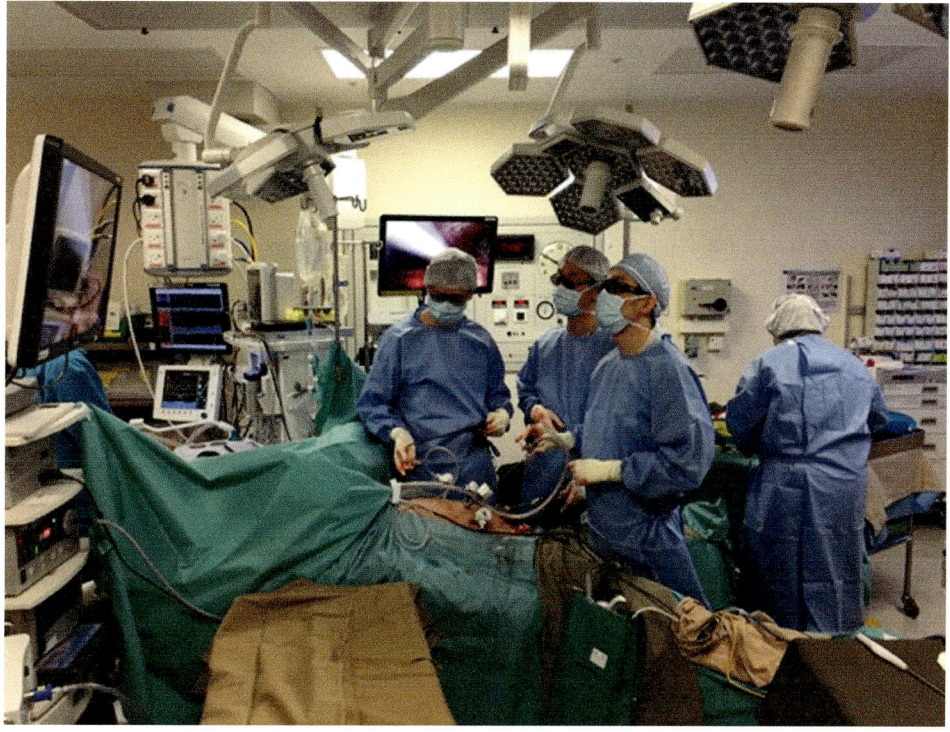

Fig. 33.1 Operating room settings for right hepatectomy by 3D laparoscopy. 3D visualization technology improves the depth perception which is beneficial for hepatic parenchymal transection in major hepatectomy

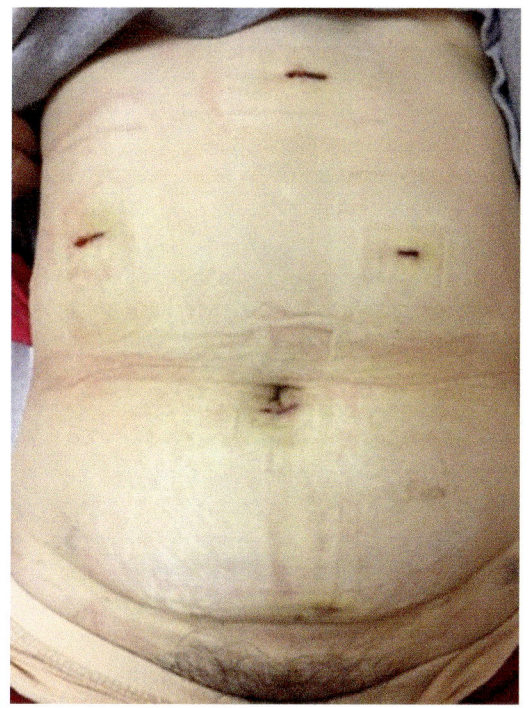

Fig. 33.2 Postoperative wounds after a 3D laparoscopic right hepatectomy. The liver specimen was retrieved via a Pfannenstiel incision

- Fewer than three retrohepatic vein tributaries
- Tumor size ≤5 cm
- Central-locating tumors or tumors located away from the paracaval region

33.4   Prognostic Factors for Overall Survival After Resection of Liver Metastasis

A resection margin free of microscopic tumor involvement remained the most important prognostic factors for survival [6, 18]. Other factors which include the size of liver metastasis, number of metastasis, lymph node status of colorectal cancer, synchronous or metachronous liver metastasis, preoperative CEA levels, and response to chemotherapy have been identified as prognostic factors in different studies [19–21]. All these parameters have been factored into formulation of different clinical scoring systems such as the Fong's score [22], Nordlinger group [23], Nagashima's system [24], Rees preoperative and postoperative risk indices [25], etc.

Nonetheless, none of these clinical scoring systems have been showed to be accurate in the determination of 10-year survival, which should be regarded as "cure" for the disease [26]. Obviously a more sophisticated system with inclusion of biomarkers to improve its prognosis prediction accuracy would be an area of interest for future research developments.

33.5   Preoperative Chemotherapy

The anticipated benefits of preoperative chemotherapy are threefolds: (1) to downsize the tumor in order to reduce the magnitude of hepatectomy, (2) to treat micrometastatic disease, and (3) to test for tumor chemosensitivity. However, the pitfalls of preoperative chemotherapy could increase the vascularity of the liver tissues, hence increasing the chance of intraoperative blood transfusion during liver resection [27], or could induce liver damage such as steatohepatitis with associated thrombocytopenia and splenomegaly that could subsequently increase the risk of postoperative liver failure. While the use of oxaliplatin of more than six cycles was associated with sinusoidal occlusive syndrome (SOS) aka veno-occlusive disease, irinotecan was known to be associated with nonalcoholic steatohepatitis (NASH), and the administration of anti-VEGF (vasoactive endothelial growth factor) predisposes to impaired wound healing. Hence, timing of the operation is important as it determined the outcome of surgery. The longer duration of preoperative chemotherapy, the more likely the liver would undergo irreversible histological changes. Previous studies have shown that the risk of postoperative complications increased when more than six cycles of chemotherapy is received [27, 28]. Prolonged liver damage in the form of NASH would increase the risk of postoperative liver failure after hepatectomy, especially in the form of major liver resection. In our center, liver resection is usually performed after the fourth or the fifth cycle of chemotherapy. Nonetheless, there was yet sufficient data to support the survival benefit of preoperative chemotherapy [29]. In the EORTC intergroup trial 40983 studying FOLFOX 4 (folinic acid, fluorouracil, and oxaliplatin) that involved 364 patients with up to 4 liver metastases in Europe, Australia, and Hong Kong, there was a lack of survival benefit between those received preoperative chemotherapy and surgery alone, with a 5-year overall survival of 51.2% and 41.8%, respectively [30]. Other studies, however, showed that preoperative chemotherapy may be beneficial when there is more extensive tumor burden with more than five liver metastases or bilobar diseases [31, 32].

33.6   Simultaneous Versus Staged Operation for Synchronous Colorectal Liver Metastasis

For patients with synchronous colorectal liver metastasis, whether simultaneous resections (i.e., resection of both liver metastasis and primary colorectal cancer within one operation) or staged operation (i.e., resection of the primary cancer first and then interval liver resection after 3–4 weeks) should be the standard approach remains controversial. There are two schools of thought behind both strategies: for simultaneous resection, patients enjoyed the benefit of complete tumor clearance in one operation within one hospitalization; proponents for staged resection argued that the interval waiting period allowed time for any occult metastasis to become apparent, and, more importantly, the waiting period in itself is deployed as a selection test for tumor biology. Recent meta-analyses in fact showed simultaneous resection did not confer inferior results to staged resections in terms of postoperative morbidity and mortality, hospital stay, and disease-free and overall survival [33, 34]. Our experience, however, showed that simultaneous resection conferred a worsened overall survival than staged resection despite similar postoperative morbidity and mortality, possibly due to a lack of selection for more favorable tumor biology in the simultaneous resection. However, the overall survival between two operating strategies became similar when only solitary liver metastasis was present [35]. Besides, consideration should also be given to the general condition, the presence of medical comorbidities, and types of liver resections when deciding the most appropriate strategies for the patients. Most of the studies that favored the adoption of simultaneous resections entailed minor liver resections only. In a recent meta-analysis by Yin et al., factors that favored simultaneous resection were resections of no more than three liver segments, younger than 70 years old, and no pre-existing medical comorbidities [34].

33.7 ALPPS vs. Two-Staged Hepatectomy

33.7.1 Two-Staged Hepatectomy (TSH) for Bilobar Liver Metastases

A TSH approach comprises resection of metastasis in one hemi-liver during the first hepatectomy followed by tumor clearance in the contralateral hemi-liver at a later stage with a curative intent. For instance, if the main tumor burden is in the right liver (*right first*), right hepatectomy could be first performed in the first hepatectomy followed by tumor clearance in the left remnant liver at a later stage. Alternatively, multiple wedge resection of metastasis could be first performed in the left liver followed by a right portal vein ligation if the left liver is considered small in volume (*left first*). A right hepatectomy is then undertaken at a later stage when the left liver remnant undergoes adequate hypertrophy. The first-stage hepatectomy could also be undertaken simultaneously with the colorectal resection in order to reduce the number of surgical treatments [36], and chemotherapy could be administered in between the two stages to prevent concomitant stimulation of tumor growth by the release of growth factors during liver regeneration. About 70% of the patients will be able to proceed to the second stage [37]. Morbidity rate was generally higher after the second-stage operation than the first stage probably due to the

technical challenges related to reoperation and adhesions. Postoperative morbidity and mortality rate after the second-stage operation was 40% and 3% [37]. The 5-year disease-free and overall survivals after TSH were 11–13% and 32–42%, respectively [38, 39].

33.7.2 ALPPS for Colorectal Liver Metastasis

Associating liver partition and portal vein ligation for staged hepatectomy (ALPPS) has been regarded as one of the major breakthroughs in the development of liver surgery in recent years [40, 41]. This novel procedure which was first discovered incidentally by Professor Hans Schlitt from Germany [42] during the surgical management of a patient with hilar cholangiocarcinoma was later popularized by the German surgical community for the management of bilobar colorectal liver metastasis when an insufficient future liver remnant was expected after extensive liver resections [43]. ALPPS comprises a two-stage operation [44]: the first stage entails right portal vein ligation and an in situ liver split, and tumor clearance in the future liver remnant is also performed during stage I operation (Fig. 33.3); the future liver remnant undergoes rapid hypertrophy thereafter, and the second-stage operation which usually takes place between 7 and 10 days after the stage I operation is to be performed when the future liver remnant hypertrophied to more than 40% of the standard liver volume. One of the major criticisms for this novel procedure during its early phase of clinical inception was the high incidence of sepsis due to biliary leakage and postoperative mortality rate. With cumulative experience, the postoperative morbidity and mortality rate has been reduced to 7.7–40.0% [45, 46] and 6.6–8.8% [47, 48], respectively. According to the International ALPPS registry, almost 1000 cases of ALPPS have been performed globally. The 2-year overall survival rate for ALPPS in colorectal liver metastasis was estimated to be 59% [49].

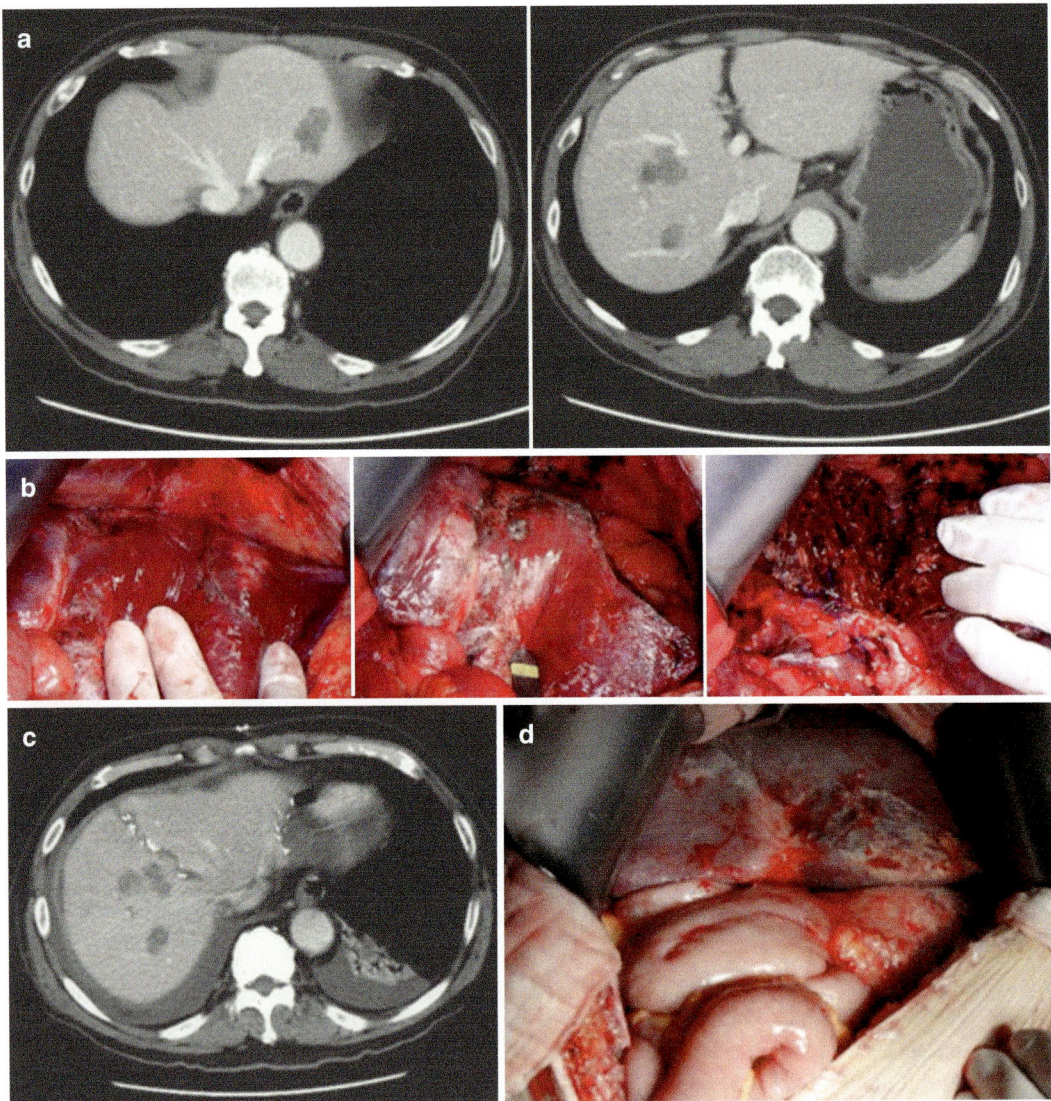

Fig. 33.3 A 69-year-old patient with bilobar liver metastasis. (**a**) S3 + S4 volumetry was 129 mL, 10.5% ESLV; (**b**) Stage I ALPPS + segment II resection; (**c**) CT volumetry S3+4 = 628 mL, 50.8% ESLV after ALPPS stage I; (**d**) right hepatectomy was completed in stage II operation

33.7.3 TSH Versus ALPPS for Bilobar Liver Metastasis

Whether there is any difference in short-term as well as long-term outcome between TSH and ALPPS for the management of bilobar liver metastasis remained largely unknown. One study of 56 patients which compared the two groups based on their own experience in France showed that while there was no significant difference in terms of postoperative morbidity and mortality, overall survival tended to be worse after ALPPS with a higher rate of intrahepatic recurrence. However, reoperation for salvage was more frequently performed for TSH than ALPPS [50].

33.8 Liver Transplantation for Unresectable Liver Metastasis

Liver transplantation for metastatic cancer from primary tumor of non-neuroendocrine origin was once regarded as an absolute contraindication due to the perceived risk of tumor recurrence as a result of prolonged immunosuppression. However, results from the Oslo group have attracted a lot of interests within the liver surgery community in recent years [51]. In this pilot study of 21 patients with non-resectable colorectal liver metastasis who have gone through a prior 6-week course of chemotherapy, a 3- and 5-year overall survival of 68% and 60% was observed. A follow-up study from the same group that compared with another cohort of patients receiving first-line chemotherapy alone showed that the 5-year overall survival rate after liver transplantation was far better than chemotherapy alone (56% vs. 9%) [51]. It was postulated that the pattern of disease recurrence attributed to the survival benefit of liver transplantation: while patients developed small and slow-growing lung metastasis after liver transplantation, patients in the chemotherapy group often died from progression of the underlying unresectable liver metastasis. Recent study showed that the survival benefit of liver transplantation even extended to include patients with liver-only metastatic lesions who failed on last-line chemotherapy with a 5-year overall survival of 44% [51]. Nonetheless, application of liver transplantation to unresectable liver metastasis remained an investigational procedure at the time of writing and should be limited to university-affiliated hospitals under a trial setting. It was worthwhile to highlight that the choice of graft for these studies were deceased whole grafts. The problem of graft shortage especially in Asia will affect the practical applicability of this procedure. Living donor liver transplantation which flourishes in Asia will provide an alternative option for graft supply, but donor expectation and the ethical issues between donor risks and early disease recurrence will need to be addressed before such program becomes feasible.

33.9 Liver Transplantation for Resectable Liver Metastasis

Whether liver transplantation offers the best hope of cure for colorectal liver metastasis remains to be seen. A randomized control trial comparing liver transplantation and liver resection (ClinialTrials.gov: NCT01311453) is being undertaken by the same group in Oslo, and the results will be eagerly awaited for.

Conclusion

Resection of colorectal liver metastasis certainly provides the only realistic hope for long-term cure, and every effort should be made to ensure a proper evaluation for resection. Different operative strategies have evolved over the years in attempt to improve the resectability of bilobar liver metastasis. Careful patient selection with regard to patient factor as well as liver and tumor factor is an essential element to ensure reasonable long-term survival after surgery. The concept of deploying liver transplantation for unresectable bilobar liver metastasis is interesting, and its role in the surgical management of this disease entity will become clearer in the coming years. A multidisciplinary approach between colorectal surgeons, liver surgeons, radiologists, and oncologists should be regarded as the standard of care for all patients with colorectal liver metastasis in the modern era.

References

1. Sharma S, Camci C, Jabbour N. Management of hepatic metastasis from colorectal cancers: an update. J Hepato-Biliary-Pancreat Surg. 2008;15(6):570–80.
2. Weiss L, Grundmann E, Torhorst J, Hartveit F, Moberg I, Eder M, et al. Haematogenous metastatic patterns in colonic carcinoma: an analysis of 1541 necropsies. J Pathol. 1986;150(3):195–203.
3. Akgul O, Cetinkaya E, Ersoz S, Tez M. Role of surgery in colorectal cancer liver metastases. World J Gastroenterol. 2014;20(20):6113–22.
4. Choti MA, Sitzmann JV, Tiburi MF, Sumetchotimetha W, Rangsin R, Schulick RD, et al. Trends in long-term

survival following liver resection for hepatic colorectal metastases. Ann Surg. 2002;235(6):759–66.

5. Brouquet A, Abdalla EK, Kopetz S, Garrett CR, Overman MJ, Eng C, et al. High survival rate after two-stage resection of advanced colorectal liver metastases: response-based selection and complete resection define outcome. J Clin Oncol. 2011;29(8):1083–90.

6. Sasaki K, Margonis GA, Andreatos N, Wilson A, Weiss M, Wolfgang C, et al. Prognostic impact of margin status in liver resections for colorectal metastases after bevacizumab. Br J Surg. 2017;104(7):926–35.

7. Jung SW, Kim DS, YD Y, Han JH, Suh SO. Risk factors for cancer recurrence or death within 6 months after liver resection in patients with colorectal cancer liver metastasis. Ann Surg Treat Res. 2016;90(5):257–64.

8. Moris D, Ronnekleiv-Kelly S, Rahnemai-Azar AA, Felekouras E, Dillhoff M, Schmidt C, et al. Parenchymal-sparing versus anatomic liver resection for colorectal liver metastases: a systematic review. J Gastrointest Surg. 2017;21(6):1076–85.

9. Pandanaboyana S, Bell R, White A, Pathak S, Hidalgo E, Lodge P, et al. Impact of parenchymal preserving surgery on survival and recurrence after liver resection for colorectal liver metastasis. ANZ J Surg. 2016. https://doi.org/10.1111/ans.13588.

10. Hibi T, Cherqui D, Geller DA, Itano O, Kitagawa Y, Wakabayashi G. Expanding indications and regional diversity in laparoscopic liver resection unveiled by the International Survey on Technical Aspects of Laparoscopic Liver Resection (INSTALL) study. Surg Endosc. 2016;30(7):2975–83.

11. Ciria R, Cherqui D, Geller DA, Briceno J, Wakabayashi G. Comparative short-term benefits of laparoscopic liver resection: 9000 cases and climbing. Ann Surg. 2016;263(4):761–77.

12. Beppu T, Wakabayashi G, Hasegawa K, Gotohda N, Mizuguchi T, Takahashi Y, et al. Long-term and perioperative outcomes of laparoscopic versus open liver resection for colorectal liver metastases with propensity score matching: a multi-institutional Japanese study. J Hepatobiliary Pancreat Sci. 2015;22(10):711–20.

13. Fretland AA, Dagenborg VJ, Bjornelv GMW, Kazaryan AM, Kristiansen R, Fagerland MW, et al. Laparoscopic versus open resection for colorectal liver metastases: the OSLO-COMET randomized controlled trial. Ann Surg. 2017. https://doi.org/10.1097/SLA.0000000000002353.

14. Martinez-Cecilia D, Cipriani F, Vishal S, Ratti F, Tranchart H, Barkhatov L, et al. Laparoscopic versus open liver resection for colorectal metastases in elderly and octogenarian patients: a multicenter propensity score based analysis of short- and long-term outcomes. Ann Surg. 2017;265(6):1192–200.

15. Wakabayashi G, Cherqui D, Geller DA, Buell JF, Kaneko H, Han HS, et al. Recommendations for laparoscopic liver resection: a report from the second international consensus conference held in Morioka. Ann Surg. 2015;261(4):619–29.

16. Polignano FM, Quyn AJ, Sanjay P, Henderson NA, Tait IS. Totally laparoscopic strategies for the management of colorectal cancer with synchronous liver metastasis. Surg Endosc. 2012;26(9):2571–8.

17. Lupinacci RM, Andraus W, De Paiva Haddad LB, Carneiro D' Albuquerque LA, Herman P. Simultaneous laparoscopic resection of primary colorectal cancer and associated liver metastases: a systematic review. Tech Coloproctol. 2014;18(2):129–35.

18. Dhir M, Lyden ER, Wang A, Smith LM, Ullrich F, Are C. Influence of margins on overall survival after hepatic resection for colorectal metastasis: a meta-analysis. Ann Surg. 2011;254(2):234–42.

19. Kato T, Yasui K, Hirai T, Kanemitsu Y, Mori T, Sugihara K, et al. Therapeutic results for hepatic metastasis of colorectal cancer with special reference to effectiveness of hepatectomy: analysis of prognostic factors for 763 cases recorded at 18 institutions. Dis Colon Rectum. 2003;46(10 Suppl):S22–31.

20. Spelt L, Andersson B, Nilsson J, Andersson R. Prognostic models for outcome following liver resection for colorectal cancer metastases: a systematic review. Eur J Surg Oncol. 2012;38(1):16–24.

21. Adam R, Pascal G, Castaing D, Azoulay D, Delvart V, Paule B, et al. Tumor progression while on chemotherapy: a contraindication to liver resection for multiple colorectal metastases? Ann Surg. 2004;240(6):1052–61. discussion 61–4.

22. Fong Y, Fortner J, Sun RL, Brennan MF, Blumgart LH. Clinical score for predicting recurrence after hepatic resection for metastatic colorectal cancer: analysis of 1001 consecutive cases. Ann Surg. 1999;230(3):309–18. discussion 18–21.

23. Nordlinger B, Guiguet M, Vaillant JC, Balladur P, Boudjema K, Bachellier P, et al. Surgical resection of colorectal carcinoma metastases to the liver. A prognostic scoring system to improve case selection, based on 1568 patients. Association Francaise de Chirurgie. Cancer. 1996;77(7):1254–62.

24. Nagashima I, Takada T, Matsuda K, Adachi M, Nagawa H, Muto T, et al. A new scoring system to classify patients with colorectal liver metastases: proposal of criteria to select candidates for hepatic resection. J Hepato-Biliary-Pancreat Surg. 2004;11(2):79–83.

25. Rees M, Tekkis PP, Welsh FK, O'Rourke T, John TG. Evaluation of long-term survival after hepatic resection for metastatic colorectal cancer: a multifactorial model of 929 patients. Ann Surg. 2008;247(1):125–35.

26. Roberts KJ, White A, Cockbain A, Hodson J, Hidalgo E, Toogood GJ, et al. Performance of prognostic scores in predicting long-term outcome following resection of colorectal liver metastases. Br J Surg. 2014;101(7):856–66.

27. Aloia T, Sebagh M, Plasse M, Karam V, Levi F, Giacchetti S, et al. Liver histology and surgical outcomes after preoperative chemotherapy with fluorouracil plus oxaliplatin in colorectal cancer liver metastases. J Clin Oncol. 2006;24(31):4983–90.

28. Karoui M, Penna C, Amin-Hashem M, Mitry E, Benoist S, Franc B, et al. Influence of preoperative chemotherapy on the risk of major hepatectomy for colorectal liver metastases. Ann Surg. 2006;243(1):1–7.

29. Nigri G, Petrucciani N, Ferla F, La Torre M, Aurello P, Ramacciato G. Neoadjuvant chemotherapy for resectable colorectal liver metastases: what is the evidence? Results of a systematic review of comparative studies. Surgeon. 2015;13(2):83–90.

30. Nordlinger B, Sorbye H, Glimelius B, Poston GJ, Schlag PM, Rougier P, et al. Perioperative FOLFOX4 chemotherapy and surgery versus surgery alone for resectable liver metastases from colorectal cancer (EORTC 40983): long-term results of a randomised, controlled, phase 3 trial. Lancet Oncol. 2013;14(12):1208–15.

31. Tanaka K, Adam R, Shimada H, Azoulay D, Levi F, Bismuth H. Role of neoadjuvant chemotherapy in the treatment of multiple colorectal metastases to the liver. Br J Surg. 2003;90(8):963–9.

32. Tanaka K, Shimada H, Ueda M, Matsuo K, Endo I, Togo S. Role of hepatectomy in treating multiple bilobar colorectal cancer metastases. Surgery. 2008;143(2):259–70.

33. Feng Q, Wei Y, Zhu D, Ye L, Lin Q, Li W, et al. Timing of hepatectomy for resectable synchronous colorectal liver metastases: for whom simultaneous resection is more suitable – a meta-analysis. PLoS One. 2014;9(8):e104348.

34. Yin Z, Liu C, Chen Y, Bai Y, Shang C, Yin R, et al. Timing of hepatectomy in resectable synchronous colorectal liver metastases (SCRLM): Simultaneous or delayed? Hepatology. 2013;57(6):2346–57.

35. She WH, Chan AC, Poon RT, Cheung TT, Chok KS, Chan SC, et al. Defining an optimal surgical strategy for synchronous colorectal liver metastases: staged versus simultaneous resection? ANZ J Surg. 2015;85(11):829–33.

36. Karoui M, Vigano L, Goyer P, Ferrero A, Luciani A, Aglietta M, et al. Combined first-stage hepatectomy and colorectal resection in a two-stage hepatectomy strategy for bilobar synchronous liver metastases. Br J Surg. 2010;97(9):1354–62.

37. Lam VW, Laurence JM, Johnston E, Hollands MJ, Pleass HC, Richardson AJ. A systematic review of two-stage hepatectomy in patients with initially unresectable colorectal liver metastases. HPB (Oxford). 2013;15(7):483–91.

38. Wicherts DA, Miller R, de Haas RJ, Bitsakou G, Vibert E, Veilhan LA, et al. Long-term results of two-stage hepatectomy for irresectable colorectal cancer liver metastases. Ann Surg. 2008;248(6):994–1005.

39. Narita M, Oussoultzoglou E, Jaeck D, Fuchschuber P, Rosso E, Pessaux P, et al. Two-stage hepatectomy for multiple bilobar colorectal liver metastases. Br J Surg. 2011;98(10):1463–75.

40. Chan AC, Poon RT, Chan C, Lo CM. Safety of ALPPS procedure by the anterior approach for hepatocellular carcinoma. Ann Surg. 2016;263(2):e14–6.

41. de Santibanes E, Clavien PA. Playing Play-Doh to prevent postoperative liver failure: the "ALPPS" approach. Ann Surg. 2012;255(3):415–7.

42. Lang SA, Loss M, Schlitt HJ. "In-situ split" (ISS) liver resection: new aspects of technique and indication. Zentralbl Chir. 2014;139(2):212–9.

43. Schnitzbauer AA, Lang SA, Goessmann H, Nadalin S, Baumgart J, Farkas SA, et al. Right portal vein ligation combined with in situ splitting induces rapid left lateral liver lobe hypertrophy enabling 2-staged extended right hepatic resection in small-for-size settings. Ann Surg. 2012;255(3):405–14.

44. Chan AC, Poon RT, Lo CM. Modified anterior approach for the ALPPS procedure: how we do it. World J Surg. 2015;39(11):2831–5.

45. Truant S, Scatton O, Dokmak S, Regimbeau JM, Lucidi V, Laurent A, et al. Associating liver partition and portal vein ligation for staged hepatectomy (ALPPS): impact of the inter-stages course on morbi-mortality and implications for management. Eur J Surg Oncol. 2015;41(5):674–82.

46. Chan ACY, Chok K, Dai JWC, Lo CM. Impact of split completeness on future liver remnant hypertrophy in associating liver partition and portal vein ligation for staged hepatectomy (ALPPS) in hepatocellular carcinoma: complete-ALPPS versus partial-ALPPS. Surgery. 2017;161(2):357–64.

47. Schadde E, Raptis DA, Schnitzbauer AA, Ardiles V, Tschuor C, Lesurtel M, et al. Prediction of mortality after alpps stage-1: an analysis of 320 patients from the international ALPPS registry. Ann Surg. 2015;262(5):780–5. discussion 5–6.

48. Alvarez FA, Ardiles V, de Santibanes M, Pekolj J, de Santibanes E. Associating liver partition and portal vein ligation for staged hepatectomy offers high oncological feasibility with adequate patient safety: a prospective study at a single center. Ann Surg. 2015;261(4):723–32.

49. Bjornsson B, Sparrelid E, Rosok B, Pomianowska E, Hasselgren K, Gasslander T, et al. Associating liver partition and portal vein ligation for staged hepatectomy in patients with colorectal liver metastases – intermediate oncological results. Eur J Surg Oncol. 2016;42(4):531–7.

50. Adam R, Imai K, Castro Benitez C, Allard MA, Vibert E, Sa Cunha A, et al. Outcome after associating liver partition and portal vein ligation for staged hepatectomy and conventional two-stage hepatectomy for colorectal liver metastases. Br J Surg. 2016;103(11):1521–9.

51. Hagness M, Foss A, Line PD, Scholz T, Jorgensen PF, Fosby B, et al. Liver transplantation for nonresectable liver metastases from colorectal cancer. Ann Surg. 2013;257(5):800–6.

Extraregional Lymph Node Metastasis

34

Jung Wook Huh and Hee Cheol Kim

Abstract

The presence of regional lymph node metastases in colorectal cancer is one of the most important prognostic factors. However, the extent of lymph node dissection in colorectal cancer surgery is still controversial. The presence of extraregional lymph node metastasis only is not a common metastatic pattern for colorectal cancer. This type of cancer is usually combined with distant metastasis or extensive regional lymph node metastasis and is categorized as M1 disease. Management of extraregional lymph node metastasis in colorectal cancer has been challenging due to lack of supportive data. Here, we summarize the approaches and managements of this category of diseases, focusing on the role of surgical treatment in colorectal cancer.

Keywords

Colorectal cancer · Stage IV · Extraregional lymph nodes · Dissection

J. W. Huh • H. C. Kim (✉)
Department of Surgery, Samsung Medical Center,
Sungkyunkwan University School of Medicine,
Seoul, South Korea
e-mail: hckim@skku.edu

34.1 Introduction

The presence or absence of lymph node metastasis in colorectal cancer is one of the most important prognostic factors. However, the extent of lymph node dissection in colorectal cancer surgery is still controversial.

Extended lymph node dissection was first described by Jamieson and Dobson in the early 1990s and is based on Halstedian principles considering mesocolic lymph node metastasis in patients without distant metastasis [1]. The current guidelines from the American Joint Conference on Cancer (AJCC) recommend a minimal assessment of 12 lymph nodes for accurate staging in colorectal cancer surgery; however, they do not consider the distribution of lymph node metastases, which is the main prognostic factor in the Japanese classification staging system [2]. The Japanese Society for Cancer of the Colon and Rectum (JSCCR) advocates careful dissection along embryologic tissue planes; however, the radicality of lymph node dissection is markedly different, being determined by preoperative radiologic imaging study [3]. The JSCCR recommends D2 resection (standard low tie) for early-stage tumors and D3 (high tie) for more advanced disease [3]. Complete mesocolic excision and D3 dissection might be associated with better survival than is conventional resection, in which mesocolic lymph nodes at the origin of the arteries are not resected [4].

© Springer Nature Singapore Pte Ltd. 2018
N. K. Kim et al. (eds.), *Surgical Treatment of Colorectal Cancer*,
https://doi.org/10.1007/978-981-10-5143-2_34

There have been concerns about potentially increased risk of perioperative morbidity and mortality associated with extended lymph node dissection [5, 6].

Extraregional lymph node metastasis only is not a common metastatic pattern for colorectal cancer. This type of cancer is usually combined with distant metastasis or extensive regional lymph node metastasis and is categorized as M1 disease, according to the AJCC staging system. Recently, complete removal of all metastatic tumor combined with effective chemotherapy based on biologic agents offers a promising oncologic outcome in patients with metastatic colorectal cancer. However, the effect of surgery itself in this situation remains controversial, and there are few studies specifically addressing and focusing on this issue [7, 8].

Thus, in this chapter, we aimed to provide a comprehensive review of the literature describing the pattern of mesocolic lymph node metastasis and to review the investigations regarding extraregional lymph node dissection.

34.2 Regional Lymph Nodes

There are between 100 and 150 lymph nodes in the mesentery of the colon. Regional lymph nodes are those located along the colon, plus the nodes along the major arteries that supply blood to that particular colon segment. It has been generally accepted that lymphatic drainage of colorectal tumors tends to follow the blood-supplying arteries. The classification of the lymph nodes related to the ileocolic and inferior mesenteric arteries is relatively consistent, but that of the lymph nodes associated with the right colic and middle colic arteries is not straightforward due to their variations [9–11]. The right colic artery is usually able to be defined as a separate artery between the ileocolic artery and trunk of the middle colic artery running inferior to the avascular mesocolic window as one of two to three separate middle colic arteries with a separate origin from the superior mesenteric artery or the right branch of the middle colic artery [12]. It can often be difficult to distinguish between the potentially different classifications used.

The JSCCR classification staging system is based on the distribution rather than the absolute number of metastatic lymph nodes. Whether the distribution of lymph node metastasis is a better predictor than the current TNM staging system focusing on the number of lymph node metastases remains unclear. Some authors have suggested that the N categorization including the distribution of lymph node metastasis can enhance the prognostic value of the current TNM classification [13–15]. However, the JSCCR classification has not been widely adopted because of its complexity and the controversial results as to oncologic outcomes [14–17].

34.3 Paraaortic Lymph Node Dissection

It is well known that the complete removal of metastatic tumors can improve survival in patients with stage IV colorectal cancers. An aggressive surgical approach combined with modern chemotherapy with biologic agents offers a promising strategy for treatment of colorectal cancer patients with liver metastasis [18, 19]. In contrast to liver or lung metastasis, there is no consensus on the treatment strategy for extraregional lymph node metastasis in patients with colorectal cancer [20]. It is not yet established whether upfront chemotherapy followed by surgical resection or surgery before chemotherapy is the better treatment strategy in this disease entity. In cases of clinically suspicious lymph nodes, NCCN guidelines recommend biopsy or excision, not prophylactic dissection due to the possible complications, including urinary and sexual impairment as well as intraoperative morbidities.

Paraaortic lymph node metastasis has been frequently confused with retroperitoneal recurrence in the literature [7, 21]. This means that an ambiguous definition can include heterogeneous

Table 34.1 Clinical data regarding paraaortic lymph node dissection in colorectal cancer. These two studies are only comparative clinical trials of oncologic outcomes between paraaortic lymph node dissection and chemotherapy

Authors	Study design	Study group	Sample size (dissection group vs. CTx.)	Outcomes (5-year OS)	Comments
Min et al. [23]	Retrospective	Recurrent	38 (6 vs. 24)	Median survival: 34 vs. 12 months ($p = 0.034$)	
Choi et al. [22]	Retrospective	Primary	77 (24 vs. 53)	5-year overall survival: 53.4 vs. 12.0% ($p = 0.045$)	Enrolled only metastasis below renal hilum

recurrence patterns, such as a local recurrence in the tumor bed and paraaortic lymph node metastasis. Isolated paraaortic lymph node metastasis is a relatively rare metastatic pattern in colorectal cancer patients, and it is categorized as M1 disease according to the AJCC staging classification. The rate of isolated paraaortic lymph node metastasis was reported to be very low, in the range 1.0–1.3%, and paraaortic node metastasis is usually accompanied by other distant metastases, such as liver, lung, or peritoneal metastases [22, 23].

New biologic chemotherapeutic agents (e.g., irinotecan, bevacizumab) in patients with metastatic colorectal cancer have recently been well recognized [24, 25]. Some authors have recommended chemotherapy as an initial treatment option for colorectal cancer patients with paraaortic lymph node metastasis [26, 27]. It is plausible that paraaortic node dissection has not been widely performed as an initial treatment due to a high postoperative morbidity and recent advancement in chemotherapeutic agents. Miyazawa et al. reported a complete response of paraaortic lymph node metastasis in rectosigmoid colon cancer following chemotherapy with capecitabine/oxaliplatin plus bevacizumab [28].

In contrary to this, evidence supporting extensive paraaortic lymph node dissection has been recently published (Table 34.1) [7, 22, 23]. Although most of the studies are a retrospective analysis from a single center and therefore have a limitation of selection bias, they emphasized the surgical role of isolated paraaortic lymph node metastasis with evidence (Figs. 34.1 and 34.2). Min et al. [23] reviewed the clinical outcomes of

38 patients with isolated paraaortic lymph node recurrence: 6 (15.8%) patients with curative surgical resection, 19 (50%) with chemoradiotherapy, and 13 (34.2%) with chemotherapy only. They reported that the median survival of the six patients who had undergone surgical resection after isolated paraaortic lymph node recurrence was 34 months, whereas it was only 14 months in those who did not. Choi et al. [22] analyzed 77 patients with isolated paraaortic lymph node metastasis from colorectal cancer below the renal vein. The authors reported a 5-year survival rate of 53.4% in 24 patients who underwent paraaortic lymph node dissection and of 12% for the 53 patients who did not. Shibata et al. [7] also demonstrated a significant survival benefit of resection of isolated retroperitoneal recurrences over surgical exploration alone (median survival, 40 months vs. 3 months) The authors also suggested that the presence of two or fewer paraaortic lymph node metastases might be a good indication for resection using univariate analysis, although no significant prognostic factors were identified by multivariate analysis.

A recent retrospective analysis analyzed the extent of lymphadenectomy in 181 patients with advanced rectal cancer located below the peritoneal reflection with extraregional lymph node metastasis [29]. The authors divided the patients into two groups: 81 patients who underwent lateral pelvic lymph node dissection only and 100 patients who underwent lateral pelvic node and paraaortic lymph node dissection (total lymph node dissection). They concluded that total lymph node dissection, compared with pelvic dissection, improved disease-free survival in

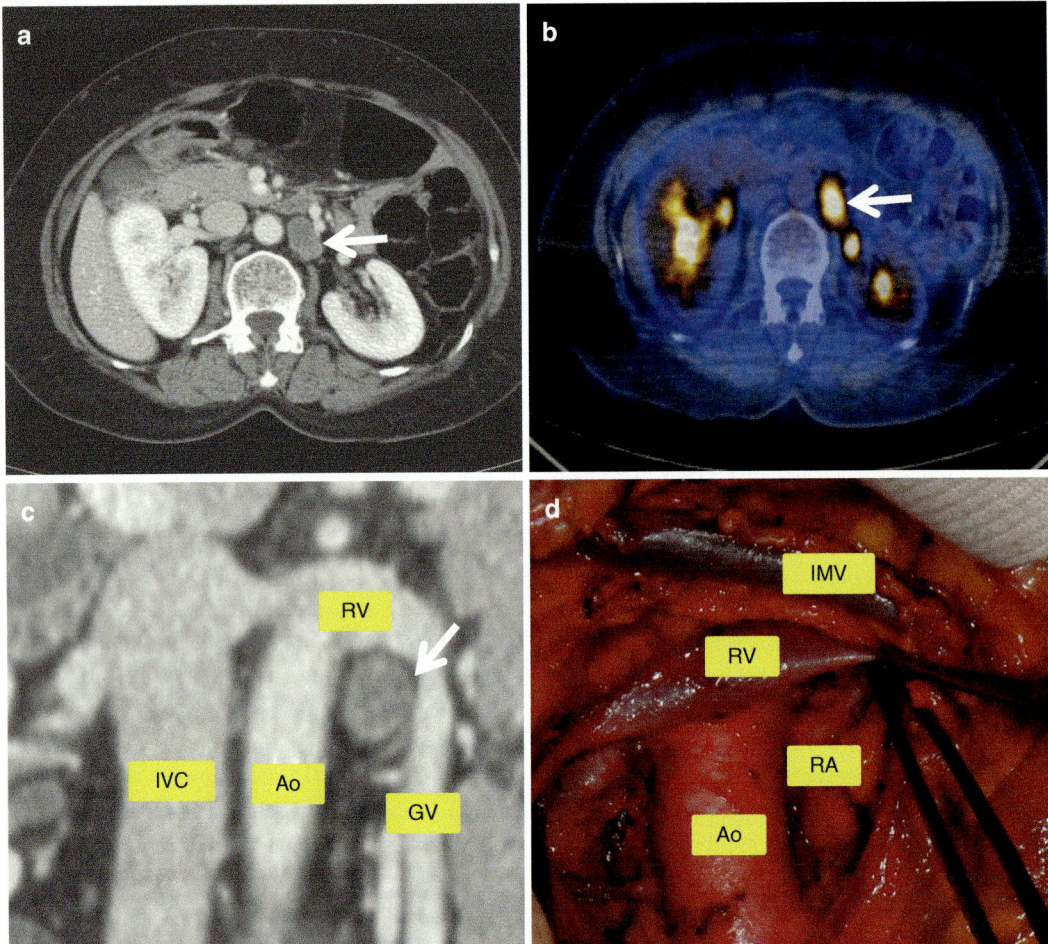

Fig. 34.1 Solitary paraaortic lymph node metastasis below the level left renal vein (**a**) in CT scan and (**b**) in PET scan. Arrow indicates the enlarged lymph node. (**c**) The metastatic lymph node was located between the aorta, left renal vein, and left gonadal vein. (**d**) Surgical removal was performed with preservation of the renal vein, artery, and inferior mesenteric vein. *Ao* Aorta, *IVC* inferior vena cava, *RV* renal vein, *RA* renal artery, *GV* gonadal vein, *IMV* inferior mesenteric vein

patients with noninfiltrating type, stage III rectal cancer and less than two positive pelvic lymph node sites. Bae et al. [8] reported oncologic outcomes of 129 colorectal cancer patients with paraaortic node metastasis who underwent tumor resection. Interestingly, they showed that only 45 patients (34.8%) had been revealed to have true positive paraaortic lymph node metastasis by final histology, among the 129 patients suspected to have positive nodes using radiologic evaluation. These findings suggest that

surgical resection in selected cases appears to be the optimal treatment strategy for isolated paraaortic lymph node metastasis from colorectal cancer, but further well-designed studies should be needed to justify this surgical approach in the current era of modern chemotherapy. Therefore, the role of paraaortic lymph node dissection in patients with isolated paraaortic lymph node metastasis has not been clearly established.

The incidence of postoperative morbidities after colorectal cancer surgery is relatively high

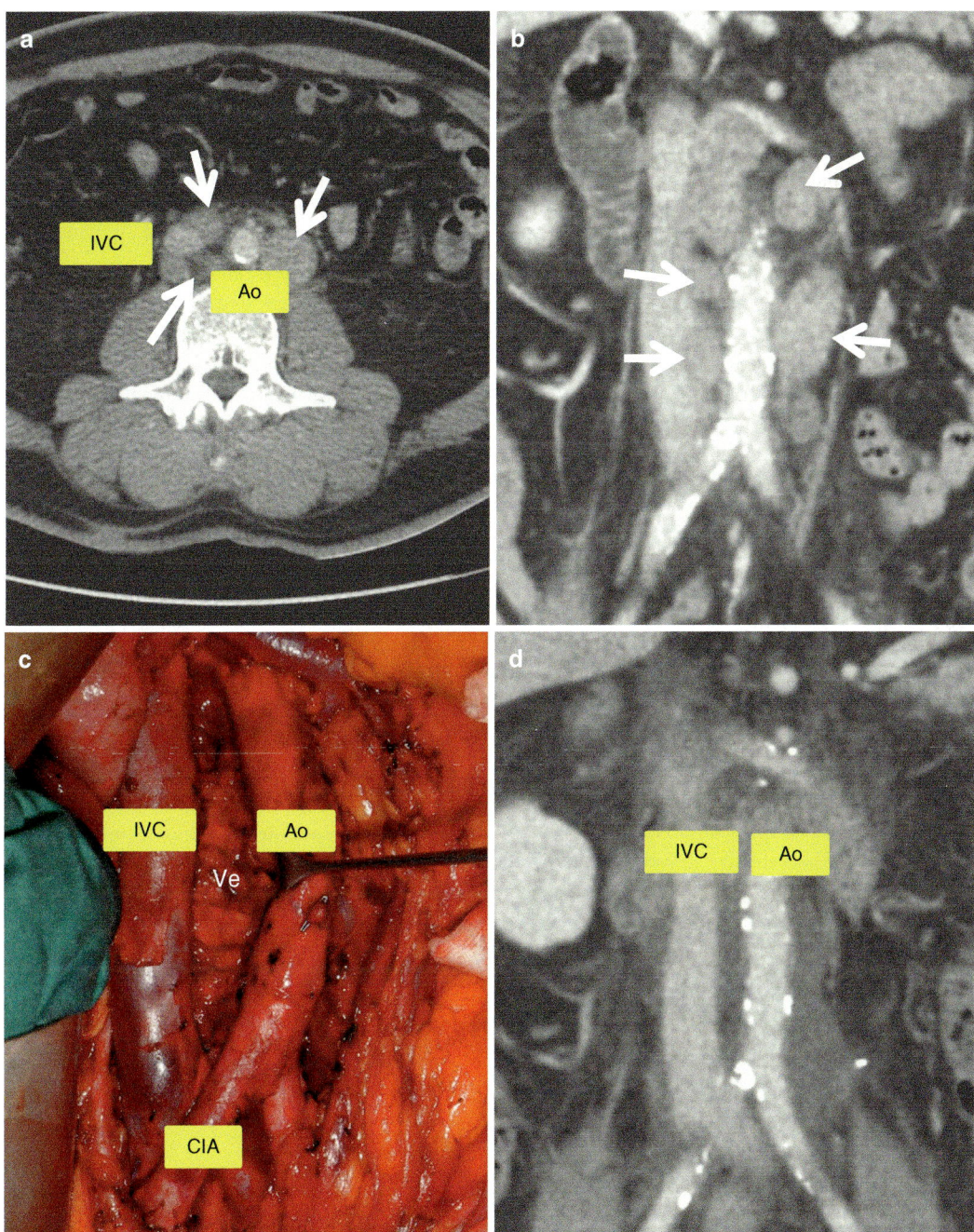

Fig. 34.2 Multiple paraaortic lymph node metastases at left side of the aorta, aortocaval space, and retrocaval area (**a**) in axial cut and (**b**) coronal cut of CT scan. Arrows indicate the multiple conglomerated lymph nodes. (**c**) Picture and (**d**) CT scan after meticulous paraaortic lymph node dissection. *Ao* Aorta, *IVC* inferior vena cava, *CIA* common iliac artery, *Ve* vertebra

and ranges between 30% and 69% depending on the extent of lymph node dissection [30–32]. Paraaortic lymph node dissection is usually performed to clear the lymphatics in the paraaortic and iliac areas, from the level of renal vessels down to the iliac bifurcation [22, 30, 33]. This aggressive surgery unavoidably increases the incidence of postoperative complications due to the difficulty in identifying sympathetic structures, such as small bowel obstruction and sexual/urinary dysfunctions. Recently, improved surgical techniques with advanced operative devices and better understanding of anatomy enabled a decrease in postoperative complications after paraaortic lymph node dissection, ranging from 7.8% to 27.8% in tertiary center hospitals [8, 22]. The surgical removal of paraaortic lymph node metastasis might be feasible and safe in selected patients with skilled surgeons.

New radiation techniques such as intensity-modulated radiotherapy and tomotherapy have made it possible to accurately deliver high-dose radiation to focused areas without scarifying adjacent normal structures [34]. However, the application of this approach to paraaortic lymph nodes metastasis with colorectal cancer is not usual, and its survival benefits remain unknown. Kim et al. [35] evaluated seven patients with paraaortic lymph node recurrence in rectal cancer after curative resection. One patient remained disease-free for 26 months, and another is still alive with recurrence after 70 months. Their initial report warranted a need of highly selection criteria that enable patients to potentially be salvaged by radiotherapy.

34.4 Inguinal Lymph Node Metastasis

Inguinal lymph node metastasis from rectal cancer is classified as distant metastasis even though inguinal lymph node metastasis from anal squamous cell ca is classified as regional metastasis (N1a) in AJCC staging system eighth edition. Solitary inguinal node metastasis is rare condition occurring in about less than 1% of rectal cancer [36, 37]. However, the patients with isolated inguinal lymph node metastasis tended to show better oncologic outcomes.

Treatment for inguinal node metastasis in rectal cancer is basically non-curative consisting of chemotherapy and sometimes combined radiotherapy. Surgical treatment can be considered for symptom control. The role of meticulous lymphadenectomy of inguinal area to improved survival has been rarely reported. Adachi et al. [38] reported better survival after inguinal lymph node excision but it was only case series.

In the future, treatment strategy may be discussed based on the reconsideration of prognosis and staging of isolated inguinal lymph node metastasis.

Conclusion

Extraregional lymph node metastasis or recurrence in patients with colorectal cancer is a relatively rare disease entity. A prospective and standardized treatment strategy for paraaortic lymph node metastasis has not been tested in a well-designed trial. It is still challenging to determine whether surgical resection of paraaortic lymph node metastasis can improve the oncologic outcomes in colorectal cancer patients with paraaortic lymph node metastasis. Although a few reports have supported a benefit of extensive lymph node dissection in this condition, the approaches seem to have a potential to increase survival with acceptable morbidities in strictly selected patients with skilled surgical teams.

References

1. Jamieson JK, Dobson JFVII. Lymphatics of the colon: with special reference to the operative treatment of cancer of the colon. Ann Surg. 1909;50(6):1077–90.
2. Nelson H, Petrelli N, Carlin A, Couture J, Fleshman J, Guillem J, et al. Guidelines 2000 for colon and rectal cancer surgery. J Natl Cancer Inst. 2001;93(8):583–96.
3. Huh JW, Lee WY, Kim SH, Park YA, Cho YB, Yun SH, et al. Immunohistochemical detection of p53 expression in patients with preoperative chemoradiation for rectal cancer: association with prognosis. Yonsei Med J. 2015;56(1):82–8.

4. Bertelsen CA, Neuenschwander AU, Jansen JE, Wilhelmsen M, Kirkegaard-Klitbo A, Tenma JR, et al. Disease-free survival after complete mesocolic excision compared with conventional colon cancer surgery: a retrospective, population-based study. Lancet Oncol. 2015;16(2):161–8.

5. Killeen S, Mannion M, Devaney A, Winter DC. Complete mesocolic resection and extended lymphadenectomy for colon cancer: a systematic review. Color Dis. 2014;16(8):577–94.

6. Rosenberg J, Fischer A, Haglind E, Scandinavian Surgical Outcomes Research Group. Current controversies in colorectal surgery: the way to resolve uncertainty and move forward. Color Dis. 2012;14(3):266–9.

7. Shibata D, Paty PB, Guillem JG, Wong WD, Cohen AM. Surgical management of isolated retroperitoneal recurrences of colorectal carcinoma. Dis Colon Rectum. 2002;45(6):795–801.

8. Bae SU, Han YD, Cho MS, Hur H, Min BS, Baik SH, et al. Oncologic outcomes of colon cancer patients with extraregional lymph node metastasis: comparison of isolated paraaortic lymph node metastasis with resectable liver metastasis. Ann Surg Oncol. 2016;23(5):1562–8.

9. Spasojevic M, Stimec BV, Dyrbekk AP, Tepavcevic Z, Edwin B, Bakka A, et al. Lymph node distribution in the d3 area of the right mesocolon: implications for an anatomically correct cancer resection. A postmortem study. Dis Colon Rectum. 2013;56(12):1381–7.

10. Garcia-Ruiz A, Milsom JW, Ludwig KA, Marchesa P. Right colonic arterial anatomy. Implications for laparoscopic surgery. Dis Colon Rectum. 1996;39(8):906–11.

11. Mike M, Kano N. Reappraisal of the vascular anatomy of the colon and consequences for the definition of surgical resection. Dig Surg. 2013;30(4–6):383–92.

12. Bertelsen CA, Kirkegaard-Klitbo A, Nielsen M, Leotta SM, Daisuke F, Gogenur I. Pattern of colon cancer lymph node metastases in patients undergoing central mesocolic lymph node excision: a systematic review. Dis Colon Rectum. 2016;59(12):1209–21.

13. Huh JW, Kim YJ, Kim HR. Distribution of lymph node metastases is an independent predictor of survival for sigmoid colon and rectal cancer. Ann Surg. 2012;255(1):70–8.

14. Suzuki O, Sekishita Y, Shiono T, Ono K, Fujimori M, Kondo S. Number of lymph node metastases is better predictor of prognosis than level of lymph node metastasis in patients with node-positive colon cancer. J Am Coll Surg. 2006;202(5):732–6.

15. Tang R, Wang JY, Chen JS, Chang-Chien CR, Tang S, Lin SE, et al. Survival impact of lymph node metastasis in TNM stage III carcinoma of the colon and rectum. J Am Coll Surg. 1995;180(6):705–12.

16. Kobayashi H, Ueno H, Hashiguchi Y, Mochizuki H. Distribution of lymph node metastasis is a prognostic index in patients with stage III colon cancer. Surgery. 2006;139(4):516–22.

17. Wong JH, Bowles BJ, Bueno R, Shimizu D. Impact of the number of negative nodes on disease-free survival in colorectal cancer patients. Dis Colon Rectum. 2002;45(10):1341–8.

18. Blazer DG 3rd, Kishi Y, Maru DM, Kopetz S, Chun YS, Overman MJ, et al. Pathologic response to preoperative chemotherapy: a new outcome end point after resection of hepatic colorectal metastases. J Clin Oncol. 2008;26(33):5344–51.

19. Nordlinger B, Sorbye H, Glimelius B, Poston GJ, Schlag PM, Rougier P, et al. Perioperative chemotherapy with FOLFOX4 and surgery versus surgery alone for resectable liver metastases from colorectal cancer (EORTC Intergroup trial 40983): a randomised controlled trial. Lancet. 2008;371(9617):1007–16.

20. Albandar MH, Cho MS, Bae SU, Kim NK. Surgical management of extra-regional lymph node metastasis in colorectal cancer. Expert Rev Anticancer Ther. 2016;16(5):503–13.

21. Bowne WB, Lee B, Wong WD, Ben-Porat L, Shia J, Cohen AM, et al. Operative salvage for locoregional recurrent colon cancer after curative resection: an analysis of 100 cases. Dis Colon Rectum. 2005;48(5):897–909.

22. Choi PW, Kim HC, Kim AY, Jung SH, CS Y, Kim JC. Extensive lymphadenectomy in colorectal cancer with isolated para-aortic lymph node metastasis below the level of renal vessels. J Surg Oncol. 2010;101(1):66–71.

23. Min BS, Kim NK, Sohn SK, Cho CH, Lee KY, Baik SH. Isolated paraaortic lymph-node recurrence after the curative resection of colorectal carcinoma. J Surg Oncol. 2008;97(2):136–40.

24. Cunningham D, Humblet Y, Siena S, Khayat D, Bleiberg H, Santoro A, et al. Cetuximab monotherapy and cetuximab plus irinotecan in irinotecan-refractory metastatic colorectal cancer. N Engl J Med. 2004;351(4):337–45.

25. Hurwitz H, Fehrenbacher L, Novotny W, Cartwright T, Hainsworth J, Heim W, et al. Bevacizumab plus irinotecan, fluorouracil, and leucovorin for metastatic colorectal cancer. N Engl J Med. 2004;350(23):2335–42.

26. Fujii S, Ota M, Ichikawa Y, Yamagishi S, Osada S, Suwa H, et al. Paraaortic lymph node metastasis showed CR to UFT/LV therapy in elderly rectal cancer. Hepato-Gastroenterology. 2010;57(99-100):472–6.

27. Takenoue T, Yamada Y, Miyagawa S, Akiyama Y, Koyama K, Nagawa H. Cisplatin-5-fluorouracil therapy with remarkable effect and 5-year survival for paraaortic lymph node metastases of rectal carcinoma in females: a case report. Jpn J Clin Oncol. 1999;29(11):582–6.

28. Miyazawa T, Ebe K, Koide N, Fujita N. Complete response of isolated para-aortic lymph node recurrence from rectosigmoid cancer treated by chemoradiation therapy with capecitabine/oxaliplatin plus bevacizumab: a case report. Case Rep Oncol. 2012;5(2):216–21.

29. Liu YL, Wang YH, Yang YM, Li MQ, Jiang SX, Wang XS. The role of para-aortic lymphadenectomy in surgical management of patients with stage N+ rectal cancer below the peritoneal reflection. Cell Biochem Biophys. 2012;62(1):41–6.

30. Glass RE, Ritchie JK, Thompson HR, Mann CV. The results of surgical treatment of cancer of the rectum by radical resection and extended abdomino-iliac lymphadenectomy. Br J Surg. 1985;72(8):599–601.

31. Bokey EL, Chapuis PH, Hughes WJ, Koorey SG, Hinder JM, Edwards R. Morbidity, mortality and survival following resection for carcinoma of the rectum at Concord Hospital. Aust N Z J Surg. 1990;60(4):253–9.

32. Enker WE, Pilipshen SJ, Heilweil ML, Stearns MW Jr, Janov AJ, Hertz RE, et al. En bloc pelvic lymphadenectomy and sphincter preservation in the surgical management of rectal cancer. Ann Surg. 1986;203(4):426–33.

33. Leggeri A, Roseano M, Balani A, Turoldo A. Lumboaortic and iliac lymphadenectomy: what is the role today? Dis Colon Rectum. 1994;37(2 Suppl):S54–61.

34. Fenwick JD, Tome WA, Soisson ET, Mehta MP, Rock Mackie T. Tomotherapy and other innovative IMRT delivery systems. Semin Radiat Oncol. 2006;16(4):199–208.

35. Kim MS, Cho CK, Yang KM, Lee DH, Moon SM, Shin YJ. Stereotactic body radiotherapy for isolated paraaortic lymph node recurrence from colorectal cancer. World J Gastroenterol. 2009;15(48):6091–5.

36. Graham RA, Hohn DC. Management of inguinal lymph node metastases from adenocarcinoma of the rectum. Dis Colon Rectum. 1990;33:212–6.

37. Bardia A, Greeno E, Miller R, Alberts S, Dozois E, Haddock M, Limburg P. Is a solitary inguinal lymph node metastasis from adenocarcinoma of the rectum really a metastasis? Color Dis. 2010;12:312–5.

38. Adachi T, Hinoi T, Egi H, Ohdan H. Surgical treatment for isolated inguinal lymph node metastasis in low rectal adenocarcinoma patients improves outcome. Int J Color Dis. 2013;28:1675–80.

Dae Joon Kim

Abstract

Lung metastases from colorectal cancer occur in approximately 10–20% of patients. In the absence of extrapulmonary metastases, the surgical removal of lung metastases can be curative treatment in selected patients. The actuarial survival after completed resection was 36% at 5 years according to the International Registry of Lung Metastases, and Thomford criteria for pulmonary metastasectomy have been widely accepted by thoracic surgeons. The standard procedure for peripherally located lesion is wedge resection, but lobectomy can be done for central lesion in highly selected patients. However, there have been controversies in the optimal timing of surgery, the role of mediastinal lymphadenectomy, and the survival benefit after repeated pulmonary metastasectomy. The nonsurgical intervention such as RFA or SABR can be applied to the patients who are not physiologically unfit for surgery.

Keywords

Colorectal cancer · Lung metastasis · Surgical resection

D. J. Kim
Department of Thoracic and Cardiovascular Surgery,
Yonsei University College of Medicine,
Seoul, South Korea
e-mail: KDJCOOL@yuhs.ac

35.1 Introduction

Lung metastases from colorectal cancer occur in approximately 10–20% of patients [1, 2]. Although the liver has been regarded as the first site of metastases, metastases bypassing the liver have been reported over the years. Unlike bone or lymph node metastases, lung metastasis is influenced by the primary site. Rectal cancers are more likely to present the lung metastasis than colon cancers, and even in rectal cancers, lung metastases are more common in patients with mid- or distal rectal cancers [3]. The isolated lung metastases were observed in 1–5.9% of colon cancer and in up to 11.7% in rectal cancer [1]. It is unclear why rectal cancers show more frequent lung metastases and anatomical factors as well as molecular genetics play an important role. Considering that lung metastases are thought to occur via hematogenous spread rather than via lymphogenous spread, vascular anatomy might be particularly important. The distal rectum drains into the inferior rectal vein which drains directly into the inferior vena cava and reaches the lung quickly. On the contrary, the colon and upper rectum drain into the portal venous system, and cancer cells arising from these areas reach the liver as the first site of metastases [4].

In the absence of extrapulmonary metastases, the surgical removal of lung metastases can be curative treatment in some patients. The multidisciplinary approach with surgical resection,

© Springer Nature Singapore Pte Ltd. 2018
N. K. Kim et al. (eds.), *Surgical Treatment of Colorectal Cancer*,
https://doi.org/10.1007/978-981-10-5143-2_35

chemotherapy, and interventional procedures provides the best treatment option in this subset of patients, and it should begin with the assessment of resectability. Although there is no prospective, randomized trial comparing the pulmonary metastasectomy to control, the surgical resection of lung metastases from colorectal cancer has been accepted in selected patients since the International Registry of Lung Metastases reported the result of pulmonary metastasectomy in 1997 [5]. This chapter will discuss the current surgical strategies with special reference to some debates in management of lung metastases from colorectal cancers.

35.2 Criteria for Lung Metastasectomy

The International Registry of Lung Metastases was established in 1991 by the European Society of Thoracic Surgeons (ESTS). This registry is a large prospective study of 5206 patients, and they reported that the actuarial survival at 5 years was 36% after complete resection and 13% after incomplete resection, respectively [5]. Multivariate analysis revealed a better prognosis in patients with a disease-free interval of more than 36 months and a single lung metastasis. Although the level of evidence to support the role of pulmonary metastasectomy is not enough so far, it is uncertain whether prospective randomized controlled trials could be conducted in near future because of heterogeneity of study population and ethical issues. Currently, thoracic surgeons have been adopting the so-called Thomford criteria [6], updated by Kondo et al. [7], for pulmonary metastasectomy:

- The complete resection of all LM must be achieved with respect to the remaining lung tissue and an adequate pulmonary function [8].
- The primary tumor has been radically (R0) resected or is under therapeutic control.
- Further extrapulmonary tumor manifestations are not present or are resectable.
- Therapeutic alternatives are not available.
- The therapeutic strategy was set up by interdisciplinary consensus.

35.3 Imaging Study

The standard and accepted imaging modality for preoperative imaging in patients with a high suspicion of pulmonary metastasis is chest computed tomography. Ideally, a multislice detector CT (CT) scan with a reconstruction thickness of up to 3 mm should be used for diagnosis. The number and size of the metastases and the infiltration of central structures are important parameters for the evaluation of the surgical procedure and extent of surgical resection. In case of solitary lung nodule in patient with colorectal cancer, the possibility of primary lung cancer or another pulmonary pathology has to be considered [9].

The value of positron emission tomography (PET) in the diagnosis of pulmonary metastasis is well studied. The sensitivity, as well as the specificity of PET CT in the detection of lung nodule, is approximately 90% for nodules larger than 10 mm. In metastases measuring less than 10 mm, the accuracy of the method decreases to less than 50% [10, 11]. According to Detterbeck et al., PET should be performed prior to metastasectomy in order to rule out extrathoracic disease rather than to detect intrathoracic lesions [12]. Pastorino et al. analyzed 86 patients and reported the improved detection of extrathoracic disease in 21% of the patients, an advantage in identifying nodal metastases larger than 10 mm and an increased accuracy of differential diagnosis of benign from malignant lung lesions [11]. Magnetic resonance imaging is not usually indicated in thoracic imaging, and it has no benefits over chest CT [13, 14].

Another application of imaging study in pulmonary metastasectomy is CT-guided localization. With advance of resolution of chest CT, the small nodule which is difficult to find even with palpation is sometimes documented in chest CT. If the suspicious pulmonary nodule is too small and thought to be difficult to find and palpate during the operation, surgeon can apply the localization technique before operation.

35.4   Surgical Resection

In general, the metastasis should be removed while preserving as much healthy lung parenchyma as possible. The standard procedure for peripherally located nodules is the simple wedge resection. Usually the metastatic lung nodule can be safely and completely removed with sufficient resection margin with the aid of a stapling device. The minimum resection margin has to be at least 0.5 cm. If several metastatic nodules are detected in a lung section, either wedge resection for every single metastasis or a segmental resection or lobectomy can be applied. If the metastatic lung nodule is centrally located, an extended resection or even a pneumonectomy may be required. However, the need for pneumonectomy to achieve complete resection is considered as a contraindication for lung metastasectomy based on the result of survey among members of the ESTS [15].

The changes of pulmonary function have to be also considered before planning the operation. The spirometric changes after pulmonary metastasectomy were found to be affected by total volume parenchyma resected within the first 90 days. According to the Italian working group by Petrella et al., the functional loss after three or more nonanatomical resections is comparable with that recorded after lobectomy [16]. If the patient has no enough lung function before pulmonary metastasectomy, the operation cannot be done due to pulmonary function.

Many surgeons prefer the open approach such as open thoracotomy or median sternotomy because this procedure allows for the manual examination of the lung parenchyma and, thus, detection of the smallest nodules which could not be detected in preoperative chest CT [15]. For the bilateral pulmonary metastasectomy, bilateral open thoracotomy, sequential unilateral open thoracotomy, or median sternotomy could be considered as possible surgical approaches. Because of recent advance in imaging modalities, minimally invasive surgery such as video-assisted thoracoscopic surgery (VATS) has been applied in metastasectomy [17, 18]. The potential advantages of VATS procedures include smaller incisions,

decreased surgical morbidity, reduced pleural adhesions, and shorter duration of hospitalization [19]. In spite of these advantages of VATS metastasectomy, smaller metastases may easily escape the surgeon's notice during the VATS metastasectomy. In Cerfolio's study with 57 patients with pulmonary metastasectomy, he found up to 38% malignant pulmonary nodules by performing bimanual palpation, despite the use of the newest generation of CT scan and integrated PET/CT. These patients were initially candidates for VATS metastasectomy but were switched to open thoracotomy due to the radiologic findings [20]. Other concerns remain regarding VATS, including the larger amount of lung parenchyma sacrificed by removing wedges of the lung using straight staplers compared with the parenchyma-sparing precision resection techniques. This problem becomes even more pronounced the deeper a lesion is lying from the surface of the lung and the larger its size is. Contrary to a precision resection, where anatomical intrapulmonary dissection allows complete removal of a central deposit while preserving normal adjacent vessels or airways and hence lung function, a VATS wedge resection being essentially a blind technique does not allow for this. Finally, the presence of metal staple lines and the resulting distortion of the normal lung anatomy can create significant technical challenges, potentially limiting the ability to perform a repeat metastasectomy if required in the future [21].

Therefore, it must be stated that the use of VATS for the resection of metastases is not internationally standardized, and VATS could be an option for patients with no more than two lung metastases, all in superficial locations [21]. In the guidelines recommended by the Eastern Canadian Colorectal Cancer Consensus Conference, VATS is the method of choice, whereas the German Society for Thoracic Surgery Education continues to propagate the open metastasectomy [22]. Regarding the relationship between survival and surgical approach, there is no proven difference in survival between thoracoscopic and thoracotomy approaches, although this was based on nonrandomized retrospective studies [19, 23–25].

35.5 Timing of Surgery

There are still controversies about the optimal timing of metastasectomy. An immediate operation has the theoretical advantages of avoiding later unresectability or spread of disease, whereas delayed surgery can potentially avoid repeated operations and/or invasive procedures in patients who progress rapidly, and delayed operation also can provide a window of time for the administration of neoadjuvant chemotherapy. The oncologist preferred the neoadjuvant chemotherapy in case of numerous pulmonary metastasis. However, after neoadjuvant chemotherapy for pulmonary metastasis, sometimes it is technically difficult to find the decreased size of metastatic nodule, and it can be a limitation to complete resection. The authors usually performed the open thoracotomy after neoadjuvant chemotherapy to palpate the decreased small nodules completely. Ideally, the therapeutic strategy and timing of operation have to be determined by an interdisciplinary consensus and any therapeutic alternatives considered.

35.6 Role of Hilar and Mediastinal Lymphadenectomy

The metastatic pulmonary nodule from colorectal cancer can be drained via pulmonary lymphatics; therefore hilar and mediastinal lymph node metastasis can occur. The lymph node metastasis in the mediastinum has been reported as a poor risk factor for survival in colorectal cancer. The 5-year OS of patients with lymph node metastases is poor (0–34%), compared to 38–79% for patients without mediastinal lymph node metastases [26, 27]. In one study of routine mediastinal lymph node dissection in colorectal cancer, mediastinal lymph node metastasis was found in 33% of patients [28], whereas the lymph node metastasis may not be apparent on preoperative imaging, as one study demonstrated mediastinal lymph node metastasis in 14% of patients with normal preoperative imaging [29]. Based on these results, several surgeons recommend the simultaneous radical mediastinal lymph node dissection in patients who underwent pulmonary metastasectomy for colorectal carcinoma. Loehe et al. performed the routine mediastinal lymph node dissection in patients with unremarkable CT findings, and they reported a trend (not statistically significant) toward a longer postoperative survival in patients without mediastinal lymph node metastasis [29]. Furthermore, prospective, randomized studies on the necessity for lymphadenectomy have not yet been carried out. In summary, whether lymphadenectomy leads to an improvement in survival has not yet been proven, and in a survey of ESTS members, only 13% of respondents routinely perform complete mediastinal lymphadenectomy [26].

Another technical concern regarding hilar and mediastinal lymphadenectomy in colorectal cancer is that it is actually impossible to dissect the hilar lymph nodes after wedge resection or segmentectomy. Even though mediastinal lymph node can be completely dissected after wedge resection, the hilar lymph nodes can be completely dissected only after lobectomy or above.

35.7 Repeated Lung Metastasectomy

The recurrence rate for patients with lung metastases is high, with up to 68% of patients developing recurrence following initial pulmonary metastasectomy and the lung being the commonest site of recurrence [30, 31]. If the metastases are operable, selected patients may benefit from multiple re-resections, with a 5-year overall survival of 25–58% for patients undergoing repeat metastasectomy and some patients having surgery two to four times [32–35]. Studies by Welter et al. [32] and Kim et al. [36] reported a 5-year overall survival of 54 and 29% in 39 and 69 patients with repeated resections, respectively. The mortality rate in both groups was zero. The working group led by Riquet et al. even found an improved 5-year survival for recurrence interventions—probably owing to positive patient selection [37]. The previous studies on repeated metastasectomy have the lack of a comparison with a prospective, controlled study, and it can be criticized. However, it has been thought that regular follow-up for the early detection of recurrence combined with parenchyma-saving resection might improve results after pulmonary metastasectomy.

There is no clear guidance on which patients may benefit from re-resection; however factors to consider include the disease-free interval, number of metastases, the presence of extrapulmonary disease, the technical challenges involved, the amount of residual lung tissue, and the patient's lung function. The short disease-free survival reflects the tumor characteristics such as aggressiveness or responsiveness. Patients with fast-growing tumors may not benefit from recurrent thoracotomies owing to the aggressive biological behavior. Therefore, various studies showed that the disease-free interval is the most important prognostic factor in patients with recurrent pulmonary disease regardless of tumor histology. Although the histology of the primary tumor is important for first-line metastasectomy [38], its influence seems to decrease in recurrent metastatic disease. For the planning of the reoperation, the pulmonary function has to be also considered, and another surgical approach such as (trans-sternal or posterior approach) has to be considered due to pleural adhesion which is related to previous operation. The surgical sheet which prevents pleural adhesion can be routinely inserted when closing the chest wall at the first operation.

35.8 Combined Lung and Liver Resection

Patients with both liver and lung metastases may benefit from resection of both sites of disease and are usually considered for surgical resection. In general, the technically more challenging operation is performed first, and that is usually the liver resection, particularly as the liver disease may be more likely to progress [23, 39]. However, there is also an argument that the lung surgery should be performed first as the recovery time is shorter [39]. The simultaneous liver and lung metastasectomy also can be tried, but it is usually avoided because it is too stressful for patients. It is important to note that many patients with potentially resectable disease may not subsequently undergo the second operation due to disease progression or recurrence [39]; therefore surgeons should always keep in mind the recovery time after operation. Also deciding the first operation depends on the more prognostically significant lesion.

A retrospective review of 73 patients with both liver and lung metastases demonstrated that the 17 patients who had metastasectomies had a significantly higher OS than the 56 patients who did not have surgery ($p < 0.01$) [40]. This result is consistent with data from the LiverMetSurvey registry, which reported that patients with resected lung and liver metastases had a higher 5-year OS than patients who underwent liver resection but not lung resection (45 vs. 14%) [41]. The 3-, 5-, and 10-year OS rates for patients having both liver and lung metastasectomies are approximately 77, 18–54, and 15% in retrospective series [40, 42–45]. In spite of all these encouraging data on survival, comparative randomized studies have not been reported.

35.9 Intervention

The various interventions have been tried as an alternative for pulmonary metastasectomy. Radiofrequency ablation (RFA) is one of alternative treatment option for selected patients with lung metastases. RFA is a minimally invasive procedure which delivers a high frequency electrical current through a needle electrode to cause tissue heating and necrosis [46]. RFA appears to be more effective in metastases with a maximum tumor diameter of ≤ 3 cm [47–50]. The possible complications of RFA include pneumothorax (up to 30–67% of cases), as well as rarer complications such as infection, nerve damage, bronchopleural fistulae, pleural effusion, and parenchymal bleeding leading to severe hemoptysis [49].

The most important limitation of RFA is the lack of histology to confirm the diagnosis and difficulty in radiological assessment of the adequacy of the ablation, because the lesion can appear larger in size as it includes the ablated parenchyma around the lesion [46, 49]. Various retrospective case series of patients undergoing RFA have been reported, with OS rates of 84–95% at 1 year and 35–56% at 5 years [46–50]. Most of the evidences and articles support operation as the most effective treatment option, but a systematic review was unable to draw firm conclusions on this issue due to the lack of phase III trials and differences in data reporting [51].

Stereotactic ablative radiotherapy (SABR) is a technique that enables the delivery of high-dose radiotherapy in a fewer number of fractions than conventional radiotherapy. A prospective study evaluated SABR in 82 patients with colorectal cancer (including 60 patients with lung metastases) who had 1–3 metastases confined to 1 organ (liver or lung) and reported a complete response in 37% of patients and a partial response in 18% of patients [52]. Local control rates at 1, 3, and 5 years were 85, 75, and 70%, and another study reported 1-, 2-, and 5-year survival rates of 84, 73, and 39% [52, 53]. In addition to RFA and SABR, a number of other interventional techniques have also been tried in the treatment of lung metastases, such as microwave ablation, high-intensity focussed ultrasound, transpulmonary chemoembolization, isolated lung perfusion, magnetic targeting, intravascular devices, brachytherapy, and cryoablation [54–56]. However, the evidence for these strategies is currently limited, and they are not routinely used in clinical practice. The critical limitation of all interventional technique is the absence of pathologic confirmation. In some cases, suspicious pulmonary metastasis has different pathology such as benign lung nodule or primary lung cancer. The exact pathologic cases in all cases are cornerstone of proper treatment. Therefore, these interventions are only suitable for patients who are not physiologically unfit for operation.

Conclusion

In conclusion, the pulmonary metastasectomy for colorectal cancer might lead to prolonged survival and sometimes even cure with low operative morbidity and mortality, in carefully selected patients treated in a multidisciplinary setting. The PulMiCC trial which is a randomized controlled trial testing the effect of pulmonary metastasectomy on survival of patients with colorectal cancer started in 2015, and its results will hopefully provide further clarity on the benefits of surgery for technically resectable lung metastases [57]. The use of nonsurgical interventions such as RFA and SABR has to be considered under the strict indications.

References

1. Tan KK, de Lima Lopes G Jr, Sim R. How uncommon are isolated lung metastases in colorectal cancer? A review from database of 754 patients over 4 years. J Gastrointest Surg. 2009;13(4):642–8.
2. Mitry E, Guiu B, Cosconea S, Jooste V, Faivre J, Bouvier A-M. Epidemiology, management and prognosis of colorectal cancer with lung metastases: a 30-year population-based study. Gut. 2010;59(10):1383–8.
3. Chiang JM, Hsieh PS, Chen JS, Tang R, You JF, Yeh CY. Rectal cancer level significantly affects rates and patterns of distant metastases among rectal cancer patients post curative-intent surgery without neoadjuvant therapy. World J Surg Oncol. 2014;12(1):197.
4. Gupta G, Minn A, Kang Y, Siegel P, Serganova I, Cordon-Cardo C, et al., editors. Identifying site-specific metastasis genes and functions. Cold Spring Harbor symposia on quantitative biology. Cold Spring Harbor Laboratory Press; 2005.
5. Pastorino U, Buyse M, Friedel G, Ginsberg RJ, Girard P, Goldstraw P, et al. Long-term results of lung metastasectomy: prognostic analyses based on 5206 cases. J Thorac Cardiovasc Surg. 1997;113(1):37–49.
6. Thomford NR. The surgical treatment of metastatic tumors in the lungs. J Thorac Cardiovasc Surg. 1965;49:357–63.
7. Kondo H, Okumura T, Ohde Y, Nakagawa K. Surgical treatment for metastatic malignancies. Pulmonary metastasis: indications and outcomes. Int J Clin Oncol. 2005;10(2):81–5.
8. Zollinger A, Hofer CK, Pasch T. Preoperative pulmonary evaluation: facts and myths. Curr Opin Anesthesiol. 2001;14(1):59–63.
9. Quint LE, Park CH, Iannettoni MD. Solitary pulmonary nodules in patients with extrapulmonary neoplasms. Radiology. 2000;217(1):257–61.
10. Lucas J, O'Doherty M, Wong J, Bingham J, McKee P, Fletcher C, et al. Evaluation of fluorodeoxyglucose positron emission tomography in the management of soft-tissue sarcomas. J Bone Joint Surg Br. 1998;80(3):441–7.
11. Pastorino U, Veronesi G, Landoni C, Leon M, Picchio M, Solli P, et al. Fluorodeoxyglucose positron emission

tomography improves preoperative staging of resectable lung metastasis. J Thorac Cardiovasc Surg. 2003;126(6):1906–10.

12. Detterbeck FC, Grodzki T, Gleeson F, Robert JH. Imaging requirements in the practice of pulmonary metastasectomy. J Thorac Oncol. 2010;5(6):S134–S9.

13. Feuerstein I, Jicha D, Pass H, Chow C, Chang R, Ling A, et al. Pulmonary metastases: MR imaging with surgical correlation – a prospective study. Radiology. 1992;182(1):123–9.

14. Kersjes W, Mayer E, Buchenroth M, Schunk K, Fouda N, Cagil H. Diagnosis of pulmonary metastases with turbo-SE MR imaging. Eur Radiol. 1997;7(8):1190–4.

15. Internullo E, Cassivi SD, Van Raemdonck D, Friedel G, Treasure T, Group EPMW. Pulmonary metastasectomy: a survey of current practice amongst members of the European Society of Thoracic Surgeons. J Thorac Oncol. 2008;3(11):1257–66.

16. Petrella F, Chieco P, Solli P, Veronesi G, Borri A, Galetta D, et al. Which factors affect pulmonary function after lung metastasectomy? Eur J Cardiothorac Surg. 2009;35(5):792–6.

17. Nakas A, Klimatsidas MN, Entwisle J, Martin-Ucar AE, Waller DA. Video-assisted versus open pulmonary metastasectomy: the surgeon's finger or the radiologist's eye? Eur J Cardiothorac Surg. 2009;36(3):469–74.

18. Carballo M, Maish MS, Jaroszewski DE, Holmes CE. Video-assisted thoracic surgery (VATS) as a safe alternative for the resection of pulmonary metastases: a retrospective cohort study. J Cardiothorac Surg. 2009;4(1):13.

19. Perentes JY, Krueger T, Lovis A, Ris H-B, Gonzalez M. Thoracoscopic resection of pulmonary metastasis: current practice and results. Crit Rev Oncol Hematol. 2015;95(1):105–13.

20. Cerfolio RJ, McCarty T, Bryant AS. Non-imaged pulmonary nodules discovered during thoracotomy for metastasectomy by lung palpation. Eur J Cardiothorac Surg. 2009;35(5):786–91.

21. Moorcraft SY, Ladas G, Bowcock A, Chau I. Management of resectable colorectal lung metastases. Clin Exp Metastasis. 2016;33(3):285–96.

22. Vickers M, Samson B, Colwell B, Cripps C, Jalink D, El-Sayed S, et al. Eastern Canadian Colorectal Cancer Consensus Conference: setting the limits of resectable disease. Curr Oncol. 2010;17(3):70–7.

23. Limmer S, Unger L. Optimal management of pulmonary metastases from colorectal cancer. Expert Rev Anticancer Ther. 2011;11(10):1567–75.

24. Berry MF. Role of segmentectomy for pulmonary metastases. Ann Cardiothoracic Surg. 2014;3(2):176–82.

25. Greenwood A, West D. Is a thoracotomy rather than thoracoscopic resection associated with improved survival after pulmonary metastasectomy? Interact Cardiovasc Thorac Surg. 2013;17(4):720–4.

26. Pfannschmidt J, Dienemann H, Hoffmann H. Surgical resection of pulmonary metastases from colorectal cancer: a systematic review of published series. Ann Thorac Surg. 2007;84(1):324–38.

27. Welter S, Jacobs J, Krbek T, Poettgen C, Stamatis G. Prognostic impact of lymph node involvement in pulmonary metastases from colorectal cancer. Eur J Cardiothorac Surg. 2007;31(2):167–72.

28. Szöke T, Kortner A, Neu R, Grosser C, Sziklavari Z, Wiebe K, et al. Is the mediastinal lymphadenectomy during pulmonary metastasectomy of colorectal cancer necessary? Interact Cardiovasc Thorac Surg. 2010;10(5):694–8.

29. Loehe F, Kobinger S, Hatz RA, Helmberger T, Loehrs U, Fuerst H. Value of systematic mediastinal lymph node dissection during pulmonary metastasectomy. Ann Thorac Surg. 2001;72(1):225–9.

30. Inoue M, Ohta M, Iuchi K, Matsumura A, Ideguchi K, Yasumitsu T, et al. Benefits of surgery for patients with pulmonary metastases from colorectal carcinoma. Ann Thorac Surg. 2004;78(1):238–44.

31. Mori M, Tomoda H, Ishida T, Kido A, Shimono R, Matsushima T, et al. Surgical resection of pulmonary metastases from colorectal adenocarcinoma: special reference to repeated pulmonary resections. Arch Surg. 1991;126(10):1297–302.

32. Welter S, Jacobs J, Krbek T, Krebs B, Stamatis G. Long-term survival after repeated resection of pulmonary metastases from colorectal cancer. Ann Thorac Surg. 2007;84(1):203–10.

33. Salah S, Watanabe K, Park JS, Addasi A, Park JW, Zabaleta J, et al. Repeated resection of colorectal cancer pulmonary oligometastases: pooled analysis and prognostic assessment. Ann Surg Oncol. 2013;20(6):1955–61.

34. Kandioler D, Krömer E, Tüchler H, End A, Müller MR, Wolner E, et al. Long-term results after repeated surgical removal of pulmonary metastases. Ann Thorac Surg. 1998;65(4):909–12.

35. Saito Y, Omiya H, Kohno K, Kobayashi T, Itoi K, Teramachi M, et al. Pulmonary metastasectomy for 165 patients with colorectal carcinoma: a prognostic assessment. J Thorac Cardiovasc Surg. 2002;124(5):1007–13.

36. Kim AW, Faber LP, Warren WH, Saclarides TJ, Carhill AA, Basu S, et al. Repeat pulmonary resection for metachronous colorectal carcinoma is beneficial. Surgery. 2008;144(4):712–8.

37. Riquet M, Foucault C, Cazes A, Mitry E, Dujon A, Barthes FLP, et al. Pulmonary resection for metastases of colorectal adenocarcinoma. Ann Thorac Surg. 2010;89(2):375–80.

38. Robert JH, Ambrogi V, Mermillod B, Dahabreh D, Goldstraw P. Factors influencing long-term survival after lung metastasectomy. Ann Thorac Surg. 1997;63(3):777–84.

39. Dave R, Pathak S, White A, Hidalgo E, Prasad K, Lodge J, et al. Outcome after liver resection in patients presenting with simultaneous hepatopulmonary colorectal metastases. Br J Surg. 2015;102(3):261–8.

40. Limmer S, Oevermann E, Killaitis C, Kujath P, Hoffmann M, Bruch H-P. Sequential surgical resection of hepatic and pulmonary metastases from colorectal cancer. Langenbeck's Arch Surg. 2010;395(8):1129–38.

41. Andres A, Mentha G, Adam R, Gerstel E, Skipenko O, Barroso E, et al. Surgical management of patients with colorectal cancer and simultaneous liver and lung metastases. Br J Surg. 2015;102(6):691–9.

42. Schüle S, Dittmar Y, Knösel T, Krieg P, Albrecht R, Settmacher U, et al. Long-term results and prognostic factors after resection of hepatic and pulmonary metastases of colorectal cancer. Int J Color Dis. 2013;28(4):537–45.

43. Sakamoto Y, Sakaguchi Y, Oki E, Minami K, Toh Y, Okamura T. Surgical outcomes after resection of both hepatic and pulmonary metastases from colorectal cancer. World J Surg. 2012;36(11):2708–13.

44. Mineo TC, Ambrogi V, Tonini G, Bollero P, Roselli M, Mineo D, et al. Longterm results after resection of simultaneous and sequential lung and liver metastases from colorectal carcinoma. J Am Coll Surg. 2003;197(3):386–91.

45. Salah S, Ardissone F, Gonzalez M, Gervaz P, Riquet M, Watanabe K, et al. Pulmonary metastasectomy in colorectal cancer patients with previously resected liver metastasis: pooled analysis. Ann Surg Oncol. 2015;22(6):1844–50.

46. Petre EN, Jia X, Thornton RH, Sofocleous CT, Alago W, Kemeny NE, et al. Treatment of pulmonary colorectal metastases by radiofrequency ablation. Clin Colorectal Cancer. 2013;12(1):37–44.

47. Yamakado K, Inoue Y, Takao M, Takaki H, Nakatsuka A, Uraki J, et al. Long-term results of radiofrequency ablation in colorectal lung metastases: single center experience. Oncol Rep. 2009;22(4):885.

48. Yan TD, King J, Sjarif A, Glenn D, Steinke K, Al-Kindy A, et al. Treatment failure after percutaneous radiofrequency ablation for nonsurgical candidates with pulmonary metastases from colorectal carcinoma. Ann Surg Oncol. 2007;14(5):1718–26.

49. Hiraki T, Gobara H, Iguchi T, Fujiwara H, Matsui Y, Kanazawa S. Radiofrequency ablation as treatment for pulmonary metastasis of colorectal cancer. World J Gastroenterol. 2014;20(4):988–96.

50. De Baere T, Aupérin A, Deschamps F, Chevallier P, Gaubert Y, Boige V, et al. Radiofrequency ablation is a valid treatment option for lung metastases: experience in 566 patients with 1037 metastases. Ann Oncol. 2015;26(5):987–91.

51. Schlijper RC, Grutters JP, Houben R, Dingemans A-MC, Wildberger JE, Van Raemdonck D, et al. What to choose as radical local treatment for lung metastases from colo-rectal cancer: surgery or radiofrequency ablation? Cancer Treat Rev. 2014;40(1):60–7.

52. Comito T, Cozzi L, Clerici E, Campisi MC, Liardo RLE, Navarria P, et al. Stereotactic ablative radiotherapy (SABR) in inoperable oligometastatic disease from colorectal cancer: a safe and effective approach. BMC Cancer. 2014;14(1):619.

53. Filippi AR, Badellino S, Ceccarelli M, Guarneri A, Franco P, Monagheddu C, et al. Stereotactic ablative radiation therapy as first local therapy for lung oligometastases from colorectal cancer: a single-institution cohort study. Int J Radiat Oncol Biol Phys. 2015;91(3):524–9.

54. Bar J, Herbst RS, Onn A. Targeted drug delivery strategies to treat lung metastasis. Exp Opin Drug Deliv. 2009;6(10):1003–16.

55. Yamauchi Y, Izumi Y, Kawamura M, Nakatsuka S, Yashiro H, Tsukada N, et al. Percutaneous cryoablation of pulmonary metastases from colorectal cancer. PLoS One. 2011;6(11):e27086.

56. Shi S, Yang J, Sun D. CT-guided 125I brachytherapy on pulmonary metastases after resection of colorectal cancer: a report of six cases. Oncol Lett. 2015;9(1):375–80.

57. Migliore M, Milošević M, Lees B, Treasure T, Di Maria G. Finding the evidence for pulmonary metastasectomy in colorectal cancer: the PulMicc trial. Future Oncol. 2015;11(2s):15–8.

Salvage Surgery

36

Jeremy Yip

Abstract

With increasing prevalence of colorectal cancer, local recurrence is becoming part of every colorectal surgeon's practice. Treatment options has been limited in the past, and mainly limited to palliative intent. A recent advance in surgical technique has opened new options with curative intent. Extended resection allows for R0 resection with clear margins with acceptable morbidities.

Keywords

Rectal cancer · Recurrence · Salvage surgery · Exenteration · Sacrectomy · Multidisciplinary team · Flap reconstruction

36.1 Introduction

Local recurrence in rectal cancer has reduced dramatically since the adoption of total mesorectal excision and neoadjuvant chemoradiation [1, 2]. However despite widespread adoption of these techniques, local recurrence still occurs in up to 30% of patients [3–5]. This may be due to technical factors associated with proctectomy.

J. Yip
Division of Colorectal Surgery, Department of Surgery, Queen Mary Hospital, University of Hong Kong, Hong Kong, China
e-mail: yipjeremy@hku.hk

Du et al. demonstrated that anastomotic leak and low lymph node sampling are associated with recurrence over the posterior and lateral compartments [6]. Leakage often results in a collection over the posterior compartment, and low lymph node sampling may be due to inadequate lateral lymph node dissection. If there is extensive unresectable distant metastasis, these patients are unsalvageable. However up to 50% of recurrences occur without the presence of distant metastasis [7]. This poses a significant dilemma. Historically pelvic recurrence has been difficult to treat. Surgery is extensive and potentially mutilating. It is associated with high morbidity. Patients with lateral pelvic sidewall recurrence and sacral involvement were often deemed unresectable. Yet without surgery, patients with recurrent disease have very limited survival with poor quality of life. They experience significant pain, intractable tenesmus, and vaginal or perineal malodorous discharge. Mean survival of patients without treatment is 7 months [3, 6]. Palliative treatment with chemotherapy and radiotherapy has limited response [4]. Survival may be extended to 9.3–15.1 months with radiotherapy alone or together with chemotherapy [8]. The outcome of salvage surgery is determined primarily by resection margin with R0 resection being the most important factor [4, 6, 9–11]. In the past the R0 resection rate is low. However, with improved surgical techniques, there is increasing hope for this group of patients. There is a growing body of evidence to suggest extended

© Springer Nature Singapore Pte Ltd. 2018
N. K. Kim et al. (eds.), *Surgical Treatment of Colorectal Cancer*,
https://doi.org/10.1007/978-981-10-5143-2_36

pelvic exenteration with en bloc partial sacrectomy, en bloc lateral compartment dissection, and even en bloc complete pubic bone excision can extend patient survival with a meaningful quality of life. A comparison between pelvic exenteration and abdominoperineal resection showed no statistical difference in perceived functional status between the two groups of patients [12]. Quality of life scores initially were lower in the pelvic exenteration group, but at 3 months after operation, the two groups were comparable [12]. A more recent systematic review on quality of life following pelvic exenteration showed quality of life returns to baseline in 2–9 months following exenteration for locally advanced and recurrent rectal cancers [13].

36.2   Assessment

Detection of recurrence can be difficult. This group of patients may have had previous irradiation and distorted anatomy from previous surgery making interpretation of imaging difficult. Recurrence can be totally asymptomatic, picked up during a routine surveillance scan/colonoscopy or an elevated carcinoembryonic antigen level. Patients can also present with a variety of symptoms depending on the location of the recurrence. This includes minor discomfort around the perineum, wound sinuses, fistulation, urinary problems, and neurological and bone pain. They had previous operations ranging from local excision to abdominoperineal resection (APR), which may make access to the pelvis difficult especially when bowel continuity is not restored. Obtaining histology is not always possible. Frequently recurrence after APR is a radiological diagnosis, and there is no histological proof prior to operation. In one series, histological confirmation was only possible in 75.2% of patients [6]. If there is no histology to confirm the recurrence, it is important to assess whether the MRI, PET, and CEA level correlates with the clinical suspicion of recurrence, especially when pelvic exenteration is a major undertaking. Multidisplinary meeting with an experienced radiologist, oncolo-

gist and colorectal surgeon is extremely important to determine whether the suspected lesion is a genuine recurrence or fibrotic changes from previous surgery or radiation. Given the extent of the surgery, assessment of patient's fitness for surgery is of utmost importance. A Delphi study conducted among a group of international colorectal surgery experts showed the presence of ascites, jaundice, portal hypertension, cachexia, and deep vein thrombosis as a poor prognostic factor to pelvic exenterative surgery and is considered a relative contraindication to surgery [14]. As with any colonic workup, a full colonoscopy is necessary to rule out metachronous tumor. Where necessary, a cystoscopy and a complete urogynecological examination should be performed when anterior compartment involvement is suspected. Positron emission tomography helps to rule out distant metastasis which is a relative contraindication for salvage surgery [14]. Pelvic exenteration in locally recurrent rectal cancer is difficult because of the effects of previous operations and irradiation leading to extensive fibrosis. It is extremely difficult to differentiate between tumor and fibrotic tissue. Often, to achieve R0 resection, preoperative imaging is the only reliable road map to success, making a good MRI irreplaceable in determining the local resectability of the tumor [14]. However due to prior operation and irradiation, it is often extremely difficult to interpret. Every patient should have a discussion with the expert radiologist, oncologist and surgeon to determine the operability of each patient. If the patient is radiotherapy naïve, long-course chemoradiation should be considered prior to salvage surgery.

36.2.1 Classification

An effective classification system conveys the most pertinent information in a straightforward manner. There are a few classification systems developed over the years by different centers. Memorial Sloan Kettering proposed a system by anatomical location, axial/perineal, anterior, posterior, and lateral [15]. The Leeds Group proposed a similar classification based on the

Table 36.1 Mayo Clinic classification

Presence of pain
S0 = asymptomatic
S1 = symptomatic without pain
S2 = symptomatic with pain
Degree of fixation
F0 = not fixed
F1 = fixed to one site
F2 = fixed at two sites
F3 = fixed at three or more sites

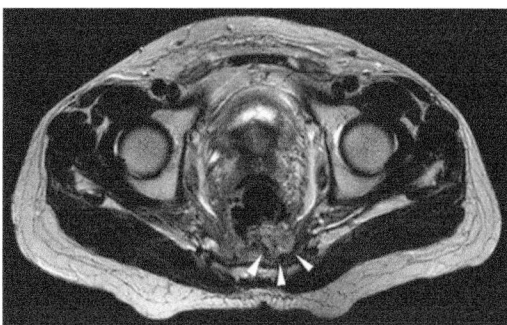

Fig. 36.1 MRI: isolated pelvic recurrence over the left piriformis (white arrow)

predominant location of the tumor, central, side-wall, sacral, or composite [5]. Axial recurrence includes local recurrence after local excision and clinical complete response after neoadjuvant therapy and anastomotic recurrence without invasion into the surrounding organs. Anterior recurrences invade into the genitourinary system. Posterior recurrence invades into the presacral space and the sacrum. Lateral recurrence involves the lateral compartment including the internal iliac vessels, ureters, piriformis, the obturator internus muscle, ischium, and the sacrotuberous and sacrospinous ligaments. The alternative classification is from Mayo Clinic, which is based on the presence of pain and the degree of fixation (Table 36.1) [16]. Classification by anatomical location is more widely adopted because surgical resection is planned according to the anatomical location of the recurrence and the organs involved. Through the anatomical classification, the intended resection is conveyed. It is also important to note that the anatomical location of the recurrence carries a heavy bearing to the rate of R0 resection. Moore et al. reported the presence of lateral compartment involvement adversely affects the rate of R0 resection when compared with the other three compartments. Isolated axial compartment recurrence is associated with significantly higher R0 resection rate (90%) [15].

36.2.2 Imaging

Previous studies have demonstrated both CT and MRI are accurate in detecting abdominal recurrences [4] (Fig. 36.1). MRI has an advantage over CT in the pelvic region providing a highly detailed soft tissue image which aids the resection as it may be difficult to differentiate between fibrosis and tumor intraoperatively. Hence MRI is the preferred modality to assess resectability [14, 17]. Because patient outcome is governed by the margin status, it is important to have a clear road map preoperatively to guide the resection. Without the MRI, it is difficult to have a good appreciation of the surgical planes, especially in the pelvis which has been operated on and irradiated on previously. Brown et al. retrospectively reviewed the correlation between MRI findings and the final pathology result and demonstrated a high sensitivity (73–100%) and specificity (50–100%) in detecting involvement of the anterior and posterior compartment [17]. However, there is some limitation in detecting lateral compartment involvement with a sensitivity of 46% and specificity of 91% [17]. Salvage surgery is always a major undertaking associated with significant morbidity. It would be devastating for the patient and the surgeon to discover after an extensive salvage surgery that there are distant metastases. A good-quality positron emission tomography (PET) helps to exclude distant metastasis which will affect the outcome of the patient. PET scan also compliments the MRI when it may be difficult for the MRI to differentiate fibrosis, postoperative changes from an actual recurrence with an overall accuracy of 87% [4]. Whether a contrast computer tomography can be a substitute if PET scan is not available remains a controversy. But given the magnitude of the surgery, it is advisable to obtain a PET scan as there is currently limited evidence to support the role of salvage surgery in patients with metastatic disease. However there is growing interest in patients with limited visceral metastases amendable with limited resection [14]. Whether pelvic exenteration should be extended to this group of patient remains to be studied.

36.3 Surgery

Without surgery, patients with pelvic recurrence often have limited survival which is also associated with an extremely poor quality of life. They experience significant pain and wound complications which can be debilitating severely limiting their quality of life. Chemotherapy and external beam radiation therapy have limited efficacy in treating isolated pelvic recurrence. Salvage surgery offers the only chance of cure in this group of patients. Salvage surgery is safe with a low perioperative mortality 0–1.6% [5, 10, 18, 19]. With surgery, overall 5-year survival can be as high as 65–68.3% [6, 19]. However there is significant morbidity from pelvic exenterative surgery for recurrence disease, 21–82% [4, 9, 18, 19]. These include but not limited to pelvis sepsis, enterocutaneous fistula, wound complications, and urinary complications. As a result, before any attempt in salvage surgery, a detailed discussion with the patient and careful surgical planning are important. Salvage surgery often involves multiple specialties including radiologist, oncologist, urologist, plastic surgeons, orthopedic surgeons, and intensivist. These patients should be referred to a dedicated tertiary center which has experience in operating on these patients. Often the operating field has been operated on and irradiated on prior to salvage surgery making it extremely difficult to differentiate scar tissue from tumor tissue. Therefore, every patient should have a discussion in a multidisciplinary meeting with an experienced radiologist and oncologist to determine the resection margin. Other involved subspecialties should also be included in the discussion as surgery frequently involves urologists, plastic surgeons, and orthopedic surgeons if a sacral transection above S3 is required. Once the margin is decided, the subsequent surgery should follow the decision at the multidisciplinary meeting as much as possible, as any deviation may result in a positive margin jeopardizing the ultimate outcome. If there is any doubt as to the margin, it is often worthwhile to obtain further margin for frozen section.

36.3.1 Axial Compartment

Axial recurrence includes anastomotic recurrence, mesorectal recurrence, and more recently recurrence after local excision or cCR after neoadjuvant treatment. Fortunately, anastomotic recurrence and failure after local excision and neoadjuvant treatment are usually detected early when patients are surveilled according to established guidelines. They are relatively easy to detect as there is still access via endoscopy. Surgery involves resecting the neo-rectum together with the surrounding soft tissue. Surgery is usually straightforward if the anastomosis is above the prostate. Difficulty arises when the previous anastomosis is at the level of the prostate in the male. The comparatively narrower pelvis in Asians, together with the dense adhesions due to lack of soft tissue between the prostate and anastomosis, makes dissection in this anterior plane extremely difficult especially with the limited visual field in the pelvis. This area runs the highest risk of positive margin. Dissection may end up in the bowel lumen, perforating the tumor. This risk needs to be balanced with the morbidity associated with a total exenteration with an ileal conduit. If this margin is threatened, it may be more prudent to treat it as an anterior recurrence. To reduce the morbidity from a total exenteration, some authors advocate an en bloc prostatectomy instead of total exenteration [20]. However, this is extremely challenging. Posteriorly, dissection follows the holy plane but can include the presacral fascia if necessary.

36.3.2 Posterior Compartment

Involvement of the sacrum or the presacral space can be effectively dealt with by en bloc sacrectomy. Preoperative imaging with MRI to plan the level of sacral resection is important. Brown et al. reported a sensitivity and specificity of S1–S2 involvement of 100% when comparing the MRI findings to the pathology findings. Sensitivity and specificity of S3 or below is slightly lower at 83% and 96%, respectively [17]. Historically, posterior compartment recurrence necessitating a sacrectomy is divided into the abdominal phase, the perineal phase, and the prone phase. The operation starts with an exploratory laparotomy and abdominal mobilization. After the abdominal and perineal parts are completed, the wound is closed and the patient is turned prone for the sacrectomy. During the prone phase, there is loss of proximal vascular control from the abdomen. In addition, turning the patient prone mid-operation is time-consuming. For low sacral (S3 or below) or coccygeal involvement, sacrectomy via an abdominal approach is possible. This procedure was proposed by Prof. Michael Solomon [21]. This is done with the patient in modified Lloyd-Davis position with the sacrum lifted off the surgical table with support over the lumbosacral joint. The first abdominal phase is completed by abdominal mobilization of the ureters, the neo-rectum, and the bladder if necessary. Preemptively dissecting the internal iliac vessels and controlling with vessel loop is advisable. Control of the internal iliac may be necessary if torrential bleeding is encountered. When ligation of the internal iliac vessels is necessary, it is preferred to preserve the first branch of the internal iliac to improve perfusion to the skin and muscle flap [20]. The need for lateral dissection is dictated by the preoperatively imaging. It is advisable to include the lateral compartment lymph nodes in the resection if it was not previously excised. Posteriorly, dissection follows presacral fascia down to the intended level of sacral transection. While the abdominal surgeon is completing the dissection, the perineal phase can begin after the anus is closed with suture to prevent tumor cell spillage. After standard ellipti-

cal incision around the anus, the ischiorectal fat can be partially or completely removed depending on the lateral extension. Entry to the pelvic cavity is guided by the abdominal surgeon. Depending on the required lateral margin, the levator ani, obturator internus, and the piriformis can be included in the resection. The dissection continues posterior to the coccyx, disconnecting the gluteus maximus from the coccyx and sacrum until the intended transection level is reach. This is not possible if the sacrum is not lifted off the table with support at the lumbosacral joint, hence the importance of good positioning before the operation. An osteotome is hammered into the sacrum posteriorly to protect the skin from a potential through and through puncture when the abdominal surgeon hammers down the osteotome anteriorly. Once the posterior osteotome is in position, the abdominal surgeon hammers an osteotome anteriorly at the level of transection until the two osteotomes meet. This approach has the benefit of not requiring repositioning the patient mid-procedure, decreasing the operative time. It also allows access to the abdomen for proximal vascular control if torrential bleeding is encountered during the sacrectomy and construction of ileal conduit, vertical rectus abdominis muscle flap, and colostomy. For tumors that require sacrectomy above the S3 level, the dissection is first completed down to the level of intended transection, and then a large radiopaque pin is applied to mark the level of transection. The pin must be large enough to be easily spotted on the image intensifier. An extra-large metallic liga-clip is usually too small to be visualized on the image intensified; hence, an orthopedic fixation pin is used instead to ensure clear visualization. The pelvis is packed with large swabs to protect the peritoneal contents when the patient is operated in a prone position. The sacrectomy is then performed in the prone position with the nerve root identified and protected (Fig. 36.2). In a recent systemic review focused on pelvic exenteration with en bloc sacrectomy, Sasikumar et al. reported R0 resection was achieved in 78% of patients, and disease-free survival of R0 patients was 55% at a median follow-up period of 33 months [9].

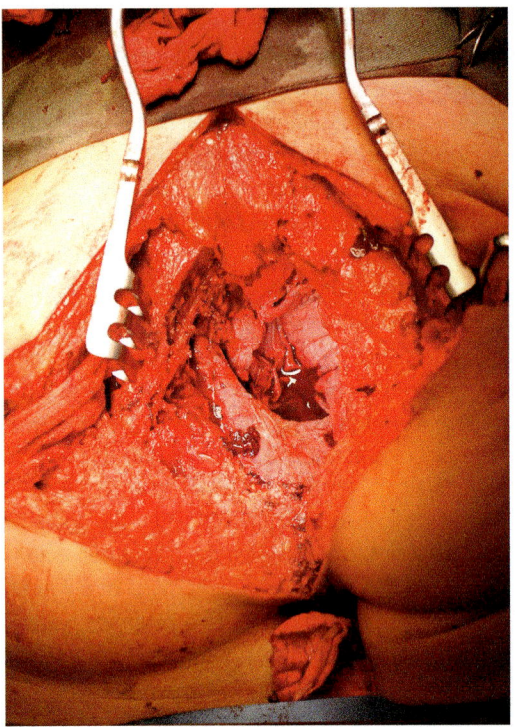

Fig. 36.2 Pelvic exenteration with en bloc sacrectomy at S2

36.3.3 Anterior Compartment

Anterior recurrence can be dealt with effectively with anterior exenteration. In the female, the vagina and uterus are the most common site of involvement. It is uncommon for primary rectal tumors to involve the pubic symphysis anteriorly although if involved an en bloc resection of the pubic symphysis is possible [22]. In one series, pathologies that may require an en bloc resection of the pubic symphysis include osteosarcoma, prostate carcinoma, squamous and transitional cell carcinoma of the bladder, anal squamous cell carcinoma, and cervical squamous cell carcinoma [22]. In male, the prostate and the urethra just distal to the prostate can be involved. If the urethra is divided just distal to the prostate after division of the dorsal venous plexus, this may expose the recurrence threatening the anterior margin. Another option would be to perform a perineal urethrectomy to extend the anterior margin [23]. This is performed at the level of the symphysis pubis. This method described by Solomon et al. begins with dissection along the inferior border of the inferior pubic rami toward the symphysis pubis and then lifting the bulbospongiosus muscle off the symphysis pubis before ligating and dividing the bulbospongiosus muscle, the urethra, and the dorsal venous plexus [23]. Besides increasing the anterior margin, this also neglects the necessity of having to transect the dorsal venous plexus at the retropubic space which can be difficult in patients with a large pelvic tumor and heavily irradiated tissue where stitches might not hold. If required, after mobilization of the bladder and perineal urethrectomy, the resection can include en bloc complete or partial pubic bone excision. This is more commonly required in patients with tumors from the anterior pelvic organs rather than from rectal recurrences [22].

36.3.4 Lateral Compartment

Direct invasion into the lateral compartment previously meant patient was unsalvageable. With the increased experience from lateral pelvic lymph node dissection, this is no longer an absolute contraindication to surgery. However, lateral compartment involvement is still associated with the worst outcome compared with all the different compartments [14, 15, 18]. R0 resection is more difficult and often limited by the bony pelvic sidewall. Operation in this region is often made even more difficult by previous radiation and surgery. In 2004, Moore et al. reported a R0 resection rate of 19% when the pelvic sidewall was involved radiologically [15]. This contrasts with 66.5% reported in a more recent publication [19]. In a retrospective review of one of the largest series of lateral pelvic compartment excision, R0 resection is again demonstrated as the only predictor of overall and disease-free survival ($p = 0.030$ and 0.014, respectively) [19]. Preoperative MRI is imperial in determining the extent of resection; however, authors reported difficulty when there are extensive postoperative or post-radiotherapy changes limiting the sensitivity. Brown et al.

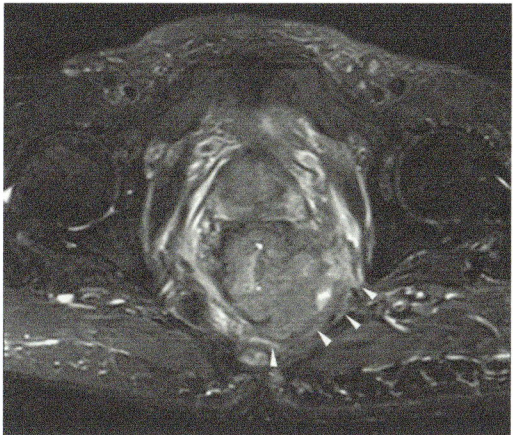

Fig. 36.3 MRI: locally advanced rectal cancer with left pelvic sidewall involvement

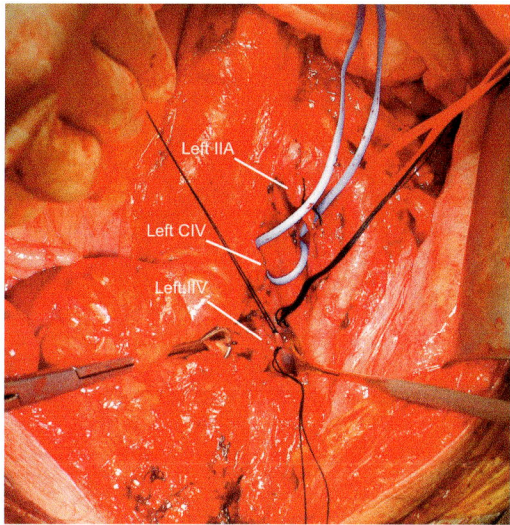

Fig. 36.4 Anatomy of lateral sidewall after the left ureter has been divided. IIA, Internal iliac artery (transected); CIV, common iliac vein; IIV, internal iliac vein

reported MRI sensitivity and specificity of 46% and 91% in determining pelvic sidewall involvement [17] (Fig. 36.3). Where MRI findings alone are inconclusive, PET scan may be of help in differentiating recurrence and scar tissue. Again, this demonstrates the importance of a multidisciplinary meeting with a dedicated experienced radiologist. To obtain a wide margin for R0 resection, the dissection should start beyond the TME plane. After ureterolysis and division of the ureter proximal to the tumor, the common iliac and internal iliac vessels are dissected and slung with vascular loops (Fig. 36.4). The beyond total mesorectal excision collaborative considers encasement of external or common iliac vessels a relative contraindication to surgery [24]. However, Solomon et al. reported excision of the common or external iliac vessels did not confer an inferior survival when compared to those who do not have common or external iliac vessel involvement [19]. Depending on the involvement by the tumor, the common and external iliac vessels may be resected and reconstructed by vascular surgeons using either autologous or synthetic graft before continuing with further dissection (Fig. 36.5). With the patient in modified Lloyd-Davies position, the deep pelvic fascia is identified by ligating and dividing the internal iliac vessels preferably distal to the first branch. Entering this plane allows dissection along the lumbosacral trunk and

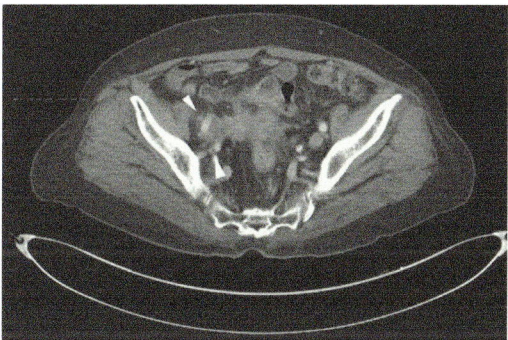

Fig. 36.5 Involvement of the left external iliac [white arrow]

the sacral nerve. Through this dissection, the piriformis muscle, obturator interns, and the levator muscles can be clearly visualized. The muscles can be dissected free from the pelvic sidewall allowing for maximal lateral margin. With this method described by Solomon et al., R0 resection rate improved from 21% to 66.5%, and a 35% 5-year survival rate was achieved by this experience group [19]. Shaikh et al. proposed a method of lateral wall dissection using a transgluteal approach in a prone position [25]. In their series of six patients, R0 resection was achieved in all

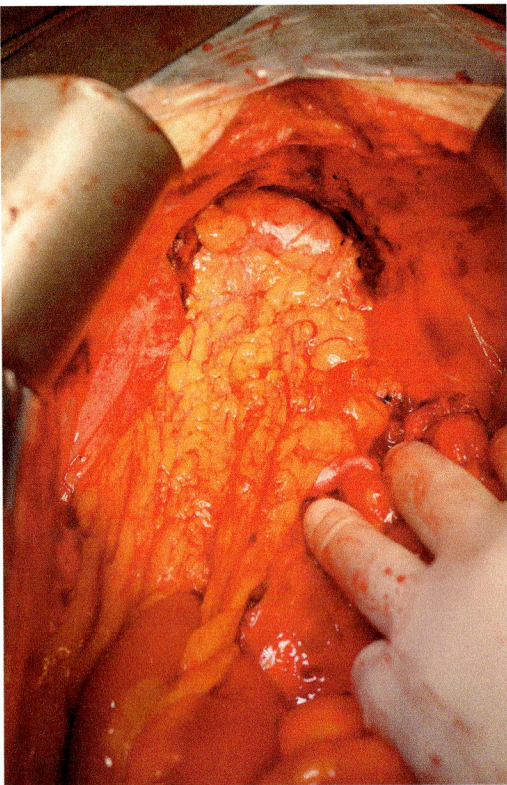

Fig. 36.6 Omentoplasty

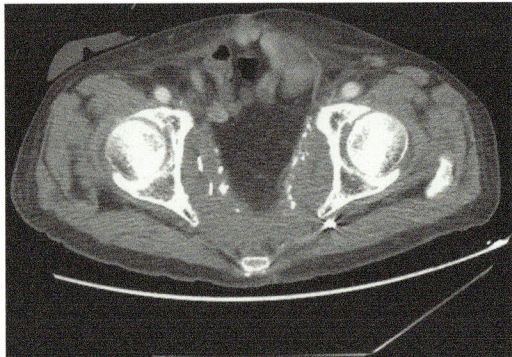

Fig. 36.7 CT image after omentoplasty with a large bulk of soft tissue in the pelvis

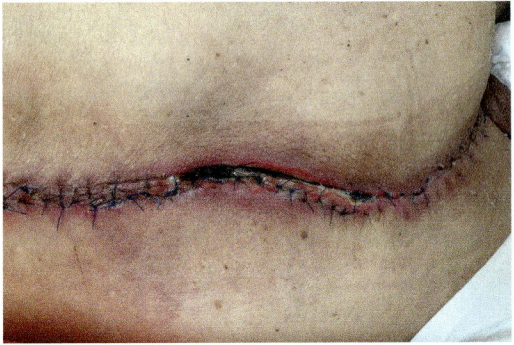

Fig. 36.8 Wound edge necrosis after ligation of the internal iliac artery at origin

six patients. This approach requires patient to be in a prone position at the start of the procedure and limits access to the abdomen to assess for metastatic disease. Transgluteal approach may also be unfamiliar to many colorectal surgeons, and an abdominal approach is preferred.

36.3.5 Flap Reconstructions

Pelvic exenterative surgery is often associated with a large perineal defect in terms of soft tissue space and skin. This large pelvic cavity is a reservoir for collections which results in pelvic sepsis. Although the bowel will drop down to fill up this space, it may not be able to completely obliterate the space, and also the bowel may adhere to sharp bony edges after bone resection. This may potentially lead to adhesive intestinal obstruction or bowel fistulation. It is the author's practice to as much as possible fill up the space with vascularized tissue. The most common method would be

to perform an omentoplasty (Fig. 36.6). A large tongue of omentum is mobilized based on a left or right gastroepiploic artery and vein and rotated along the paracolic gutter down to the pelvis to fill up the void rather than leaving the bowel to drop into the pelvis. This omental flap provides a large bulk of vascular soft tissue to fill up the potential space which helps to reduce the incidence of pelvic sepsis and prevents bowel obstruction due to adhesion in the pelvis (Fig. 36.7). This vascular soft tissue is resistant to infection and allows reabsorption of fluid in the pelvis. Perineal skin in patients with recurrent cancers is often heavily irradiated and may have impaired perfusion after exenterative surgery especially if the internal iliac vessels have been resected. In addition to bridging the skin defect, using a flap helps to reduce the wound complications such as wound edge necrosis (Fig. 36.8) and dehiscence [20]. A variety of flaps has been described to close the perineal

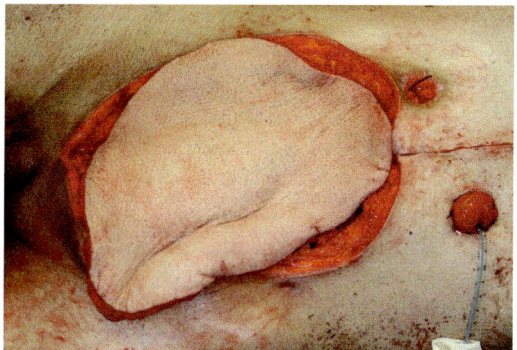

Fig. 36.9 Large ALT flap for abdominal wall reconstruction

defect. This includes anterolateral thigh flap, vertical rectus abdominis muscle flap, gracilis myocutaneous flap, and gluteal myocutaneous flap. Flap selection depends on the preference of the plastic surgeons. The anterolateral thigh flap has an advantage over vertical rectus abdominis flap in leaving the rectus muscle intact for stoma creation, potentially reducing the incidence of stoma related complication especially hernia. Another benefit of using an anterolateral thigh flap is that the plastic surgeon can work simultaneously on the thigh as it does not block access to the perineum or the abdomen and does not require reposition of the patient. This potentially saves operative time in an already long operation. The size of the anterolateral thigh flap can be as large as 10 cm by 25 cm [26]. The resulting defect in the anterolateral thigh can be closed primarily if the defect is small or with split-thickness skin graft from the contralateral thigh if necessary [26]. Before placing the flap, it is important to ensure the bony sacral transection surface is not causing excessive pressure on the wound as to cause skin necrosis and dehiscence. In cases where resection of the anterior abdominal wall is necessary, the anterolateral thigh flap can also be used for reconstruction (Fig. 36.9). Since the development of biological mesh, there has been interest in using biological mesh to repair the perineal defect. To this day, there is no strong evidence to support the routine use of biological mesh to improve wound healing after exenteration. The BIOPEX study showed limited evidence that it may reduce the incidence of perineal hernia after extralevator abdominoperineal resection [27].

36.4 Complications

There is no doubt that salvage surgery is associated with a high rate of morbidity. Bhangu et al. reported a major complication rate of 51% in a meta-analysis of 22 studies representing 1460 patients receiving surgery for recurrent rectal cancer [11]. Complication rate in each study ranges from 27% to 81%. The most common complications include pelvic collection and wound dehiscence. Other complications include enterocutaneous fistula, chest infection, ileal conduit leak, urinary sepsis, and stoma complications. Solomon et al. reported sepsis as the most common cause of morbidity, including urinary sepsis, intra-abdominal collection, and wound related. Pelvic collection occurs in as many as 29.5% of patients in their series about half of which requires reoperation [19].

36.5 Summary

Locally recurrent rectal cancer remains a challenging problem faced by many colorectal surgeons. Despite advances in the management of rectal cancer, recurrence still occurs. Although challenging, it is potentially curable with a meaningful quality of life [12, 13]. Patients with suspected recurrence require a thorough assessment with MRI and PET and discussion in a multidisciplinary meeting to determine the resectability. R0 resection is the goal in all salvage surgery and is the major determinant of outcome after operation. Because salvage surgery is associated with significant morbidity, a careful patient selection and thorough discussion with the patient are warranted.

References

1. Heald RJ, RDH R. Recurrence and survival after total mesorectal excision for rectal cancer. Lancet. 1986;327(8496):1479–82.
2. Kapiteijn E, Marijnen CAM, Nagtegaal ID, Putter H, Steup WH, Wiggers T, et al. Preoperative radiotherapy combined with total mesorectal excision for resectable rectal cancer. https://doi.org/10.1056/NEJMoa010580. Massachusetts Medical Society; 2009.

3. Sagar PM, Pemberton JH. Surgical management of locally recurrent rectal cancer. Br J Surg. 1996;83(3):293–304.

4. Heriot AG, Tekkis PP, Darzi A, Mackay J. Surgery for local recurrence of rectal cancer. Colorectal Dis. 2006;8(9):733–47.

5. Boyle KM, Sagar PM, Chalmers AG, Sebag-Montefiore D, Cairns A, Eardley I. Surgery for locally recurrent rectal cancer. Dis Colon Rectum. 2005;48(5):929–37.

6. Du P, Burke JP, Khoury W, Lavery IC, Kiran RP, Remzi FH, et al. Factors associated with the location of local rectal cancer recurrence and predictors of survival. Int J Colorectal Dis. 2016;31(4):825–32.

7. Hogan NM, Joyce MR. Surgical management of locally recurrent rectal cancer. Int J Surg Oncol. 2012;2012(12):1–6.

8. Ito Y. Efficacy of chemoradiotherapy on pain relief in patients with intrapelvic recurrence of rectal cancer. Jpn J Clin Oncol. 2003;33(4):180–5.

9. Sasikumar A, Bhan C, Jenkins JT, Antoniou A, Murphy J. Systematic review of pelvic exenteration with en bloc sacrectomy for recurrent rectal adenocarcinoma: R0 resection predicts disease-free survival. Dis Colon Rectum. 2017;60(3):346–52.

10. Rizzuto A, Palaia I, Vescio G, Serra R, Malanga D, Sacco R. Multivisceral resection for occlusive colorectal cancer: is it justified? Int J Surg. 2016;33:S142–7.

11. Bhangu A, Ali SM, Darzi A, Brown G, Tekkis P. Meta-analysis of survival based on resection margin status following surgery for recurrent rectal cancer. Colorectal Dis. 2012;14(12):1457–66.

12. Radwan RW, Codd RJ, Wright M, Fitzsimmons D, Evans MD, Davies M, et al. Quality-of-life outcomes following pelvic exenteration for primary rectal cancer. Br J Surg. 2015;102(12):1574–80.

13. Rausa E, Kelly ME, Bonavina L, O'Connell PR, Winter DC. A systematic review examining quality of life following pelvic exenteration for locally advanced and recurrent rectal cancer. Colorectal Dis. 2017;19(5):430–6.

14. Chew M-H, Brown WE, Masya L, Harrison JD, Myers E, Solomon MJ. Clinical, MRI, and PET-CT criteria used by surgeons to determine suitability for pelvic exenteration surgery for recurrent rectal cancers. Dis Colon Rectum. 2013;56(6):717–25.

15. Moore HG, Shoup M, Riedel E, Minsky BD, Alektiar KM, Ercolani M, et al. Colorectal cancer pelvic recurrences: determinants of resectability. Dis Colon Rectum. 2004;47(10):1599–606.

16. Suzuki K, Dozois RR, Devine RM, Nelson H, Weaver AL, Gunderson LL, et al. Curative reoperations for locally recurrent rectal cancer. Dis Colon Rectum. 1996;39(7):730–6.

17. Brown WE, Koh CE, Badgery-Parker T, Solomon MJ. Validation of MRI and surgical decision making to predict a complete resection in pelvic exenteration for recurrent rectal cancer. Dis Colon Rectum. 2017;60(2):144–51.

18. Heriot AG, Byrne CM, Lee P, Dobbs B, Tilney H, Solomon MJ, et al. Extended radical resection: the choice for locally recurrent rectal cancer. Dis Colon Rectum. 2008;51(3):284–91.

19. Solomon MJ, Brown KGM, Koh CE, Lee P, Austin KKS, Masya L. Lateral pelvic compartment excision during pelvic exenteration. Br J Surg. 2015;102(13):1710–7.

20. Mirnezami AH, Sagar PM, Kavanagh D, Witherspoon P, Lee P, Winter D. Clinical algorithms for the surgical management of locally recurrent rectal cancer. Dis Colon Rectum. 2010;53(9):1248–57.

21. Solomon MJ, Tan K-K, Bromilow RG, Al-mozany N, Lee PJ. Sacrectomy via the abdominal approach during pelvic exenteration. Dis Colon Rectum. 2014;57(2):272–7.

22. Austin KKS, Herd AJ, Solomon MJ, Ly K, Lee PJ. Outcomes of pelvic exenteration with en bloc partial or complete pubic bone excision for locally advanced primary or recurrent pelvic cancer. Dis Colon Rectum. 2016;59(9):831–5.

23. Solomon MJ, Austin KKS, Masya L, Lee P. Pubic bone excision and perineal urethrectomy for radical anterior compartment excision during pelvic exenteration. Dis Colon Rectum. 2015;58(11):1114–9.

24. The Beyond TME Collaborative. Consensus statement on the multidisciplinary management of patients with recurrent and primary rectal cancer beyond total mesorectal excision planes. Br J Surg. 2013;100(8):1009–14.

25. Shaikh I, Aston W, Hellawell G, Ross D, Littler S, Burling D, et al. Extended lateral pelvic sidewall excision (ELSiE): an approach to optimize complete resection rates in locally advanced or recurrent anorectal cancer involving the pelvic sidewall. Tech Coloproctol. 2014;18(12):1161–8.

26. Ali RS, Bluebond-Langner R, Rodriguez ED, Cheng M-H. The versatility of the anterolateral thigh flap. Plast Reconstr Surg. 2009;124(6S):e395.

27. Musters GD, Klaver CEL, Bosker RJI, Burger JWA, van Duijvendijk P, van Etten B, et al. Biological mesh closure of the pelvic floor after extralevator abdominoperineal resection for rectal cancer: a multicenter randomized controlled trial (the BIOPEX-study). Ann Surg. 2016;265(6):1074–81.

Palliative Management for Advanced Colorectal Cancer

37

Seung Yoon Yang, Jong Min Lee, and Nam Kyu Kim

Abstract

Over the last two decades, the concept of "palliative" has changed due to the pivotal role of multidisciplinary approach and chemotherapy. Incurable CRC patients may be asymptomatic or present various symptoms from dyspepsia to life-threatening conditions such as malignant obstruction, perforation, and lower gastrointestinal bleeding which needs emergency surgical intervention. The overall survival is still the main endpoint of palliative management in CRC patients. But the quality of residual life affected by surgery, chemotherapy, and any other palliative treatment should not be underestimated but should be an immensely important issue. Multidisciplinary approach is needed for appropriate management to control the symptoms and to improve the quality of life of patients with disease progression and incurable CRC.

Keywords

Colorectal cancer · Palliative care · Multimodal treatment · Surgery · Chemotherapy

37.1 Introduction

Colorectal cancer (CRC) is a common neoplasia in the world, and every fifth patient with CRC presents with metastatic disease which is not curable with radical intent in roughly 80% of cases [1, 2]. Traditionally palliative approach to incurable stage IV CRC patients was surgery by resection of the primary tumor, intestinal bypass, or stoma. Over the last two decades, concept of "palliative" has changed due to the progress of surgery and systemic therapy of CRC and distant metastasis [3–5]. Especially by a pivotal role of multidisciplinary approach and chemotherapy, the management of incurable stage IV CRC patients has significantly changed and increased the oncological outcomes [6]. For unresectable colorectal cancers, the most important issue is whether the disease is symptomatic or asymptomatic. Unresectable CRC patients may be asymptomatic or present various symptoms from dyspepsia to life-threatening conditions such as malignant obstruction, perforation, and lower gastrointestinal bleeding which needs emergency management. This may not only prolong survival and enable to receive palliative systemic treatment but also impact patient's quality of life [7]. The treatment goal for asymptomatic patients is to decelerate cancer progression to prolong survival and prevent cancer-related modalities. Recent guidelines do not recommend primary tumor resection in asymptomatic unresectable

S. Y. Yang · J. M. Lee · N. K. Kim (✉)
Department of Surgery, Yonsei University College of Medicine, Seoul, South Korea
e-mail: syjeong@snu.ac.kr; NAMKYUK@yuhs.ac

© Springer Nature Singapore Pte Ltd. 2018
N. K. Kim et al. (eds.), *Surgical Treatment of Colorectal Cancer*,
https://doi.org/10.1007/978-981-10-5143-2_37

patients [6–8]. Modern systemic chemotherapeutic agents have been shown to be more effective and reduced the need of palliative surgery when compared to conventional 5-fluorouracil-based chemotherapy [9, 10]. The overall survival is still the main endpoint of palliative management in CRC patients. But the quality of residual life affected by surgery, chemotherapy, and any other palliative treatment should not be underestimated but should be an immensely important issue.

37.2 Palliative Surgery of the Symptomatic Incurable CRC

Palliative surgery for symptomatic incurable CRC is aimed for symptom relief and recommended on complications such as obstruction or significant bleeding by international guidelines [11]. Otherwise it would be better to avoid surgical intervention, but if needed, the extent of surgery, the type of surgery, and timing of surgical intervention should be considered. And also surgical plans to effectively achieve that goal must balance the potential benefit of durable symptom relief with the inherent risk of postoperative morbidity and mortality, with already nutritionally replete patients [12]. For patients with advanced incurable malignancy, complications, along with their required additional care, are not as well tolerated. This morbidity diminishes the potential benefit of a palliative procedure by negatively impacting the patient's quality of life. The appropriated application of palliative surgery in well-selected patients can provide effective symptom relief [13].

37.2.1 Stomas

Loop stomas are preferred than end stomas by pulling the ileum or the colon through a full-thickness incision passing through the rectus muscle. Choosing an appropriate position on the abdominal wall for the stoma is one of the most important things to consider. A stoma that is lateral to the rectus sheath can predispose the patient to a parastomal hernia and prolapse. Colostomy

is more favorable for palliation for having the advantage of lower volume, solid stools, and lower morbidity and is easier to manage the stomas than ileostomy [14]. Colostomy formation is a procedure particularly well suited to laparoscopic techniques since there is no requirement for specimen extraction. For most indications, a sigmoid colostomy is superior to a colostomy created from more proximal colon. The ease with which the transverse colon can be delivered as a stoma is more than offset by the difficulty of ostomy care experienced by patients [15, 16].

37.2.2 Internal Bypass

Internal bypasses are usually performed for colon cancer through laparotomy by side-to-side anastomosis between the ileum/colon proximal to obstructing tumor and the colon distal to tumor. Since colonic obstruction is normally associated to bowel distension, performing laparoscopic anastomosis should be considered a very demanding procedure and reserved to experienced laparoscopic surgeons [17].

37.3 Tumor-Related Emergency

When surgeons are confronted with colorectal cancer patients who are suffering from life-threatening complication, the first decision point should be whether this complication could be managed surgically or not. In addition to surgery, non-operative approaches such as stent insertion and laser therapy have been applied recently. Surgery is the last step in solving this situation, but we should make a careful assessment of whether patients can withstand surgical stress. And we must determine the best way to manage the problem (Fig. 37.1).

37.3.1 Obstruction

Obstruction is reported in 10–26% of metastatic CRC, the most frequent condition requiring an aggressive and emergent management of patients

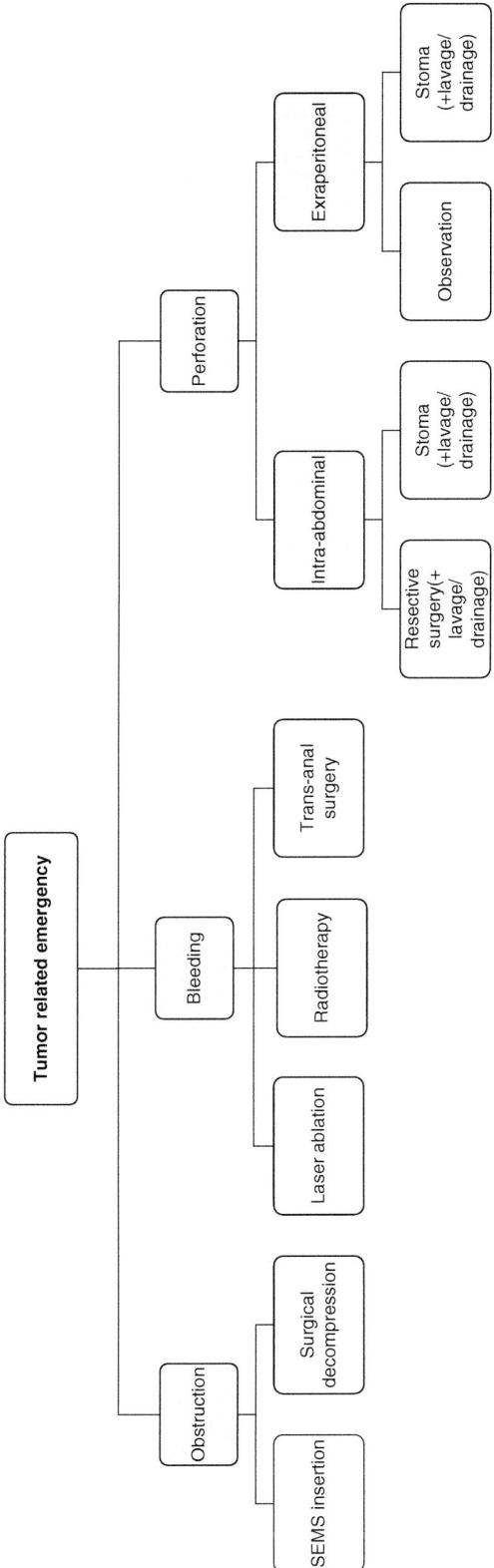

Fig. 37.1 Algorithm for management of tumor-related emergency for incurable colorectal cancer patients

with incurable CRC [18, 19]. The management of obstructing CRCs varies according to the site of primary tumor. Mostly resection is preferred in proximal tumors, whereas other treatment options may be preferred in the case of CRCs located in the sigmoid or rectum including stenting [20, 21].

37.3.1.1 Colonic Stent

After the first being used by Dohmoto et al. [22], self-expanding metallic stent (SEMS) placement became an alternative approach to emergency surgical interventions for patients with inoperable malignant colonic obstruction. The colonic stent insertion showed clear advantages of lower postoperative mortality, reduced intensive and overall hospital stay, and earlier start of chemotherapy than emergency surgery in previous research [20, 23]. However the clinical success rate was higher in emergency surgery, and there was no difference in the postoperative complications. There are concerns about chemotherapy raising complication rates of stent placement, especially of colonic perforation especially with anti-angiogenic agents. Colonic stenting is not recommended in patients who are considered for treatment with anti-angiogenic agents such as bevacizumab, regorafenib, and aflibercept due to increased stent-related colonic perforation [24–26]. Although complications associated with colonic stent insertion such as perforation, stent failure, re-obstruction, and stent migration were major concerns, colonic stents obviously have a role in the palliation. Stent-related complications may need reinterventions either with re-stenting or palliative surgery [27].

37.3.1.2 Surgical Palliation

Traditionally, resection (LAR, APR, Hartmann's operation) has been advocated to prevent later complication such as bleeding or pelvic pain and ureteral obstruction. Resective surgery is usually preferred in proximal CRC, where colostomy is not an option. Internal bypass by ileo-colonic (transverse or sigmoid) anastomosis is performed. For obstructing distal tumors, diversion with a proximal colostomy and loop ileostomy is likely still the safest and most durable option.

Colostomy or ileostomy has the advantage that it can also be done by laparoscopy. Laparoscopic surgery is associated with less postoperative pain and shorter hospital stay, which enable the resumption of palliative [28]. A primary anastomosis can be considered in select, low-risk patients. This should be weighed very carefully when performing surgical palliation, as an anastomotic leakage after primary anastomosis may delay chemotherapy and other palliative treatments [29].

37.3.2 Bleeding

37.3.2.1 Laser Ablation

The most commonly used nonsurgical treatment in this situation is the neodymium-doped yttrium aluminum garnet (Nd: YAG) laser. The energy delivered by the laser causes coagulative necrosis to stop the bleeding. It can be tried several times thanks to the advantage of being easy to perform without any anesthesia. It is also used for the obstruction but is said to be particularly effective in controlling bleeding. Coagulation was achieved in 80–90% of patients, with complications occurring in 2–15% [30]. It is known to be relatively ineffective for cancer involving long-segment colon or circumferential tumor. Despite these limitations, laser ablation is an acceptable modality for palliation of bleeding in high-risk patients.

37.3.2.2 Radiotherapy

Radiotherapy is a treatment that can reduce the pain caused by nerve involvement as well as bleeding, with relief in about 75% of patients [31]. However, the survival benefit due to radiotherapy is unexpected and is useful for patients with short life expectancy because the symptoms recur within 6 months of approximately half of the patients [32].

37.3.3 Perforation

Colonic perforation is the most life-threatening condition requiring emergent surgery. There are various mechanisms that can cause perforation, such as the distension of the large bowel due to obstruction, tumor necrosis, the complication of stent insertion, and laser therapy [33]. However, regardless of the mechanism, the most important part in determining the direction of surgery is the location of the perforation and the presence of diffuse peritonitis.

If the perforation causes signs of diffuse peritonitis or severe sepsis, emergency surgery with laparotomy should usually be performed. The aim of surgery in this case should be to focus on eliminating septic focus and preventing future peritonitis by resecting the perforated segment and cleaning contaminated intra-abdominal cavity. The removal of perforated colon and anastomosis can be performed simultaneously, but it is accompanied with the risk of postoperative leakage. Instead, creating a temporary stoma without anastomosis is a safer option. Although performing anastomosis with protective stoma can be executed at the same time, this is rarely performed unless the patient is expected to have longer survival.

If the location of the perforated tumor is extraperitoneal rectum or the perforation is sealed off to cause localized peritonitis, it is possible to manage with drainage of abscess with broad-spectrum antibiotics.

37.4 Role of Radiotherapy

Radiotherapy is a successful, time-efficient, well-tolerated, and cost-effective intervention that is crucial for the appropriate delivery of palliative oncology care. Goals of palliative radiotherapy are symptom relief at the site of primary tumor or from metastatic lesions [34].

Rectal can be successfully palliated with external beam radiotherapy (EBRT). Patients with rectal cancer who are unable to or unwilling to undergo palliative resection can be treated with aggressive palliative dose regimens totaling 40–60 Gy, although those with poor performance status or prognosis can gain relief with courses as short as 30 Gy in six fractions over 3 weeks with concurrent fluorouracil chemotherapy [35]. Recurrent rectal cancers frequently cause pelvic morbidity including pain, bleeding, and mass effect (Fig. 37.2). Palliative pelvic radiotherapy is also used to relieve these symptoms and delay local progression [36]. Bone metastasis from colorectal cancer is reported in 7–10% of cases [37]. Symptoms from bone metastases may commonly include pain, pathologic fracture, or spinal cord compression. When combined with the appropriate use of other measures such as a pain medicine regimen, surgical

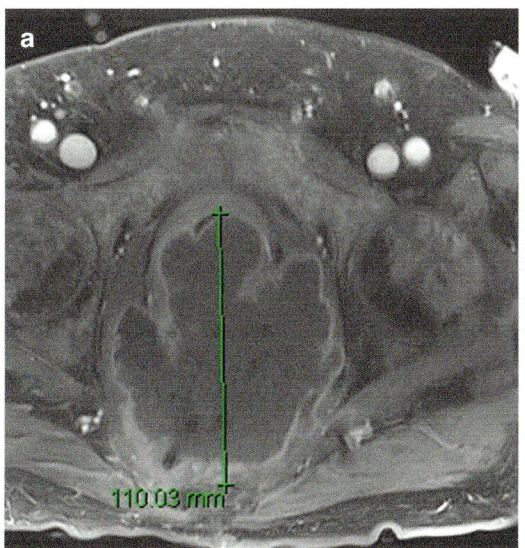
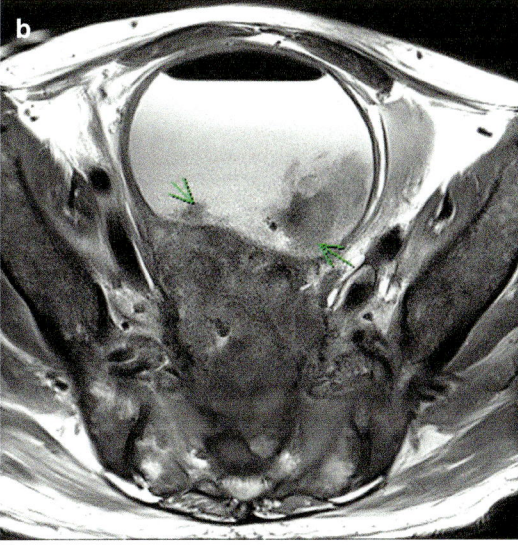

Fig. 37.2 A 56-year-old man with rectal cancer recurrence. The recurrence involves the urinary bladder and bilateral ureter. (**a**) About 11 cm recurrent presacral mass causing severe pain. (**b**) Rectal cancer recurrence invading posterior wall of urinary bladder

stabilization, systemic treatments including bone-strengthening agents, and radiopharmaceuticals, external beam radiotherapy constitutes the most effective and well-tolerated treatment for painful bone metastasis [38].

37.5 Role of Chemotherapy and Target Therapy

Traditionally, chemotherapy was considered as a palliative treatment and was administered only in unresectable metastatic colorectal cancers. After years of attempts and modulation of approaches with chemotherapy on metastatic colorectal cancer patients with the development of new targeted drugs, the shift on decision making emerged [39–42]. Such development of chemotherapy and targeted therapy improves the oncological outcome of selected patients with good performance status and converting metastatic disease from non-operable to operable [43].

Conclusion

Diverse therapeutic options, such as open surgery to minimally invasive techniques, new chemotherapeutic regimens, and molecular target agents, have increased the survival of incurable CRC patients. The role of surgery in the palliative management of asymptomatic patients is changing following the impressive results of chemotherapy. Other than survival prolongation, disease control and better quality of life are gaining importance as primary endpoints of palliative management of incurable CRC. Palliative treatment for end-stage colorectal cancer including recurrent patients should be provided by a multidisciplinary team of surgeons, medical oncologists, pathologists, radiation oncologists, and radiologists not only for disease control but also for better quality of life.

References

1. Cirocchi R, Trastulli S, Abraha I, Vettoretto N, Boselli C, Montedori A, et al. Non-resection versus resection for an asymptomatic primary tumour in patients with unresectable stage IV colorectal cancer. Cochrane Database Syst Rev. 2012;(8):Cd008997. https://doi.org/10.1002/14651858.CD008997.pub2.
2. Golan T, Urban D, Berger R, Lawrence YR. Changing prognosis of metastatic colorectal adenocarcinoma: differential improvement by age and tumor location. Cancer. 2013;119(16):3084–91. https://doi.org/10.1002/cncr.28143.
3. Petrelli N, Herrera L, Rustum Y, Burke P, Creaven P, Stulc J, et al. A prospective randomized trial of 5-fluorouracil versus 5-fluorouracil and high-dose leucovorin versus 5-fluorouracil and methotrexate in previously untreated patients with advanced colorectal carcinoma. J Clin Oncol Off J Am Soc Clin Oncol. 1987;5(10):1559–65. https://doi.org/10.1200/jco.1987.5.10.1559.
4. Saltz LB, Douillard JY, Pirotta N, Alakl M, Gruia G, Awad L, et al. Irinotecan plus fluorouracil/leucovorin for metastatic colorectal cancer: a new survival standard. Oncologist. 2001;6(1):81–91.
5. Zisis C, Tsakiridis K, Kougioumtzi I, Zarogoulidis P, Darwiche K, Machairiotis N, et al. The management of the advanced colorectal cancer: management of the pulmonary metastases. J Thorac Dis. 2013;5(Suppl 4):S383–8. https://doi.org/10.3978/j.issn.2072-1439.2013.06.23.
6. van de Velde CJ, Boelens PG, Borras JM, Coebergh JW, Cervantes A, Blomqvist L, et al. EURECCA colorectal: multidisciplinary management: European consensus conference colon & rectum. Eur J Cancer. 2014;50(1):1.e1–1.e34. https://doi.org/10.1016/j.ejca.2013.06.048.
7. Van Cutsem E, Cervantes A, Adam R, Sobrero A, Van Krieken JH, Aderka D, et al. ESMO consensus guidelines for the management of patients with metastatic colorectal cancer. Ann Oncol Off J Eur Soc Med Oncol. 2016;27(8):1386–422. https://doi.org/10.1093/annonc/mdw235.
8. Chang GJ, Kaiser AM, Mills S, Rafferty JF, Buie WD. Practice parameters for the management of colon cancer. Dis Colon Rectum. 2012;55(8):831–43. https://doi.org/10.1097/DCR.0b013e3182567e13.
9. Saltz LB, Cox JV, Blanke C, Rosen LS, Fehrenbacher L, Moore MJ, et al. Irinotecan plus fluorouracil and leucovorin for metastatic colorectal cancer. N Engl J Med. 2000;343(13):905–14. https://doi.org/10.1056/nejm200009283431302.
10. Venook AP, Niedzwiecki D, Lenz H-J, Innocenti F, Mahoney MR, O'Neil BH, et al. CALGB/SWOG 80405: phase III trial of irinotecan/5-FU/leucovorin (FOLFIRI) or oxaliplatin/5-FU/leucovorin (mFOLFOX6) with bevacizumab (BV) or cetuximab (CET) for patients (pts) with KRAS wild-type (wt) untreated metastatic adenocarcinoma of the colon or rectum (MCRC). Proc Am Soc Clin Oncol. 2014;32(5s):LBA3.
11. Benson AB 3rd, Bekaii-Saab T, Chan E, Chen YJ, Choti MA, Cooper HS, et al. Metastatic colon cancer, version 3.2013: featured updates to the NCCN guidelines. J Natl Compr Cancer Netw. 2013;11(2):141–52.
12. Folkert IW, Roses RE. Value in palliative cancer surgery: a critical assessment. J Surg Oncol.

2016;114(3):311–5. https://doi.org/10.1002/jso.24303.

13. Miner TJ, Cohen J, Charpentier K, McPhillips J, Marvell L, Cioffi WG. The palliative triangle: improved patient selection and outcomes associated with palliative operations. Arch Surg. 2011;146(5):517–22. https://doi.org/10.1001/archsurg.2011.92.

14. Law WL, Choi HK, Chu KW, Ho JW, Wong L. Bowel preparation for colonoscopy: a randomized controlled trial comparing polyethylene glycol solution, one dose and two doses of oral sodium phosphate solution. Asian J Surg. 2004;27(2):120–4. https://doi.org/10.1016/s1015-9584(09)60324-9.

15. Marquis P, Marrel A, Jambon B. Quality of life in patients with stomas: the Montreux study. Ostomy Wound Manage. 2003;49(2):48–55.

16. Fuhrman GM, Ota DM. Laparoscopic intestinal stomas. Dis Colon Rectum. 1994;37(5):444–9.

17. Fleshman JW, Nelson H, Peters WR, Kim HC, Larach S, Boorse RR, et al. Early results of laparoscopic surgery for colorectal cancer. Retrospective analysis of 372 patients treated by clinical outcomes of surgical therapy (COST) study group. Dis Colon Rectum. 1996;39(10 Suppl):S53–8.

18. Rosen SA, Buell JF, Yoshida A, Kazsuba S, Hurst R, Michelassi F, et al. Initial presentation with stage IV colorectal cancer: how aggressive should we be? Arch Surg. 2000;135(5):530–4.

19. Law WL, Chan WF, Lee YM, Chu KW. Non-curative surgery for colorectal cancer: critical appraisal of outcomes. Int J Color Dis. 2004;19(3):197–202. https://doi.org/10.1007/s00384-003-0551-7.

20. Zhao XD, Cai BB, Cao RS, Shi RH. Palliative treatment for incurable malignant colorectal obstructions: a meta-analysis. World J Gastroenterol. 2013;19(33):5565–74. https://doi.org/10.3748/wjg.v19.i33.5565.

21. Sagar J. Role of colonic stents in the management of colorectal cancers. World J Gastrointest Endosc. 2016;8(4):198–204. https://doi.org/10.4253/wjge.v8.i4.198.

22. Dohmoto M, Hunerbein M, Schlag PM. Application of rectal stents for palliation of obstructing rectosigmoid cancer. Surg Endosc. 1997;11(7):758–61.

23. Liang TW, Sun Y, Wei YC, Yang DX. Palliative treatment of malignant colorectal obstruction caused by advanced malignancy: a self-expanding metallic stent or surgery? A system review and meta-analysis. Surg Today. 2014;44(1):22–33. https://doi.org/10.1007/s00595-013-0665-7.

24. Small AJ, Coelho-Prabhu N, Baron TH. Endoscopic placement of self-expandable metal stents for malignant colonic obstruction: long-term outcomes and complication factors. Gastrointest Endosc. 2010;71(3):560–72. https://doi.org/10.1016/j.gie.2009.10.012.

25. van Halsema EE, van Hooft JE, Small AJ, Baron TH, Garcia-Cano J, Cheon JH, et al. Perforation in colorectal stenting: a meta-analysis and a search for risk factors. Gastrointest Endosc. 2014;79(6):970-82.e7. https://doi.org/10.1016/j.gie.2013.11.038.

26. Cennamo V, Fuccio L, Mutri V, Minardi ME, Eusebi LH, Ceroni L, et al. Does stent placement for advanced colon cancer increase the risk of perforation during bevacizumab-based therapy? Clin Gastroenterol Hepatol Off Clin Pract J Am Gastroenterol Assoc. 2009;7(11):1174–6. https://doi.org/10.1016/j.cgh.2009.07.015.

27. Lo SK. Metallic stenting for colorectal obstruction. Gastrointest Endosc Clin N Am. 1999;9(3):459–77.

28. Gash K, Chambers W, Ghosh A, Dixon AR. The role of laparoscopic surgery for the management of acute large bowel obstruction. Colorectal Dis Off J Assoc Coloproctol G B Irel. 2011;13(3):263–6. https://doi.org/10.1111/j.1463-1318.2009.02123.x.

29. Smithers BM, Theile DE, Cohen JR, Evans EB, Davis NC. Emergency right hemicolectomy in colon carcinoma: a prospective study. Aust N Z J Surg. 1986;56(10):749–52.

30. Kimmey MB. Endoscopic methods (other than stents) for palliation of rectal carcinoma. J Gastrointest Surg. 2004;8(3):270–3. https://doi.org/10.1016/j.gassur.2003.11.017.

31. Saltz LB. Palliative management of rectal cancer: the roles of chemotherapy and radiation therapy. J Gastrointest Surg. 2004;8(3):274–6. https://doi.org/10.1016/j.gassur.2003.11.016.

32. Stelzner S, Hellmich G, Koch R, Ludwig K. Factors predicting survival in stage IV colorectal carcinoma patients after palliative treatment: a multivariate analysis. J Surg Oncol. 2005;89(4):211–7. https://doi.org/10.1002/jso.20196.

33. Costi R, Leonardi F, Zanoni D, Violi V, Roncoroni L. Palliative care and end-stage colorectal cancer management: the surgeon meets the oncologist. World J Gastroenterol. 2014;20(24):7602–21. https://doi.org/10.3748/wjg.v20.i24.7602.

34. Lutz ST, Jones J, Chow E. Role of radiation therapy in palliative care of the patient with cancer. J Clin Oncol Off J Am Soc Clin Oncol. 2014;32(26):2913–9. https://doi.org/10.1200/jco.2014.55.1143.

35. Janjan NA, Breslin T, Lenzi R, Rich TA, Skibber J. Avoidance of colostomy placement in advanced colorectal cancer with twice weekly hypofractionated radiation plus continuous infusion 5-fluorouracil. J Pain Symptom Manag. 2000;20(4):266–72.

36. Allum WH, Mack P, Priestman TJ, Fielding JW. Radiotherapy for pain relief in locally recurrent colorectal cancer. Ann R Coll Surg Engl. 1987;69(5):220–1.

37. Santini D, Tampellini M, Vincenzi B, Ibrahim T, Ortega C, Virzi V, et al. Natural history of bone metastasis in colorectal cancer: final results of a large Italian bone metastases study. Ann Oncol Off J Eur Soc Med Oncol. 2012;23(8):2072–7. https://doi.org/10.1093/annonc/mdr572.

38. Lutz S, Berk L, Chang E, Chow E, Hahn C, Hoskin P, et al. Palliative radiotherapy for bone metastases: an ASTRO evidence-based guideline. Int J Radiat Oncol Biol Phys. 2011;79(4):965–76. https://doi.org/10.1016/j.ijrobp.2010.11.026.

39. Cunningham D, Lang I, Marcuello E, Lorusso V, Ocvirk J, Shin DB, et al. Bevacizumab plus capecitabine versus capecitabine alone in elderly patients with previously untreated metastatic colorectal cancer (AVEX): an open-label, randomised phase 3 trial. Lancet Oncol. 2013;14(11):1077–85. https://doi.org/10.1016/s1470-2045(13)70154-2.

40. Loupakis F, Cremolini C, Masi G, Lonardi S, Zagonel V, Salvatore L, et al. Initial therapy with FOLFOXIRI and bevacizumab for metastatic colorectal cancer. N Engl J Med. 2014;371(17):1609–18. https://doi.org/10.1056/NEJMoa1403108.

41. Gruenberger T, Bridgewater J, Chau I, Garcia Alfonso P, Rivoire M, Mudan S, et al. Bevacizumab plus mFOLFOX-6 or FOLFOXIRI in patients with initially unresectable liver metastases from colorectal cancer: the OLIVIA multinational randomised phase II trial. Ann Oncol Off J Eur Soc Med Oncol. 2015;26(4):702–8. https://doi.org/10.1093/annonc/mdu580.

42. Cremolini C, Loupakis F, Antoniotti C, Lupi C, Sensi E, Lonardi S, et al. FOLFOXIRI plus bevacizumab versus FOLFIRI plus bevacizumab as first-line treatment of patients with metastatic colorectal cancer: updated overall survival and molecular subgroup analyses of the open-label, phase 3 TRIBE study. Lancet Oncol. 2015;16(13):1306–15. https://doi.org/10.1016/s1470-2045(15)00122-9.

43. Adam R, de Gramont A, Figueras J, Kokudo N, Kunstlinger F, Loyer E, et al. Managing synchronous liver metastases from colorectal cancer: a multidisciplinary international consensus. Cancer Treat Rev. 2015;41(9):729–41. https://doi.org/10.1016/j.ctrv.2015.06.006.